Death Receptors in Cancer Therapy

Cancer Drug Discovery and Development

Beverly A. Teicher, Series Editor

Death Receptors in Cancer Therapy, edited by *Wafik S. El-Deiry,* 2005

Bone Metastasis: *Experimental and Clinical Therapeutics,* edited by *Gurmit Singh and Shafaat A. Rabbani,* 2005

The Oncogenomics Handbook, edited by *William J. LaRochelle and Richard A. Shimkets,* 2005

Camptothecins in Cancer Therapy, edited by *Thomas G. Burke and Val R. Adams,* 2005

Combination Cancer Therapy: *Modulators and Potentiators,* edited by *Gary K. Schwartz,* 2005

Cancer Chemoprevention, Volume 2: *Strategies for Cancer Chemoprevention,* edited by *Gary J. Kelloff, Ernest T. Hawk, and Caroline C. Sigman,* 2005

Cancer Chemoprevention, Volume 1: *Promising Cancer Chemopreventive Agents,* edited by *Gary J. Kelloff, Ernest T. Hawk, and Caroline C. Sigman,* 2004

Proteasome Inhibitors in Cancer Therapy, edited by *Julian Adams,* 2004

Nucleic Acid Therapeutics in Cancer, edited by *Alan M. Gewirtz,* 2004

DNA Repair in Cancer Therapy, edited by *Lawrence C. Panasci and Moulay A. Alaoui-Jamali,* 2004

Hematopoietic Growth Factors in Oncology: *Basic Science and Clinical Therapeutics,* edited by *George Morstyn, MaryAnn Foote, and Graham J. Lieschke,* 2004

Handbook of Anticancer Pharmacokinetics and Pharmacodynamics, edited by *William D. Figg and Howard L. McLeod,* 2004

Anticancer Drug Development Guide: *Preclinical Screening, Clinical Trials, and Approval, Second Edition,* edited by *Beverly A. Teicher and Paul A. Andrews,* 2004

Handbook of Cancer Vaccines, edited by *Michael A. Morse, Timothy M. Clay, and Kim H. Lyerly,* 2004

Drug Delivery Systems in Cancer Therapy, edited by *Dennis M. Brown,* 2003

Oncogene-Directed Therapies, edited by *Janusz Rak,* 2003

Cell Cycle Inhibitors in Cancer Therapy: *Current Strategies,* edited by *Antonio Giordano and Kenneth J. Soprano,* 2003

Chemoradiation in Cancer Therapy, edited by *Hak Choy,* 2003

Fluoropyrimidines in Cancer Therapy, edited by *Youcef M. Rustum,* 2003

Targets for Cancer Chemotherapy: *Transcription Factors and Other Nuclear Proteins,* edited by *Nicholas B. La Thangue and Lan R. Bandara,* 2002

Tumor Targeting in Cancer Therapy, edited by *Michel Pagé,* 2002

Hormone Therapy in Breast and Prostate Cancer, edited by *V. Craig Jordan and Barrington J. A. Furr,* 2002

Tumor Models in Cancer Research, edited by *Beverly A. Teicher,* 2002

Tumor Suppressor Genes in Human Cancer, edited by *David E. Fisher,* 2001

Matrix Metalloproteinase Inhibitors in Cancer Therapy, edited by *Neil J. Clendeninn and Krzysztof Appelt,* 2001

Farnesyltransferase Inhibitors in Cancer, edited by *Saïd M. Sebti and Andrew D. Hamilton,* 2001

Platinum-Based Drugs in Cancer Therapy, edited by *Lloyd R. Kelland and Nicholas P. Farrell,* 2000

Apoptosis and Cancer Chemotherapy, edited by *John A. Hickman and Caroline Dive,* 1999

Signaling Networks and Cell Cycle Control: *The Molecular Basis of Cancer and Other Diseases,* edited by *J. Silvio Gutkind,* 1999

Antifolate Drugs in Cancer Therapy, edited by *Ann L. Jackman,* 1999

Antiangiogenic Agents in Cancer Therapy, edited by *Beverly A. Teicher,* 1999

Death Receptors in Cancer Therapy

Edited by

Wafik S. El-Deiry, MD, PhD

University of Pennsylvania School of Medicine, Philadelphia, PA

Humana Press
Totowa, New Jersey

999 Riverview Drive, Suite 208
Totowa, New Jersey 07512

www.humanapress.com

Production Editor: Tracy Catanese
Cover design by Patricia F. Cleary

This publication is printed on acid-free paper. ∞
ANSI Z39.48-1984 (American National Standards Institute)
Permanence of Paper for Printed Library Materials

For additional copies, pricing for bulk purchases, and/or information about other Humana titles, contact Humana at the above address or at any of the following numbers: Tel:973-256-1699; Fax: 973-256-8341; Email: humana@humanapr.com; or visit our Website: www.humanapress.com

Printed in the United States of America. 10 9 8 7 6 5 4 3 2 1

e-ISBN: 1-59259-851-X

Library of Congress Cataloging-in-Publication Data

Death receptors in cancer therapy / edited by Wafik S. El-Deiry.
p. ; cm. -- (Cancer drug discovery and development)
Includes bibliographical references and index.
ISBN 1-58829-172-3 (alk. paper)
1. Apoptosis. 2. Cell receptors. 3. Cancer--Molecular aspects. 4. Cellular signal transduction.
[DNLM: 1. Neoplasms--immunology. 2. Neoplasms--therapy. 3. Cell Death--immunology. 4. Gene Therapy--methods. 5. Receptors, Tumor Necrosis Factor. QZ 266 D285 2005] I. El-Deiry, Wafik S. II. Series.
QH671.D43 2005
571.9'36--dc22

2004006682

PREFACE

The study of cell death, or apoptosis, has turned into a very large field. Both the extrinsic and intrinsic cell-death pathways appear to have fundamental importance to tumor progression and cancer therapy. It has become clear that the extrinsic pathway provides a number of mechanisms for host immune surveillance of tumors and their suppression. Because this is a fast-moving area that is generating a huge literature, there is an ongoing need in the scientific community to distill the knowledge and to organize it so that students as well as experienced investigators can both learn it and build upon it.

The chapters comprising *Death Receptors in Cancer Therapy* have been written by experts in the field of cell-death research, particularly those interested in death receptors and their relevance to cancer and cancer therapy. The basic information about signaling, as well as conservation of the pathways in *Drosophila* or *Caenorhabditis elegans*, can be found herein. There is information on the role of death domains and receptors in development, and there is secondary and tertiary structural information about receptors and ligands. One of the important aspects of the text that will be of use for experts is the cross-talk in signal transduction pathways. It is clear that pathways are networked and cross-regulated through other signaling pathways that may be on or off depending on physiological or cellular state. Finally, with a firm foundation in the understanding of the molecular events in cell death, the major emphasis of *Death Receptors in Cancer Therapy* is on both alterations in cancer as well as therapeutic strategies and combination therapies.

It is important to note that, although there is a great deal of preclinical translational research on death receptors and ligands, the history of drug development is complex and subject to many forces and hurdles. As such, it is important to mention that the opinions or conclusions of the contributors to this text are theirs, and not necessarily endorsed by the editor or the publisher. However, it is very important in a fast-moving field with exciting possibilities for new cancer therapies to provide readers with the views of leaders in the field from their own perspectives.

One of the chapters in this book was a contribution from Dr. Vincent Kidd and colleagues at St. Jude Children's Research Hospital. In reviewing the proofs, I became aware that Dr. Kidd passed away suddenly on May 7, 2004. His colleagues have dedicated the chapter on caspase methylation, to which he made a major contribution, to his memory. We will all miss him.

I wish to take this opportunity to personally thank each and every contributor to this volume. I believe a useful resource has been created that will serve as a reference in the field and will also provide an excellent introduction of the cell death field to the beginner. There are many acronyms in this field, and this text describes the many molecules involved in death signaling and allows the reader to get a handle on their many names. The extrinsic death pathway and death receptors are of great interest to cancer biologists, immunologists, developmental biologists, medical oncologists, hematologists, radiation therapists, and rheumatologists as well as to those in the biotech and pharmaceutical industries.

W. El-Deiry

Contents

Contributors

Alex Almasan, PhD • *Department of Cancer Biology, Lerner Research Institute, and Department of Radiation Oncology, Cleveland Clinic Foundation, Cleveland, OH*

Atul Bedi, MD • *The Sidney Kimmel Comprehensive Cancer Center at Johns Hopkins, The Johns Hopkins University School of Medicine, Baltimore, MD*

Alicja Bielawska, PhD • *Department of Biochemistry and Molecular Biology, Medical University of South Carolina, Charleston, SC*

Mahaveer Swaroop Bhojani, PhD • *Center for Molecular Imaging, Departments of Radiology and Radiation Oncology, University of Michigan, Ann Arbor, MI*

Charles Chalfant, PhD • *Department of Biochemistry and Molecular Biology, Medical University of South Carolina, Charleston, SC*

Preet M. Chaudhary, MD, PhD • *Departments of Internal Medicine and Molecular Biology, University of Texas Southwestern Medical Center, Dallas, TX*

Nien-Jung Chen, PhD • *Advanced Medical Discovery Institute, University Health Network, and Department of Medical Biophysics, University of Toronto, Toronto, Ontario, Canada*

Youhai H. Chen, MD, PhD • *Department of Pathology and Laboratory Medicine, University of Pennsylvania School of Medicine, Philadelphia, PA*

Klaus-Michael Debatin, MD • *University Children's Hospital, Ulm, Germany*

Abraham M. de Vos, PhD • *Department of Protein Engineering, Genentech Inc, South San Francisco, CA*

Jian-Yun Dong, MD, PhD • *Department of Microbiology and Immunology, Medical University of South Carolina, Charleston, SC*

Wafik S. El-Deiry, MD, PhD • *Departments of Medicine, Genetics, and Pharmacology, University of Pennsylvania School of Medicine, Philadelphia, PA*

Ahmed El-Zawahry, MD • *Department of Microbiology and Immunology, Medical University of South Carolina, Charleston, SC*

Bingliang Fang, MD • *Department of Thoracic and Cardiovascular Surgery, The University of Texas MD Anderson Cancer Center, Houston, TX*

Simone Fulda, MD • *University Children's Hospital, Ulm, Germany*

Rüdiger Göke • *Clinical Research Unit for Gastrointestinal Endocrinology, University of Marburg, Marburg, Germany*

Yusuf A. Hannun, MD • *Department of Biochemistry and Molecular Biology, Medical University of South Carolina, Charleston, SC*

Peter Hersey, FRACP, DPhil • *Immunology and Oncology Unit, David Maddison Building, University of Newcastle, Newcastle, New South Wales, Australia*

John G. Hissong, MD, PhD • *Department of Cancer Biology, Lerner Research Institute, Cleveland, OH*

DAVID H. HOLMAN, BS • *Department of Microbiology and Immunology, Medical University of South Carolina, Charleston, SC*

MARC L. HYER, PhD • *The Burnham Institute, La Jolla, CA*

SARAH G. HYMOWITZ, PhD • *Department of Protein Engineering, Genentech Inc, South San Francisco, CA*

VINCENT J. KIDD, PhD (DECEASED) • *Department of Genetics and Tumor Cell Biology, St. Jude Children's Research Hospital, Memphis, TN*

MI-HYANG KIM • *Department of Surgery, University of Pittsburgh School of Medicine, Pittsburgh, PA*

UDO KONTNY, MD • *Division of Pediatric Hematology and Oncology, University Children's Hospital, Freiburg, Germany*

HEINRICH KOVAR, PhD • *Children's Cancer Research Institute, St. Anna Kinderspital, Vienna, Austria*

JILL M. LAHTI, PhD • *Department of Genetics and Tumor Cell Biology, St. Jude Children's Research Hospital, Memphis, TN*

CHARLES LANDEN, MD • *Department of Microbiology and Immunology, Medical University of South Carolina, Charleston, SC*

JUNG YOUNG LEE • *Department of Pathology, College of Medicine, The Catholic University of Korea, Seoul, Korea*

SUG HYUNG LEE • *Department of Pathology, College of Medicine, The Catholic University of Korea, Seoul, Korea*

E. ROBERT McDONALD III, PhD • *Laboratory of Molecular Oncology and Cycle Cell Regulation, Howard Hughes Medical Institute, Chevy Chase, MD*

DAVID J. McCONKEY, PhD • *Department of Cancer Biology, University of Texas MD Anderson Cancer Center, Houston, TX*

JAMES S. NORRIS, PhD • *Department of Microbiology and Immunology, Medical University of South Carolina, Charleston, SC*

MARCELA OANCEA • *Department of Cancer Biology, Lerner Research Institute, and Department of Chemistry, Cleveland State University, Cleveland, OH*

LINA M. OBEID, MD • *Department of Medicine, Medical University of South Carolina, Charleston, SC*

SUBRATA RAY, PhD • *Department of Cancer Biology, Lerner Research Institute, Cleveland, OH*

RAJANI RAVI, PhD • *The Sidney Kimmel Comprehensive Cancer Center at Johns Hopkins, The Johns Hopkins University School of Medicine, Baltimore, MD*

ALNAWAZ REHEMTULLA, PhD • *Center for Molecular Imaging, Departments of Radiation Oncology and Radiology, University of Michigan, Ann Arbor, MI*

BRIAN D. ROSS, PhD • *Center for Molecular Imaging, Departments of Radiology and Biological Chemistry, University of Michigan, Ann Arbor, MI*

DAI-WU SEOL, PhD • *Department of Surgery, University of Pittsburgh School of Medicine, Pittsburgh, PA*

SHI-YONG SUN, PhD • *Winship Cancer Institute, Emory University School of Medicine, Atlanta, GA*

RISHU TAKIMOTO, MD, PhD • *Fourth Department of Internal Medicine, Sapporo Medical University School of Medicine, Sapporo, Japan*

TAL TEITZ, PhD • *Department of Genetics and Tumor Cell Biology, St. Jude Children's Research Hospital, Memphis, TN*

TANYA TEKAUTZ, MD • *Departments of Hematology and Oncology and Genetics and Tumor Cell Biology, St. Jude Children's Research Hospital, Memphis, TN*

STEPHEN TOMLINSON, PhD • *Department of Microbiology and Immunology, Medical University of South Carolina, Charleston, SC*

CHRISTINA VOELKEL-JOHNSON, PhD • *Department of Microbiology and Immunology, Medical University of South Carolina, Charleston, SC*

XIAOLU YANG, PhD • *Abramson Family Cancer Research Institute, Department of Cancer Biology, University of Pennsylvania School of Medicine, Philadelphia, PA*

WEN-CHEN YEH, MD, PhD • *Advanced Medical Discovery Institute, University Health Network, and Department of Medical Biophysics, University of Toronto, Toronto, Ontario, Canada*

NAM JIN YOO • *Department of Pathology, College of Medicine, The Catholic University of Korea, Seoul, Korea*

LIDONG ZHANG, MD • *Department of Thoracic and Cardiovascular Surgery, The University of Texas MD Anderson Cancer Center, Houston, TX*

SI YI ZHANG, PhD • *David Maddison Building, University of Newcastle, Newcastle, New South Wales, Australia*

XU DONG ZHANG, MD, PhD • *David Maddison Building, University of Newcastle, Newcastle, New South Wales, Australia*

1 Mammalian Cell Death Pathways

Intrinsic and Extrinsic

E. Robert McDonald III, PhD
and Wafik S. El-Deiry, MD, PhD

SUMMARY

Programmed cell death results from a conserved cascade of events essential in the development and maintenance of tissue homeostasis. "Extrinsic" cell-death pathways initiate at the cell surface, leading to execution through substrate cleavage, and may involve mitochondrial amplification. Multiple "intrinsic" death pathways converge and require signaling through the mitochondria. Extrinsic cell death is integral to cell-mediated immunity and host immune surveillance/suppression of cancer. Caspase activation is highly regulated and defects at virtually all levels of death regulation are observed in cancer. This chapter focuses on the cell biology, biochemistry, and genetics of programmed cell death.

ORIGINS OF APOPTOSIS IN *CAENORHABDITIS ELEGANS*

Even after numerous reports in the early to mid-1900s of "programmed cell death" with characteristic morphological changes such as cell shrinkage and nuclear condensation and fragmentation, the importance of this process in normal cellular physiology went largely unexplored *(1)*. However, with the description of the genetically controlled deletion of a subset of cells within the nematode *C. elegans* and the subsequent cloning of the genes responsible for this process, the field of programmed cell death or apoptosis gained popularity *(2)*. The realization that apoptosis is an evolutionarily conserved, genetic event has sparked interest in understanding the regulation of the process in various model systems. Furthermore the deregulation of apoptosis in human disorders such as neurodegenerative disease and cancer has lead to the manipulation of these pathways in order to combat these diseases *(3)*. It was, however, seminal work in *C. elegans* that laid the foundation for the central themes of apoptosis found throughout the animal kingdom.

While Richard Lockshin coined the term programmed cell death in 1964 *(4)*, John Kerr is credited with early microscopic observations of cell death distinct from necrosis called "apoptosis" which he, Wyllie, and Currie perceived to be controlled by a series of con-

From: *Cancer Drug Discovery and Development: Death Receptors in Cancer Therapy*
Edited by: W. S. El-Deiry

served events *(1)*. However, Robert Horvitz was responsible for providing the first molecular clues of how apoptosis is controlled *(5)*. The identification of *C. elegans* cell death abnormal or *ced* mutants with defective development *(5,6)* established three families of highly conserved proteins, which oversee apoptosis in most organisms (Fig. 1): caspases (ced-3), caspase-activating adaptor proteins (ced-4) and the bcl-2 family of proteins (ced-9). Caspases are the enzymes responsible for dismantling the cell and for eliciting the cellular phenotypes first described by Kerr, therefore their regulation is paramount when considering apoptotic pathways. In the worm, these three gene products act in a linear fashion to either suppress or activate ced-3, with ced-9 acting as the only antiapoptotic protein in the pathway. ced-9 inhibits ced-4 function, which is required for ced-3 caspase activation *(7)*. Whereas the loss of ced-3 or ced-4 did not compromise the longevity of the organism, suppression of apoptosis by ced-9 was crucial for its long-term survival *(6)*. Subsequently, the lone BH3-only protein, egl-1, was placed genetically upstream of ced-9 due to the ability of egl-1 to bind and negatively regulate ced-9 *(8)*. These four genes constitute the core apoptotic machinery in *C. elegans* required for the execution phase of cell death.

INCREASED APOPTOTIC COMPLEXITY OF HIGHER EUKARYOTES

Cloning of the core apoptotic genes in *C. elegans* led to the discovery that higher eukaryotes adhered to this basic blueprint but had predictably evolved to include novel gene families to regulate further complexity (Fig. 1). Mammalian systems, being the most complex, contain 14 caspases (ced-3), 2 proapoptotic adaptor proteins (ced-4), at least 10 bcl-2 family proteins (ced-9), and a similar number of BH3-only proteins (egl-1) to date *(9,10)*. BH3-only proteins antagonize the antiapoptotic members of the bcl-2 family in order to facilitate downstream adaptor-mediated caspase activation *(11)*. However, unlike *C. elegans*, antiapoptotic bcl-2 proteins do not directly interact with adaptors but rather regulate adaptor assembly by influencing mitochondrial homeostasis *(12)*. This pathway involving mitochondria and subsequent caspase activation is referred to as the intrinsic pathway and is the functional equivalent of the *C. elegans* cell death pathway (Fig. 1).

Following mitochondrial dysfunction, formation of a caspase activation complex known as the apoptosome initiates the death program. The apoptosome is comprised of the ced-4 homolog, Apaf-1, along with procaspase-9, ATP, and cytochrome c, which has been extruded from the mitochondria. Activation of caspase-9 within the apoptosome in turn leads to the activation of caspase-3, the true mammalian ced-3 homolog, committing the cell to death *(13)*. The basic principle from *C. elegans* of bcl-2 mediated inhibition of adaptor-driven caspase activation is therefore represented at the mammalian level by the intrinsic pathway. In addition to the intrinsic pathway, however, mammals have evolved an alternative pathway—the extrinsic pathway—which is initiated at the cell surface by death receptor/death ligand interactions *(14)*. Activation of this pathway also results in adaptor-driven caspase activation. The adaptor, FADD, and caspase-8 and -10, through a series of protein interactions with the death ligand-associated receptors, form a death-inducing signaling complex (DISC) which is sufficient for caspase activation *(15)*. The last major difference between *C. elegans* and higher eukaryotes is the creation of another protein family, the inhibitor of apoptosis proteins, or IAPs *(16)*. These proteins have evolved to bind to and negatively regulate caspases and will be discussed in more detail in a subsequent section (Fig. 1).

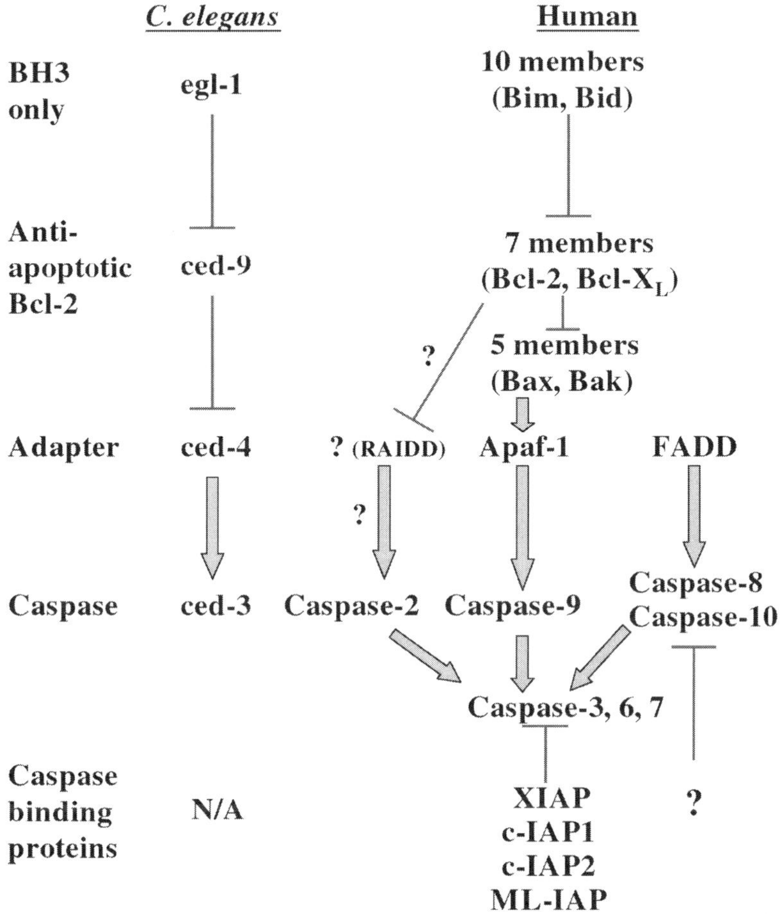

Fig. 1. Increased apoptotic complexity of Higher Eukaryotes as compared to the *Caenorhabitis elegans* system. Although the linear system of adaptor-mediated caspase activation is conserved in higher eukaryotes, a number of important differences exist. The expansion of each gene family is dramatic in addition to a new family of proapoptotic Bcl-2 proteins that regulate mitochondrial homestasis in mammalian systems. The death receptor pathway and caspase binding proteins are completely absent in the worm. Unanswered points within a putative mitochondrial-independent, caspase-2-dependent pathway are denoted by a question mark.

THE GENETICS OF THE *DROSOPHILA* APOPTOTIC RESPONSE

Another genetically tractable organism used for the study of cell death regulation is *Drosophila melanogaster*. As would be expected, the complexity of the apoptotic program of this organism is intermediate between that of *C. elegans* and humans. The intrinsic pathway mediated by mitochondrial homeostasis and apoptosome formation in humans has conserved elements in *Drosophila* (Fig. 2). Dark, the *Drosophila* Apaf-1 homolog, and Dronc, the *Drosophila* caspase-9 homolog, are able to interact consistent with a model using adaptor-driven caspase activation *(17)*, and furthermore, cytochrome c interacts with Dark in *Drosophila* tissue culture cells *(18)*. Despite these similarities with higher organisms, initial studies suggest that cytochrome c is not released from

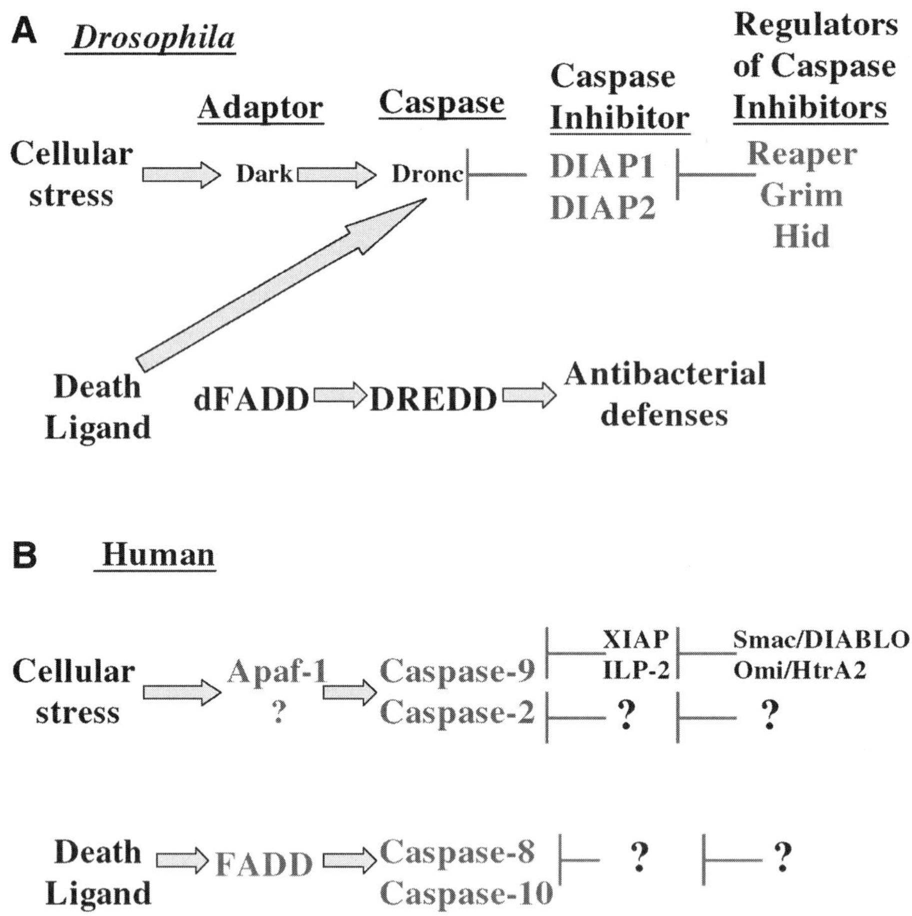

Fig. 2. Differences between the *Drosophila* and mammalian cell death pathways. **(A)** The main regulators of apoptosis in *Drosophila* are Reaper, Grim, and Hid that negatively regulate IAP function. The IAPs in turn control caspase activity that is a triggered in cytochrome c-independent manner. The only "putative" death ligand described in *Drosophila* activates a Dark, Dronc pathway while FADD and caspase-8 homologs regulate antibacterial defenses. **(B)** The human pathways are dominated by caspase regulation and activation. Caspase inhibitory proteins only delay the death process which is highly regulated by adaptor-mediated caspase activation. Cytochrome c-dependent caspase-9 activation and cytochrome c-independent caspase-2 regulation both contribute to death in response to cellular stress.

mitochondria in *Drosophila* and is not required for Dronc or downstream Drice activation *(19,20)* inconsistent with a role for cytochrome c in cell death. Further experiments must be carried out, but this preliminary evidence suggests that mechanistically the core machinery of the intrinsic pathway may not require cytochrome c and therefore may more closely resemble *C. elegans*.

Unlike *C. elegans* however, *Drosophila* contains FADD (dFADD) and caspase-8 (DREDD) homologs consistent with the existence of an extrinsic pathway in *Drosophila*. Despite the absence of recognizable death receptors in the genome, an apoptosis-inducing death ligand, Eiger, was recently cloned *(21)*. Surprisingly however, this ligand did not require DREDD (caspase-8) for cell death but rather used a DRONC/DARK-mediated pathway induced by JNK activation *(21)*. Furthermore, recent experiments with both dFADD and DREDD demonstrate that they play a role in the antibacterial response to Gram-negative bacteria *(22,23)*. These studies imply that the extrinsic death pathway exists in *Drosophila* but that caspase-8 (DREDD) may not be necessary; instead, it may be required for antibacterial defenses (Fig. 2). The identification of putative death receptors for the *Drosophila* death ligand should assist in determining the biological relevance of the extrinsic pathway in *Drosophila*.

IAPs are also found in *Drosophila* and appear to play a more significant role in apoptotic regulation than any other system studied (Fig. 2). Loss of DIAP1 leads to embryonic lethality due to constitutive caspase activation *(24)*, reinforcing the role of IAPs in the negative regulation of caspases. Furthermore, the lethality due to DIAP1 loss is suppressed by subsequent loss of Dark or DRONC *(20,25)*, suggesting that DIAP1 plays a crucial role in regulating the apoptosome in *Drosophila*, an observation not made in mammalian systems. The importance of IAPs in *Drosophila* is further supported by the presence of three genes— rpr, hid, *and* grim (collectively known as the RHG proteins)— that inhibit IAPs to induce apoptosis *(26)*. Interestingly, rpr, hid, *and* grim control almost all apoptosis in the fly, as was initially described by a deletion mutant, deficiency H99 *(27)*. However, structural homologs of RHG proteins appear to be absent in other species, although functional homologs (Smac/DIABLO and HtrA2/Omi) in mammals have recently been described *(28–34)*. More recent experiments suggest that select RHG proteins can promote the degradation of DIAP1 as a means to promote cell death *(35)*. Therefore, *Drosophila*, despite their acquistion of components of the extrinsic pathway and IAPs, differ from mammals significantly in the control of apoptosis by relying on a novel group of proteins, the RHG family, to regulate IAP function which is critical in controlling an intrinsic pathway devoid of cytochrome c involvement (Fig. 2). All further discussions of the apoptotic pathways will focus on the mammalian systems garnered over the past twenty years.

CASPASES—STRUCTURE, CLASSIFICATION, AND ACTIVATION

The first mammalian homolog of *C. elegans* ced-3 identified was the interleukin (IL)-1-converting enzyme, or ICE *(36)*. This protease, responsible for the processing and subsequent maturation of IL-1β, was then demonstrated to possess apoptotic potential when expressed in rat fibroblasts *(37)*. This was the first demonstration that the overexpression of a ced-3 -like protease could cause programmed cell death in mammalian cells. The identification of numerous mammalian ced-3-like proteins led to the adoption of a common nomenclature for the family. Due to the presence of a *c*ysteine residue within the active site of the protease coupled with the substrate specificity following *asp*artic acid residues, the proteins were designated as the *caspase* family *(38)*. All caspases are synthesized as inactive precursors (procaspases) containing a regulatory prodomain of varying length and a large subunit (p20) as well as a small subunit (p10). Activation of procaspases (with the exception of initiator caspases) requires cleavage to form the active enzyme, which is a tetramer of two large subunits and two small subunits creating two active sites *(39)* (Fig. 3). Examination of cleavage sites within procaspases reveals that they adhere to caspase substrate sites, suggesting that caspases are activated in a sequential fashion forming a caspase cascade *(40)*.

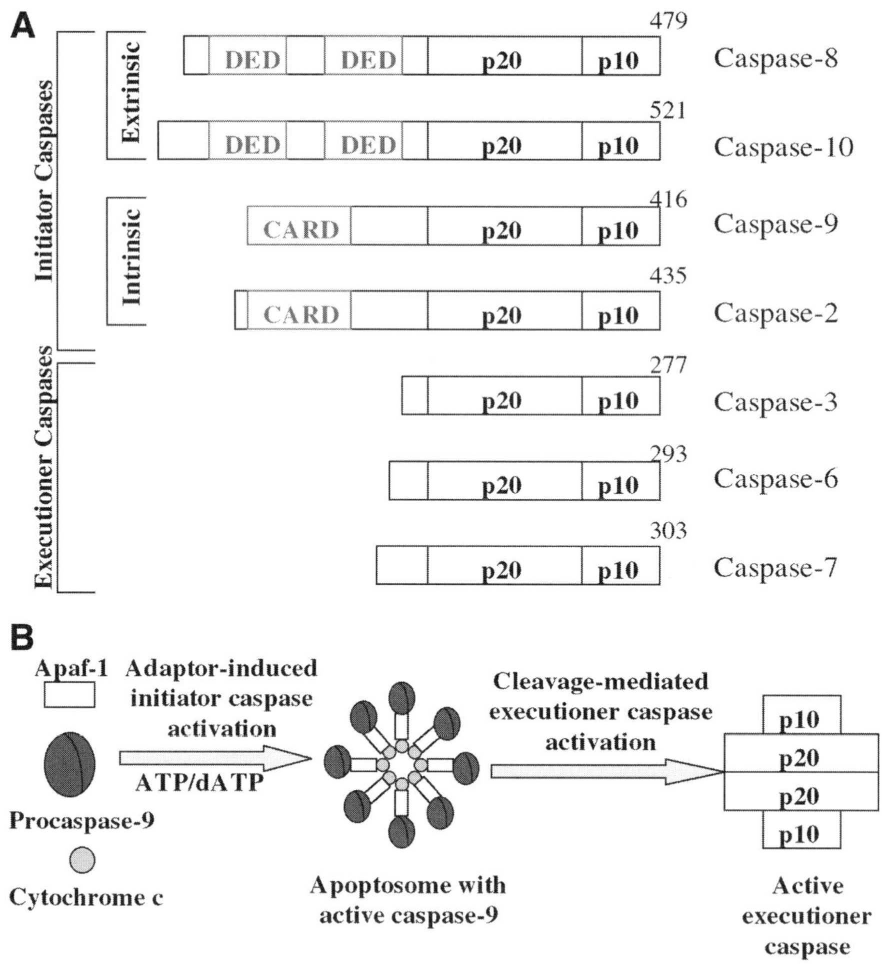

Fig. 3. Mammalian apoptotic caspase classification and activation mechanisms. **(A)** Caspases are divided into initiator and executioner caspases based on mechanism of activation and the presence or absence of a prodomain. Initiator caspases of the extrinsic pathway contain DEDs to allow FADD interaction while initiator caspases of the intrinsic pathway utilize a CARD for adaptor interaction. **(B)** Initiator caspase activation is driven by adaptor-mediated oligomerization that in turn leads to cleavage-induced executioner caspase activation. In this example, procaspase-9 is activated within the apoptosome after CARD-mediated recruitment by Apaf-1 and cytochrome c in a process driven by ATP. Apoptosome formation leads to cleavage and activation of executioner caspase-3.

To date, 14 mammalian caspases have been cloned and belong to one of two functional subgroups: inflammation or apoptosis. Incidentally, the first mammalian caspase cloned, ICE or caspase-1, is involved in inflammation *(41)*, not apoptosis as was originally suggested *(37)*. The expansion of the caspase family can be explained by the increase in the number and complexity of the pathways as well as the different substrate specificity of each caspase defined by the tetrapeptide recognition motif with an aspartic acid requirement in the first position *(42)*. The apoptotic caspases have more recently been subdivided into two categories: initiator and executioner (Fig. 3A). This distinction reflects the caspase's overall structure, which determines at what point in the pathway it participates *(39)*. Initiator caspases are activated by adaptor-mediated processes and, as the name implies, begin the caspase cascade. These caspases include caspase-9 and -2 as well as caspase-8 and -10. The adaptor-driven activation of these caspases depends on conserved motifs within their long prodomains. The caspase activation and recruitment domain (CARD) of caspase-9 and -2 and the death effector domain (DED) of caspase-8 and -10 facilitate their interactions with CARD- or DED-containing adaptor proteins, leading to the local aggregation and activation of these initiator caspases *(41)* (Fig. 3B). Knockout studies in mice have demonstrated a requirement in signaling for caspase-8 downstream of all known death receptors *(43)*, whereas caspase-9 is required for most death stimuli using the intrinsic pathway, with a few notable exceptions *(44,45)*.

Once activated, the main function of initiator caspases is in targeting the specific cleavage and activation of the second set of apoptotic caspases, the executioner caspases including caspase-3, -6, and -7 (Fig. 3A,B). Executioner caspases are mainly responsible for cleaving various intracellular target proteins containing consensus caspase cleavage sites in order to dismantle the cell as quickly as possible, avoiding an inflammatory response *(46)*. Similar to observations with caspase-9, caspase-3 knockout mice display gross brain malformations and die prematurely, suggesting a role for caspase-3 in normal development of the brain *(47,48)*. Furthermore, apoptotic defects are stimulus- and tissue-dependent, as seen with the caspase-9 knockout, but death in response to most stimuli of the intrinsic and extrinsic pathways display a defect in some cell type with the loss of caspase-3. Therefore caspase-3 has been proposed to be the crucial executioner caspase responsible for most of the nuclear phenotypes associated with apoptosis *(48)*. Lesser roles are postulated for the remaining executioner caspases; however, caspase-7 likely plays a more predominant role in the execution phase of cell death than caspase-6 based on knockout studies *(49)*.

CASPASE ACTIVATING ADAPTOR PROTEINS—APAF-1 AND FADD

Initiator caspases become activated in response to a number of apoptotic stimuli including death ligands, serum withdrawal, and DNA damage due to replication dysfunction, irradiation, or exposure to chemotherapeutic agents. Initiator caspase activation is contingent on their local aggregation via adaptor proteins. DED-containing initiator caspase-8 and -10 function in the extrinsic pathway and undergo autoproteolytic cleavage due to induced aggregation *(50–52)*. Aggregation is a result of the ligation of death ligands to their cognate receptors, leading to recruitment of the adaptor protein FADD followed by DED-caspase recruitment (Fig. 4A). A conserved motif termed the death domain (DD) *(53)*, present in both the receptor and the adaptor, is responsible for their interaction *(54,55)*. FADD, in turn via its DED, is able to recruit and concentrate DED-caspases at the cell surface; thus, the compilation of these factors (ligand, receptor, adaptor, and caspases) are the minimal requirements within the DISC *(56,57)*. Formation of the DISC is sufficient to increase the local concentration of DED-caspases, leading to their cleavage *(15)* (Fig. 4A). This cleavage event was considered the DED-caspase activating event; however, more recent studies suggest that dimerization, not cleavage, leads to DED-caspase activation, with the cleavage event serving a stabilizing role *(58–60)*. Knockout studies in human and mouse cells demonstrate an absolute requirement for FADD and caspase-8 in death receptor-mediated apoptosis *(61–64)*.

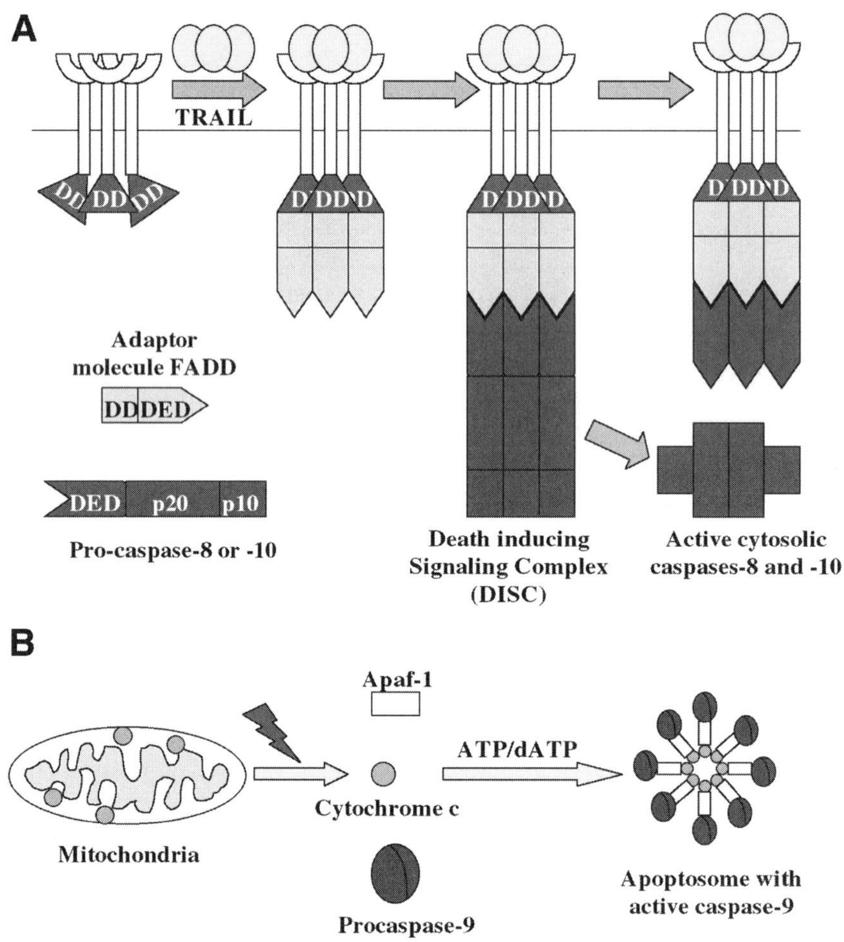

Fig. 4. Adaptor-mediated initiator caspase activation. **(A)** FADD-mediated procaspase-8 and -10 recruitment following death ligand exposure leads DISC formation and subsequent DED-caspase activation. **(B)** Following cellular stress, cytochrome c release from mitochondria in conjunction with ATP, Apaf-1, and procaspase-9 leads to apoptosome formation and subsequent caspase-9 activity. Apaf-1 undergoes a conformational change to allow binding to procaspase-9.

The other adaptor protein responsible for initiator caspase activation is Apaf-1 *(65)*, the ced-4 homolog, which functions in the intrinsic pathway leading to procaspase-9 activation *(66)* (Fig. 4B). Besides Apaf-1, other cofactors are necessary for the activation of caspase-9. Following mitochondrial dysfunction in response to growth factor withdrawal or DNA damage, cytochrome c is released from the mitochondria *(67)*. Cytosolic cytochrome c interacts with the WD-40 repeats of Apaf-1, enhancing the recruitment of ATP *(68)*. This causes a conformational change within Apaf-1, exposing the CARD and allowing for adaptor-mediated procaspase-9 recruitment via CARD/CARD interactions. Cytochrome c in conjunction with ATP, Apaf-1, and procaspase-9 form the holoenzyme known as the apoptosome *(66)* (Fig. 4B). Unlike other known caspases, active caspase-9 remains associated with the apoptosome without undergoing cleavage events to achieve its maximal activity *(69)*. The apoptosome is then competent to activate executioner caspases such as caspase-3 *(66)*. The phenotype and death characteristics of Apaf-1 knockout mice *(70,71)* support a pathway from Apaf-1 to caspase-9 to caspase-3, regulating the intrinsic pathway.

CASPASE INHIBITORY PROTEINS—MAMMALIAN AND VIRAL

Due to the central role that caspases play in apoptosis, mammals as well as *Drosophila* regulate caspase activity in part by a family of caspase binding proteins called IAPs. The first IAP was identified by Lois Miller in baculovirus as a protein that increases host cell survival following infection *(72)*. Initial studies suggested that two features of these genes were necessary for antiapoptotic function: the baculovirus IAP repeat (BIR) domain and the RING domain *(73)*. Subsequently, a number of mammalian IAP genes were recognized and cloned based on homology *(16)*. A number of these genes, including the first human IAP discovered (NAIP) *(74)*, survivin, and Bruce, contain only BIR domains. Although when overexpressed they inhibit apoptosis to varying degrees, they are not considered classical IAPs but rather BIR-containing proteins (BIRPs) *(75)*and will not be discussed further. The five remaining IAPs—namely, XIAP (ILP-1), ILP-2 (not found in mouse), c-IAP1 (hIAP2), c-IAP2 (hIAP1), and ML-IAP (Livin)—contain a variable number of BIR domains (anywhere from one to three) with intervening linker regions as well as a C-terminal RING domain (Fig. 5).

The most studied family member, XIAP *(76)*, provided the first clues as to how IAPs inhibit cell death. XIAP directly interacts with executioner caspase-3 and -7 to inhibit caspase function *(77)*. Caspase-9 was subsequently identified as an XIAP target for inhibition as well *(78)*. These effects are mediated in part by the BIR domains that have different caspase specificity, BIR2 for caspase-3 and -7 and BIR3 for caspase-9 *(79)*. Surprisingly, subsequent crystal structure analysis revealed a role for linker binding directly to caspase-3 and -7, preventing substrate binding and allowing only a limited number of contacts between caspase and the actual BIR domain *(80–83)*. Therefore, the linker region between the BIR1 and 2 domains directly binds caspase-3 and -7 and helps in determining the caspase specificity along with the BIR2 domain. Recently the crystal structure of the BIR3 domain of XIAP complexed with caspase-9 revealed the mechanism behind the inhibition. Due to the necessity of initiator caspase dimerization for activation *(59,84)*, the BIR3 domain acts to prevent caspase dimerization, trapping the caspase in an inactive monomeric state *(85)*.

XIAP is generally considered the most potent of the IAP family due to its ability to bind and inhibit caspase-9, -3, and -7. On the other hand, a recently cloned, highly homologous human protein, ILP-2, has specificity for only caspase-9 due to the presence of only one BIR domain, most similar to BIR 3 of XIAP *(86)*. Interestingly this gene is absent in mice, does not contain any introns, and is only expressed in the testis. Other family members, c-IAP1 and c-IAP2, distinguish themselves based on their cloning as tumor necrosis factor (TNF) receptor 2-associated proteins which interact with TRAF1 and TRAF2 *(87)*. These two proteins were subsequently shown to inhibit caspase-3 and -7 *(88)* in studies similar to those initially performed with XIAP. c-IAP1 and c-IAP2, two highly similar proteins, also contain a CARD, the significance of which is still not understood. Despite their recruitment to the TNF receptor complex that contains caspase-8, c-IAP1 and c-IAP2 do not demonstrate any specificity for this caspase *(78,88)*. The same can be said for all

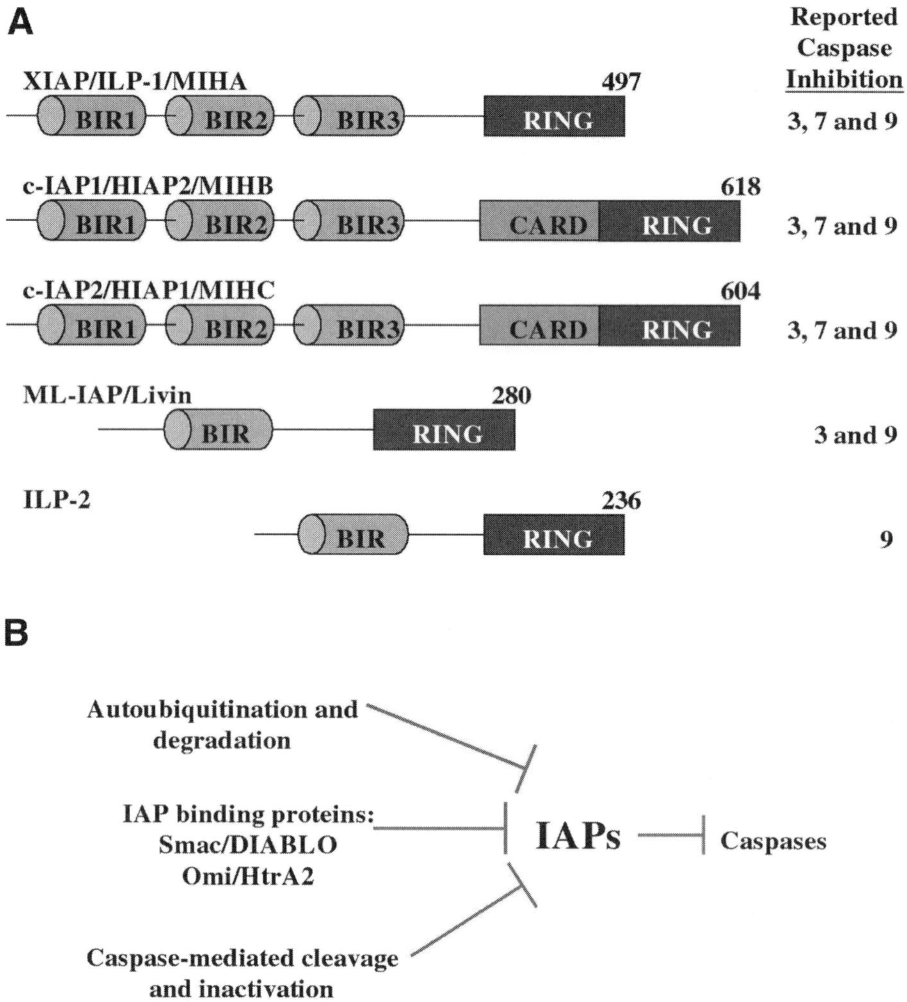

Fig. 5. The human antiapoptotic IAP family members and mechanisms of IAP inhibition. **(A)** The five human IAP proteins thought to directly bind caspases are listed above along with their cellular caspase targets. Conserved motifs include the BIR domain, the RING domain and the CARD. The BIR domain of ILP-2 most closely resembles the BIR3 domain of XIAP while the BIR domain of ML-IAP looks like a hybrid between XIAP's BIR2 and BIR3 domain. **(B)** The IAPs are inhibited by three distinct mechanisms: auto-ubiquitination and degradation, caspase-mediated cleavage and sequestration by IAP binding proteins, Smac/DIABLO and Omi/HtrA2.

other IAP family members. No IAP has been found to bind or inhibit the DED-caspases of the extrinsic pathway. Lastly, ML-IAP was recently identified as a single BIR domain containing IAP with a RING domain and is overexpressed in a majority of melanoma cell lines *(89)*.

Despite the controversy surrounding its requirement for the suppression of apoptosis *(90)*, the IAP RING domain has recently been recognized as a regulator of IAP and associated protein stability *(91)*. The realization that RING domains, in a variety of unrelated proteins, serve as E3 ubiquitin ligases in the ubiquitin-mediated proteolytic pathway *(92)* initiated subsequent work on the IAPs. Both XIAP and c-IAP1 were demonstrated to contain ubiquitin ligase activity that was dependent on their RING domains. This activity was shown to mediate the autoubiquitination of both proteins in response to glucocorticoids or etoposide in thymocytes, suggesting that the degradation of both proteins was necessary for death progression *(93)*. Recent studies have attempted to identify targets of IAP-mediated ubiquitination and degradation. In vitro data with c-IAP2 suggests that it promotes the monoubiquitination of caspase-3 and -7 *(94)*. Similarly, XIAP has been shown to ubiquitinate caspase-3 in vitro and a constitutively active caspase-3 mutant could be degraded by XIAP in a RING-domain dependent manner *(95)*. Both of these studies suggest that caspases could be a target of IAP-mediated ubiquitination and degradation, supplying another means by which IAPs inhibit cell death. These observations suggest that the E3 ligase function is crucial for the ability of IAPs to suppress cell death. The identification of more physiologic E3 IAP targets will further our understanding of IAP biology.

With the creation of the IAP family of proteins in higher organisms to inhibit caspase activity also comes the necessity to counteract this inhibition when a death stimulus is received (Fig. 5B). As was discussed above, the ubiquitin ligase activity of the IAPs is one mechanism by which the cell targets IAPs for degradation to allow death progression *(93)*. Furthermore, caspase-dependent IAP cleavage provides another means by which the cell eliminates IAP function *(96,97)*. Lastly, IAP binding proteins, functionally homologous to the *Drosophila* RHG proteins, have been discovered in mammals *(28–34)*. Unlike their *Drosophila* counterparts, Smac/DIABLO and HtrA2/Omi are resident mitochondrial proteins that are released upon mitochondrial dysfunction in order to bind and sequester IAPs. Despite the lack of overall amino acid conservation between the *Drosophila* and mammalian genes, all of the IAP binding proteins including caspase-9 contain a common tetrapeptide sequence or an IAP-binding motif (IBM) that is either constitutively exposed (RHG proteins) or exposed following posttranslational processing (mammalian proteins), which mediates IAP binding *(98)*. Although their relative contribution in different physiological settings remains unclear, these three mechanisms of IAP inhibition cooperate to eliminate IAP function following an apoptotic signal (Fig. 5B).

In addition to the IAPs, baculoviruses encode a second protein, p35, that appears to be required for host cell survival *(99)*. p35 encodes a broad spectrum caspase inhibitor whose cleavage generates a tight inhibitor/caspase complex *(100,101)*. With the evolution of an extrinsic pathway in mammalian cells, viruses began to develop inhibitors of caspase-8 in order to subvert the host's immune response. The cowpox virus utilizes the gene product CrmA to target caspase-8 as means to shut down the extrinsic pathway *(102–104)*. Two other recently described viral caspase-8 binding proteins include vICA from cytomegalovirus *(105)* and the 14.7kDa adenovirus protein *(106)*. A more indirect means of caspase-8 inhibition can be seen with some herpesviruses as well as with molluscipoxvirus. These viruses encode DED-containing proteins termed viral FLICE-inhibitory proteins (v-FLIPs) that compete with cellular caspase-8 and -10 for recruitment to the DISC *(107–109)*. This competition leads to decreased DED-caspase activation and cell survival. All of the aforementioned viral strategies have evolved to target apoptosis at its core, the caspase, in order to allow viral propagation in the face of an attacking immune system.

CELLULAR CASPASE SUBSTRATES

The morphological changes associated with programmed cell death are a direct result of the systematic cleavage of intracellular proteins by caspases. In the initiation phase, the apical caspases begin the caspase cascade by directly cleaving and activating executioner caspases *(41)*. The executioner caspases are therefore responsible for dismantling the cell by cleaving specific substrates leading to DNA fragmentation, membrane blebbing, and cell shrinkage *(110)* (Fig. 6). However, besides executioner caspases, there are two notable noncaspase substrates of caspase-8: the BH3-only protein, Bid, as well as plectin involved in cytoskeletal integrity. Bid was initially described as a proapoptotic BH3-only protein that interacted with both pro- and antiapoptotic Bcl-2 family members *(111)*. The identification of Bid as a caspase-8 target established a link between the extrinsic pathway and the intrinsic pathway, resulting in cytochrome c release following death ligand treatment *(112,113)*. Cleavage of Bid by caspase-8 results in the subsequent myristoylation of an exposed glycine that assists in the translocation to mitochondrial membranes *(114)*. This mitochondrial amplification step through Bid serves to further activate caspases, which in some cell types is absolutely necessary for cell death.

Plectin is the only known cytoskeletal protein that is targeted by initiator caspases, namely caspase-8. Cleavage of plectin is thought to be important for cytoskeletal reorganization because plectin-deficient mouse embryonic fibroblasts (MEFs) do not undergo the characteristic actin rearrangements seen in response to death stimuli *(115)*. Additional cytoskeletal and cytosolic caspase cleavage targets involved in the cell reshaping, blebbing, and shrinkage process include gelsolin *(116)*, keratins *(117,118)*, PAK2 *(119)*, α-fodrin *(120)*, and ROCK I *(121,122)*; however, these proteins are among a growing list of over 100 proteins which are targeted by the executioner caspase group, caspase-3, -6, and -7 *(9)* (Fig. 6). The executioner caspases can further amplify the death signal through further caspase activation. Caspase-3 has been shown to be necessary for the activation of caspase-6 in response to cytochrome c release *(123)* while caspase-6 has the ability to activate caspase-3 *(124)*.

One of the most characteristic changes associated with apoptosis is chromatin condensation and DNA fragmentation creating a laddering effect due to cleavage between nucleosomes *(125)*. The identification of the caspase-activated DNase (CAD) revealed that CAD was latent in undamaged cells due to the association of an inhibitor (ICAD) *(126–128)*. An apoptotic stimulus then led to a caspase-3 dependent cleavage of ICAD, releasing CAD to cleave cellular DNA. More recent experiments have also attributed roles for the cleavage/degradation of cellular DNA to endoG *(129)* released from mitochondria and DNase II contributed by phagocytic cells *(130)*. Apoptotic chromatin condensation is both a caspase-dependent and -independent process. The caspase-3 target, acinus *(131)*, as well as the apoptosis inducing factor (AIF) *(132)*, normally sequestered in the mitochondria, have the capacity to trigger chromatin condensation following cellular insult. Elimination of DNA repair enzymes such as PARP *(133,134)* and DNA-PK *(135)* through executioner caspase-mediated cleavage prevents the cell from attempting to fix apoptotic DNA fragmentation.

Caspase-3 was originally identified as the enzyme responsible for the majority of the cellular phenotypic changes due to mouse knockout studies that demonstrate impaired PARP cleavage and DNA fragmentation *(47,48)*. However, compensatory mechanisms mediated by caspase-6 and -7 may exist in cells that lose caspase-3 expression *(136,137)*.

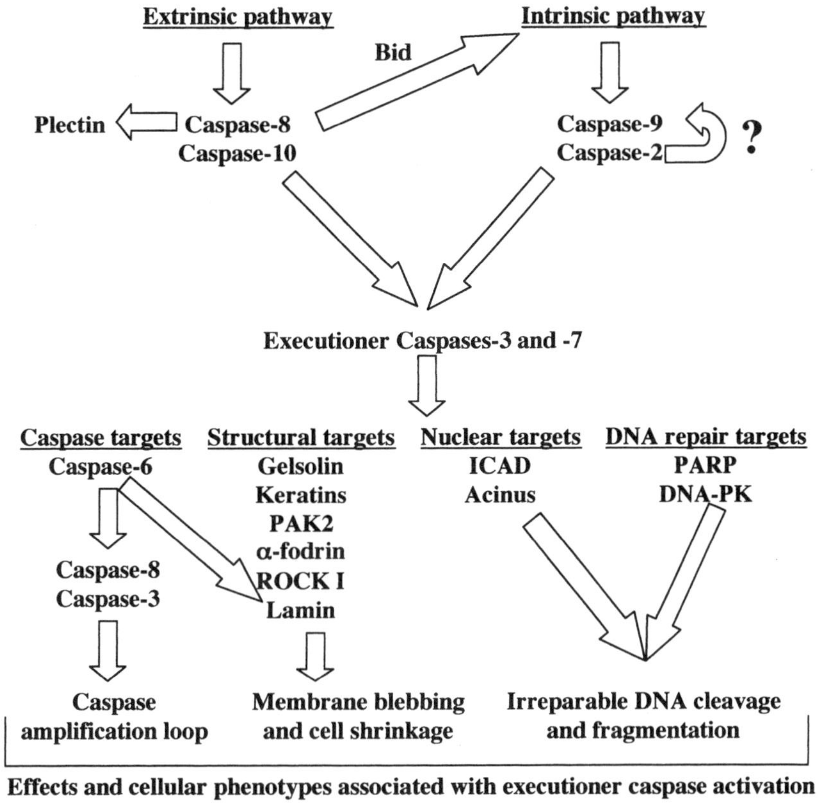

Fig. 6. The caspase cascade of the intrinsic and extrinsic pathways and the relevant caspase targets mediating cellular breakdown. Following death stimuli, initiator caspases are activated and primarily function to activate executioner caspases. Two relevant noncaspase-8 targets are shown which participate in the cell reshaping process (Plectin) as well as initiating the mitochondrial amplification loop (Bid). Activation of the executioner caspases however are primarily responsible for the large scale phenotypic changes associated with programmed cell death.

Due to the substrate specificity similarities between caspase-3 and -7 *(42)*, they are believed to act on a similar substrates with caspase-3 being the predominant effector. Caspase-6, however, has a different substrate specificity than the other executioner caspases *(42)*. Besides caspase-3 *(124)*, Lamin A/C is also recognized as a caspase-6 target for cleavage involved in nuclear breakdown *(138)*. Recently, caspase-6 was biochemically purified as the caspase-8 activating enzyme in response to cytochrome c release *(139)*, identifying the mechanism by which the intrinsic pathway activates the caspases of the extrinsic pathway.

CLEARANCE OF APOPTOTIC CELLS BY PHAGOCYTOSIS

Elimination of cells via apoptosis avoids an immune response that is contingent on the apoptotic cell being cleared via phagocytosis *(140)*. In mammalian cells, macrophages (professional phagocytes) or neighboring cells (nonprofessional phagocytes) carry out this function. One active area of research focuses on identifying "eat me" signals on dying cells. Although a number of signals probably cooperate to initiate phagocytosis *(141)*, the phospholipid, phosphatidylserine (PS) is the best characterized signal to date. PS is normally only exposed on the inner leaflet of the plasma membrane but becomes permanently externalized when aminophopholipid translocase is switched off in apoptotic cells *(142)*. With the discovery of the phosphatidylserine receptor (PSR) on macrophages, fibroblasts, and epithelial cells *(143)*, one component of the mechanism by which phagocytes recognize apoptotic cells was elucidated. More recently, a protein produced and secreted by macrophages, MFG-E8, binds apoptotic cells via aminophospholipids such as PS and serves to assist in engulfment by macrophages *(144)*. Roles for additional extracellular proteins such as lectins, integrins, and scavenger receptors on the surface of phagocytes in the recognition of dying cells are still ongoing *(141)*.

Following the recognition of "eat me" signals on dying cells, understanding the cytoskeletal rearrangements involved in carrying out the engulfment process is a major task. The use of phagocytosis mutants from *C. elegans* has identified a Rac-dependent cell reshaping process involving ELMO-1, DOCK180, and Crk11 that is conserved in mammalian cells *(145)*. Experiments on this pathway in *C. elegans* have led to the theory of "assisted cell suicide." The idea stems from data in ced-3 partial loss of function mutant worms (caspase compromised) in which engulfment genes were also mutated leading to an increase in cell survival. This supports the idea that cells surrounding apoptotic cells can actively participate in the life or death decision of that cell (i.e., assisted suicide) via phagocytosis *(146,147)*. Evidence of a similar phenomenon is being studied in mammalian cells as well *(148)*.

REGULATION OF THE INTRINSIC PATHWAY BY THE BCL-2 FAMILY OF PROTEINS

Recent studies have revealed that mitochondria function at the core of the intrinsic pathway by not only sensing cellular stress but also by responding to this stress by releasing necessary components of the pathway into the cytosol. Therefore, understanding the maintenance and subsequent disruption of mitochondrial integrity has become paramount in delineating these pathways. Even though the mechanism(s) involved in altering mitochondrial integrity are not completely understood, the importance of pro- and antiapoptotic Bcl-2 family members in apoptosis is irrefutable *(11)* (Fig. 7). The genesis of the field dates back to the realization that Bcl-2, a gene overexpressed in follicular lymphoma due to a translocation, promoted cell survival without affecting cell proliferation directly *(149)*. This was the first demonstration that alteration of an apoptotic pathway could lead to tumor development. Similar to the revelation that *C. elegans* ced-3 represented the primordial caspase gene, subsequent studies demonstrated that Bcl-2 could functionally substitute for the loss of ced-9 in *C. elegans (150)*. In the case of *C. elegans* where one pro- (egl-1) and one antiapoptotic (ced-9) Bcl-2-like genes exist, the pathway seems straightforward; however, when considering that multiple pro- and antiapoptotic Bcl-2 members, including at least 10 BH3-only proteins, exist in humans, the situation becomes more complex.

Classification as a Bcl-2 family protein requires the presence of at least one Bcl-2 homology (BH) domain. The Bcl-2 family is divided into three groups based on BH structure/function: one antiapoptotic family with three to four BH domains (Bcl-2, Bcl-X_L, BCL-w, A1, Mcl-1, Bcl-B and Boo), and two proapoptotic families, the Bcl-2-like (Bax) group with two to three BH domains (Bax, Bak, Bok, Bcl-G_L, $_a$nd Bcl-X_S) and the BH3-

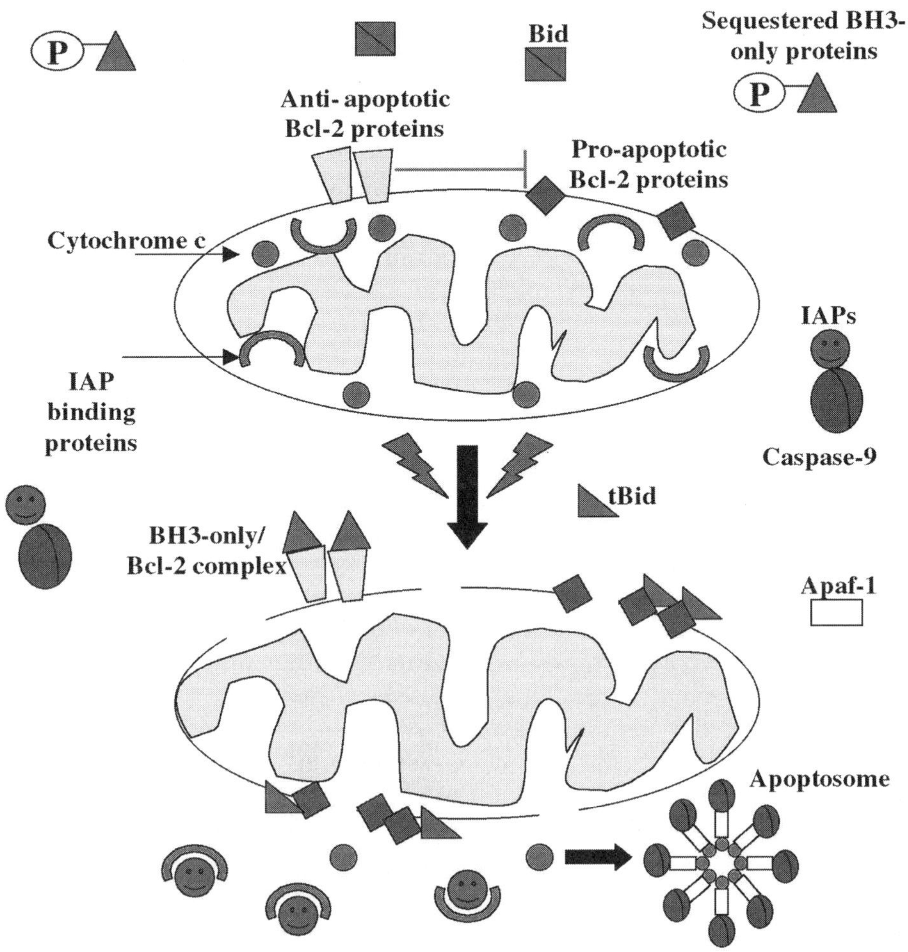

Fig. 7. Intrinsic pathway mediated by mitochondrial homeostasis. Although the exact mechanism by which mitochondria become permeabilized is of much debate, Bcl-2 proteins impact this decision. In the absence of stress, BH3-only proteins are sequestered and thereby inactivated by a number of posttranslational mechanisms. Antiapoptotic Bcl-2 proteins inhibit the pro-apoptotic members on the surface of the mitochondria. Following stress, BH3-only proteins target the antiapoptotic proteins on the surface of the mitochondria. This relieves the inhibition on proapoptotic members such as Bax and Bak allowing multimerization in conjunction with membrane targeted tBid. These events can lead to membrane disruption by a number of mechanims resulting in the release of cytochrome c, IAP binding proteins and subsequent apoptosome formation.

only group (Bid, Bad, Bik, Bim, Hrk, Blk, Bmf, Noxa, Puma, and Bcl-G_S) *(10)*. The antiapoptotic group relies on its ability to either inducibly or constitutively localize to intracellular membranes (mitochondria, ER, and nucleus) via a C-terminal transmembrane tail to prevent cell death *(13)*. Evidence for their importance comes from mouse knockout studies as well as transgenic animals. Bcl-2, the prototype member, causes enhanced hematopoetic cell survival when overexpressed in different lineages *(151–153)* or leads to kidney and mature lymphocyte cell loss when deleted *(154)*.

Similar to *C. elegans*, the BH3-only proteins are upstream of and negatively regulate the antiapoptotic Bcl-2 members through direct protein/protein interactions (Fig. 7). The conserved BH3 domain, consisting of only nine amino acids, is sufficient to interact with the antiapoptotic family, nullifying their protective effects *(155)*. The large expansion of this group in mammalian cells has led to the hypothesis that the different members respond in a stimulus-dependent, tissue-specific manner, which is being tested in BH3-only knockout mice *(10)*. For instance, the Bim knockout mice respond normally to DNA damage but are partially resistant to cytokine withdrawal while displaying increased numbers of only lymphoid and myeloid cells *(156)*. The combined knockout of Bim and Bcl-2 also confirms that BH3-only proteins regulate the activity of the antiapoptotic members because loss of only one Bim allele in a Bcl-2 –/– background rescues the degenerative kidney disease in these mice *(157)*. Because the BH3-only proteins are the most upstream regulators within this family, their regulation has become an active area of research. Transcriptional mechanisms of increasing cellular protein levels as well as posttranslational modifications affecting subcellular localization and/or conformation has begun to unravel the signaling pathways upstream of the mitochondria *(10)*.

The remaining family of multi-BH domain proapoptotic Bcl-2 proteins appears to act most distally in the mitochondrial pathway, based on studies of mice lacking two of these proteins, Bax and Bak. Single gene knockout of either protein yielded no dramatic (or lethal) organismal phenotype; however, deletion of both genes rendered most animals nonviable due to a variety of developmental defects stemming from loss of apoptosis *(158)*. Subsequent studies demonstrated that overexpression of BH3-only proteins was unable to induce apoptosis in the absence of Bax and Bak, placing these two genes most downstream genetically in the Bcl-2 pathway *(159–161)*. Cytosolic Bax and mitochondrial Bak both undergo conformational changes and oligomerize in the mitochondrial membrane upon activation of the pathway, relieving inhibition by the antiapoptotic family members *(11)* (Fig. 7). Nevertheless, how oligomerization of Bax family members contributes to mitochondrial dysfunction and effects the permeability transition (PT), and whether it occurs directly through pore formation or other means, is still under investigation *(162)*. Regardless of the mechanism(s) involved, mitochondrial dysfunction leads to the release of proapoptotic factors from the mitochondrial intermembrane space that serves to activate procaspase-9 through apoptosome formation (Fig. 7).

MITOCHONDRIA—INITIATOR OR AMPLIFIER OF THE INTRINSIC PATHWAY?

Recently, the classical view of the mammalian intrinsic pathway, as described above, has been challenged as a few inconsistencies have become apparent *(155)*. Despite the fact that *C. elegans* and mammalian systems contain the same basic core machinery (namely a BH3-only protein, Bcl-2 protein, an adaptor, and a caspase), mechanistically the two systems operate very differently. In *C. elegans*, after a death signal is received, the BH3-only protein binds to and negatively regulates the Bcl-2 protein (similar to what is observed in the mammalian systems). However, Bcl-2 sequestration in *C. elegans* releases the adaptor protein, leading directly to caspase activation, unlike what is observed in mammalian systems. In addition, the mitochondria play no active role in this process in *C. elegans* or *Drosophila*. This has led to the hypothesis that Bcl-2 proteins may play a similar role in sequestering unknown adaptors in mammalian cells *(155)*. Such adaptor

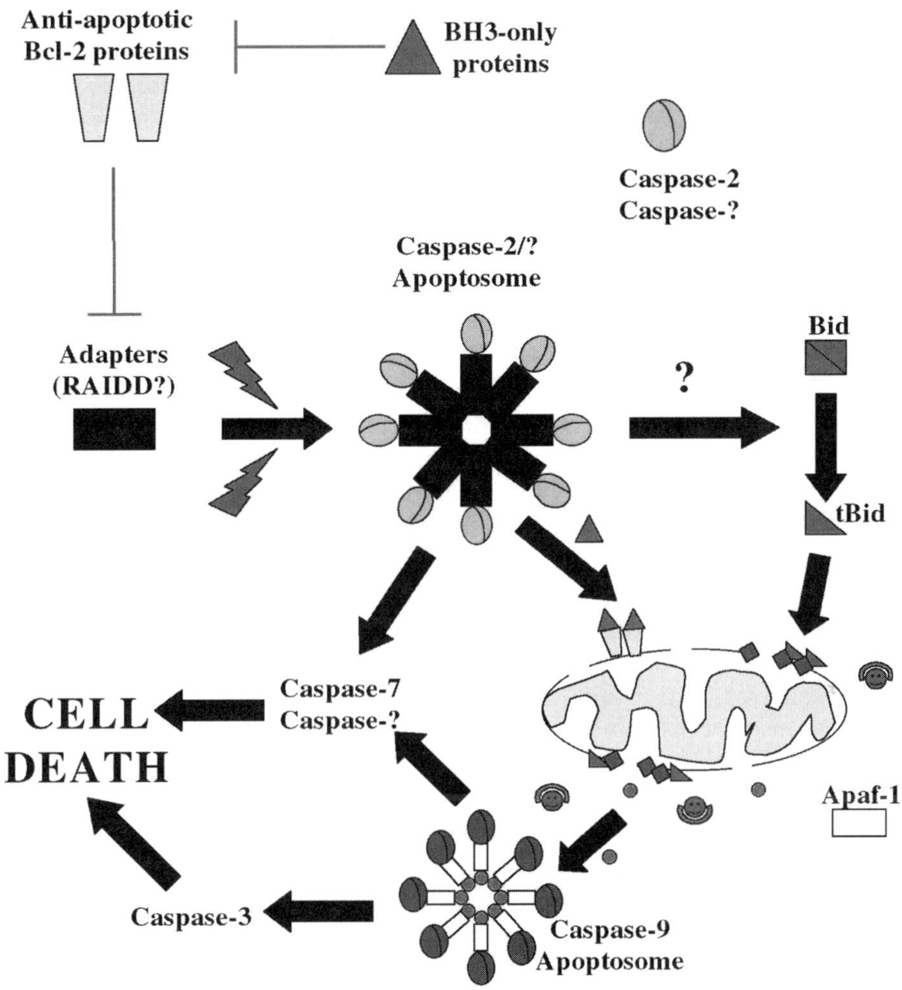

Fig. 8. Alternative model of the intrinsic pathway. This model more closely reflects the basic cell death machinery of C. elegans in which antiapoptotic Bcl-2 family members antagonize an adaptor molecule necessary for caspase activation. A role for caspase-2 upstream of the mitochondria has recently been suggested in which an unknown adaptor molecule triggers its activation. Caspase-2 activation (and potentially other unidentified caspases) simultaneously activates the mitochondrial pathway as well as an alternative pathway not requiring caspase-9. In this model, mitochondrial involvement only serves as an amplification loop, as is seen in the death receptor pathway. The other pathway activated by caspase-2 is sufficient to carry out the death program via the intrinsic pathway in the absence of Apaf-1 or caspase-9.

proteins in turn may activate caspase(s) upstream of mitochondrial engagement. Mitochondrial dysfunction therefore may be a consequence of this upstream caspase activation rather than the event responsible for caspase activation, similar to what is seen after activation of the extrinsic pathway (Fig. 8). Two recent reports give support to this model *(163,164)*; however, many questions still remain.

One study to support this idea comes from observations comparing wild-type mice reconstituted with fetal liver stem cells from Bcl-2 transgenic mice, Bim –/– mice, Apaf-1 –/– mice, or caspase-9 –/– mice *(163)*. The survival of thymocytes from a Bcl-2 transgenic mouse or a Bim –/– mouse is enhanced compared with Apaf-1 –/– or caspase-9 –/– mice when challenged with cytokine withdrawal. In addition, thymocytes isolated directly from Bcl-2 transgenic mice or Apaf-1 or caspase-9 knockout mice demonstrate that Bcl-2 plays a major role in their clonogenic survival after cytokine withdrawal, whereas the loss of Apaf-1 or caspase-9 does not rescue their survival. These observations suggest that Bcl-2 and Bim play a major role in the apoptotic process of hematopoetic cells whereas caspase-9 and Apaf-1 are largely dispensible *(163)*. In contrast to previous reports *(44,45,70,71)*, the Apaf-1 –/– and caspase-9 –/– thymocytes undergo caspase-mediated cell death with traditional hallmarks (PARP cleavage, DNA fragmentation) in response to cytokine withdrawal and irradiation *(163)*. The kinetics of death are delayed, presumably as a result of the lack of a mitochondrial amplification loop, but cytochrome c is released in a caspase-dependent manner ultimately leading to caspase-7 activation followed by PARP and ICAD cleavage *(163)*. These observations are consistent with a model in which an initiator caspase acts upstream of the mitochondria, possibly inhibited by antiapoptotic bcl-2 family members (Fig. 8).

One potential initiator caspase to serve this role upstream of the mitochondria has recently been identified through the use of RNAi technology. The knockdown of caspase-2 protein levels by RNAi resulted in resistance to etoposide, cisplatin, and ultraviolet (UV) irradiation as robustly as knockdown of Apaf-1 protein *(164)*. However, depletion of caspase-2 results in a lack of cytochrome c and Smac release from the mitochondria and loss of Bax translocation, whereas Apaf-1 ablation does not effect these events. Caspase-2 activation in the absence of Apaf-1 in response to etoposide suggests that it may occur upstream of the mitochondria in an initiator caspase role. The lack of a significant phenotype in the caspase-2 knockout mouse does not support a major role in the intrinsic pathway *(165)*; however, another caspase may compensate for the loss of caspase-2 in the mouse or it may represent a difference between humans and mice. Preliminary experiments with caspase-2 suggest that it may also form a multiprotein complex leading to activation upstream of cytochrome c release, but the constituents of the activating complex have not been identified *(166)* (Fig. 8). More experiments are required to discern what initiator caspase(s) and cofactors form upstream of the mitochondria and which substrates contribute to mitochondrial dysfunction.

RELEASE OF PROAPOPTOTIC FACTORS FROM THE MITOCHONDRIA

Regardless of whether the intrinsic pathway initiates at the mitochondria or upstream of it, mitochondrial dysfunction occurs in response to both the intrinsic and extrinsic pathway and this leads to the release of proapoptotic proteins from the intermembrane space *(167)*. The first to be identified was cytochrome c *(67)*, previously known to function only within the electron transport chain. Subsequently it was shown to play a crucial role in the activation of caspase-9. Caspase-9 is monomeric in unstimulated cells *(84)*, however all caspase-9 activity following cytochrome c release is associated with a large molecular weight complex *(69)*. Activation of caspase-9 minimally requires dimerization *(59,84)*, therefore oligomerization is mediated via complex formation with released cytochrome c, Apaf-1, and ATP (or dATP) to create the holoenzyme known as the apoptosome *(66)* (Fig. 7). Apoptosome formation leads to the activation of executioner caspase-3, -6, and -7 *(66)*. Activation of caspase-3 by the apoptosome leads to a positive caspase feedback loop as caspase-3-mediated caspase-9 cleavage results in more active apoptosome *(168)*.

Because caspase activation and amplification is crucial for cell death, the elimination of caspase inhibitory proteins, such as IAPs, will further enhance the process. The mitochondria sequester two known IAP binding proteins, Smac/DIABLO and HtrA2/Omi (Fig. 7). Smac/DIABLO was simultaneously cloned through its ability to biochemically enhance caspase-3 activation and by its ability to bind to XIAP *(28,29)*. HtrA2/Omi also acts by binding and inhibiting IAPs, but additionally contains serine protease activity which also contributes to its proapoptotic function *(30–34)*. When overexpressed, HtrA2/Omi mutants, which are unable to bind IAPs, can still potentiate death by virtue of this serine protease activity. Consequently, this death is not inhibitable by zVAD, XIAP, or a dominant negative caspase-9. The identification of HtrA2/Omi as a mediator in the apoptotic process could potentially reveal a novel role for serine proteases in apoptosis. IAP binding of both Smac/DIABLO and HtrA2/Omi is mediated by an IAP binding motif (AVPI for SMAC/Diablo and AVPS for Omi) that is revealed once the mitochondrial targeting sequence is removed, thereby preventing IAP binding during their translocation to the mitochondria. Elimination of IAP function by these two proteins serves to release caspase-9, -3, and -7, allowing for their activation.

Activation of caspases leads to DNA fragmentation, one of the earliest recognized hallmarks of programmed cell death, and subsequent work provided evidence that the activation of the nuclease (CAD) by caspase-3 was responsible for this phenotype *(126–128)*; however, the absence of significant defects in mice lacking CAD activity *(169)* prompted the search for another apoptotic nuclease activity. Two mitochondrially localized proteins that cause DNA fragmentation were subsequently discovered, endonuclease G (endoG) and AIF. EndoG was identified as a mitochondrial protein which induces nuclear DNA fragmentation upon release from the mitochondria even in the absence of CAD *(170)*. This pathway appears to be evolutionarily conserved in *C. elegans* because cps6 mutants can be rescued with the murine endonuclease G *(132)*. AIF is also released from the mitochondria, and microinjection of AIF in resting cells results in caspase-independent chromatin condensation and degradation, loss of mitochondrial membrane potential, and phosphatidylserine exposure *(132,171)*. While the mechanism(s) behind these effects remain elusive due to an early embryonic lethality in the knockout (an apparent necessity for AIF in the first wave of developmental apoptosis) *(172)*, an interaction with Hsp70 may begin to shed light on this pathway *(173)*. Nevertheless, EndoG and AIF represent two caspase-independent mechanisms by which the cell can undergo DNA degradation upon mitochondrial disruption. All of the aforementioned proteins released from the mitochondria either serve to enhance caspase activation or directly lead to DNA fragmentation in order to propagate the death signal.

THE EXTRINSIC PATHWAY

The intrinsic cell death pathway involving the mitochondria with the interplay of Bcl-2 family members leading to apoptosome formation and subsequent executioner caspase activation is considered to be the ancestral apoptotic pathway with conservation of its core components in *C. elegans (9)*. A more recently evolved cell death cascade, termed the extrinsic pathway, employs a ligand/receptor interaction to transduce a death signal inside the cell in order to activate an independent set of initiator caspases (-8 and -10) *(174)* (Fig. 9). Specific ligand/receptor interactions evoke the formation of a DISC that is comprised of a trimeric ligand, trimeric receptor, an adaptor molecule (such as FADD) and caspases (-8 and -10). DISC formation has been postulated to occur due to protein/protein interactions mediated by conserved modules such as the death domain (receptor/adaptor) and death effector domain (adaptor/caspase) *(175)*. DISC formation leads to oligomerization of initiator caspase-8 and -10 that results in caspase activation via induced proximity *(176)*. Initiator caspase activation can either directly activate downstream executioner caspases to lead to cell death or employ the mitochondria through the cleavage of Bid to amplify the signal from the receptors *(177)* (Fig. 9). The intrinsic and extrinsic pathways ultimately converge to use the same executioner caspases to dismantle the cell; therefore, the gross phenotypic changes brought about by programmed cell death are the same regardless of which pathway is employed.

DEATH LIGANDS FROM THE TNF SUPERFAMILY (TNF-α, FAS, AND TRAIL)

Observations from the 1800s that acute bacterial infections caused tumor shrinkage in patients led to the description of a TNF that could kill tumor cells in patients *(178)* and in culture *(179)*. Cloning of the molecule *(180)* marked the beginning of an era that has identified members of the TNF superfamily of ligands, now numbering 18 *(177)*. This superfamily mainly evolved to regulate immune homeostasis *(181)*. Discussions will only focus on three of these ligands that cause cell death in which the molecular mechanisms are fairly well understood: TNF, FasL (CD95L, APO1L), and TNF-related apoptosis-inducing ligand (TRAIL or APO2L) (Fig. 10). Despite having "tumor necrosis" activity and the ability to cause cell death, TNF engages multiple pathways that regulate cell proliferation and inflammatory responses as well, depending on the cellular environment *(182)*. Conversely, FasL and TRAIL primarily mediate cell death when bound to their cognate receptors, although situations in which FasL and TRAIL promote cell proliferation have been described *(183,184)*. The evolution of death ligands was thought to occur specifically in order to respond to threats to the host (bacterial/viral infections and injured/cancerous cells) as well as to regulate immune homeostasis *(177)*. These type II transmembrane proteins are active as trimers with homology of TNF family members restricted to the residues necessary for trimerization *(185)*. Nonconserved residues between family members account for ligand/receptor specificity.

The biological activities of these death ligands in vivo have been explored through the use of neutralizing antibodies and knockout animals as well as studies of hereditary syndromes with defects in these pathways. Bacterial pathogens are recognized by Toll receptors, leading to TNF production in order to mount appropriate inflammatory responses *(181)*. TNF is produced from a variety of hematopoetic cell types in response to inflammation, injury, and environmental stresses. The biological responses to TNF treatment include cell proliferation, differentiation, apoptosis, and necrosis. Deregulation of TNF can lead to conditions such as septic shock, arthritis, irritable bowel disorder, and cachexia *(186)*. Unlike TNF, FasL, due to its propensity to primarily initiate cell death, leads to lymphoproliferation when the signaling pathway is compromised. Physiologic roles of

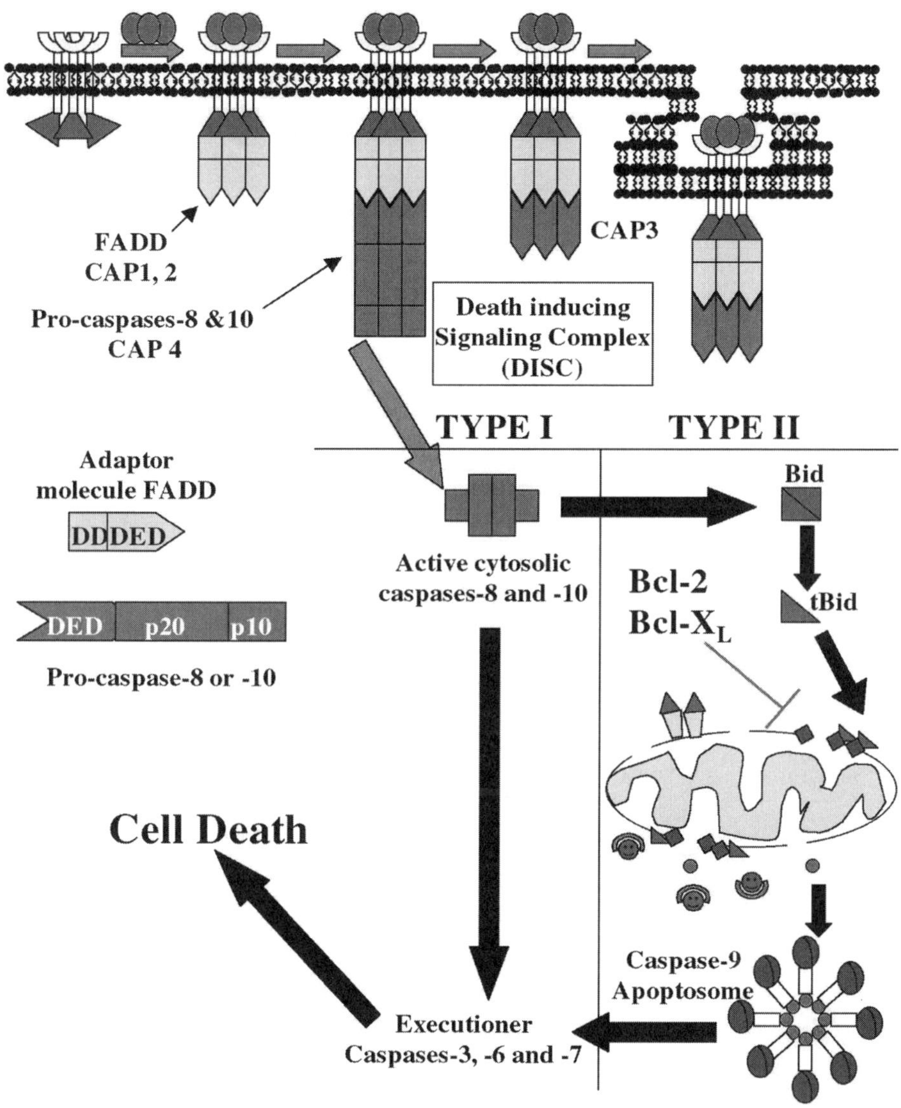

Fig. 9. The extrinsic death pathway. Trimeric death ligand binding leads to a conformational change within the cytoplasmic domains of the receptors allowing for FADD and caspase recruitment completing DISC formation. Release of large amounts of active caspases from the DISC in type I cells directly activates executioner caspases. Alternatively, Type II cells generate little DED-caspase activity and require mitochondrial amplification (which is inhibitable by Bcl-2) through caspase-8-mediated Bid cleavage. Ligand/receptor complexes are internalized into endosomes.

FasL in the elimination of cells include activation-induced cell death following immune responses, the deletion of self-reactive lymphocytes, and elimination of lymphocytes within immune privileged sites *(187)*. Inherited mutations of Fas ligand can lead to lymphadenopathy, enlarged T cell populations, and autoimmunity, consistent with the aforementioned biological roles *(14)*.

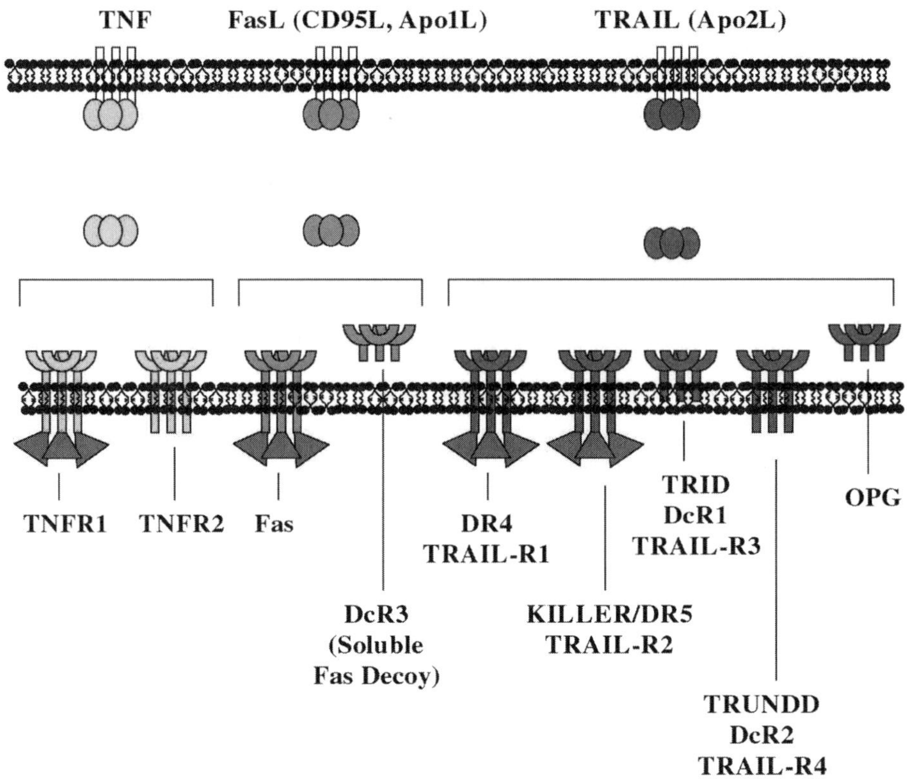

Fig. 10. Associations between members of the TNF and TNF Receptor superfamilies known to induce apoptosis upon ligand binding to cognate receptors. Death ligands are depicted as either type II membrane bound proteins or as shed soluble ligands. Receptors with the ability to transduce a death signal contain a death domain on the cytoplasmic face depicted by a triangle. All other receptors (with the exception of TNFR2) with the ability to bind ligand but unable to signal death are termed decoys. The TRAIL signaling pathway is most complex containing two proapoptotic receptors along with three putative decoys. Other members of the TNFR superfamily are known to induce apoptosis when overexpressed but either the ligand is unknown or the mechanism by which death is signaled is unclear.

Despite the ability of TNF and FasL to kill cells in vitro and in vivo, systemic administration of TNF or FasL is not a viable therapeutic option for cancer patients due to dangerous, potentially fatal systemic effects (i.e., inflammatory responses and liver failure) *(14)*. TRAIL, on the other hand, has represented a promising cancer therapy since its cloning owing to the observation that TRAIL has specificity for transformed cells but not normal cells in culture *(188,189)*. Experiments in mouse and primate models demonstrated that TRAIL could induce tumor regression without the systemic toxicity seen with FasL or TNF *(190,191)*. Given the antitumor activity seen with exogenous TRAIL, more recent studies have focused on the contribution of endogenous TRAIL to immune surveillance of tumor cells. TRAIL neutralizing antibodies have demonstrated a role for TRAIL (along with FasL and perforin) on liver natural killer (NK) cells against tumors in vivo as well as in the suppression of liver metastases *(192,193)*. These results were dependent on NK cells and interferon (IFN)-γ, which induces the expression of TRAIL on a variety of cell types *(192,193)*. These results coupled with studies from TRAIL knockout mice demonstrating increased tumor initiation and formation in response to chemical challenge *(194,195)* suggest that IFN-γ-mediated upregulation of TRAIL plays a role in the innate surveillance against tumors and metastases. The use of TRAIL or agonist antibodies against TRAIL receptors to combat cancer is currently being explored with promising results using an anti-DR5 monoclonal antibody against liver tumors *(196)* and an anti-DR4 monoclonal antibody in Phase I clinical trials *(197)*. Manipulation of the TRAIL pathway may also be beneficial in allogenic hematopoetic cell transplantation as recent studies suggest a role for TRAIL in the graft-vs-tumor (GVT) response, but not graft-vs-host disease (GVHD) *(198)*.

DEATH RECEPTORS AND DECOYS

The TNF receptor (TNFR) superfamily with 28 members is characterized by the presence of cysteine rich domains (CRDs), which mediate contacts between ligand and these type I transmembrane domain receptors *(177)*. Members of the TNF receptor superfamily that initiate cell death constitute a subgroup and are termed death receptors (DRs): TNF receptor 1 (TNFR1), Fas/Apo1 (CD95), DR3, DR4, KILLER/DR5, and DR6 *(181)*. The ability to cause cell death is contingent on the presence of an intracellular "death domain" *(53,199)*, a conserved motif within receptors and adaptor proteins that mediates their interaction leading to caspase activation and cell death *(174)*. Death ligands may interact with more than one cognate receptor with TRAIL being the most complex to date containing five described receptors in humans *(177)* (Fig. 10). Various receptors for each ligand can modulate the cell's response to ligand binding, either death or survival. Receptors that bind death ligands but do not trigger cell death are often called decoys and are easily identifiable due to the lack of a functional death domain (Fig. 10).

The existence of the Fas receptor was first realized through the generation of monoclonal antibodies against cell surface antigens *(200,201)*, and the receptor was subsequently cloned and shown to induce apoptosis *(202)*. DcR3, a soluble decoy receptor for Fas that is capable of binding FasL but not inducing apoptosis due to its lack of membrane localization and lack of death domain, was then found *(203)*. TRAIL has two proapoptotic death receptors, DR4 and KILLER/DR5, as well as three decoys, DcR1 (TRID), DcR2 (TRUNDD), and osteoprotegerin (OPG) *(177)*. Lastly, TNF has two receptors, TNFR1 with a death domain and TNFR2 without one, and these two molecules cooperate to determine the physiological outcome depending on the cellular context with TNFR1 being responsible for most of the responses to ligand *(182)* (Fig. 10).

Similar to their ligand counterparts, these death receptors associate as trimers to form an active ligand/receptor complex competent for recruitment of signaling molecules. It was believed that a trimeric ligand actively recruited receptors, which then trimerized due to their local aggregation *(185)*. However the discovery of an extracellular preligand assembly domain ([PLAD], distinct from the ligand binding domain) established that these complexes are preformed as trimers within the plasma membrane before ligand binding *(204)*. Mutation of death receptors such as Fas results in the formation of signaling-incompetent receptor trimers in the absence of ligand, and leads to lymphoproliferative disorders *(205)*. Because death receptors exist in a preformed state, ligand binding must induce conformational changes within the cytoplasmic death domains in order to trigger DISC formation, but the mechanism is still unclear. The silencer of death domain

(SODD) protein acts to hold TNFR1 in a signaling incompetent state in the absence of ligand *(206)*, yet no such mechanism has been described for Fas or the TRAIL receptors.

DEATH INDUCING SIGNALING COMPLEX (DISC) FORMATION AND DED-CASPASE ACTIVATION

The formation of a DISC was originally dissected using the Fas/FasL system to determine what proteins were recruited to receptor complexes following ligand binding *(207)*. Treatment of metabolically labeled Fas-sensitive lymphoid cell lines with agonist Fas antibodies demonstrated the recruitment of four cytotoxicity-dependent APO-1-associated proteins (CAP). The recruitment of these proteins was dependent on receptor aggregation and a functional death domain but only occurred in FasL-sensitive cell lines *(207)*. Identification of the adaptor protein that interacted with the death domain of Fas was accomplished earlier that year through the use of yeast two hybrid screening. The adaptor protein called FADD or MORT1 also contained a death domain that mediated its interaction with the receptor *(54,55)*. FADD accounted for two of the CAP proteins (CAP1 and CAP2), an unphosphorylated and phosphorylated form, originally identified in the Fas DISC *(207)* (Fig. 9).

CAP3 and CAP4 were identified as proteolytic products of the same protein, FLICE or MACH, through direct protein sequencing of CAP proteins using mass spectrometry as well as through yeast two hybrid by virtue of its interaction with FADD *(56,57)* (Fig. 9). The interaction between FADD and FLICE/MACH is mediated by the DED, another protein/protein interaction motif, which resides in both proteins. Overexpression of FLICE/MACH, which has homology to caspases, led to its proteolytic processing and cell death that was inhibited by CrmA and ZVAD-fmk *(56,57)*. FLICE processing was deemed to occur at the level of the DISC in a two-step mechanism as measured by cleavage into three fragments: the prodomain, the large subunit (p18), and the small subunit (p10) *(15)*. FLICE/MACH was recognized as the most proximal caspase protein in the death receptor pathway capable of initiating cell death and was then renamed caspase-8 *(38)*. Mouse knockout studies have verified that FADD and caspase-8 are required for Fas-induced cell death *(43,62,63)*.

The mechanism of caspase-8 activation at the DISC was proposed to result from induced proximity activation of the proenzymes *(50–52)*. These studies demonstrated that removal of the DEDs followed by their replacement with artificial inducible dimerization domains could result in the processing of caspase-8 in the presence of the dimerization agent. This processing was attributed to the low amount of enzymatic activity of the caspase that could be harnessed when dimerized to lead to local aggregation-induced processing and activation. This model has been recently updated to explain a previous finding that a noncleavable mutant retains a small but measurable amount of caspase activity *(51)*. The recent studies suggest that dimerization of the caspase-8 molecules themselves leads to their activation, and processing is a secondary but not a necessary event for this activation and only serves to stabilize activated dimers *(58–60)*. This new model would suggest that cleavage of caspase-8 therefore is not necessarily a marker for its activation *(59)*; however, previous findings have shown that release of caspase-8 from the membrane is required to induce cell death *(52)*.

A highly homologous caspase protein, caspase-10 (FLICE2), was also postulated to play a similar enzymatic role as caspase-8 *(208)*, but its verification as a true DISC component was not realized until the generation of caspase-10 specific antibodies *(209,210)*. The need for two DED-containing initiator caspases (caspase-8 and -10) is unclear at this point and the absence of a caspase-10 homolog in mouse raises further questions regarding its role in death receptor-mediated apoptosis *(211)*. Nevertheless, the identification of caspase-10 mutations in autoimmune lymphoproliferative syndrome type II suggests that wild-type caspase-10 function may be needed for some aspects of immune system homeostasis, possibly TRAIL-mediated apoptosis *(212)*. A number of other proteins have been described to interact with Fas or its DISC. Receptor-interacting protein (RIP) was originally isolated as a Fas- and TNFR1-associated protein by yeast two hybrid screening, with its overexpression in mammalian cells leading to cell death suggesting a role in death receptor-mediated apoptosis *(213)*. However, subsequent knockout studies showed that RIP was dispensible for cell death in response to death ligands but instead was necessary for prosurvival NF-κB signaling in response to TNF *(214)*. FLASH *(215)* and SADS *(216)* were both described as caspase-8 interacting proteins that were recruited to the Fas DISC that promoted cell death; however, the description of SADS was subsequently retracted *(217)* and a role for FLASH in promoting cell death remains questionable given recent evidence of a possible role in TNF-induced NF-κB activation *(218)*.

The last verified member of the Fas DISC is the cellular FLICE inhibitory protein (c-FLIP), which was cloned simultaneously by a number of independent groups *(219–226)*. c-FLIP is differentially spliced leading to a short form (c-$FLIP_S$) containing only two DEDs that resembles the v-FLIP proteins and a long form (c-$FLIP_L$) that is DED-caspase-like in its domain structure despite a lack of critical residues that renders it enzymatically inactive. As the name implies, c-FLIP was cloned as a cell death inhibitory molecule based on its homology to v-FLIP proteins and its ability to inhibit death receptor-induced apoptosis *(219,222,225,226)*. However, a number of groups have reported that c-$FLIP_L$ also has a proapoptotic function in certain cellular contexts that requires its enzymatically inactive caspase like domain *(220,221,223,224)*. These seemingly contradictory findings were recently rectified by the finding that physiological levels of c-$FLIP_L$ function as a caspase-8 activator in the context of the DISC and high levels of c-$FLIP_L$ induced by overexpression or found in tumors leads to inhibition of death *(227,228)*. These findings are also consistent with the recent model of dimer-induced caspase activation *(58–60)* because FLIP is able to act as a dimerization partner for caspase-8 without contributing any enzymatic activity.

The constituents of the Fas DISC (FADD, caspase-8, caspase-10, and c-FLIP) have been verified as components of the TRAIL DISC as well *(177)*. The TNF receptor complex following TNF binding is more complicated, however. The ability of TNF to cause proliferation as well as apoptosis suggests that other proteins are involved in the signaling cascades downstream of the receptor. TNFR1 uses the adaptor protein TRADD mediated by an adaptor DD/receptor DD interaction *(229)* to create a platform onto which signaling molecules are recruited. Apoptosis was believed to be initiated by TRADD-mediated recruitment of FADD *(230)* leading to caspase activation and cell death; however, recent studies demonstrate that FADD and caspase-8, despite being required for TNF-induced cell death, are not recruited to the membrane bound TNF-R1 signaling complex, suggesting an alternate mechanism of caspase-8 activation as compared to FasL or TRAIL *(231)*. Proliferative and inflammatory responses to TNF recruit an alternate set of proteins to receptor-associated TRADD leading to NF-κB and AP-1 activation *(232)*. Activation of these transcription factors promotes the upregulation of prosurvival genes leading to proliferation, explaining the observation that protein synthesis inhibitors are usually required for TNF-induced cell death *(174)*. Some NF-κB target genes are direct inhibitors of the basal apoptotic machinery, including IAPs, FLIP, Bcl-X_L, and A1 *(233)*. TRADD-associated TRAF2 is required for TNF-induced AP-1 activation, whereas it is only partially responsible for NF-κB activation *(234,235)*. Meanwhile, RIP, recruited via TRADD or directly by TNFR1 *(236)*, is required for NF-κB activation *(214)*. TRAF2 may also transmit prosurvival signals through its ability to recruit the IAPs, c-IAP1 and c-IAP2 *(87)*. The relative recruitment of these proteins to TNFR1 as well as contributions made by TNFR2 regulate the cell's response to TNF, proliferation or death *(182)*.

CROSS-TALK BETWEEN THE INTRINSIC AND EXTRINSIC PATHWAY

Despite the classification of ligands into the extrinsic pathway and cellular stresses into the intrinsic pathway, cross-talk between the pathways has been observed. The involvement of the mitochondria in response to death ligands has been debated with little evidence for such a role in hematopoetic cells *(183)*. However, studies based on the overexpression of bcl-2 have demonstrated that two types (types I and II) of cells exist with differential requirements for mitochondrial involvement *(237)* (Fig. 9). Type I cells, in response to Fas ligand, generate functional DISCs that activate caspase-8 and -10, leading to direct activation of downstream caspases (-3, -6, and -7). In contrast, Type II cells recruit small amounts of FADD and caspase-8 to the DISC, resulting in inefficient caspase-8 activation. This signal is not sufficient to directly activate downstream caspases; rather, the death signal must be amplified through the mitochondria by caspase-8-mediated cleavage of cytosolic Bid. tBID then translocates to the mitochondria and, with the help of Bax or Bak, leads to mitochondrial dysfunction and apoptosome formation (Fig. 9). Therefore, type II cell death can be inhibited by overexpression of antiapoptotic Bcl-2 family members. The evidence that these two cell types occur physiologically comes from Bid –/– mice in which hepatocytes respond to Fas in a Type II manner and thymocytes in a Type I manner *(238)*. Similar observations have been made in cell lines and hepatocytes in terms of Type I versus II in response to TRAIL as well *(239)*.

In the intrinsic pathway, the involvement of CARD-containing caspases in mediating cell death is not disputed, regardless of whether caspase-2 is activated upstream of the mitochondria *(164)*. The role of components of the extrinsic pathway in the execution phase following intrinsic pathway activation is less clear. The tumor suppressor p53 mediates its effects through the transcriptional upregulation of target proteins involved in cell cycle arrest and apoptosis in response to DNA damage, nucleotide depletion, and other cellular stresses consistent with the intrinsic pathway *(240)*. Despite the clear involvement of Apaf-1 and caspase-9 in p53-mediated apoptosis *(241)*, a number of genes upregulated in a p53-dependent manner are involved in the extrinsic pathway, including Fas *(242)* and the TRAIL receptor KILLER/DR5 *(243)* (Fig. 11). Recent experiments with Fas suggest that it may play a role in p53-dependent death in the testis in

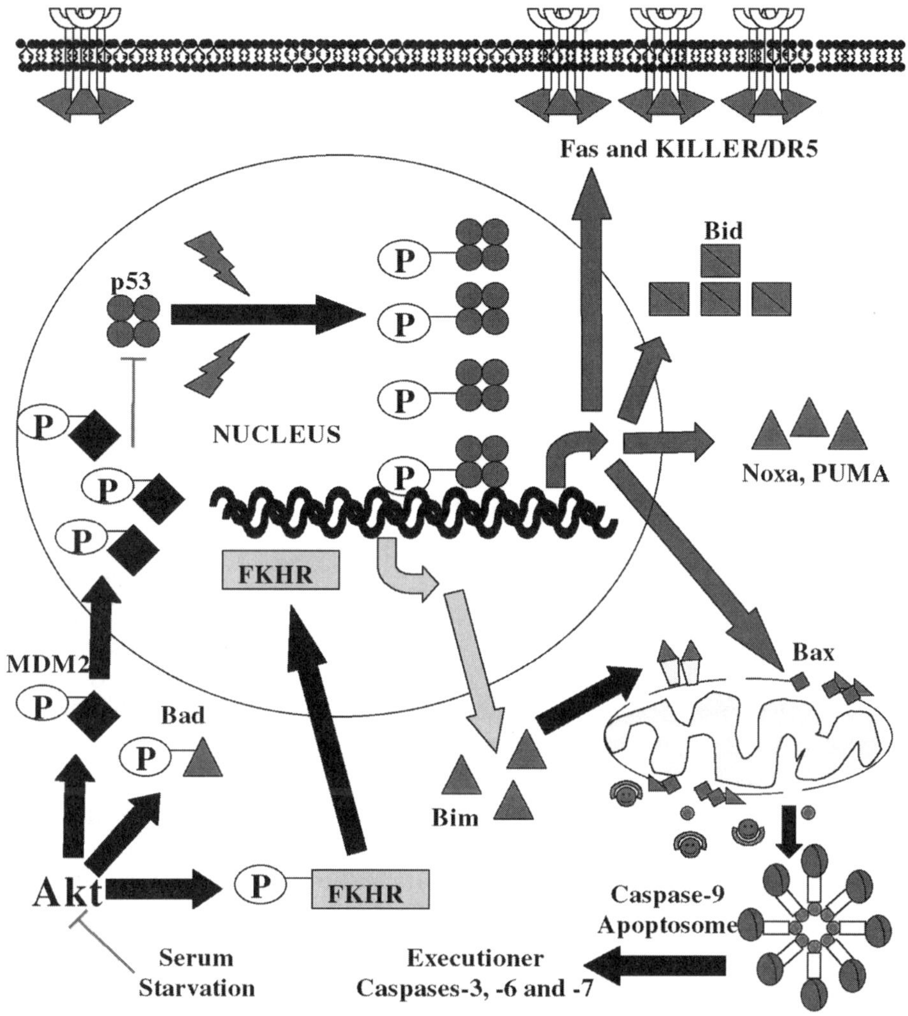

Fig. 11. Upstream Regulators of the Apoptotic machinery. The tumor suppressor p53 is a transcription factor which is induced upon cellular stress. Activation of p53 via phosphorylation leads to its accumulation in the nucleus and an increase in its transactivation function. Transcriptional targets include Fas, KILLER/DR5, Bid, Noxa, PUMA, and Bax. Furthermore the survival kinase Akt regulates sequestration of Bad, mdm2 and FKHR via phosphorylation. Serum starvation allows translocation of Bad to the mitochondria and FKHR to the nucleus. Nuclear translocation of FKHR results in Bim and FasL upregulation. Interruption of the nuclear accumulation of mdm2 also allows p53 accumulation and transactivation.

response to ionizing radiation *(244)*. Besides the role of death receptors in the p53-dependent apoptotic response, numerous studies have implicated caspase-8 in the response to chemotherapeutic agents potentially acting in order to enhance further caspase activation and accelerate death kinetics *(245–247)*. Although the loss of caspase-8 in mouse did not have profound effects on cell survival, the kinetics of death were not studied *(43)*. Similar studies in human cells lacking caspase-8 demonstrated delayed death kinetics in response to cytotoxic agents *(61)*. Lastly, caspase-8 and -10 cleavage in cell free extracts in response to cytochrome c addition demonstrates activation downstream of the mitochondria *(123)* and caspase-6 was recently isolated as the caspase-8-activating enzyme in this circumstance *(139)*. These findings suggest that cross-talk between the intrinsic and extrinsic pathways may occur in a tissue-specific and stimulus-specific manner.

UPSTREAM REGULATORS OF THE APOPTOTIC MACHINERY

The core apoptotic machinery of the extrinsic and intrinsic pathways is regulated at the transcriptional and posttranslational levels in response to pro- and antiapoptotic signals. p53 is the most commonly mutated gene in human cancers and alteration of some component of the pathway leading to deregulation occurs in most cancer cells. The reason for this selectivity against p53 function in tumors is due to its roles in cell cycle regulation, genome stability, and cell death during the DNA damage or stress response *(240)*. DNA damage is somehow "sensed" by the cell leading to activation of signal transducing kinases such as ATM and ATR, followed by the activation of the Chk kinases. Activation of p53 ensues due to phosphorylation and acetylation events on the p53 protein that leads to increased protein half-life *(248)*. Tetramerization of p53 allows it to bind DNA in a sequence-specific manner and to transactivate target genes involved in a variety of cellular processes. p53 target genes involved in cell death can be grouped into the intrinsic (Bax, Noxa, PUMA, Apaf-1) or extrinsic (Fas, KILLER/DR5) pathways as well as those common to both (Bid, caspase-6) *(249–251)* (Fig. 11). Loss of p53's transactivation function results in chemoresistance mainly due to a lack of p53-dependent cell death *(252)*.

Forkhead (FKHR) is another transcription factor that responds to cellular signals to positively regulate cell death progression. The localization of FKHR is controlled by phosphorylation events by the survival kinase, Akt, resulting in cytoplasmic sequestration of FKHR by 14-3-3 proteins *(253)* (Fig. 11). Absence of survival signals such as growth factors leads to the nuclear translocation of FKHR due to the absence of Akt signaling. Nuclear FKHR can then bind DNA in a sequence-specific manner and lead to transactivation of Fas ligand as well as the BH3-only protein, Bim *(253,254)*. Akt also promotes FKHR-independent survival events including the phosphorylation of Bad leading to its cytoplasmic sequestration by 14-3-3 *(255,256)* (Fig. 11). Furthermore, Akt can phosphorylate human caspase-9 promoting inhibition *(257)*; however, this mechanism has been questioned due to the lack of conservation of the phosphorylation site in mouse caspase-9 *(258)*. Lastly, Akt can inhibit the tumor suppressor p53 by directly phosphorylating its negative regulator, mdm2, and increasing its nuclear localization resulting in decreased p53 protein levels and function *(259,260)*. Continued study of survival mechanisms will no doubt uncover more proteins within the apoptotic pathways that undergo regulation by survival signals.

DISEASE STATES AND MECHANISMS OF TUMOR RESISTANCE

The need for developmental programmed cell death is obvious when considering issues of tissue remodeling and the deletion of unnecessary structures *(2)*; however, the prominent role of cell death in various human disease states including neurodegenerative diseases, AIDS, and cancer is becoming more apparent as alterations in the pathways are identified *(3,261)*. Alterations in the extrinsic pathway range from ligand to caspase in the case of the autoimmune lymphoproliferative syndrome (ALPS) in humans where mutations define the classification: type Ia (Fas), Ib (FasL), II (caspase-10) and III (undefined) *(212,262–265)*. The importance of the Fas/FasL system in controlling immune homeostasis was originally recognized with the naturally occurring mutations in lpr and gld mice resulting in lymphoproliferation, due to mutations in Fas and FasL, respectively *(266,267)*. Alterations in the Fas pathway including Fas, FADD, and caspase-10 have also been detected in human cancer *(268–271)*.

Mutations in receptors and ligands extend beyond the Fas/FasL system to include TNFR1 mutations in the TNFR1 associated periodic syndrome (TRAPS) resulting in periods of fever and inflammation *(272)* as well as TRAIL receptor mutations in cancer *(273–277)*. In addition to inactivating receptor mutations, amplification or overexpression of decoy receptors is another mechanism employed by tumors to escape immune surveillance. DcR3, the Fas decoy receptor, was originally recognized as being amplified in colon and lung tumors and subsequently shown to be overexpressed in a variety of other malignancies *(203,278–281)*. The identification of the TRAIL decoys, DcR1 and DcR2, coupled with their expression in normal but not transformed cells, led to the hypothesis that decoy receptors determine a cell's sensitivity to TRAIL *(282–285)*. Other mechanisms including FLIP expression and the relative cell surface expression of the different TRAIL receptors are now known to contribute to TRAIL sensitivity *(286–289)*. High levels of FLIP, both cellular and viral, have been correlated with increased resistance to FasL and TRAIL in tumor cells, and interestingly a potential role for FLIP in multiple sclerosis and Graves disease has recently been postulated *(290)*.

Caspase-8 and -10 of the extrinsic pathway also represent targets for inactivation resulting in disease progression. Methylation of both caspase-8 and -10 in neuroblastoma is an effective means to eliminate both proximal caspases of the extrinsic pathway simultaneously since both proteins are on chromosome 2q33 *(291–294)*. Treatment of these cells with methyltransferase inhibitors restores sensitivity to death ligands. Methylation of caspase-10 has also been reported in lung cancer *(271)*. Mutations in both caspase-8 and -10 have also been described that directly effect their enzymatic activity *(295,296)*. Interestingly, patients with an inherited mutation in caspase-8 have recently been described and in addition to defective lymphocyte apoptosis, they exhibit defects in the activation of T cells and B cells as well *(297)*. This supports the idea that in some circumstances Fas can lead to proliferation/costimulation of hematopoetic cells in vivo *(183)*. With the exception of caspase-8 and -10, inactivation of caspases appears to be a rare event in genetic disorders probably due to irreversible developmental miscues *in utero*.

Despite the overall lack of caspase mutations, a number of proteins within the intrinsic pathway that regulate caspase activity are targeted for deregulation to provide cells with a selective growth advantage. Mutations that target the intrinsic pathway are particularly important to consider due to their relevance in determining a cell's response to chemotherapy. The caspase-9 adaptor, Apaf-1, is a methylation target in melanomas leading to chemoresistance *(298)*. Furthermore, the caspase-binding IAP family is also a target for deregulation in a variety of tumor types *(299)*. Deregulation of antiapoptotic Bcl-2 proteins can provide long-term chemoresistance *(252)*. In addition to the translocation in follicular lymphoma that led to the discovery of Bcl-2, overexpression of Bcl-2 and Bcl-X_L has been detected in breast and pancreatic tumors as well as leukemias *(11)*. Homologs of antiapoptotic Bcl-2 proteins have been discovered in a number of viruses including adenovirus (E1B 19K), Epstein–Barr (BHRF), and Herpes virus (v-Bcl-2-KSHV) in order to promote host cell survival *(300)*. The proapoptotic Bcl-2 proteins, Bax and Bak, are both targets for mutational inactivation in colon cancer *(301,302)* leading to increased drug resistance in vivo *(303–305)*.

Acquired chemoresistance of tumors is the most dramatic, however, after the loss of p53 function presumably because the regulation of both extrinsic and intrinsic pathways is compromised. p53 inactivation can occur through a variety mechanisms including: p53 mutation or deletion, inactivation of p53 by viral oncoproteins, overexpression of the negative regulator mdm2 or loss of the positive p53 regulator, p19ARF *(240)*. Hereditary loss of p53 function or the p53 pathway through the upstream regulator Chk2 results in a familial cancer syndrome called Li–Fraumeni, characterized by the early onset of tumors *(306)*. The loss of apoptotic pathways is now considered a requisite event for tumor formation *(261)*, often leading to chemoresistance. The rational design of cancer therapies targeting the intrinsic pathway (bcl-2 antagonists) and the extrinsic pathway (TRAIL) or downstream molecules (IAPs) have started to show promise in the clinic *(197)* as our understanding of these pathways continues to grow. It will be important to identify the apoptotic molecular lesions of different tumor types in order to appropriately tailor cancer regimens. Studies from a variety of genetic organisms as well as humans over the past ten years has helped elucidate the basal apoptotic machinery and application of this information should improve therapy.

REFERENCES

1. Rich T, Watson CJ, Wyllie A. Apoptosis: the germs of death. Nat Cell Biol 1999;1:E69–E71.
2. Jacobson MD, Weil M, Raff MC. Programmed cell death in animal development. Cell 1997;88:347–354.
3. Thompson CB. Apoptosis in the pathogenesis and treatment of disease. Science 1995;267:1456–1462.
4. Lockshin RA, Zakeri Z. Programmed cell death and apoptosis: origins of the theory. Nat Rev Mol Cell Biol 2001;2:545–550.
5. Ellis HM, Horvitz HR. Genetic control of programmed cell death in the nematode *C. elegans*. Cell 1986;44:817–829.
6. Hengartner MO, Ellis RE, Horvitz HR. Caenorhaditis elegans gene ced-9 protects cells from programmed cell death. Nature 1992;356:494–499.
7. Liu QA, Hengartner MO. The molecular mechanism of programmed cell death in *C. elegans*. Ann N Y Acad Sci 1999;887:92–104.
8. Conradt B, Horvitz HR. The *C. elegans* protein EGL-1 is required for programmed cell death and interacts with the Bcl-2-like protein CED-9. Cell 1998;93:519–529.
9. Hengartner MO. The biochemistry of apoptosis. Nature 2000;407:770–776.
10. Puthalakath H, Strasser A. Keeping killers on a tight leash: transcriptional and post-translational control of the pro-apoptotic activity of BH3-only proteins. Cell Death Differ 2002;9:505–512.20
11. Cory S, Adams JM. The Bcl2 family: regulators of the cellular life-or-death switch. Nat Rev Cancer 2002;2:647–656.
12. Meier P, Finch A, Evan G. Apoptosis in development. Nature 2000;407:796–801.
13. Vander Heiden MG, Thompson CB. Bcl-2 proteins: regulators of apoptosis or of mitochondrial homeostasis? Nat Cell Biol 1999;1:E209–E216.
14. Nagata S. Apoptosis by death factor. Cell 1997;88:355–365.
15. Medema JP, Scaffidi C, Kischkel FC, et al. FLICE is activated by association with the CD95 death-inducing signaling complex (DISC). EMBO J 1997;16:2794–2804.
16. Salvesen GS, Duckett CS. IAP proteins: blocking the road to death's door. Nat Rev Mol Cell Biol 2002;3:401–410.
17. Quinn LM, Dorstyn L, Mills K, et al. An essential role for the caspase dronc in developmentally programmed cell death in *Drosophila*. J Biol Chem 2000;275:40,416–40,424.
18. Rodriguez A, Oliver H, Zou H, Chen P, Wang X, Abrams JM. Dark is a *Drosophila* homologue of Apaf-1/CED-4 and functions in an evolutionarily conserved death pathway. Nat Cell Biol 1999;1:272–279.

19. Dorstyn L, Read S, Cakouros D, Huh JR, Hay BA, Kumar S. The role of cytochrome c in caspase activation in *Drosophila* melanogaster cells. J Cell Biol 2002;156:1089–1098.
20. Zimmermann KC, Ricci JE, Droin NM, Green DR. The role of ARK in stress-induced apoptosis in *Drosophila* cells. J Cell Biol 2002;156:1077–1087.
21. Moreno E, Yan M, Basler K. Evolution of TNF signaling mechanisms: JNK-dependent apoptosis triggered by Eiger, the *Drosophila* homolog of the TNF superfamily. Curr Biol 2002;12:1263–1268.
22. Leulier F, Vidal S, Saigo K, Ueda R, Lemaitre B. Inducible expression of double-stranded RNA reveals a role for dFADD in the regulation of the antibacterial response in *Drosophila* adults. Curr Biol 2002;12:996–1000.
23. Leulier F, Rodriguez A, Khush RS, Abrams JM, Lemaitre B. The *Drosophila* caspase Dredd is required to resist gram-negative bacterial infection. EMBO Rep 2000;1:353–358.
24. Wang SL, Hawkins CJ, Yoo SJ, Muller HA, Hay BA. The *Drosophila* caspase inhibitor DIAP1 is essential for cell survival and is negatively regulated by HID. Cell 1999;98:453–463.
25. Rodriguez A, Chen P, Oliver H, Abrams JM. Unrestrained caspase-dependent cell death caused by loss of Diap1 function requires the *Drosophila* Apaf-1 homolog, Dark. EMBO J 2002;21:2189–2197.
26. Richardson H, Kumar S. Death to flies: *Drosophila* as a model system to study programmed cell death. J Immunol Methods 2002;265:21–38.
27. White K, Grether ME, Abrams JM, Young L, Farrell K, Steller H. Genetic control of programmed cell death in *Drosophila*. Science 1994;264:677–683.
28. Du C, Fang M, Li Y, Li L, Wang X. Smac, a mitochondrial protein that promotes cytochrome c-dependent caspase activation by eliminating IAP inhibition. Cell 2000;102:33–42.
29. Verhagen AM, Ekert PG, Pakusch M, et al. Identification of DIABLO, a mammalian protein that promotes apoptosis by binding to and antagonizing IAP proteins. Cell 2000;102:43–53.
30. Suzuki Y, Imai Y, Nakayama H, Takahashi K, Takio K, Takahashi R. A serine protease, HtrA2, is released from the mitochondria and interacts with XIAP, inducing cell death. Mol Cell 2001;8:613–621.
31. Hegde R, Srinivasula SM, Zhang Z, et al. Identification of Omi/HtrA2 as a mitochondrial apoptotic serine protease that disrupts inhibitor of apoptosis protein-caspase interaction. J Biol Chem 2002;277:432–438.
32. Verhagen AM, Silke J, Ekert PG, et al. HtrA2 promotes cell death through its serine protease activity and its ability to antagonize inhibitor of apoptosis proteins. J Biol Chem 2002;277:445–454.
33. van Loo G, van Gurp M, Depuydt B, et al. The serine protease Omi/HtrA2 is released from mitochondria during apoptosis. Omi interacts with caspase-inhibitor XIAP and induces enhanced caspase activity. Cell Death Differ 2002;9:20–26.
34. Martins LM, Iaccarino I, Tenev T, et al. The serine protease Omi/HtrA2 regulates apoptosis by binding XIAP through a reaper-like motif. J Biol Chem 2002;27:439–444.
35. Palaga T, Osborne B. The 3D's of apoptosis: death, degradation and DIAPs. Nat Cell Biol 2002; 4:E149–E151.
36. Yuan J, Shaham S, Ledoux S, Ellis HM, Horvitz HR. The *C. elegans* cell death gene ced-3 encodes a protein similar to mammalian interleukin-1 beta-converting enzyme. Cell 1993;75:641–652.
37. Miura M, Zhu H, Rotello R, Hartwieg EA, Yuan J. Induction of apoptosis in fibroblasts by IL-1 beta-converting enzyme, a mammalian homolog of the *C. elegans* cell death gene ced-3. Cell 1993;75:653–660.
38. Alnemri ES, Livingston DJ, Nicholson DW, et al. Human ICE/CED-3 protease nomenclature. Cell 1996;87:171.
39. Salvesen GS, Dixit VM. Caspases: intracellular signaling by proteolysis. Cell 1997;91:443–446.
40. Raff M. Cell suicide for beginners. Nature 1998;396:119–122.
41. Thornberry NA, Lazebnik Y. Caspases: enemies within. Science 1998;281:1312–1316.
42. Thornberry NA, Rano TA, Peterson EP, et al. A combinatorial approach defines specificities of members of the caspase family and granzyme B. Functional relationships established for key mediators of apoptosis. J Biol Chem 1997;272:17,907–17,911.
43. Varfolomeev EE, Shuchmann M, Luria V, et al. Targeted disruption of the mouse Caspase 8 gene ablates cell death induction by the TNF receptors, Fas/Apo1, and DR3 and is lethal prenatally. Immunity 1998;9:267–276.
44. Hakem R, Hakem A, Duncan GS, et al. Differential requirement for caspase 9 in apoptotic pathways in vivo. Cell 1998;94:339–352.
45. Kuida K, Haydar TF, Kuan CY, et al. Reduced apoptosis and cytochrome c-mediated caspase activation in mice lacking caspase 9. Cell 1998;94:325–337.

46. Nicholson DW, Thornberry NA. Caspases: killer proteases. Trends Biochem Sci 1997;22:299–306.
47. Kuida K, Zheng TS, Na S, et al. Decreased apoptosis in the brain and premature lethality in CPP32-deficient mice. Nature 1996;384:368–372.
48. Woo M, Hakem R. Soengas MS, et al. Essential contribution of caspase 3/CPP32 to apoptosis and its associated nuclear changes. Genes Dev 1998;12:806–819.
49. Zheng TS, Flavell RA. Divinations and surprises: genetic analysis of caspase function in mice. Exp Cell Res 2000;256:67–73.
50. Yang X, Chang HY, Baltimore D. Autoproteolytic activation of pro-caspases by oligomerization. Mol Cell 1998;1:319–325.
51. Muzio M, Stockwell BR, Stennicke HR, Salvesen GS, Dixit VM. An induced proximity model for caspase-8 activation. J Biol Chem 1998;273:2926–2930.
52. Martin DA, Sigel RM, Zheng L, Lenardo MJ. Membrane oligomerization and cleavage activates the caspase-8 (FLICE/MACHalpha1) death signal. J Biol Chem 1998;273:4345–4349.
53. Tartaglia LA, Ayres TM, Wong GH, Goeddel DV. A novel domain within the 55 kd TNF receptor signals cell death. Cell 1993;74:845–853.
54. Chinnaiyan AM, O'Rourke K, Tewari M, Dixit VM. FADD, a novel death domain-containing protein, interacts with the death domain of Fas and initiates apoptosis. Cell 1995;81:505–512.
55. Boldin MP, Varfolomeev EE, Pancer Z, Mett IL, Camonis JH, Wallach D. A novel protein that interacts with the death domain of Fas/APO1 contains a sequence motif related to the death domain. J Biol Chem 1995;270:7795–7798.
56. Muzio M, Chinnaiyan AM, Kischkel FC, et al. FLICE, a novel FADD-homologous ICE/CED-3-like protease, is recruited to the CD95 (Fas/APO-1) death-inducing signaling complex. Cell 1996;85:817–827.
57. Boldin MP, Goncharov TM, Goltsev YV, Wallach D. Involvement of MACH, a novel MORT1/FADD-interacting protease, in Fas/APO- and TNF receptor-induced cell death. Cell 1996;85:803–815.
58. Chen M, Orozco A, Spencer DM, Wang J. Activation of initiator caspases through a stable dimeric intermediate. J Biol Chem 2002;277:50,761–50,767.
59. Boatright KM, Renatus M, Scott FL, et al. A unified model for apical caspase activation. Mol Cell 2003; 11:529–541.
60. Donepudi M, Sweeney AM, Briand C, Grutter MG. Insights into the regulatory mechanism for caspase-8 activation. Mol Cell 2003;11:543–549.
61. Juo P, Kuo CJ, Yuan J, Blenis J. Essential requirement for caspase-8/FLICE in the initiation of the Fas-induced apoptotic cascade. Curr Biol 1998;8:1001–1008.
62. Yeh WC, Pompa JL, McCurrach ME, et al. FADD: essential for embryo development and signaling from some, but not all, inducers of apoptosis. Science 1998;279:1954–1958.
63. Zhang J, Cado D, Chen A, Kabra NH, Winoto A. Fas-mediated apoptosis and activation-induced T-cell proliferation are defective in mice lacking FADD/Mort1. Nature 1998;392:296–300.
64. Kuang AA, Diehl GE, Zhang J, Winoto A. FADD is required for DR4- and DR5-mediated apoptosis: lack of trail-induced apoptosis in FADD-deficient mouse embryonic fibroblasts. J Biol Chem 2000;275:25,065–25,068.
65. Zou H, Henzel WJ, Liu X, Lutschg A, Wang X. Apaf-1, a human protein homologous to *C. elegans* CED-4, participates in cytochrome c-dependent activation of caspase-3. Cell 1997;90:405–413.
66. Li P, Nijhawan D, Budihardjo I, et al. Cytochrome c and dATP-dependent formation of Apaf-1/caspase-9 complex initiates an apoptotic protease cascade. Cell 1997;91:479–489.
67. Liu X, Kim CN, Yang J, Jemmerson R, Wang X. Induction of apoptotic program in cell-free extracts: requirement for dATP and cytochrome c. Cell 1996;86:147–157.
68. Jiang X, Wang X. Cytochrome c promotes caspase-9 activation by inducing nucleotide binding to Apaf-1. J Biol Chem 2000;275:31,199–31,203.
69. Rodriguez J, Lazebnik Y. Caspase-9 and APAF-1 form an active holoenzyme. Genes Dev 1999; 13:3179–3184.
70. Cecconi F, Alvarez-Bolado G, Meyer BI, Roth KA, Gruss P. Apaf1 (CED-4 homolog) regulates programmed cell death in mammalian development. Cell 1998;94:727–737.
71. Yoshida H, Kong YY, Yoshida R, et al. Apaf1 is required for mitochondrial pathways of apoptosis and brain development. Cell 1998;94:739–750.
72. Crook NE, Clem RJ, Miller LK. An apoptosis-inhibiting baculovirus gene with a zinc finger-like motif. J Virol 1993;67:2168–2174.
73. Clem RJ, Miller Lk. Control of programmed cell death by the baculovirus genes p35 and iap. Mol Cell Biol 1994;14:5212–5222.

74. Roy N, Mahadevan MS, McLean M, et al. The gene for neuronal apoptosis inhibitory protein is partially deleted in individuals with spinal muscular atrophy. Cell 1995;80:167–178.
75. Verhagen AM, Coulson EJ, Vaux DL. Inhibitor of apoptosis proteins and their relatives: IAPs and other BIRPs. Genome Biol 2001;2:REVIEWS3009.
76. Liston P, Roy N, Tamai K, et al. Suppression of apoptosis in mammalian cells by NAIP and a related family of IAP genes. Nature 1996;379:349–353.
77. Deveraux QL, Takahashi R, Salvesen GS, Reed JC. X-linked IAP is a direct inhibitor of cell-death proteases. Nature 1997;388:300–304.
78. Deveraux QL, Roy N, Stennicke HR, et al. IAPs block apoptotic events induced by caspase-8 and cytochrome c by direct inhibition of distinct caspases. EMBO J 1998;17:2215–2223.
79. Takahashi R, Deveraux Q, Tamm I, et al. A single BIR domain of XIAP sufficient for inhibiting caspases. J Biol Chem 1998;273:7787–7790.
80. Sun C, Cai M, Gunasekera AH, et al. NMR structure and mutagenesis of the inhibitor-of-apoptosis protein XIAP. Nature 1999;401:818–822.
81. Huang Y, Park YC, Rich RL, Segal D, Myszka DG, Wu H. Structural basis of caspase inhibition by XIAP: differential roles of the linker versus the BIR domain. Cell 2001;104:781–790.
82. Chai J, Shiozaki E, Srinivasula SM, et al. Structural basis of caspase-7 inhibition by XIAP. Cell 2001;104:769–780.
83. Riedl SJ, Renatus M, Schwarzenbacher R, et al. Structural basis for the inhibition of caspase-3 by XIAP. Cell 2001:104:791–800.
84. Renatus M, Stennicke HR, Scott FL, Liddington RC, Salvesen GS. Dimer formation drives the activation of the cell death protease caspase 9. Proc Natl Acad Sci U S A 2001;98:14,250–14,255.
85. Shiozaki EN, Chai J, Rigotti DJ, et al. Mechanism of XIAP-mediated inhibition of caspase-9. Mol Cell 2003;11:519–527.
86. Richter BW, Mir SS, Eiben LJ, et al. Molecular cloning of ILP-2, a novel member of the inhibitor of apoptosis protein family. Mol Cell Biol 2001;21:4292–4301.
87. Rothe M, Pan MG, Henzel WJ, Ayres TM, Goeddel DV. The TNFR2-TRAF signaling complex contains two novel proteins related to baculoviral inhibitor of apoptosis proteins. Cell 1995;83:1243–1252.
88. Roy N, Deveraux QL, Takahashi R, Salvesen Gs, Reed JC. The c-IAP-1 and c-IAP-2 proteins are direct inhibitors of specific caspases. EMBO J 1997;16:6914–6925.
89. Vucic D, Stennicke HR, Pisabarro MT, Salvesen GS, Dixit VM. ML-IAP, a novel inhibitor of apoptosis that is preferentially expressed in human melanomas. Curr Biol 2000;10:1359–1366.
90. Deveraux QL, Reed JC. IAP family proteins—suppressors of apoptosis. Genes Dev 1999;13:239–252.
91. Martin SJ. Destabilizing influences in apoptosis: sowing the seeds of IAP destruction. Cell 2002;109:793–796.
92. Joazeiro CA, Weissman AM. RING finger proteins: mediators of ubiquitin ligase activity. Cell 2000;102:549–552.
93. Yang Y, Fang S, Jensen JP, Weissman AM, Ashwell JD. Ubiquiting protein ligase activity of IAPs and their degradation in proteasomes in response to apoptotic stimuli. Science 2000;288:874–877,
94. Huang H, Joazeiro CA, Bonfoco E, Kamada S, Leverson JD, Hunter T. The inhibitor of apoptosis, cIAP2, functions as a ubiquitin-protein ligase and promotes in vitro monoubiquitination of caspases 3 and 7. J Biol Chem 2000;275:26,661–26,664.
95. Suzuki Y, Nakabayashi Y, Takahashi R. Ubiquitin-protein ligase activity of X-linked inhibitor of apoptosis protein promotes proteasomal degradation of caspase-3 and enhances its anti-apoptotic effect in Fas-induced cell death. Proc Natl Acad Sci U S A 2001;98:8662–8667.
96. Deveraux QL, Leo E, Stennicke HR, Welsh K, Salvesen GS, Reed JC. Cleavage of human inhibitor of apoptosis protein XIAP results in fragments with distinct specificities for caspases. EMBO J 1999;18:5242–5251.
97. Clem RJ, Sheu TT, Richter BW, et al. c-IAP1 is cleaved by caspases to produce a proapoptotic C-terminal fragment. J Biol Chem 2001;276:7602–7608.
98. Srinivasula SM, Hegde R, Saleh A, et al. A conserved XIAP-interaction motif in caspase-9 and Smac/DIABLO regulates caspase activity and apoptosis. Nature 2001;410:112–116.
99. Clem RJ, Fechheimer M, Miller LK. Prevention of apoptosis by a baculovirus gene during infection of insect cells. Science 1991;254:1388–1390.
100. Xue D, Horvitz HR. Inhibition of the Caenorhabditis elegans cell-death protease CED-3 by a CED-3 cleavage site in baculovirus p35 protein. Nature 1995;377:248–251.

101. Bump NJ, Hackett M, Hugunin M, et al. Inhibition of ICE family proteases by baculovirus antiapoptotic protein p35. Science 1995;269:1885–1888.
102. Srinivasula SM, Ahmad M, Fernandes-Alnemri T, Litwack G, Alnemri ES. Molecular ordering of the Fas-apoptotic pathway: the Fas/APO-1 protease Mch5 is a CrmA-inhibitable protease that activates multiple Ced-3/ICE-like cysteine proteases. Proc Natl Acad Sci U S A 1996;93:14,486–14,491.
103. Muzio M, Salvesen GS, Dixit VM. FLICE induced apoptosis in a cell-free system. Cleavage of caspase zymogens. J Biol Chem 1997;272:2952–2956.
104. Zhou Q, Snipas S, Orth K, Muzio M, Dixit VM, Salvesen GS. Target protease specificity of the viral serpin CrmA. Analysis of five caspases. J Biol Chem 1997;272:7797–7800.
105. Skaletskaya A, Bartle LM, Chittenden T, McCormick AL, Mocarski ES, Goldmacher VS. A cytomegalovirus-encoded inhibitor of apoptosis that suppresses caspase-8 activation. Proc Natl Acad Sci U S A 2001;98:7829–7834.
106. Chen P, Tian J, Kovesdi I, Bruder JT. Interaction of the adenovirus 14. 7-kDa protein with FLICE inhibits Fas ligand-induced apoptosis. J Biol Chem 1998;273:5815–5820.
107. Thome M, Schneider P, Hofmann K, et al. Viral FLICE-inhibitory proteins (FLIPs) prevent apoptosis induced by death receptors. Nature 1997;386:517–521.
108. Bertin J, Armstrong RC, Ottilie S, et al. Death effector domain-containing herpesvirus and poxvirus proteins inhibit both Fas- and TNFR1-induced apoptosis. Proc Natl Acad Sci U S A 1997;94:1172–1176.
109. Wang GH, Bertin J, Wang Y, et al. Bovine herpesvirus 4 BORFE2 protein inhibits Fas- and tumor necrosis factor receptor 1-induced apoptosis and contains death effector domains shared with other gamma-1 herpesviruses. J Virol 1997;71:8928–8932.
110. Zimmerman KC, Bonzon C, Green DR. The machinery of programmed cell death. Pharmacol Ther 2001;92:57–70.
111. Wang K, Yin XM, Chao DT, Milliman CL, Korsmeyer SJ. BID: a novel BH3 domain-only death agonist. Genes Dev 1996;10:2859–2869.
112. Luo X, Budihardjo I, Zou H, Slaughter C, Wang X. Bid, a Bcl2 interacting protein, mediates cytochrome c release from mitochondria in response to activation of cell surface death receptors. Cell 1998;94:481–490.
113. Li H, Zhu H, Xu CJ, Yuan J. Cleavage of BID by caspase 8 mediates the mitochondrial damage in the Fas pathway of apoptosis. Cell 1998;94:491–501.
114. Zha J, Weiler S, Oh KJ, Wei MC, Korsmeyer SJ. Posttranslational N-myristoylation of BID as a molecular switch for targeting mitochondria and apoptosis. Science 2000;290:1761–1765.
115. Stegh AH, Herrmann H, Lampel S, et al. Identification of the cytolinker plectin as a major early in vivo substrate for caspase 8 during CD95- and tumor necrosis factor receptor-mediated apoptosis. Mol Cell Biol 2000;20:5665–5679.
116. Kothakota S, Azuma T, Reinhard C, et al. Caspase-3-generated fragment of gelsolin: effector of morphological change in apoptosis. Science 1997;278:294–298.
117. Ku NO, Liao J, Omary MB. Apoptosis generates stable fragments of human type I keratins. J Biol Chem 1997;272:33,197–33,203.
118. Caulin C, Salvesen GS, Oshima RG. Caspase cleavage of keratin 18 and reorganization of intermediate filaments during epithelial cell apoptosis. J Cell Biol 1997;138:1379–1394.
119. Rudel T, Bokoch GM. Membrane and morphological changes in apoptotic cells regulated by caspase-mediated activation of PAK2. Science 1997;276:1571–1574.
120. Martin SJ, O'Brien GA, Nishioka WK, et al. Proteolysis of fodrin (non-erythroid spectrin) during apoptosis. J Biol Chem 1995;270:6425–6428.
121. Coleman ML, Sahai EA, Yeo M, Bosch M, Dewar A, Olson MF. Membrane blebbing during apoptosis results from caspase-mediated activation of ROCK I. Nat Cell Biol 2001;3:339–345.
122. Sebbagh M, Renvoize C, Hamelin J, Riche N, Bertoglio J, Breard J. Caspase-3-mediated cleavage of ROCK I induces MLC phosphorylation and apoptotic membrane blebbing. Nat Cell Biol 2001;3: 346–352.
123. Slee EA, Harte MT, Kluck RM, et al. Ordering the cytochrome c-initiated caspase cascade: hierarchical activation of caspases-2, -3, -6, -7, -8, and -10 in a caspase-9-dependent manner. J Cell Biol 1999;144:281–292.
124. Kawahara A, Enari M, Talanian RV, Wong WW, Nagata S. Fas-induced DNA fragmentation and protelysis of nuclear proteins. Genes Cells 1998;3:297–306.
125. Wyllie AH. Glucocorticoid-induced thymocyte apoptosis is associated with endogenous endonuclease activation. Nature 1980;284:555–556.

126. Sakahira H, Enari M, Nagata S. Cleavage of CAD inhibitor in CAD activation and DNA degradation during apoptosis. Nature 1998;391:96–99.
127. Enari M, Sakahira H, Yokoyama H, Okawa K, Iwamatsu A, Nagata S. A caspase-activated DNase that degrades DNA during apoptosis, and its inhibitor ICAD. Nature 1998;391:43–50.
128. Liu X, Zou H, Slaughter C, Wang X. DFF, a heterodimeric protein that functions downstream of caspase-3 to trigger DNA fragmentation during apoptosis. Cell 1997;89:175–184.
129. Li LY, Luo X, Wang X. Endonuclease G is an apoptotic DNase when released from mitochondria. Nature 2001;412:95–99.
130. McIlroy D, Tanaka M, Sakahira H, et al. An auxiliary mode of apoptotic DNA fragmentation provided by phagocytes. Genes Dev 2000;14:549–558.
131. Sahara S, Aoto M, Eguchi Y, Imamoto N, Yoneda Y, Tsujimoto Y. Acinus is a caspase-3-activated protein required for apoptotic chromatin condensation. Nature 1999;401:168–173.
132. Susin SA, Lorenzo HK, Zamzami N, et al. Molecular characterization of mitochondrial apoptosis-inducing factor. Nature 1999;397:441–446.
133. Lazebnik YA, Kaufmann SH, Desnoyers S, Poirier GG, Earnshaw WC. Cleavage of poly(ADP-ribose) polymerase by a proteinase with properties like ICE. Nature 1994;371:346–347.
134. Tewari M, Quan LT, O'Rourke K, et al. Yama/CPP32 beta, a mammalian homolog of CED-3, is a CrmA-inhibitable protease that cleaves the death substrate poly(ADP-ribose) polymerase. Cell 1995;81:801–809.
135. Casciola-Rosen LA, Anhalt GJ, Rosen A. DNA-dependent protein kinase is one of a subset of autoantigens specifically cleaved early during apoptosis. J Exp Med 1995;182:1625–1634.
136. Zheng TS, Hunot S, Kuida K, et al. Deficiency in caspase-9 or caspase-3 induces compensatory caspase activation. Nat Med 2000;6:1241–1247.
137. Janicke RU, Ng P, Sprengart ML, Porter AG. Caspase-3 is required for alpha-fodrin cleavage but dispensable for cleavage of other death substrates in apoptosis. J Biol Chem 1998;273:15,540–15,545.
138. Ruchaud S, Korfali N, Villa P, et al. Caspase-6 gene disruption reveals a requirement for lamin A cleavage in apoptotic chromatin condensation. EMBO J 2002;21:1967–1977.
139. Cowling V, Downward J. Caspase-6 is the direct activator of caspase-8 in the cytochrome c-induced apoptosis pathway: absolute requirement for removal of capsase-6 prodomain. Cell Death Differ 2002;9:1046–1056.
140. Ren Y, Savill J. Apoptosis: the importance of being eaten. Cell Death Differ 1998;5:563–568.
141. Savill J, Fadok V. Corpse clearance defines the meaning of cell death. Nature 2000;407:784–788.
142. Fadok VA, Bratton DL, Frasch SC, Warner ML, Henson PM. The role of phospatidylserine in recognition of apoptotic cells by phagocytes. Cell Death Differ 1998;5:551–562.
143. Fadok VA, Bratton DL, Rose DM, Pearson A, Ezekewitz RA, Henson PM. A receptor for phosphatidylserine-specific clearance of apoptotic cells. Nature 2000;405:85–90.
144. Hanayama R, Tanaka M, Miwa K, Shinohara A, Iwamatsu A, Nagata S. Identification of a factor that links apoptotic cells to phagocytes. Nature 2002; 417:182–187.
145. Hengartner MO. Apoptosis: corralling the corpses. Cell 2001;104:325–328.
146. Reddien PW, Cameron S, Horvitz HR. Phagocytosis promotes programmed cell death in *C. elegans*. Nature 2001;412:198–202.
147. Hoeppner DJ, Hengartner MO, Schnabel R. Engulfment genes cooperate with ced-3 to promote cell death in Caenorhabditis elegans. Nature 2001;412:202–206.
148. Conradt B. With a little help form your friends: cells don't die alone. Nat Cell Biol 2002;4:E139–E143.
149. Vaux DL, Cory S, Adams JM. Bcl-2 gene promotes haemopoietic cell survival and cooperates with c-myc to immortalize pre-B cells. Nature 1988;335:440–442.
150. Vaux DL, Weissman IL, Kim SK. Prevention of programmed cell death in Caenorhabditis elegans by human bcl-2. Science 1992;258:1955–1957.
151. McDonnell TJ, Deane N, Platt FM, et al. bcl-2-immunoglobulin transgenic mice demonstrate extended B cell survival and follicular lymphoproliferation. Cell 1989;57:79–88.
152. Strasser A, Harris AW, Cory S. bcl-2 transgene inhibits T cell death and perturbs thymic self-censorship. Cell 1991;67:889–899.
153. Sentman CL, Shutter JR, Hockenbery D, Kanagawa O, Korsmeyer SJ. bcl-2 inhibits multiple forms of apoptosis but not negative selection in thymocytes. Cell 1991;67:879–888.
154. Veis DJ, Sorenson CM, Shutter JR, Korsmeyer SJ. Bcl-2-deficient mice demonstrate fulminant lymphoid apoptosis, polycystic kidneys, and hypopigmented hair. Cell 1993;75:229–240.

155. Huang DC, Strasser A. BH3-Only proteins-essential initiators of apoptotic cell death. Cell 2000;103:839–842.
156. Bouillet P, Metcalf D, Huang DC, et al. Proapoptotic Bcl-2 relative Bim required for certain apoptotic responses, leukocyte homeostasis, and to preclude autoimmunity. Science 1999;286:1735–1738.
157. Bouillet P, Cory S, Zhang LC, Strasser A, Adams JM. Degenerative disorders caused by Bcl-2 deficiency prevented by loss of its BH3-only antagonist Bim. Dev Cell 2001;1:645–653.
158. Lindsten T, Ross AJ, King A, et al. The combined functions of proapoptotic Bcl-2 family members bak and bax are essential for normal development of multiple tissues. Mol Cell 2000;6:1389–1399.
159. Zong WX, Lindsten T, Ross AJ, MacGregor GR, Thompson CB. BH3-only proteins that bind-pro-survival Bcl-2 family members fail to induce apoptosis in the absence of Bax and Bak. Genes Dev 2001;15:1481–1486.
160. Wei MC, Zong WX, Cheng EH, et al. Proapoptotic BAX and BAK: a requisite gateway to mitochondrial dysfunction and death. Science 2001;292:727–730.
161. Cheng EH, Wei MC, Weiler S, et al. BCL-2, BCL-X(L) sequester BH3 domain-only molecules preventing BAX- and BAK-mediated mitochondrial apoptosis. Mol Cell 2001;8:705–711.
162. Newmeyer DD, Ferguson-Miller S. Mitochondria. Releasing power for life nad unleashing the machineries of death. Cell 2003;112:481–490.
163. Marsden VS, O'Connor L, O'Reilly LA, et al. Apoptosis initiated by Bcl-2-regulated caspase activation independently of the cytochrome c/Apaf-1/caspase-9 apoptosome. Nature 2002;419:634–637.
164. Lassus P, Opitz-Araya X, Lazebnik Y. Requirement for caspase-2 in stress-induced apoptosis before mitochondrial permeabilization. Science 2002;297:1352–1354.
165. Bergeron L, Perez GI, Macdonald G, et al. Defects in regulation of apoptosis in caspase-2-deficient mice. Genes Dev 1998;12:1304–1314.
166. Read SH, Baliga BC, Ekert PG, Vaux DL, Kumar S. A novel Apaf-2-independent putative capsase-2 activation complex. J Cell Biol 2002;159:739–745.
167. Wang X. The expanding role of mitochondria in apoptosis. Genes Dev 2001;15:2922–2933.
168. Zou H, Yang R, Hao J, et al. Regulation of the Apaf-1/caspase-9 apoptosome by caspase-3 and XIAP. J Biol Chem 2003;278:8091–8098.
169. Kawane K, Fukuyama H, Yoshida H, et al. Impaired thymic development in mouse embryos deficient in apoptotic DNA degradation. Nat Immunol 2003:4:138–144.
170. Parrish J, Li L, Klotz K, Ledwich D, Wang X, Xue D. Mitochondrial endonuclease G is important for apoptosis in *C. elegans*. Nature 2001;412:90–94.
171. Susin SA, Daugas E, Ravagnan L, et al. Two distinct pathways leading to nuclear apoptosis. J Exp Med 2000;192:571–580.
172. Joza N, Susin SA, Daugas E, et al. Essential role of the mitochondrial apoptosis-inducing factor in programmed cell death. Nature 2001;410:549–554.
173. Ravagnan L, Gurbuxani S, Susin SA, et al. Heat-shock protein 70 antagonizes apoptosis-inducing factor. Nat Cell Biol 2001;3:839–843.
174. Ashkenazi A, Dixit VM. Death receptors: signaling and modulation. Science 1998;281:1305–1308.
175. Igney FH, Krammer PH. Death and anti-death: tumour resistance to apoptosis. Nat Rev Cancer 2002;2:277–288.
176. Stennicke HR, Salvesen GS. Caspases—controlling intracellular signals by protease zymogen activation. Biochim Biophys Acta 2000;1477:299–306.
177. Ashkenazi A. Targeting death and decoy receptors of the tumour-necrosis factor superfamily. Nat Rev Cancer 2002;2:420–430.
178. Carswell EA, Old LJ, Kassel RL, Green S, Fiore N, Williamson B. An endotoxin-induced serum factor that causes necrosis of tumors. Proc Natl Acad Sci U S A 1975;72:3666–3670.
179. Helson L, Green S, Carswell E, Old LJ. Effect of tumour necrosis factor on cultured human melanoma cells. Nature 1975;258:731–732.
180. Pennica D, Nedwin GE, Hayflick JS, et al. Human tumour necrosis factor: precursor structure, expression and homology to lymphotoxin. Nature 1984;312:724–729.
181. Locksley RM, Killeen N, Lenardo MJ. The TNF and TNF receptor superfamilies: integrating mammalian biology. Cell 2001;104:487–501.
182. Chen G, Goeddel DV. TNF-R1 signaling: a beautiful pathway. Science 2002;296:1634–1635.
183. Rathmell JC, Thompson CB. Pathways of apoptosis in lymphocyte development, homeostasis, and disease. Cell 2002;109(Suppl):S97–S107.

184. Chou AH, Tsai HF, Lin LL, Hsieh SL, Hsu PI, Hsu PN. Enhanced proliferation and increased IFN-gamma production in T cells by signal transduced through TNF-related apoptosis-inducing ligand. J Immunol 2001;167:1347–1352.
185. Fesik SW. Insights into programmed cell death through structural biology. Cell 2000;103:273–282.
186. MacEwan DJ. TNF receptor subtype signalling: differences and cellular consequences. Cell Signal 2002;14:477–492.
187. Krammer PH. CD95's deadly mission in the immune system. Nature 2000;407:789–795.
188. Wiley SR, Schooley K, Smolak PJ, et al. Identification and characterization of a new member of the TNF family that induces apoptosis. Immunity 1995;3:673–682.
189. Pitti RM, Marsters SA, Ruppert S, Donahue CJ, Moore A, Ashkenazi A. Induction of apoptosis by Apo-2 ligand, a new member of the tumor necrosis factor cytokine family. J Biol Chem 1996;271:12,687–12,690.
190. Walczak H, Miller RE, Ariail K, et al. Tumoricidal activity of tumor necrosis factor-related apoptosis-inducing ligand in vivo. Nat Med 1999;5:157–163.
191. Ashkenazi A, Pai RC, Fong S, et al. Safety and antitumor activity of recombinant soluble Apo2 ligand. J Clin Invest 1999;104:155–162.
192. Takeda K, Hayakawa Y, Smyth MJ, et al. Involvement of tumor necrosis factor-related apoptosis-inducing ligand in surveillance of tumor metastasis by liver natural killer cells. Nat Med 2001;7:94–100.
193. Smyth MJ, Cretney E, Takeda K, et al. Tumor necrosis factor-related apoptosis-inducing ligand (TRAIL) contributes to interferon gamma-dependent natural killer cell protection from tumor metastasis. J Exp Med 2001;193:661–670.
194. Cretney E, Takeda K, Yagita H, Glaccum M, Peschon JJ, Smyth MJ. Increased susceptibility to tumor initiation and metastasis in TNF-related apoptosis-inducing ligand-deficient mice. J Immunol 2002;168:1356–1361.
195. Takeda K, Smyth MJ, Cretney E, et al. Critical role for tumor necrosis factor-related apoptosis-inducing ligand in immune surveillance against tumor development. J Exp Med 2002;195:161–169.
196. Ichikawa K, Liu W, Zhao L, et al. Tumoricidal activity of a novel anti-human DR5 monoclonal antibody without hepatocyte cytotoxicity. Nat Med 2001;7:954–960.
197. Reed JC. Apoptosis-targeted therapies for cancer. Cancer Cell 2003;3:17–22.
198. Schmaltz C, Alpdogan O, Kappel BJ, et al. T cells require TRAIL for optimal graft-versus-tumor activity. Nat Med 2002;8:1433–1437.
199. Itoh N, Nagata S. A novel protein domain required for apoptosis. Mutational analysis of human Fas antigen. J Biol Chem 1993;268:10,932–10,937.
200. Trauth BC, Klas C, Peters AM, et al. Monoclonal antibody-mediated tumor regression by induction of apoptosis. Science 1989;245:301–305.
201. Yonehara S, Ishii A, Yonehara M. A cell-killing monoclonal antibody (anti-Fas) to a cell surface antigen co-downregulated with the receptor of tumor necrosis factor. J Exp Med 1989;169:1747–1756.
202. Itoh N, Yonehara S, Ishii A, et al. The polypeptide encoded by the cDNA for human cell surface antigen Fas can mediate apoptosis. Cell 1991;66:233–243.
203. Pitti RM, Marsters SA, Lawrence DA, et al. Genomic amplification of a decoy receptor for Fas ligand in lung and colon cancer. Nature 1998;396:699–703.
204. Chan FK, Chun HJ, Zheng L, Siegel RM, Bui KL, Lenardo MJ. A domain in TNF receptors that mediates ligand-independent receptor assembly and signaling. Science 2000;288:2351–2354.
205. Siegel RM, Frederiksen JK, Zacharias DA, et al. Fas preassociation required for apoptosis signaling and dominant inhibition by pathogenic mutations. Science 2000;288:2354–2357.
206. Jiang Y, Woronicz JD, Liu W, Goeddel DV. Prevention of constitutive TNF receptor 1 signaling by silencer of death domains. Science 1999;283:543–546.
207. Kischkel FC, Hellbardt S, Behrmann I, et al. Cytotoxicity-dependent APO-1 (Fas/CD95)-associated proteins form a death-inducing signaling complex (DISC) with the receptor. EMBO J 1995;14:5579-5588.
208. Vincenz C, Dixit VM. Fas-associated death domain protein interleukin-1beta-converting enzyme 2 (FLICE2), and ICE/Ced-3 homologue, is proximally involved in CD95- and p55-mediated death signaling. J Biol Chem 1997;272:6578–6583.
209. Wang J, Chun HJ, Wong W, Spencer DM, Lenardo MJ. Caspase-10 is an initiator caspase in death receptor signaling. Proc Natl Acad Sci USA 2001;98:13,884–13,888.
210. Kischkel FC, Lawrence DA, Tinel A, et al. Death receptor recruitment of endogenous caspase-10 and apoptosis initiation in the absence of caspase-8. J Biol Chem 2001;276:46,639–46,646.

211. Sprick MR, Rieser E, Stahl H, Grosse-Wilde A, Weigand MA, Walczak H. Caspase-10 is recruited to and activated at the native TRAIL and CD95 death-inducing signalling complexes in a FADD-dependent manner but can not functionally substitute caspase-8. EMBO J 2002;21:4520–4530.
212. Wang J, Zheng L, Lobito A, et al. Inherited human Caspase 10 mutations underlie defective lymphocyte and dendritic cell apoptosis in autoimmune lymphoprolierative syndrome type II. Cell 1999;98:47–58.
213. Stanger BZ, Leder P, Lee TH, Kim E, Seed B. RIP: a novel protein containing a death domain that interacts with Fas/APO-1 (CD95) in yeast and causes cell death. Cell 1995;81:513–523.
214. Kelliher MA, Grimm S, Ishida Y, Kuo F, Stanger BZ, Leder P. The death domain kinase RIP mediates the TNF-induced NF-kappaB signal. Immunity 1998;8:297–303.
215. Imai Y, Kimura T, Murakami A, Yajima N, Sakamaki K, Yonehara S. The CED-4-homologous protein FLASH is involved in Fas-mediated activation of caspase-8 during apoptosis. Nature 1999;398:777–785.
216. Suzuki A, Obata S, Hayashida M, Kawano H, Nakano T, Shiraki K. SADS: A new component of Fas-DISC is the accelerator for cell death signaling and is downregulated in patients with colon carcinoma. Nat Med 2001;7:88–93.
217. Suzuki A, Obata S, Hayashida M, Kawano H, Nakano T, Shiraki K. Retraction: SADS: A new component of Fas-DISC is the accelerator for cell death signaling and is downregulated in patients with colon carcinoma. Nat Med 2001;7:749.
218. Choi YH, Kim KB, Kim HH, et al. FLASH coordinates NF-kappa B activity via TRAF2. J Biol Chem 2001;276:25,073–25,077.
219. Irmler M, Thome M, Hahne M, et al. Inhibition of death receptor signals by cellular FLIP. Nature 1997;388:190–195.
220. Goltsev YV, Kovalenko AV, Arnold E, Varfolomeev EE, Brodianskii VM, Wallach D. CASH, a novel caspase homologue with death effector domains. J Biol Chem 1997;272:19,641–19,644.
221. Han DK, Chaudhary PM, Wright ME, et al. MRIT, a novel death-effector domain-containing protein, interacts with caspases and BclXL and initiates cell death. Proc Natl Acad Sci USA 1997;94: 11,333–11,338.
222. Hu S, Vincenz C, Ni J, Gentz R, Dixit VM. I-FLICE, a novel inhibitor of tumor necrosis factor receptor-1- and CD-95-induced apoptosis. J Biol Chem 1997;272:17,255–17,257.
223. Inohara N, Koseki T, Hu Y, Chen S, Nunez G. CLARP, a death effector domain-containing protein interacts with caspase-8 and regulates apoptosis. Proc Natl Acad Sci U S A 1997;94:10,717–10,722.
224. Shu HB, Halpin DR, Goeddel DV. Casper is a FADD- and caspase-related inducer of apoptosis. Immunity 1997;6:751–763.
225. Srinivasula SM, Ahmad M, Ottilie S, et al. FLAME-1, a novel FADD-like anti-apoptotic molecule that regulates Fas/TNFR1-induced apoptosis. J Biol Chem 1997;272:18,542–18,545.
226. Rasper DM, Vaillancourt JP, Hadano S, et al. Cell death attenuation by ‚ÄòUsurpin', a mammalian DED-caspase homologue that precludes caspase-8 recruitment and activation by the CD-95 (Fas, APO-1) receptor complex. Cell Death Differ 1998;5:271–288.
227. Chang DW, Xing Z, Pan Y, et al. c-FLIP(L) is a dual function regulator for caspase-8 activation and CD95-mediated apoptosis. EMBO J 2002;21:3704–3714.
228. Micheau O, Thome M, Schneider P, et al. The long form of FLIP is an activator of caspase-8 at the Fas death-inducing signaling complex. J Biol Chem 2002;277:45,162–45,171.
229. Hsu H, Xiong J, Goeddel DV. The TNF receptor 1-associated protein TRADD signals cell death and NF-kappa B activation. Cell 1995;81:495–504.
230. Hsu H, Shu HB, Pan MG, Goeddel DV. TRADD-TRAF2 and TRADD-FADD interactions define two distinct TNF receptor 1 signal transduction pathways. Cell 1996;84:299–308.
231. Harper N, Hughes M, MacFarlane M, Cohen GM. Fas-associated death domain protein and caspase-8 are not recruited to the tumor necrosis factor receptor 1 signaling complex during tumor necrosis factor-induced apoptosis. J Biol Chem 2003;278:25,534–25,541.
232. Liu ZG, Hsu H, Goeddel DV, Karin M. Dissection of TNF receptor 1 effector functions: JNK activation is not linked to apoptosis while NF-kappaB activation prevents cell death. Cell 1996;87:565–576.
233. Karin M, Cao Y, Greten FR, Li ZW. NF-kappaB in cancer: from innocent bystander to major culprit. Nat Rev Cancer 2002;2:301–310.
234. Devin A, Cook A, Lin Y, Rodriguez Y, Kelliher M, Liu Z. The distinct roles of TRAF2 and RIP in IKK activation by TNF-R1: TRAF2 recruits IKK to TNF-R1 while RIP mediates IKK activation. Immunity 2000;12:419–429.
235. Lee SY, Reichlin A, Santana A, Sokol KA, Nussenzweig MC, Choi Y. TRAF2 is essential for JNK but not NF-kappaB activation and regulates lymphocyte proliferation and survival. Immunity 1997;7:703–713.

236. Hsu H, Huang J, Shu HB, Baichwal V, Goedel DV. TNF-dependent recruitment of the protein kinase RIP to the TNF receptor-1 signaling complex. Immunity 1996;4:387–396.
237. Scaffidi C, Fulda S, Srinivasan A, et al. Two CD95 (APO-1/Fas) signaling pathways. EMBO J 1998;17:1675–1687.
238. Yin XM, Wang K, Gross A, et al. Bid-deficient mice are resistant to Fas-induced hepatocellular apoptosis. Nature 1999;400:886–891.
239. Ozoren N, Kim K, Burns TF, Dicker DT, Moscioni AD, El-Deiry WS. The caspase 9 inhibitor Z-LEHD-FMK protects human liver cells while permitting death of cancer cells exposed to tumor necrosis factor-related apoptosis-inducing ligand. Cancer Res 2000;60:6259–6265.
240. Vogelstein B, Lane D, Levine AJ. Surfing the p53 network. Nature 2000;408:307–310.
241. Soengas MS, Alarcon RM, Yoshida H, et al. Apaf-1 and caspase-9 in p53-dependent apoptosis and tumor inhibition. Science 1999;284:156–159.
242. Bennett M, Macdonald K, Chan SW, Luzio JP, Simari R, Weissberg P. Cell suface trafficking of Fas: a rapid mechanism of p53-mediated apoptosis. Science 1998;282:20–293.
243. Wu GS, Burns TF, McDonald ER, 3rd, et al. KILLER/DR5 is a DNA damag-inducible p53-regulated death receptor gene. Nat Genet 1997;17:141–143.
244. Embree-Ku M, Venturini D, Boekelheide K. Fas is involved in the p53-dependent apoptotic response to ionizing radiation in mouse testis. Biol Reprod 2002;66:1456–1461.
245. Engels IH, Stepczynska A, Stroh C, et al. Caspase-8/FLICE functions as an executioner caspase in anticancer drug-induced apoptosis. Oncogene 2000;19:4563–4573.
246. Wesselborg S, Engels IH, Rossmann E, Los M, Schulze-Osthoff K. Anticancer drugs induce caspase-8/FLICE activation and apoptosis in the absence of CD95 receptor/ligand interaction. Blood 1999;93:3053–3063.
247. Tang D, Lahti JM, Kidd VJ. Caspase-8 activation and bid cleavage contribute to MCF7 cellular execution in a caspase-3-dependent manner during staurosporine-mediated apoptosis. J Biol Chem 2000;275:9303–9307.
248. Zhou BB, Elledge SJ. The DNA damage response: putting checkpoints in perpective. Nature 2000;408:433–439.
249. Vousden KH, Lu X. Live or let die: the cell's response to p53. Nat Rev Cancer 2002;2:594–604.
250. Sax JK, Fei P, Murphy ME, Bernhard E, Korsmeyer SJ, El-Deiry WS. BID regulation by p53 contributes to chemosensitivity. Nat Cell Biol 2002;4:842–849.
251. MacLachlan TK, El-Deiry WS. Apoptotic threshold is lowered by p53 transactivation of caspase-6. Proc Natl Acad Sci U S A 2002;99:9492–9497.
252. Johnstone RW, Ruefli AA, Lowe SW. Apoptosis: a link between cancer genetics and chemotherapy. Cell 2002;108:153–164.
253. Brunet A, Bonni A, Zigmond MJ, et al. Akt promotes cell survival by phosphorylating and inhibiting a Forkhead transcription factor. Cell 1999;96:857–868.
254. Dijkers PF, Medema RH, Lammers JW, Koenderman L, Coffer PJ. Experssion of the pro-apoptotic Bcl-2 family member Bim is regulated by the forkhead transcription factor FKHR-L1. Curr Biol 2000;10:1201–1204.
255. Datta SR, Dudek H, Tao X, et al. Akt phosphorylation of BAD couples survival signals to the cell-intrinsic death machinery. Cell 1997;91:231–241.
256. del Peso L, Gonzalez-Garcia M, Page C, Herrera R, Nunez G. Interleukin-3-induced phosphorylation of BAD through the protein kinase Akt. Science 1997;278:687–689.
257. Cardone MH, Roy N, Stennicke HR, et al. Regulation of cell death protease caspase-9 by phosphorylation. Science 1998;282:1318–1321.
258. Fujita E, Jinbo A, Matuzaki H, Konishi H, Kikkawa U, Momoi T. Akt phosphorylation site found in human caspase-9 is absent in mouse caspase-9. Biochem Biophys Res Commun 1999;264:550–555.
259. Mayo LD, Donner DB. A phosphatidylinositol 3-kinase/Akt pathway promotes translocation of Mdm2 from the cytoplasm to the nucleus. Proc Natl Acad Sci U S A 2001;98:11,598–11,603.
260. Zhou BP, Liao Y, Xia W, Zou Y, Spoh B, Hung MC. HER-2/neu induces p53 ubiquitination via Akt-mediated MDM2 phosphorylation. Nat Cell Biol 2001;3:973–982.
261. Hanahan D, Weinberg RA. The hallmarks of cancer. Cell 2000;100:57–70.
262. Fisher GH, Rosenberg FJ, Straus SE, et al. Dominant interfering Fas gene mutations impair aopoptosis in a human autoimmune lymphoproliferative syndrome. Cell 1995;81:935–946.
263. Rieux-Laucat F, Le Deist F, Hivroz C, et al. Mutations in Fas associated with human lymphoproliferative syndrome and autoimmunity. Science 1995;268:1347–1349.

264. Wu J, Wilson J, He J, Xiang L, Schur PH, Mountz JD. Fas ligand mutation in a patient with systemic lupus erythematosus and lymphoproliferative disease. J Clin Invest 1996;98:1107–1113.
265. Jackson CE, Puck JM. Autoimmune lymphoproliferative syndrome, a disorder of apoptosis. Curr Opin Pediatr 1999;11:521–527.
266. Watanabe-Fukunaga R, Brannan CI, Copeland NG, Jenkins NA, Nagata S. Lymphoproliferation disorder in mice explained by defects in Fas antigen that mediates apoptosis. Nature 1992;356:314–317.
267. Takahashi T, Tanaka M, Branna CI, et al. Generalized lymphoproliferative disease in mice, caused by a point mutation in the Fas ligand. Cell 1994;76:969–976.
268. Lee SH, Shin MS, Park WS, et al. Alterations of Fas (APO-1/CD95) gene in transitional cell carcinomas of urinary bladder. Cancer Res 1999;59:3068–3072.
269. Lee SH, Shin MS, Park WS, et al. Alterations of Fas (APO-1/CD95) gene in non-small cell lung cancer. Oncogene 1999;18:3754–3760.
270. Lee SH, Shin MS, Park WS, et al. Alterations of Fas (Apo-1/CD95) gene in cutaneous malignant melanoma. Am J Pathol 1999;154:1785–1791.
271. Shin MS, Kim HS, Lee SH, et al. Alterations of Fas-pathway genes associated with nodal metastasis in non-small cell lung cancer. Oncogene 2002;32:4129–4136.
272. McDermott MF, Aksentijevich I, Galon J, et al. Germline mutations in the extracellular domains of the 55 kDa TNF receptor, TNFR1, define a family of dominantly inherited autoinflammatory syndromes. Cell 1999;97:133–144.
273. Pai SI, Wu GS, Ozoren N, et al. Rare loss-of-function mutation of a death receptor gene in head and neck cancer. Cancer Res 1998;59:3513–3518.
274. Lee SH, Shin MS, Kim HS, et al. Alterations of the DR5/TRAIL receptor 2 gene in non-small cell lung cancers. Cancer Res 1999;59:5683–5686.
275. Ozoren N, Fisher MJ, Kim K, et al. Homozygous deletion of the death receptor DR4 gene in a nasopharyngeal cancer cell line is associated with TRAIL resistance. Int J Oncol 2000;16:917–925.
276. Shin MS, Kim HS, Lee SH, et al. Mutations of tumor necrosis factor-related apoptosis-inducing ligand receptor 1 (TRAIL-R1) and receptor 2 (TRAIL-R2) genes in metastatic breast cancers. Cancer Res 2001;61:4942–4946.
277. Lee SH, Shin MS, Kim HS, et al. Somatic mutations of TRAIL-receptor 1 and TRAIL-receptor 2 genes in non-Hodgkin's lymphoma. Oncogene 2001;20:399–403.
278. Bai C, Connolly B, Metzker ML, et al. Overexpression of M68/DcR3 in human gastrointestinal tract tumors independent of gene amplification and its location in a four-gene cluster. Proc Natl Acad Sci U S A 2000;160:89–97.
279. Ohshima K, Haraoka S, Sugihara M, et al. Amplification and expression of a decoy receptor for fas ligand (DcR3) in virus (EBV or HTLV-I) associated lymphomas. Cancer Lett 2000;160:89–97.
280. Roth W, Isenmann S, Nakamura M, et al. Soluble decoy receptor 3 is expressed by malignant gliomas and suppresses CD95 ligand-induced apoptosis and chemotaxis. Cancer Res 2001;61:2759–2765.
281. Takahama Y, Yamada Y, Emoto K, et al. The prognostic significance of overexpression of the decoy receptor for Fas ligand (DcR3) in patients with gastric carcinomas. Gastric Cancer 2002;5:61–68.
282. Pan G, Ni J, Wei YF, Yu G, Gentz R, Dixit VM. An antagonist decoy receptor and a death domain-containing receptor for TRAIL. Science 1997;277:815–818.
283. Sheridan JP, Marsters SA, Pitti RM, et al. Control of TRAIL-induced apoptosis by a family of signaling and decoy receptors. Science 1997;277:818–821.
284. Marsters SA, Sheridan JP, Pitti RM, et al. A novel receptor for Apo2L/TRAIL contains a truncated death domain. Curr Biol 1997;7:1003–1006.
285. Pan G, Ni J, Yu G, Wei YF, Dixit VM. TRUNDD, a new member of the TRAIL receptor family that antagonizes TRAIL signalling. FEBS Lett 1998;424:41–45.
286. Rieger J, Naumann U, Glaser T, Ashkenazi A, Weller M. APO2 ligand: a novel lethal weapon against malignant glioma? FEBS Lett 1998;427:124–128.
287. Griffith TS, Chin WA, Jackson GC, Lynch DH, Kubin MZ. Intracellular regulation of TRAIL-induced apoptosis in human melanoma cells. J Immunol 1998;161:2833–2840.
288. Zhang XD, Franco A, Myers K, Gray C, Nguyen T, Hersey P. Relation of TNF-related apoptosis-inducing ligand (TRAIL) receptor and FLICE-inhibitory protein expression to TRAIL-induced apoptosis of melanoma. Cancer Res 1999;59:2747–2753.
289. Kim K, Fisher MJ, Xu SQ, El-Deiry WS. Molecular determinants of response to TRAIL in killing of normal and cancer cells. Clin Cancer Res 2000;6:335–346.

290. Thome M, Tschopp J. Regulation of lymphocyte proliferation and death by FLIP. Nat Rev Immunol 2001;1:50–58.
291. Teitz T, Wei T, Valentine MB, et al. Caspase 8 is deleted or silenced preferentially in childhood neuroblastaomas with amplification of MYCN. Nat Med 2000;6:529–535.
292. Hopkins-Donaldson S, Bodmer JL, Bourloud KB, Brognara CB, Tschopp J, Gross N. Loss of caspase-8 expression in highly malignant human neuroblastoma cells correlates with resistance to tumor necrosis factor-related apoptosis-inducing ligand-induced apoptosis. Cancer Res 2000;60:4315–4319.
293. Grotzer MA, Eggert A, Zuzak TJ, et al. Resistance to TRAIL-induced apoptosis in primitive neuroectodermal brain tumor cells correlates with a loss of caspase-8 expression. Oncogne 2000; 19:4606–4610.
294. Eggert A, Grotzer MA, Zuzak TJ, et al. Resistance to tumor necrosis factor-related apoptosis-inducing ligand (TRAIL)-induced apoptosis in neuroblastoma cells correlates with a loss of caspase-8 expression. Cancer Res 2001;61:1314–1319.
295. Liu B, Pend D, Lu Y, Jin W, Fan Z. A novel single amino acid deletion caspase-8 mutant in cancer cells that lost proapoptotic activity. J Biol Chem 2002;277:30,159–30,164.
296. Park WS, Lee JH, Shin MS, et al. Inactivating mutations of the caspase-10 gene in gastric cancer. Oncogene 2002;21:2919–2925.
297. Chun HJ, Zheng L, Ahmad M, et al. Pleiotropic defects in lymphocyte activation caused by caspase-8 mutations lead to human immunodeficiency. Nature 2002;419:395–399.
298. Soengas MS, Capodieci P, Polsky D, et al. Inactivation of the apoptosis effector Apaf-1 in malignant melanoma. Nature 2001;409:207–211.
299. LaCasse EC, Baird S, Korneluk RG, MacKenzie AE. The inhibitors of apoptosis (IAPs) and their emerging role in cancer. Oncogene 1998;17:3247–3259.
300. Adams JM, Cory S. The Bcl-2 protein family: arbiters of cell survival. Science 1998;281:1322–1326.
301. Rampino N, Yamamoto H, Ionov Y, et al. Somatic fameshift mutations in the BAX gene in colon cancers of the microsatellite mutator phenotype. Science 1997;275:967–969.
302. Kondo S, Shinomura Y, Miyazaki Y, et al. Mutations of the bak gene in human gastric and colorectal cancers. Cancer Res 2000;60:4328–4330.
303. McCurrach ME, Connor TM, Knudson CM, Korsmeyer SJ, Lowe SW. bax-deficiency promotes drug resistance and oncogenic transformation by attenuating p53-dependent apoptosis. Proc Natl Acad Sci U S A 1997;94:2345–2349.
304. Yin C, Knudson CM, Korsmeyer SJ, Van Dyke T. Bax suppresses tumorigenesis and stimulates apoptosis in vivo. Nature 1997;385:637–640.
305. Ionov Y, Yamamoto H, Krajewski S, Reed JC, Perucho M. Mutational inactivation of the proapoptotic gene BAX confers selective advantage during tumor clonal evolution. Proc Natl Acad Sci USA 2000;97:10,872–10,877.
306. Mullauer L, Gruber P, Sebinger D, Buch J, Wohlfart S, Chott A. Mutations in apoptosis genes: a pathogenetic factor for human disease. Mutat Res 2001;488:211–231.

2 Resistance to Apoptosis in Cancer Therapy

David J. McConkey, PhD

SUMMARY

An enormous body of work has established that conventional cancer therapies induce apoptosis in tumor cell lines and preclinical models of human disease. Parallel efforts have defined the evolutionarily conserved components of the apoptotic pathway, inspiring efforts to characterize the functional status of these components in human tumor cells. Although core pathway defects have been documented, the apoptotic pathway appears to be intact in most tumors, perhaps because disruption of the core machinery inhibits cell proliferation or interferes with other processes that are essential for tumor progression. On the other hand, it is clear that the selective pressures encountered by tumor cells do increase apoptosis resistance, most often via disruption of upstream mechanisms that produce parallel decreases in apoptosis sensitivity and increases in cell proliferation. Two of the most common examples of this type of disruption are inactivation of the p53 pathway and activation of PI-3 kinase/AKT/NF-κB, and aggressive efforts to specifically target these defects are underway. A major challenge for the immediate future is to validate the concept that apoptosis plays a crucial role in tumor response to therapy in patients receiving conventional and "designer" drugs, and more specifically, to confirm that the latter effectively hit their targets and produce the desired biological responses.

APOPTOSIS AND TUMOR PROGRESSION

Most conventional cancer therapies kill tumor cells by directly or indirectly damaging DNA, and DNA "breaks" are clearly important in triggering tumor cell death *(1)*. Thus, many investigators have assumed that the preferential cell killing observed in tumor cells as compared to their normal counterparts (the "therapeutic window") is attributable to the higher rates of cell proliferation displayed by the former. This should make the tumor cells more vulnerable to agents that interrupt DNA synthesis and/or other processes

From: *Cancer Drug Discovery and Development: Death Receptors in Cancer Therapy*
Edited by: W. S. El-Deiry © Humana Press Inc., Totowa, NJ

associated with cell division (i.e., cytokinesis), and tumor cells might die as a result of either permanent mitotic arrest or mitotic "crisis" caused by the failure to successfully complete division. This model also provides an explanation for why the death of normal cells with relatively high rates of proliferation (bone marrow hematopoietic precursors and epithelial cells in the gastrointestinal tract) is usually responsible for the dose-limiting toxicities associated with these agents. In addition, this model would predict that drug resistance would be due largely to increased drug efflux and/or DNA repair capacity.

The recognition that most (if not all) cancer therapies trigger apoptosis in models of human cancer *(1–4)* has prompted a reappraisal of this paradigm. Apoptosis is an energy-dependent evolutionarily conserved pathway that is regulated by a very diverse array of factors *(5)*, any of which could be disrupted by selection mechanisms associated either with natural tumor progression or prior exposure to therapy. At the core is a family of cysteine proteases known as caspases *(6)*, whose activation is controlled by pro- and antiapoptotic members of the BCL-2 family *(7)*. Thus, as will be described in more detail below, indirect interference with caspase activation, most likely via indirect effects on the BCL-2 family, now appears to be a common theme in the development of therapeutic resistance in cancer *(8,9)*. However, data accumulated over the past decade strongly suggest that direct inactivation of the core machinery for apoptosis (for example, via massive overexpression of BCL-2 or mutational inactivation of caspases) is not nearly as common indirect inactivation of apoptosis, commonly in a pathway-specific manner.

Why is this the case? Returning to the idea that tumor cell susceptibility to cancer therapy is associated with cell proliferation, work conducted over the past decade has also shown that apoptosis and cell division are tightly coupled *(10,11)*. The earliest report of this phenomenon came from Evan, Wyllie, and their colleagues, who showed that enforced expression of the *myc* oncogene increased levels of apoptosis in normal fibroblasts deprived of growth factors *(12)*; Jacks and Lowe refined this observation by showing that normal fibroblasts transfected with proliferation-driving oncogenes were also dramatically sensitized to cell death induced by conventional cancer chemotherapeutic agents and ionizing radiation *(13,14)*. Loss of expression of certain cell-cycle-regulating tumor suppressor proteins (for example, the Rb protein *[15,16]*) can also sensitize cells to apoptosis via deregulated activation of E2F-1 *(17,18)* (*see also* refs. *19–21* for more recent interpretations of the effects of loss of Rb on neurological development) . Indeed, recent studies have demonstrated that normal cells can be protected from the toxic effects of cancer therapy by pretreating them with cell-cycle inhibitors, thereby "parking" them in a state of reduced sensitivity to apoptosis *(22)*. Thus, a new explanation for the therapeutic window observed in cancer therapy is that early stage tumor cells display increased apoptosis sensitivity due to cell-cycle deregulation.

Considering these findings, it is easier to understand why tumor cells tend to almost always disrupt certain apoptosis regulatory mechanisms and not others. Just as deregulated cell-cycle control increases sensitivity to apoptosis, many apoptosis inhibitors also tend to inhibit cell-cycle progression. Perhaps the best example of this phenomenon has come from studies with BCL-2 itself, which delays cell-cycle progression in normal cells *(23)* as well as many different tumor cell lines *(24,25)*. Thus, BCL-2-mediated resistance to apoptosis comes at a cost in terms of cell proliferation. Even caspases themselves have been recently implicated in cell proliferation *(26–28)*, which may explain why tumor cells (and especially tumor cell lines) rarely display loss of caspases by mutation. Tumor cells that select for this type of cell death resistance must therefore also specifically overcome the inhibition of proliferation by acquiring a second genetic or epigenetic defect *(11)*. Therefore, the most common examples of acquired apoptosis resistance in tumors simultaneously promote both apoptosis resistance and cell-cycle progression *(11)*.

LOSS OF FUNCTIONAL P53 AND RESISTANCE TO CANCER THERAPY

The fact that the p53 pathway is inactivated in the vast majority of human cancers is one of the most familiar concepts in cancer biology. p53 functions as part of an increasingly complex network of proteins that mediate cellular responses to DNA damage and a variety of other stimuli *(29,30)*. It is clear that p53-induced cell-cycle arrest is mediated largely via transcriptional activation of the gene encoding p21/WAF-1 *(31,32)*, a polypeptide inhibitor of the cyclin-dependent kinases. However, p21 does not appear to play a direct role in promoting p53-mediated cell death *(33–36)* (although it does play an important indirect role, as will be discussed in more detail below). The precise mechanisms that underlie p53-mediated cell death are complex, but there is general consensus that members of the BH3-only subfamily of BCL-2 proteins *(37,38)* and death receptor pathway components *(39,40)* play predominant roles. Most of the available evidence indicates that the p53-mediated transcriptional activation is required for cell death, but there are prominent recent examples of transcription-independent effects in the literature *(41–48)*.

Other recent studies have identified some of the pressures associated with tumor progression that select for cancer cells that possess defects in the p53 pathway. Of particular importance is the observation that p53 is activated by oncogenes via p19ARF, a protein encoded within the p16 locus that inhibits MDM-2/HDM-2-mediated ubiquitination and degradation of p53 *(49,50)*. Thus, the apoptosis that results from overexpression of Myc *(51)* or inactivation of Rb *(52)* is p53-dependent in many normal cells and presumably in early-stage tumors, and loss of p53 function reverses apoptosis sensitization.

Tumor hypoxia is another important factor that selects for loss of p53 function *(53)*. As tumors grow beyond the diffusion limit of oxygen, they must acquire the capacity to stimulate new blood flow, or a crisis caused by hypoxia and hypoglycemia ensues *(54,55)*. Hanahan has termed this transition the "angiogenic switch" *(56)*, and his laboratory and others have shown that it is associated with increased expression of proangiogenic cytokines (VEGF, bFGF, IL-8) *(56–58)* and decreased cell death *(59)*. For reasons that are not entirely clear, hypoxia-induced cell death is highly sensitive to cellular p53 status, and the hypoxic microenvironment within growing solid tumors actually selects for mutational inactivation of p53 *(53)*. This phenomenon has important implications for antiangiogenic therapy, in that tumors that retain wild-type p53 appear to respond much more impressively to therapy than do cells with mutant forms of the protein *(60)*. Other tumor progression-associated mechanisms associated with the angiogenic switch include upregulation of BCL-2 family proteins (BCL-2, BCL-X_L) *(59)*.

The molecular mechanisms underlying p53-mediated apoptosis are complex and likely depend on the cell type in question. Early work demonstrated that p53 binds to and activates the Bax promoter *(61)*, leading to increased expression of this proapoptotic member of the BCL-2 family. However, it is now thought that Bax activation is a complex process involving translocation of the protein from the cytosol to the mitochondrion *(62,63)* and subsequent oligomerization of the protein within the mitochondrial membrane *(64–66)*. These events are sensitive to amino acids within the C-terminal "transmembrane" domain of Bax *(67)* and may be driven by members of the so-called "BH3-only" subfamily of BCL-2-related polypeptides *(66,68)* or p53 itself *(48)*. Indeed, recent studies have demonstrated that p53-mediated apoptosis is dependent on PUMA and/or NOXA, two BH3-only proteins identified in a screen for p53 targets *(38)*. Other work has shown that expression of the death receptor-associated protein Bid is also driven by wild-type p53, and still other studies suggest that p53-dependent induction of the BH3-only protein Bik drives apoptosis-associated disruption of the endoplasmic reticulum. Finally, very recent work from Green's laboratory demonstrated that cytosolic p53 can directly drive Bax activation *(48)*, an observation that is probably related to previous work showing that p53 localizes to mitochondria to promote cytochrome c release *(47)*.

p53 activation also increases the expression of critical components of death receptor-mediated pathways of apoptosis. Early work from Owen-Schaub's laboratory demonstrated that wild-type p53 drove expression of Fas in human osteosarcoma cells *(40)*, an observation that was subsequently confirmed in a variety of other tumors as well as normal tissues *(69)*. These effects appear to be mediated by p53 response elements located within the first intron of the Fas gene *(70)* as well as elements located >1.5 kb upstream of the transcriptional initiation site (L. Owen-Schaub, personal communication). Debatin's group extended these observations by showing that conventional chemotherapeutic agents kill some tumor cell lines via Fas-sensitive mechanisms *(71,72)*, and other work has shown that p53-induced Fas-Fas ligand interactions are required for the appearance of apoptotic "sunburn cells" in the skin *(73)*. Cells containing mutations in p53 accumulate in Fas ligand$^{-/-}$ animals (H. Ananthaswamy, personal communication), demonstrating the importance of this pathway in the elimination of damaged, potentially transformed cells.

More recent work has demonstrated that tumor necrosis factor-related apoptosis-inducing ligand (TRAIL) receptor-2/death receptor (DR)5 is also an important transcriptional target for p53 *(74)*. Interestingly, as is true for Fas, the effects of p53 on DR5 are mediated by a p53 response element localized to the first intron of the DR5 promoter *(75)*. The effects of p53 on DR5 expression are certainly involved in the synergistic effects of DNA-damaging agents and TRAIL on apoptosis *(76)*, although p53-independent mechanisms also appear to contribute to enhanced cell killing *(77)*. That synergy is sensitive to cellular p53 status has important implications for planned human clinical trials of combination therapy with conventional agents and TRAIL, in that p53 status could prove to be an important predictor of response.

Although studies in knockout mice have established that p53 is required for DNA damage-induced apoptosis in many normal tissues *(78–80)*, loss of wild-type p53 clearly does not engender absolute insensitivity to DNA damage-induced apoptosis in tumors. There are many examples of DNA damage-induced, p53-independent apoptosis in the literature, but one of the most informative studies of the relative importance of p53 status in dictating sensitivity to chemotherapy comes from a study of relative sensitivity to 5-fluorouracil (5-FU) in the National Cancer Institute's panel of 60 tumor cell lines *(81)*. The results of this work confirmed that loss of wild-type p53 was associated with resistance to 5-FU, but the mean IC_{50} observed in p53 wild-type cells was only about 3- to 10-fold lower than the mean IC_{50} observed in tumor cells lacking wild-type p53. Furthermore, since the assay employed in the screen cannot distinguish growth arrest from apoptosis, it is likely that p53-mediated cell-cycle arrest contributed significantly to the effects observed. Whether or not other members of the p53 family (p63, p73) can compensate for loss of p53 remains to be determined.

Reconstitution of wild-type p53 by gene transfer is the most direct means of restoring p53 pathway function in tumors *(82,83)*. Effective replication-incompetent adenoviral systems for p53 gene therapy were among the first gene transfer systems developed *(84)*. Promising results were obtained in several different preclinical (xenograft) models where Ad-p53 was combined with conventional modalities (radiation, DNA-damaging agents, taxanes *[85–89]*) *(90)*. However, obtaining high-level expression of p53 throughout the tumor has been a major obstacle to optimization of these approaches, and in the clinical trials performed to date, protein expression was largely confined to regions immediately adjacent to the needle entry site. The development of replication-competent viruses may provide one means of overcoming this pitfall. For example, Onyx Pharmaceuticals, Inc., developed a p53 adenovirus that selectively replicates in cells lacking p53 *(91,92)* by taking advantage of the fact that the adenoviral E1A protein (like Myc) drives both cell-cycle progression and p53-mediated apoptosis, effects that must be counteracted by two proteins encoded by the E1B locus *(93)*. Thus, by deleting E1B, Onyx produced a virus that can propagate efficiently only within a p53-null background. Clinical trials with the Onyx virus in combination with conventional therapy *(86,94)* are ongoing at present, but promising clinical activity has been observed in trials performed to date *(95–100)*. However, work still needs to be done to improve methods for systemic gene delivery to combat disseminated (metastatic) disease *(101)*, which is really the relevant target of adjuvant therapy in patients with most forms of cancer.

APOPTOSIS RESISTANCE MEDIATED BY AKT/PKB

AKT/PKB is a protein serine/threonine kinase that functions downstream of phosphoinositol 3' (PI-3) kinase to regulate cell proliferation, glycolytic metabolism, and survival *(102–105)*. Recent studies have demonstrated that AKT interferes with apoptosis at multiple levels via phosphorylation of survival-associated substrates including the BH3-only protein BAD, the forkhead family of transcription factors, the transcription factor NF-κB, and possibly caspases themselves *(103)*. In addition, AKT simultaneously promotes cell-cycle progression and apoptosis resistance by phosphorylating and activating another kinase, the molecular target of rapamycin (mTOR). mTOR drives proliferation via activation of ribosomal S6 kinase *(106)* and recent studies indicate that AKT-induced, mTOR-dependent increases in glucose, iron, and cholesterol uptake function to promote cell survival under conditions of growth factor withdrawal *(107,108)*. Thus, as is true for inactivation of p53, activation of AKT simultaneously promotes cell division and survival, making it an attractive target for disruption during tumor progression.

Two of the most common progression-associated molecular events that mediate tumor cell acquisition of active AKT are loss of the MMAC/PTEN tumor suppressor and overexpression of growth factor receptors (EGF-R, HER-2, and IGF-IR) *(109)*. PTEN is a lipid phosphatase that functions as an enzymatic antagonist of PI-3 kinase, and it is commonly inactivated at a relatively late stage in solid tumor progression, often at the point where the cells acquire an invasive and/or metastatic phenotype *(110)*. Thus, loss of PTEN interferes with detachment-induced apoptosis (anoikis), a process observed in normal epithelial and other adherent cells when they are dissociated from basement membrane or extracellar matrix *(111–113)*. Although PTEN may have other biological functions unrelated to AKT, overexpression of constitutively active forms of AKT suppresses anoikis and enhances metastasis, whereas reintroduction of wild-type PTEN into tumor cells that lack it promotes sensitivity to detachment-induced cell death and loss of metastatic potential *(114–117)*. In addition, one group demonstrated that metastatic potential and AKT activation were enhanced in squamous cell carcinomas of the oral tongue selected for an aniokis-resistant phenotype via repeated short-term suspension culture *(118)*.

The acquisition of growth factor independence is a second pressure that selects for tumor clones containing active AKT *(109,119)*. Like anoikis, apoptosis associated with growth factor withdrawal probably functions physiologically to prevent the inappropriate migration of cells away from their normal microenvironment. Tumor cells subvert this regulatory mechanism by overexpressing growth factor receptors and their ligands, thereby establishing autocrine pathways that render the tumor cell less dependent upon growth factors provided by the microenvironment. In addition, tumors may induce stromal cells within the microenvironment to express the specific growth factors the tumor requires for proliferation and survival. Wherever the mechanisms have been carefully interrogated, AKT activation plays a central role in these responses.

The growth-factor receptors that have received the most attention in studies of tumor progression to date are the members of the erbB family *(120)*. This family consists of four homologous transmembrane polypeptides (erbB1–4) that contain tyrosine kinase domains within their cytoplasmic tails *(121)*. The most familiar members of the family are erbB1 (the EGF receptor) *(122)* and erbB2 (HER-2/Neu) *(123)*, both of which are overexpressed in most solid tumors as a function of progression. Furthermore, all members of the erbB family can dimerize with one another to form signaling complexes that probably mediate distinct effects on tumor cell biology *(121)*.

Studies with primary tumors have demonstrated that the EGFR and HER-2 and their ligands (EGF, TGF-α) are overexpressed in almost all solid malignancies *(109,124–126)*. In human tumor xenograft models, selection for increased metastatic potential via orthotopic "recycling" results in increased EGFR and/or HER-2 in colon, prostate, breast, bladder, and pancreatic cancer *(127–129)*. Overexpression of HER-2 in the HER-2-negative human breast line MDA-MB-435 results in increased metastatic potential and decreased sensitivity to chemotherapy-induced apoptosis *(130–132)*, whereas down-regulation of HER-2 inhibits metastasis *(133)*. Ligand-mediated activation of EGFR and HER-2 activates AKT *(123,134–136)* and other kinases involved in cell proliferation *(137)*.

Although many different targets appear to contribute to AKT-mediated apoptosis resistance, one of the best studied within the context of therapeutic resistance is the transcription factor, NF-κB. Early studies in NF-κB (p65) knockout mice demonstrated that the transcription factor is required for a critically important cellular survival pathway that is activated by tumor necrosis factor (TNF) and other proinflammatory cytokines *(138)*. Subsequent studies revealed that NF-κB is also commonly activated in tumor cells exposed to conventional chemotherapeutic agents, and suppression of this NF-κB activation via overexpression of a molecular inhibitor of NF-κB (IκBαM) dramatically enhances tumor cell killing *(139)*. At the core of the upstream signal transduction pathway leading to NF-κB activation is IκB kinase (IKK), a large multisubunit complex that is responsible for phosphorylating IκBα and targeting it for ubiquitination and degradation by the 26S proteasome *(140,141)*. However, optimal NF-κB activation is also dependent on AKT in many different cellular systems *(142)*, either because AKT also participates in phosphorylation of IκBα *(143)* or because it directly modifies the NF-κB subunit(s) themselves (p50, p65) via serine phosphorylation.

The transcriptional targets of NF-κB are quite diverse, but its effects on cell survival appear to involve upregulation of antiapoptotic BCL-2 family proteins (BCL-2, BCL-X_L, A1) *(144–148)* and inhibitor of apoptosis proteins (IAPs) *(149)*. BCL-2 family proteins regulate caspase activation upstream of mitochondrial events leading to cytochrome c release *(147,148,150)*, whereas the IAP proteins bind directly to caspases and inhibit their activities *(151)*. These cell death inhibitory events are complementary and probably act to reinforce resistance to cell death in tumor cells that express constitutively active NF-κB. However, no systematic evaluation of the relative importance of each target in NF-κB-mediated cell death resistance in any tumor model has been performed to date. Thus, most current therapeutic strategies are aimed at inhibiting tumor cell AKT or NF-κB rather than their downstream targets.

There are several potential strategies that could be employed to block AKT activation in tumor cells, and all of them are being aggressively pursued. Excellent inhibitors of EGFR and HER-2 have been developed, including blocking antibodies and small-molecule tyrosine kinase inihibitors, which display very promising activity in preclinical models and clinical trials *(122,152)*. Furthermore, preclinical studies have demonstrated that these agents act in an additive or synergistic fashion with cytotoxic agents, although these effects are sensitive to schedule. Small-molecule inhibitors of PI-3 kinase and AKT are also being developed for human cancer therapy, and where tested preclinically, they too have displayed very promising bioactivity *(153,154)*. Trials with an inhibitor of mTOR (a rapamycin analog) are already underway in patients with prostate cancer and certain other malignancies *(155,156)*.

One fascinating approach to chemosensitization involves using proteasome inhibitors to block NF-κB activation. The first of these compounds (bortezomib, formerly PS-341, also known as Velcade*(157)*) recently received FDA approval for the treatment of patients with multiple myeloma *(158–160)*, and it is also displaying promising activity in other hematological and solid malignancies. Bortezomib prevents chemotherapy-induced activation of NF-κB in cell lines and xenograft models, and synergizes with several different agents (gemcitabine, camptothecin, radiation) to promote tumor growth inhibition *(161–164)*. Inhibition of NF-κB may also decrease invasion, metastasis, and angiogenesis by downregulating matrix metalloprotease, integrin, and angiogenic factor (VEGF, IL-8) expression by tumor cells *(165–167)*. Importantly, because the proteasome is involved in such a large number of different cellular processes, bortezomib's effects go well beyond inhibition of NF-κB. Thus, a recent side-by-side comparison study concluded that bortezomib was more active than a chemical IKK inhibitor (PS-1145) in a preclinical multiple myeloma model *(168)*. Bortezomib is a very potent inhibitor of cell-cycle progression and causes endoplasmic reticular stress by interfering with the clearance of misfolded or damaged proteins within the cell. These effects probably contribute to make bortezomib a more effective anticancer agent than compounds that are designed to exclusively target NF-κB itself.

LOSS OF DEATH RECEPTOR RESPONSIVENESS

Death receptors are a family of transmembrane proteins homologous to the tumor necrosis factor receptor 1 (TNFR1) that play key roles in the maintenance of immune homeostasis and host defense *(169)*. The most familiar members of the family are the TNFR1 itself, CD95/Fas, and two of the receptors for TRAIL (DR4 and DR5). The importance of death receptors in immunity was first demonstrated in studies of the mechanism of apoptosis induced by T-cell receptor engagement of previously activated mature T-cells, a phenomenon known as "activation-induced cell death" (AICD). These studies demonstrated that AICD is mediated by increased expression of Fas and Fas ligand *(170,171)*. As noted earlier, Fas-Fas ligand interactions also mediate apoptosis in various normal cells exposed to DNA-damaging agents, and Fas expressed by tumor cells is recognized by activated cytotoxic T-cells and natural killer cells that express Fas ligand, resulting in specific tumor cell killing. Tumor cell sensitivity to Fas is further increased by cytokines (particularly interferons) that are produced by activated T-cells and components of the innate immune system (macrophages). Antibodies to Fas are also highly cytotoxic to a subset of human tumor cells in vitro *(172)*, which at one time prompted enthusiasm for their potential use in cancer therapy. Unfortunately, normal hepatocytes are highly sensitive to Fas-mediated apoptosis *(173)*, making a systemic approach based on anti-Fas antibodies or Fas ligand itself infeasible.

Although there are substantial concerns about using TNF or Fas ligand in cancer therapy, the prospects for TRAIL appear much more promising. Initial studies demonstrated that TRAIL triggered apoptosis in most human cancer cell lines but not in their normal counterparts *(174)*, and initial in vivo studies with recombinant murine or human TRAIL in rodents or primates demonstrated little to no toxicity *(175)*. These findings prompted academic centers and industry to develop recombinant TRAIL and agonistic anti-DR4 and -DR5 antibodies for use in cancer therapy *(176)*, and clinical trials with these agents are underway. Unfortunately, the clinical development of TRAIL encountered a setback with a prominent report demonstrating that isolated human hepatocytes underwent apoptosis when they were exposed to certain preparations of recombinant TRAIL in vitro *(177)*. These concerns have been alleviated somewhat by arguments that the effects were preparation-specific and that the recombinant TRAIL and the anti-death-receptor antibodies are not cytotoxic to normal cells.

Given their central roles in host defense, it is not surprising that tumors disrupt death receptor pathways as a function of progression. The earliest examples of this phenomenon came from studies with metastatic melanoma cells, which short-circuit the Fas pathway by downregulating surface expression of the receptor *(178)* and by expressing a soluble "decoy" form of Fas that competes with the full-length molecule for binding to Fas ligand *(179)*. Subsequent studies demonstrated that colon cancer cells also downregulate Fas expression and sensitivity with progression *(180,181)*, and similar processes have been described in other solid tumor models. The selective pressures that enrich for Fas resistance are associated with innate and adaptive antitumor immunity as well as the high-level expression of Fas ligand in endothelial cells within "immune privileged sites" (lung, brain), which probably serves to prevent the inward migration of activated T-cells and tumor cells that express Fas *(182)*. Because DNA-damaging agents appear to kill certain tumor cells via p53-dependent, Fas-mediated mechanisms, it is likely that the same pressures that induce loss of p53 select for loss of Fas sensitivity as well.

Like Fas, the receptors for TRAIL are also upregulated via p53-dependent mechanisms, and the loss of TRAIL receptor inducibility that accompanies loss of functional p53 also probably contributes to chemoresistance in tumors. However, given current enthusiasm for TRAIL-based cancer therapy, the observation that many tumor cells display baseline resistance to TRAIL presents an additional challenge. The mechanisms underlying TRAIL resistance in tumors are complex and probably include expression of decoy receptors that compete for TRAIL binding and expression of cellular FLICE-inhibitory proteins (c-FLIPs) *(169)*, which are enzymatically inactive homologs of caspase-8 that compete for binding to the death-inducing signaling complex (DISC). Furthermore, recent studies have demonstrated that AKT desensitizes tumor cells to death receptor-mediated suicide, in part via effects on the FKHD family of transcription factors (which promote death receptor/ligand expression) *(183)* and in part via more direct effects on the death receptor-mediated signaling pathways that precipitate cell death.

Recent work from our laboratory has identified another tumor progression-associated event that selects for loss of TRAIL and Fas sensitivity. These studies have been conducted in bladder cancer cells, which appear to be particularly sensitive to innate immune defense systems, as exemplified by the fact that the immune modulator BCG remains frontline therapy for invasive disease, producing complete responses in a majority of patients. Thus, it is likely that inflammatory cytokines expressed by stromal elements within the bladder apply constant pressure to transformed bladder epithelial cells. We have found that interferons induce high-level TRAIL expression in approx 50% of human bladder cancer cell lines (from a panel of over 20), and a subset of these are directly sensitive to interferon (IFN)-induced apoptosis (A. Papageorgiou et al., manuscript submitted). Importantly, specific inhibitors of caspase-8 and blocking anti-TRAIL antibodies attenuate cell death, strongly suggesting that IFN-induced apoptosis is mediated in part via autocrine production of TRAIL. However, some of the lines that secrete high levels of TRAIL are not sensitive to TRAIL-induced apoptosis. Thus, the emergence of TRAIL resistance appears to be a common event in bladder cancer progression. Even though IFNs can activate p53, loss of wild-type p53 does not explain the emergence of TRAIL resistance in our panel.

Although TRAIL resistance appears to be a fairly common problem in cancer cell lines, exciting new data indicate that this resistance can be overcome by combining TRAIL with certain conventional and investigational agents. A key feature of TRAIL-mediated cell death is that, unlike many of the other pathways described above, cell-cycle arrest appears to sensitize tumor cells to TRAIL *(184,185)*. For example, some TRAIL-resistant cell lines can be dramatically sensitized with DNA-damaging agents *(186–189)*, effects that may be sensitive to wild-type p53 and its transcriptional targets *(76)*. Furthermore, a variety of different investigational agents (flavopiridol *[190]*, histone deacetylase inhibitors *[191,192]*, bortezomib *[189,193,194]*) also synergize with TRAIL to promote killing of otherwise resistant tumor cells. In our recent studies we have linked these effects to an inhibition of cyclin-dependent kinases (L. Lashinger, manuscript in preparation), and we suspect that any therapy that blocks cell-cycle progression at the G_1 to S transition *(184)* will sensitize tumor cells to TRAIL. An excellent example of this is found with our studies with EGFR antagonists, which appear to promote TRAIL sensitization in bladder cancer cells via a p27-dependent mechanism *(195)* (M. Shrader, manuscript in preparation).

OTHER RESISTANCE MECHANISMS

As discussed above, given that the core molecular machinery for apoptosis is evolutionarily conserved, one might predict that the downstream elements would represent common targets for inactivation during tumor progression. Current thinking holds that caspase activation is the key rate-limiting step in apoptosis and that in mammalian cells activation of the so-called execution-phase caspases (3, 6, and 7) correlates with irreversible commitment to death. Members of the BCL-2 and IAP families promote or inhibit cell death via direct or indirect effects on caspase activation, and in mammalian cells, mitochondrial factors (cytochrome c, SMAC) and the cytosolic adaptor protein Apaf-1 also cooperate to promote caspase activation. Thus, defects in the caspases themselves or in the regulation of BCL-2 family proteins, IAPs, SMAC, cytochrome c, or Apaf-1 would be expected to be commonly associated with drug resistance in human tumors.

There are data consistent with this hypothesis, although it is not clear why these central pathways are not disrupted even more frequently than they are. Mutational inactivation of caspase-3 has been documented in only one human cancer cell line (the breast adenocarcinoma MCF-7) *(196,197)*, and caspase-7 mutations have been identified in only a relatively small subset of human solid tumors (<3%) *(198)*. Mutational inactivation of Apaf-1 has recently been described in melanoma *(199)*, and downreglation of Apaf-1 has also been reported in ovarian cancer *(200)*. There are no reports of mutational inactivation of SMAC or cytochrome c, although disruption of the latter's ability to participate in electron transport might select against cytochrome c modification. Importantly, early studies conducted by Raff's laboratory failed to identify any mammalian tumor cell line (or for that matter primary cell type) that could not be induced to undergo apoptosis following treatment with the protein kinase inhibitor staurosporine *(201)*. (The only exception to this rule was human embryonic cells isolated before the blastomere stage of development.) Together, these observations strongly suggest that disruption of the core apoptotic machinery for apoptosis does not commonly occur in human cancer cells.

There is much more evidence available implicating alterations in BCL-2 family proteins or the IAPs in tumor progression, but the results of these studies are mixed. Early work demonstrated that follicular B-cell lymphoma is driven by a chromosomal translocation that mediates high-level expression of BCL-2 in follicular B-cells *(202)*, and subsequent work showed that the acquisition of androgen independence in prostate cancer is associated with increased BCL-2 levels *(203)*. However, in other common solid tumors the role of BCL-2 in tumor progression and response to therapy is less clear. For example, the majority of early studies showed that expression of BCL-2 correlated with expression of the estrogen and progesterone receptors and a well differentiated phenotype in primary breast adenocarcinomas *(204)*, although more recent work suggests that higher levels of BCL-2 may correlate with poor response to neoadjuvant therapy *(205)*.

There is also some evidence that BCL-2 levels increase in metastatic melanoma, but once again reports arguing against this conclusion can also be found in the literature *(206)*. Perhaps even more paradoxically, our laboratory and another group independently demonstrated that basal levels of apoptosis were significantly elevated in matched liver metastases relative to the levels observed in primary colorectal adenocarcinomas *(207,208)*, effects that were associated with significant decreases in BCL-2 expression in the metastases. Frameshift mutations in Bax or Bak have been identified in subsets of gastric and colorectal adenocarcinomas (mostly with microsatellite instability) *(209–212,213)* and in human DU-145 prostate adenocarcinoma cells, but simultaneous inactivation of both Bax and Bak has not been reported. Finally, there are numerous studies that have linked increased expression of the IAP family member survivin to progression in breast and prostate cancer and various other solid malignancies *(214)*. However, survivin's function as a caspase inhibitor appears to be more restricted than the spectra of activity of other IAP family members, whereas it appears to function as a mitotic cofactor in most cells *(214)*, raising questions about whether tumors select for increased survivin in order to block apoptosis or to increase proliferation. Even the other IAP family members display diverse intracellular functions ranging from ubiquitin ligase activity to the regulation of death receptor function. As discussed above, one attractive explanation for these observations is that BCL-2 family proteins and the IAPs also play important roles in cell division or other critical homeostatic mechanisms. Thus, a tumor that gains apoptosis resistance by disrupting one of these pathways may do so at a cost. It is possible that posttranslational modifications of the core machinery that selectively promote resistance to cell death will be more common in cancer. If this proves true, then it may be possible to target these events to reverse cell death resistance.

APOPTOSIS RESISTANCE AND CANCER THERAPY: IMPLICATIONS FOR CANCER PATIENTS

An important caveat associated with almost all of the work described above is that the experiments were conducted in models of human cancer rather than in primary human tumors themselves. Recent studies employing microarrays to survey patterns of gene expression have cast doubt concerning how accurately human cell lines reflect primary tumors. Furthermore, most of the popular transgenic mouse models rely on tissue-specific viral inactivation of key pathways (i.e., p53 and Rb) to produce solid tumors, and in most cases they do not accurately model specific processes associated with spontaneous tumorigenesis in humans. Even more important to the present discussion, apoptosis is not the only cell-death pathway that can be activated by conventional and investigational cancer therapies, and where interrogated, the effects of strong apoptosis inhibitors (overexpression of BCL-2, exposure to peptide caspase antagonists) on clonogenic survival have not been particularly impressive. It is formally possible (and many prominent investigators remain convinced) that induction of permanent growth arrest (senescence) and necrosis are just as important as apoptosis in promoting tumor regression in patients receiving cancer therapy *(1)*.

Our laboratory and others have begun to address this gap in knowledge by measuring apoptosis before and at various times after neoadjuvant or investigational therapy in patients, with the aim of determining whether or not rates of apoptosis are predictive of clinical response. A major challenge presented by these studies is that current methods for measuring apoptosis require tissue (i.e., biopsies), and in many cases acquiring these tissues may present significant risk to the patient. Furthermore, tumors are thought to be very heterogeneous, so the selection of site(s) for biopsy could have significant effects on the results obtained. Apoptosis is also a very dynamic process, and steady-state measurements of cell death at arbitrarily selected time points might not accurately reflect rates of death within the tumor as a whole.

In spite of these concerns, our recent experience strongly suggests that early, drug-induced increases in apoptosis are critically important for overall clinical response in patients receiving neoadjuvant doxorubicin and/or taxanes for advanced breast cancer *(205,215)*. In this study we obtained 18-gauge core biopsies from 14 breast tumors just prior to and 24, 48, or 72 h after the first dose of chemotherapy. We stained the tumors using a fluorescent TUNEL method and quantified percentages of positive cells using a laser scanning cytometer (LSC). The LSC functions much like a flow cytometer to quantify immunofluorescence intensities at the single-cell level using tissue sections rather than cells in suspension. Compared to manual counting methods, the LSC provides greater sensitivity and objectivity, and using combinations of fluorescent probes one can interrogate events within subpopulations of tumor cells (i.e., epithelial vs endothelial cells). Furthermore, with the LSC we are able to measure percentages of apoptosis in very large numbers of tumor cells (typically over 10,000), providing much greater accuracy. The results of our first study revealed a strongly significant correlation (p = 0.003) between chemotherapy-induced apoptosis and the clinical (pathological) responses that were observed 3 mo later, in spite of the relatively small sample size *(215)*. If these preliminary observations can be validated in a larger patient population, they confirm that apoptosis is of central importance to therapeutic outcome.

In other studies we are investigating the role of apoptosis in tumor responses to antiangiogenic agents. The tumor vasculature has become a popular therapeutic target with the appreciation that tumors absolutely depend on angiogenesis for continued growth (see above) and that endothelial cells do not appear to acquire a drug-resistant phenotype following repeated exposure to antiangiogenic agents *(216)*. By first labeling tumor sections with a marker for endothelial cells (i.e., anti-CD31), one can simultaneously determine rates of apoptosis in tumor cells as well as tumor-associated endothelial cells. In preclinical models we showed that a variety of different biology-based investigational approaches (EGFR antagonists, interferons, VEGF receptor antagonists) induce a wave of apoptosis in tumor-associated endothelial cells that then leads to increases in epithelial cell death, presumably as a consequence of hypoxia and nutrient deprivation *(217–219)*. Thus, we have argued that increased endothelial cell apoptosis represents an excellent surrogate for effective antiangiogenic therapy *(220)*. However, endothelial cell death will result in tumor growth inhibition or regression only when it triggers a subsequent wave of tumor cell death. Because susceptibility to hypoxia nutrient deprivation-induced apoptosis is determined by tumor cell properties (p53 status), some tumors will be more sensitive to vascular targeting agents than others.

Based on this preclinical experience we designed a study to determine the effects of the antiangiogenic agent endostatin on parameters of angiogenesis inhibition and apoptosis in biopsies obtained from patients enrolled on a Phase I dose escalation trial *(221,222)*. In this study, excisional biopsies were obtained just prior to initiation of therapy and again after 56 d of treatment. No objective clinical responses were observed in our trial or the two other trials performed at different institutions. However, LSC-mediated quantification of apoptosis in endothelial (CD31+) cells revealed that endostatin induced significant increases in cell death at intermediate dose levels (180–300 mg/m^2) *(223)*. Furthermore, quantitative analysis of several other markers of angiogenesis inhibition (MVD, endothelial BCL-2 content, nuclear HIF-1α localization) all revealed maximal biological effects within the same dose range *(223)*. Importantly, however, tumor cell death did not increase in parallel, strongly suggesting that the extent of angiogenesis inhibition was not sufficient to produce a meaningful therapeutic effect. We are currently performing similar studies with biopsies obtained from patients enrolled in clinical trials with other antiangiogenic agents, some of which have generated a significant number of clinical responses. Many of these compounds target growth factor receptors, so quantitative analysis of their effects on proximal and distal signal transduction pathways is an integral component of the studies.

The results of the two examples outlined above strongly suggest that meaningful biological information can be obtained from primary patient tumor tissue via the use of sensitive analytical methods. Thus, one of the major challenges for the near future is to directly test some of the conclusions generated in preclinical studies summarized above. For example, there is general consensus that DNA-damaging agents trigger apoptosis via a p53-sensitive pathway. Thus, one prediction from this model is that effective therapy with conventional DNA-damaging agents should be associated with p53 activation and perhaps accumulation of relevant p53 target proteins (BH3-only proteins, Fas, DR5). Similarly, effective inhibition of AKT activation can be readily confirmed using phosphospecific antibodies designed to detect the active form of the kinase. Thus, as PI-3 kinase/AKT inhibitors enter clinical trials in patients, it will be important to confirm that these compounds "hit" their targets, leading to decreased AKT phosphorylation and inhibition of downstream AKT targets (mTOR, NF-κB, and so on). Similar strategies should be used to confirm that inhibitors of the erbB family of receptors (EGFR, HER-2) hit their targets in tumors. Phosphospecific antibodies are commercially available that recognize the active forms of the EGFR and HER-2, and preclinical studies have demonstrated that they can be used to monitor receptor activity in tumor tissues. Therefore, the hypothesis that erbB family members drive AKT activation in some tumors can now be directly tested in primary patient tissues. Finally, as TRAIL and anti-death-receptor antibodies are developed, it will be important to measure the markers of TRAIL susceptibility or resistance identified in the preclinical studies and to monitor markers of TRAIL sensitization and apoptosis in patients treated with TRAIL-based combination therapies. Related to this issue, we are starting a clinical trial with recombinant interferon-α in which we will measure IFN-induced signal transduction (phosphorylation of STAT-1, accumulation of IRF-1), accumulation of TRAIL, and apoptosis in biopsies obtained just prior to and 24–72 h after the initiation of therapy. If these studies are not performed, it is likely that molecular targets will be discarded because inactive compounds failed to produce clinical responses in patients treated with them.

Although biopsy-based approaches for measuring apoptosis and apoptosis-associated molecular mechanisms are currently the most feasible, a major priority for ongoing research is to develop noninvasive strategies to measure these pharmacodynamic processes. There are already good methods available to measure blood flow and glucose metabolism by positron emission tomography or magnetic resonance (MR) imaging

(222), and it appears that the development of new contrast agents will allow for MR-based assessment of apoptosis in real time in the near future *(224)*. For example, it is possible to detect apoptotic cells by staining them with annexin V, which binds to surface-exposed phosphatidylserine on the dying cell, and it is also possible to couple annexin V to contrast-enhancing agents for in vivo imaging of cell death *(225)*. It is anticipated that new contrast agents capable of directly monitoring caspase activation and the signal transduction events that regulate it will be available soon *(226)*. Ultimately, we hope that these methods will be employed to monitor therapeutic effects long before overt tumor regression can be observed and will allow physicians to rapidly tailor therapy to optimize patient benefit.

REFERENCES

1. Brown JM, Wilson G. Apoptosis genes and resistance to cancer therapy: what does the experimental and clinical data tell us? Cancer Biol Ther 2003;2:477–490.
2. Dive C, Evans CA, Whetton AD. Induction of apoptosis—new targets for cancer chemotherapy. Semin Cancer Biol 1992;3:417–427.
3. Hickman JA, Potten CS, Merritt AJ, Fisher TC. Apoptosis and cancer chemotherapy. Philos Trans R Soc Lond B Biol Sci 1994;345:319–325.
4. Schmitt CA, Lowe SW. Apoptosis and therapy. J Pathol 1999;187:127–137.
5. Hengartner MO. The biochemistry of apoptosis. Nature 2000;407:770–776.
6. Thornberry NA, Lazebnik Y. Caspases: enemies within. Science 1998;281:1312–1316.
7. Danial NN, Korsmeyer SJ. Cell death: critical control points. Cell 2004;116:205–219.
8. Reed JC. Regulation of apoptosis by bcl-2 family proteins and its role in cancer and chemoresistance. Curr Opin Oncol 1995;7:541–546.
9. Reed JC. Bcl-2 family proteins: regulators of apoptosis and chemoresistance in hematologic malignancies. Semin Hematol 1997;34:9–19.
10. Green DR, Evan GI. A matter of life and death. Cancer Cell 2002;1:19–30.
11. Evan GI, Vousden KH. Proliferation, cell cycle and apoptosis in cancer. Nature 2001;411:342–348.
12. Evan GI, Wyllie AH, Gilbert CS, et al. Induction of apoptosis in fibroblasts by c-myc protein. Cell 1992;69:119–128.
13. Lowe SW, Ruley HE, Jacks T, Housman DE. p53-dependent apoptosis modulates the cytotoxicity of anticancer agents. Cell 1993;74:957–967.
14. Lowe SW, Jacks T, Housman DE, Ruley HE. Abrogation of oncogene-associated apoptosis allows transformation of p53-deficient cells. Proc Natl Acad Sci USA 1994;91:2026–2030.
15. Clarke AR, Maandag ER, van Roon M, et al. Requirement for a functional Rb-1 gene in murine development. Nature 1992;359:328–330.
16. Picksley SM, Lane DP. p53 and Rb: their cellular roles. Curr Opin Cell Biol 1994;6:853–858.
17. Field SJ, Tsai FY, Kuo F, et al. E2F-1 functions in mice to promote apoptosis and suppress proliferation. Cell 1996;85:549–561.
18. Johnson DG. The paradox of E2F1: oncogene and tumor suppressor gene. Mol Carcinog 2000;27:151–157.
19. MacPherson D, Sage J, Crowley D, Trumpp A, Bronson RT, Jacks T. Conditional mutation of Rb causes cell cycle defects without apoptosis in the central nervous system. Mol Cell Biol 2003;23:1044–1053.
20. de Bruin A, Wu L, Saavedra HI, et al. Rb function in extraembryonic lineages suppresses apoptosis in the CNS of Rb-deficient mice. Proc Natl Acad Sci USA 2003;100:6546–6551.
21. Wu L, de Bruin A, Saavedra HI, et al. Extra-embryonic function of Rb is essential for embryonic development and viability. Nature 2003;421:942–947.
22. Chen X, Lowe M, Herliczek T, et al. Protection of normal proliferating cells against chemotherapy by staurosporine-mediated, selective, and reversible G(1) arrest. J Natl Cancer Inst 2000;92:1999–2008.
23. Gil-Gomez G, Berns A, Brady HJ. A link between cell cycle and cell death: Bax and Bcl-2 modulate Cdk2 activation during thymocyte apoptosis. Embo J 1998;17:7209–7218.
24. Pietenpol JA, Papadopoulos N, Markowitz S, Willson JDV, Kinzler KW, Vogelstein B. Paradoxical inhibition of solid tumor cell growth by bcl-2. Cancer Res 1994;54:3714–3717.
25. Huang DC, O'Reilly LA, Strasser A, Cory S. The anti-apoptosis function of Bcl-2 can be genetically separated from its inhibitory effect on cell cycle entry. Embo J 1997;16:4628–4638.

26. Kennedy NJ, Kataoka T, Tschopp J, Budd RC. Caspase activation is required for T cell proliferation. J Exp Med 1999;190:1891–1896.
27. Mack A, Hacker G. Inhibition of caspase or FADD function blocks proliferation but not MAP kinase-activation and interleukin-2-production during primary stimulation of T cells. Eur J Immunol 2002;32:1986–1992.
28. Boissonnas A, Bonduelle O, Lucas B, Debre P, Autran B, Combadiere B. Differential requirement of caspases during naive T cell proliferation. Eur J Immunol 2002;32:3007–3015.
29. Vogelstein B, Lane D, Levine AJ. Surfing the p53 network. Nature 2000;408:307–310.
30. El-Deiry WS. The role of p53 in chemosensitivity and radiosensitivity. Oncogene 2003;22:7486–7495.
31. El-Deiry WS, Tokino T, Velculescu VE, et al. WAF1, a potential mediator of p53 tumor suppression. Cell 1993;75:817–825.
32. El-Deiry WS, Harper JW, O'Connor PM, et al. WAF1/CIP1 is induced in p53-mediated G1 arrest and apoptosis. Cancer Res 1994;54:1169–1174.
33. Gorospe M, Cirielli C, Wang X, Seth P, Capogrossi MC, Holbrook NJ. p21(Waf1/Cip1) protects against p53-mediated apoptosis of human melanoma cells. Oncogene 1997;14:929–935.
34. Martinez LA, Yang J, Vazquez ES, et al. p21 modulates threshold of apoptosis induced by DNA-damage and growth factor withdrawal in prostate cancer cells. Carcinogenesis 2002;23:1289–1296.
35. Yu J, Tiwari S, Steiner P, Zhang L. Differential apoptotic response to the proteasome inhibitor Bortezomib [VELCADE, PS-341] in Bax-deficient and p21-deficient colon cancer cells. Cancer Biol Ther 2003;2:694–699.
36. Barlow C, Brown KD, Deng CX, Tagle DA, Wynshaw-Boris, A. Atm selectively regulates distinct p53-dependent cell-cycle checkpoint and apoptotic pathways. Nat Genet 1997;17:453–456.
37. Nakano K, Vousden KH. PUMA, a novel proapoptotic gene, is induced by p53. Mol Cell 2001;7:683–694.
38. Villunger A, Michalak EM, Coultas L, et al. p53- and drug-induced apoptotic responses mediated by BH3-only proteins puma and noxa. Science 2003;302:1036–1038.
39. Wu GS, Burns TF, McDonald ER, 3rd, et al. KILLER/DR5 is a DNA damage-inducible p53-regulated death receptor gene. Nat Genet 1997;17:141–143.
40. Owen-Schaub LB, Zhang W, Cusack JC, et al. Wild-type human p53 and a temperature-sensitive mutant induce Fas/APO-1 expression. Mol Cell Biol 1995;15:3032–3040.
41. Bennett M, MacDonald K, Chan SW, Luzio JP, Simari R, Weissberg P. Cell surface trafficking of Fas: a rapid mechanism of p53-mediated apoptosis. Science 1998;282:290–293.
42. Caelles C, Helmberg A, Karin M. p53-dependent apoptosis in the absence of transcriptional activation of p53-target genes. Nature 1994;370:220–223.
43. Mihara M, Moll UM. Detection of mitochondrial localization of p53. Methods Mol Biol 2003;234: 203–209.
44. Mihara M, Erster S, Zaika A, et al. p53 has a direct apoptogenic role at the mitochondria. Mol Cell 2003;11:577–590.
45. Moll UM, Zaika A. Nuclear and mitochondrial apoptotic pathways of p53. FEBS Lett 2001;493:65–69.
46. Sansome C, Zaika A, Marchenko ND, Moll UM. Hypoxia death stimulus induces translocation of p53 protein to mitochondria. Detection by immunofluorescence on whole cells. FEBS Lett 2001;488:110–115.
47. Marchenko ND, Zaika A, Moll UM. Death signal-induced localization of p53 protein to mitochondria. A potential role in apoptotic signaling. J Biol Chem 2000;275:16,202–16,212.
48. Chipuk JE, Kuwana T, Bouchier-Hayes L, et al. Direct activation of Bax by p53 mediates mitochondrial membrane permeabilization and apoptosis. Science 2004;303:1010–1014.
49. Sherr CJ, Weber JD. The ARF/p53 pathway. Curr Opin Genet Dev 2000;10:94–99.
50. Sherr CJ. The INK4a/ARF network in tumour suppression. Nat Rev Mol Cell Biol 2001;2:731–737.
51. Hermeking H, Eick D. Mediation of c-Myc-induced apoptosis by p53. Science 1994;265:2091–2093.
52. Morgenbesser SD, Williams BO, Jacks T, DePinho RA. p53-dependent apoptosis produced by Rb-deficiency in the developing mouse lens. Nature 1994;371:72–74.
53. Graeber TG, Peterson JF, Tsai M, Monica K, Fournace AJ, Giaccia AJ. Hypoxia induces accumulation of p53 protein, but activation of a G1-phase checkpoint by low-oxygen conditions is independent of p53 status. Mol Cell Biol 1994;14:6264–6277.
54. Folkman J. Tumor angiogenesis: therapeutic implications. N Engl J Med 1971;285:1182–1186.
55. Fidler IJ, Ellis LM. The implications of angiogenesis for the biology and therapy of cancer metastasis. Cell 1994;79:185–188.

56. Hanahan D, Folkman J. Patterns and emerging mechanisms of the angiogenic switch during tumorigenesis. Cell 1996;86:353–364.
57. Ellis LM, Fidler IJ. Angiogenesis and metastasis. Eur J Cancer 1996;32A:2451–2460.
58. Kandel J, Bossy-Wetzel E, Radvanyi F, Klagsbrun M, Folkman J, Hanahan D. Neovascularization is associated with a switch to the export of bFGF in the multistep development of fibrosarcoma. Cell 1991;66:1095–1104.
59. Naik P, Karrim J, Hanahan D. The rise and fall of apoptosis during multistage tumorigenesis: down-modulation contributes to tumor progression from angiogenic progenitors. Genes Dev 1996;10: 2105–2116.
60. Yu JL, Rak JW, Coomber BL, Hicklin DJ, Kerbel RS. Effect of p53 status on tumor response to antiangiogenic therapy. Science 2002;295:1526–1528.
61. Miyashita T, Reed JC. Tumor suppressor p53 is a direct transcriptional activator of the human bax gene. Cell 1995;80:293–299.
62. Hsu YT, Wolter KG, Youle RJ. Cytosol-to-membrane redistribution of Bax and Bcl-X(L) during apoptosis. Proc Natl Acad Sci USA 1997;94:3668–3672.
63. Goping IS, Gross A, Lavoie JN, et al. Regulated targeting of BAX to mitochondria. J Cell Biol 1998;143:207–215.
64. Gross A, Jockel J, Wei MC, Korsmeyer SJ. Enforced dimerization of BAX results in its translocation, mitochondrial dysfunction and apoptosis. Embo J 1998;17:3878–3885.
65. Korsmeyer SJ, Wei MC, Saito M, Weiler S, Oh KJ, Schlesinger PH. Pro-apoptotic cascade activates BID, which oligomerizes BAK or BAX into pores that result in the release of cytochrome c. Cell Death Differ 2000;7:1166–1173.
66. Wei MC, Lindsten T, Mootha VK, et al. tBID, a membrane-targeted death ligand, oligomerizes BAK to release cytochrome c. Genes Dev 2000;14:2060–2071.
67. Nechushtan A, Smith CL, Hsu YT, Youle RJ. Conformation of the Bax C-terminus regulates subcellular location and cell death. Embo J 1999;18:2330–2341.
68. Letai A, Bassik MC, Walensky LD, Sorcinelli MD, Weiler S, Korsmeyer SJ. Distinct BH3 domains either sensitize or activate mitochondrial apoptosis, serving as prototype cancer therapeutics. Cancer Cell 2002;2:183–192.
69. Santamaria AB, Davis DW, Nghiem DX, et al. p53 and Fas ligand are required for psoralen and UVA-induced apoptosis in mouse epidermal cells. Cell Death Differ 2002;9:549–560.
70. Muller M, Wilder S, Bannasch D, et al. p53 activates the CD95 (APO-1/Fas) gene in response to DNA damage by anticancer drugs. J Exp Med 1998;188:2033–2045.
71. Friesen C, Herr I, Krammer PH, Debatin KM. Involvement of the CD95 (APO-1/Fas) receptor/ligand system in drug-induced apoptosis in leukemia cells. Nature Medicine 1996;2:574–577.
72. Fulda S, Sieverts H, Friesen C, Herr I, Debatin KM. The CD95 (APO-1/Fas) system mediates drug-induced apoptosis in neuroblastoma cells. Cancer Res 1997;57:3823–3829.
73. Hill LL, Ouhtit A, Loughlin SM, Kripke ML, Ananthaswamy HN, Owen-Schaub LB. Fas ligand: a sensor for DNA damage critical in skin cancer etiology. Science 1999;285:898–900.
74. Wu GS, Kim K, el-Deiry WS. KILLER/DR5, a novel DNA-damage inducible death receptor gene, links the p53-tumor suppressor to caspase activation and apoptotic death. Adv Exp Med Biol 2000;465:143–151.
75. Takimoto R, El-Deiry WS. Wild-type p53 transactivates the KILLER/DR5 gene through an intronic sequence-specific DNA-binding site. Oncogene 2000;19:1735–1743.
76. Wang S, El-Deiry WS. Requirement of p53 targets in chemosensitization of colonic carcinoma to death ligand therapy. Proc Natl Acad Sci USA 2003;100:15,095–15,100.
77. Vivo C, Liu W, Broaddus VC. c-Jun N-terminal kinase contributes to apoptotic synergy induced by tumor necrosis factor-related apoptosis-inducing ligand plus DNA damage in chemoresistant, p53 inactive mesothelioma cells. J Biol Chem 2003;278:25,461–25,467.
78. Lowe SW, Schmitt EM, Smith SW, Osborne BA, Jacks T. p53 is required for radiation-induced apoptosis in mouse thymocytes. Nature 1993;362:847–849.
79. Clarke AR, Purdie CA, Harrison DJ, et al. Thymocyte apoptosis induced by p53-dependent and independent pathways. Nature 1993;362:849–852.
80. Lowe SW, Schmitt EM, Smith SW, Osborne BA, Jacks T. p53 is required for radiation-induced apoptosis in mouse thymocytes. Nature 1993;362:847–849.
81. O'Connor PM, Jackman J, Bae I, et al. Characterization of the p53 tumor suppressor pathway in cell lines of the National Cancer Institute's anticancer drug screen and correlations with the growth-inhibitory potency of 123 anticancer agents. Cancer Res 1997;57:4285–4300.

82. Roth JA, Swisher SG, Meyn RE. p53 tumor suppressor gene therapy for cancer. Oncology (Huntingt) 1999;13:148–154.
83. Roth JA, Nguyen D, Lawrence DD, et al. Retrovirus-mediated wild-type p53 gene transfer to tumors of patients with lung cancer. Nat Med 1996;2:985–991.
84. Swisher SG, Roth JA, Nemunaitis J, et al. Adenovirus-mediated p53 gene transfer in advanced non-small-cell lung cancer. J Natl Cancer Inst 1999;91:763–771.
85. Advani SJ, Chung SM, Yan SY, et al. Replication-competent, nonneuroinvasive genetically engineered herpes virus is highly effective in the treatment of therapy-resistant experimental human tumors. Cancer Res 1999;59:2055–2058.
86. Heise C, Lemmon M, Kirn D. Efficacy with a replication-selective adenovirus plus cisplatin-based chemotherapy: dependence on sequencing but not p53 functional status or route of administration. Clin Cancer Res 2000;6:4908–4914.
87. Nishizaki M, Meyn RE, Levy LB, et al. Synergistic inhibition of human lung cancer cell growth by adenovirus-mediated wild-type p53 gene transfer in combination with docetaxel and radiation therapeutics in vitro and in vivo. Clin Cancer Res 2001;7:2887–2897.
88. Horowitz J. Adenovirus-mediated p53 gene therapy: overview of preclinical studies and potential clinical applications. Curr Opin Mol Ther 1999;1:500–509.
89. Geoerger B, Grill J, Opolon P, et al. Potentiation of radiation therapy by the oncolytic adenovirus dl1520 (ONYX-015) in human malignant glioma xenografts. Br J Cancer 2003;89:577–584.
90. Nielsen LL, Lipari P, Dell J, Gurnani M, Hajian G. Adenovirus-mediated p53 gene therapy and paclitaxel have synergistic efficacy in models of human head and neck, ovarian, prostate, and breast cancer. Clin Cancer Res 1998;4:835–846.
91. Bischoff JR, Kirn DH, Williams A, et al. An adenovirus mutant that replicates selectively in p53-deficient human tumor cells. Science 1996;274:373–376.
92. Heise C, Sampson-Johannes A, Williams A, McCormick F, Von Hoff DD, Kirn D. H. ONYX-015, an E1B gene-attenuated adenovirus, causes tumor-specific cytolysis and antitumoral efficacy that can be augmented by standard chemotherapeutic agents. Nat Med 1997;3:639–645.
93. McCormick F. Interactions between adenovirus proteins and the p53 pathway: the development of ONYX-015. Semin Cancer Biol 2000;10:453–459.
94. Rogulski KR, Freytag SO, Zhang K, et al. In vivo antitumor activity of ONYX-015 is influenced by p53 status and is augmented by radiotherapy. Cancer Res 2000;60:1193–1196.
95. Kirn D, Hermiston T, McCormick F. ONYX-015: clinical data are encouraging. Nat Med 1998;4: 1341–1342.
96. Ganly I, Kirn D, Eckhardt G, et al. A phase I study of Onyx-015, an E1B attenuated adenovirus, administered intratumorally to patients with recurrent head and neck cancer. Clin Cancer Res 2000;6:798–806.
97. Khuri FR, Nemunaitis J, Ganly I, et al. A controlled trial of intratumoral ONYX-015, a selectively-replicating adenovirus, in combination with cisplatin and 5-fluorouracil in patients with recurrent head and neck cancer. Nat Med 2000;6:879–885.
98. Nemunaitis J, Ganly I, Khuri F, et al. Selective replication and oncolysis in p53 mutant tumors with ONYX-015, an E1B-55kD gene-deleted adenovirus, in patients with advanced head and neck cancer: a phase II trial. Cancer Res 2000;60:6359–6366.
99. Nemunaitis J, Khuri F, Ganly I, et al. Phase II trial of intratumoral administration of ONYX-015, a replication-selective adenovirus, in patients with refractory head and neck cancer. J Clin Oncol 2001;19:289–298.
100. Post LE. Selectively replicating adenoviruses for cancer therapy: an update on clinical development. Curr Opin Investig Drugs 2002;3:1768–1772.
101. Sweeney P, Karashima T, Ishikura H, et al. Efficient therapeutic gene delivery after systemic administration of a novel polyethylenimine/DNA vector in an orthotopic bladder cancer model. Cancer Res 2003;63:4017–4020.
102. Harris TE, Lawrence JC, Jr. TOR signaling. Sci STKE 2003;2003:re15.
103. Datta SR, Brunet A, Greenberg ME. Cellular survival: a play in three Akts. Genes Dev 1999;13: 2905–2927.
104. Plas DR, Thompson CB. Cell metabolism in the regulation of programmed cell death. Trends Endocrinol Metab 2002;13:75–78.
105. Franke TF, Hornik CP, Segev L, Shostak GA, Sugimoto C. PI3K/Akt and apoptosis: size matters. Oncogene 2003;22:8983–8998.

106. Neshat MS, Mellinghoff IK, Tran C, et al. Enhanced sensitivity of PTEN-deficient tumors to inhibition of FRAP/mTOR. Proc Natl Acad Sci USA 2001;98:10,314–10,319.
107. Edinger AL, Thompson CB. Akt maintains cell size and survival by increasing mTOR-dependent nutrient uptake. Mol Biol Cell 2002;13:2276–2288.
108. Edinger AL, Linardic CM, Chiang GG, Thompson CB, Abraham RT. Differential effects of rapamycin on mammalian target of rapamycin signaling functions in mammalian cells. Cancer Res 2003;63:8451–8460.
109. Danielsen AJ, Maihle NJ. The EGF/ErbB receptor family and apoptosis. Growth Factors 2002;20:1–15.
110. Steck PA, Pershouse MA, Jasser SA, et al. Identification of a candidate tumour suppressor gene, MMAC1, at chromosome 10q23.3 that is mutated in multiple advanced cancers. Nat Genet 1997;15:356–362.
111. Tamura M, Gu J, Tran H, Yamada KM. PTEN gene and integrin signaling in cancer. J Natl Cancer Inst 1999;91:1820–1828.
112. Lu Y, Lin YZ, LaPushin R, et al. The PTEN/MMAC1/TEP tumor suppressor gene decreases cell growth and induces apoptosis and anoikis in breast cancer cells. Oncogene 1999;18:7034–7045.
113. Davies MA, Lu Y, Sano T, et al. Adenoviral transgene expression of MMAC/PTEN in human glioma cells inhibits Akt activation and induces anoikis. Cancer Res 1998;58:5285–5290.
114. Delcommenne M, Tan C, Gray V, Rue L, Woodgett J, Dedhar S. Phosphoinositide-3-OH kinase-dependent regulation of glycogen synthase kinase 3 and protein kinase B/AKT by the integrin-linked kinase. Proc Natl Acad Sci USA 1998;95:11,211–11,216.
115. Attwell S, Roskelley C, Dedhar S. The integrin-linked kinase (ILK) suppresses anoikis. Oncogene 2000;19:3811–3815.
116. Rytomaa M, Lehmann K, Downward J. Matrix detachment induces caspase-dependent cytochrome c release from mitochondria: inhibition by PKB/Akt but not Raf signalling. Oncogene 2000;19: 4461–4468.
117. Windham TC, Parikh NU, Siwak DR, et al. Src activation regulates anoikis in human colon tumor cell lines. Oncogene 2002;21:7797–7807.
118. Swan EA, Jasser SA, Holsinger FC, Doan D, Bucana C, Myers JN. Acquisition of anoikis resistance is a critical step in the progression of oral tongue cancer. Oral Oncol 2003;39:648–655.
119. Talapatra S, Thompson CB. Growth factor signaling in cell survival: implications for cancer treatment. J Pharmacol Exp Ther 2001;298:873–878.
120. Holbro T, Civenni G, Hynes NE. The ErbB receptors and their role in cancer progression. Exp Cell Res 2003;284:99–110.
121. Burgess AW, Cho HS, Eigenbrot C, et al. An open-and-shut case? Recent insights into the activation of EGF/ErbB receptors. Mol Cell 2003;12:541–552.
122. Mendelsohn J, Baselga J. Status of epidermal growth factor receptor antagonists in the biology and treatment of cancer. J Clin Oncol 2003;21:2787–2799.
123. Zhou BP, Hung MC. Dysregulation of cellular signaling by HER2/neu in breast cancer. Semin Oncol 2003;30:38–48.
124. Izawa JI, Slaton JW, Kedar D, et al. Differential expression of progression-related genes in the evolution of superficial to invasive transitional cell carcinoma of the bladder. Oncol Rep 2001;8:9–15.
125. Ziober BL, Willson JK, Hymphrey LE, Childress-Fields K, Brattain MG. Autocrine transforming growth factor-alpha is associated with progression of transformed properties in human colon cancer cells. J Biol Chem 1993;268:691–698.
126. Davies P, Eaton CL, France TD, Phillips ME. Growth factor receptors and oncogene expression in prostate cells. Am J Clin Oncol 1988;11 Suppl 2:S1–S7.
127. Radinsky R. Growth factors and their receptors in metastasis. Semin Cancer Biol 1991;2:169–177.
128. Radinsky R, Risin, Fan, et al. Level and function of epidermal growth factor receptor predict the metastatic potential of human colon carcinoma cells. Clin Cancer Res 1995;1:19–31.
129. Parker C, Roseman BJ, Bucana CD, Tsan R, Radinsky R. Preferential activation of the epidermal growth factor receptor in human colon carcinoma liver metastases in nude mice. J Histochem Cytochem 1998;46:595–602.
130. Tan M, Yao J, Yu D. Overexpression of the c-erbB-2 gene enhanced intrinsic metastasis potential in human breast cancer cells without increasing their transformation abilities. Cancer Res 1997;57: 1199–1205.
131. Yu D, Jing T, Liu B, et al. Overexpression of ErbB2 blocks Taxol-induced apoptosis by upregulation of p21Cip1, which inhibits p34Cdc2 kinase. Mol Cell 1998;2:581–591.

132. Tan M, Jing T, Lan KH, et al. Phosphorylation on tyrosine-15 of p34(Cdc2) by ErbB2 inhibits p34(Cdc2) activation and is involved in resistance to taxol-induced apoptosis. Mol Cell 2002;9:993–1004.
133. Yu D, Hung MC. The erbB2 gene as a cancer therapeutic target and the tumor- and metastasis-suppressing function of E1A. Cancer Metastasis Rev 1998;17:195–202.
134. Zhou BP, Hu MC, Miller SA, et al. C. HER-2/neu blocks tumor necrosis factor-induced apoptosis via the Akt/NF-kappaB pathway. J Biol Chem 2000;275:8027–8031.
135. Wen Y, Hu MC, Makino K, et al. HER-2/neu promotes androgen-independent survival and growth of prostate cancer cells through the Akt pathway. Cancer Res 2000;60:6841–6845.
136. Zhou BP, Liao Y, Xia W, Zou Y, Spohn B, Hung MC. HER-2/neu induces p53 ubiquitination via Akt-mediated MDM2 phosphorylation. Nat Cell Biol 2001;3:973–982.
137. Fischer OM, Hart S, Gschwind A, Ullrich A. EGFR signal transactivation in cancer cells. Biochem Soc Trans 2003;31:1203–1208.
138. Beg AA, Sha WC, Bronson RT, Ghosh S, Baltimore D. Embryonic lethality and liver degeneration in mice lacking the RelA component of NF-kappa B. Nature 1995;376:167–170.
139. Wang CY, Mayo MW, Baldwin AS, Jr. TNF- and cancer therapy-induced apoptosis: potentiation by inhibition of NF-kappaB. Science 1996;274:784–787.
140. Karin M. The beginning of the end: IkappaB kinase (IKK) and NF-kappaB activation. J Biol Chem 1999;274:27,339–27,342.
141. Rothwarf DM, Karin M. The NF-kappa B activation pathway: a paradigm in information transfer from membrane to nucleus. Sci STKE 1999;1999:RE1.
142. Ozes ON, Mayo LD, Gustin JA, Pfeffer SR, Pfeffer LM, Donner DB. NF-kappaB activation by tumour necrosis factor requires the Akt serine-threonine kinase. Nature 1999;401:82–85.
143. Madrid LV, Mayo MW, Reuther JY, Baldwin AS, Jr. Akt stimulates the transactivation potential of the RelA/p65 Subunit of NF-kappa B through utilization of the Ikappa B kinase and activation of the mitogen-activated protein kinase p38. J Biol Chem 2001;276:18,934–18,940.
144. Wu M, Lee H, Bellas RE, et al. Inhibition of NF-kappaB/Rel induces apoptosis of murine B cells. Embo J 1996;15:4682–4690.
145. Stroka DM, Badrichani AZ, Bach FH, Ferran C. Overexpression of A1, an NF-kappaB-inducible anti-apoptotic bcl gene, inhibits endothelial cell activation. Blood 1999;93:3803–3810.
146. Grad JM, Zeng XR, Boise LH. Regulation of Bcl-xL: a little bit of this and a little bit of STAT. Curr Opin Oncol 2000;12:543–549.
147. Kurland JF, Voehringer DW, Meyn RE. The MEK/ERK pathway acts upstream of NF kappa B1 (p50) homodimer activity and Bcl-2 expression in a murine B-cell lymphoma cell line. MEK inhibition restores radiation-induced apoptosis. J Biol Chem 2003;278:32,465–32,470.
148. Kurland JF, Kodym R, Story MD, Spurgers KB, McDonnell TJ, Meyn RE. NF-kappaB1 (p50) homodimers contribute to transcription of the bcl-2 oncogene. J Biol Chem 2001;276:45,380–45,386.
149. Wang CY, Mayo MW, Korneluk RG, Goeddel DV, Baldwin AS, Jr. NF-kappaB antiapoptosis: induction of TRAF1 and TRAF2 and c-IAP1 and c-IAP2 to suppress caspase-8 activation. Science 1998;281:1680–1683.
150. Yang J, Liu X, Bhalla K, et al. Prevention of apoptosis by Bcl-2: release of cytochrome c from mitochondria blocked. Science 1997;275:1129–1132.
151. Deveraux QL, Takahashi R, Salvesen GS, Reed JC. X-linked IAP is a direct inhibitor of cell-death proteases. Nature 1997;388:300–304.
152. Ross JS, Fletcher JA, Bloom KJ, et al. Targeted therapy in breast cancer: The HER-2/neu gene and protein. Mol Cell Proteomics 2004.
153. Bondar VM, Sweeney-Gotsch B, Andreeff M, Mills GB, McConkey DJ. Inhibition of the phosphatidylinositol 3'-kinase-AKT pathway induces apoptosis in pancreatic carcinoma cells in vitro and in vivo. Mol Cancer Ther 2002;1:989–997.
154. Mills GB, Kohn E, Lu Y, et al. Linking molecular diagnostics to molecular therapeutics: targeting the PI3K pathway in breast cancer. Semin Oncol 2003;30:93–104.
155. Rowinsky EK. Signal events: Cell signal transduction and its inhibition in cancer. Oncologist 2003;8 Suppl 3:5–17.
156. Mita MM, Mita A, Rowinsky EK. The molecular target of rapamycin (mTOR) as a therapeutic target against cancer. Cancer Biol Ther 2003;2:S169–177.
157. Adams J, Palombella VJ, Sausville EA, et al. Proteasome inhibitors: a novel class of potent and effective antitumor agents. Cancer Res 1999;59:2615–2622.

158. LeBlanc R, Catley LP, Hideshima T, et al. Proteasome inhibitor PS-341 inhibits human myeloma cell growth in vivo and prolongs survival in a murine model. Cancer Res 2002;62:4996–5000.
159. Anderson KC. Moving disease biology from the laboratory to the clinic. Semin Oncol 2002;29:17–20.
160. Richardson PG, Barlogie B, Berenson J, et al. A phase 2 study of bortezomib in relapsed, refractory myeloma. N Engl J Med 2003;348:2609–2617.
161. Russo SM, Tepper JE, Baldwin AS, Jr, et al. Enhancement of radiosensitivity by proteasome inhibition: implications for a role of NF-kappaB. Int J Radiat Oncol Biol Phys 2001;50:183–193.
162. Cusack JC, Jr, Liu R, Houston M, et al. Enhanced chemosensitivity to CPT-11 with proteasome inhibitor PS-341: implications for systemic nuclear factor-kappaB inhibition. Cancer Res 2001;61: 3535–3540.
163. Bold RJ, Virudachalam S, McConkey DJ. Chemosensitization of pancreatic cancer by inhibition of the 26S proteasome. J Surg Res 2001;100:11–17.
164. Nawrocki ST, Sweeney-Gotsch B, Takamori R, McConkey DJ. The proteasome inhibitor bortezomib enhances the activity of docetaxel in orthotopic human pancreatic tumor xenografts. Mol Cancer Ther 2004;3:59–70.
165. Williams S, Pettaway C, Song R, Papandreou C, Logothetis C, McConkey DJ. Differential effects of the proteasome inhibitor bortezomib on apoptosis and angiogenesis in human prostate tumor xenografts. Mol Cancer Ther 2003;2:835–843.
166. Nawrocki ST, Bruns CJ, Harbison MT, et al. Effects of the proteasome inhibitor PS-341 on apoptosis and angiogenesis in orthotopic human pancreatic tumor xenografts. Mol Cancer Ther 2002;1:1243–1253.
167. Sunwoo JB, Chen Z, Dong G, et al. Novel proteasome inhibitor PS-341 inhibits activation of nuclear factor-kappa B, cell survival, tumor growth, and angiogenesis in squamous cell carcinoma. Clin Cancer Res 2001;7:1419–1428.
168. Hideshima T, Chauhan D, Richardson P, et al. NF-kappa B as a therapeutic target in multiple myeloma. J Biol Chem 2002;277:16,639–16,647.
169. Ashkenazi A, Dixit VM. Death receptors: signaling and modulation. Science 1998;281:1305–1308.
170. Yang Y, Mercep M, Ware CF, Ashwell JD. Fas and activation-induced Fas ligand mediate apoptosis of T cell hybridomas: inhibition of Fas ligand expression by retinoic acid and glucocorticoids. J Exp Med 1995;181:1673–1682.
171. Green DR, Mahboubi A, Nishioka W, et al. Promotion and inhibition of activation-induced apoptosis in T-cell hybridomas by oncogenes and related signals. Immunol Rev 1994;142:321–342.
172. Trauth BC, Klas C, Peters AM, et al. Monoclonal antibody-mediated tumor regression by induction of apoptosis. Science 1989;245:301–305.
173. Lacronique V, Mignon A, Fabre M, et al. Bcl-2 protects from lethal hepatic apoptosis induced by an anti-Fas antibody in mice. Nat Med 1996;2:80–86.
174. Ashkenazi A, Dixit VM. Apoptosis control by death and decoy receptors. Curr Opin Cell Biol 1999;11:255–260.
175. de Jong S, Timmer T, Heijenbrok FJ, de Vries EG. Death receptor ligands, in particular TRAIL, to overcome drug resistance. Cancer Metastasis Rev 2001;20:51–56.
176. Buchsbaum DJ, Zhou T, Grizzle WE, et al. Antitumor efficacy of TRA-8 anti-DR5 monoclonal antibody alone or in combination with chemotherapy and/or radiation therapy in a human breast cancer model. Clin Cancer Res 2003;9:3731–3741.
177. Lawrence D, Shahrokh Z, Marsters S, et al. Differential hepatocyte toxicity of recombinant Apo2L/TRAIL versions. Nat Med 2001;7:383–385.
178. Owen-Schaub LB, van Golen KL, Hill LL, Price JE. Fas and Fas ligand interactions suppress melanoma lung metastasis. J Exp Med 1998;188:1717–1723.
179. Owen-Schaub L. Soluble Fas and cancer. Clin Cancer Res 2001;7:1108–1109.
180. Ryu BK, Lee MG, Chi SG, Kim YW, Park JH. Increased expression of cFLIP(L) in colonic adenocarcinoma. J Pathol 2001;194:15–19.
181. Backus HH, Van Groeningen CJ, Vos W, et al. Differential expression of cell cycle and apoptosis related proteins in colorectal mucosa, primary colon tumours, and liver metastases. J Clin Pathol 2002;55:206–211.
182. Walsh K, Sata M. Is extravasation a Fas-regulated process? Mol Med Today 1999;5:61–67.
183. Brunet A, Bonni A, Zigmond MJ, et al. Akt promotes cell survival by phosphorylating and inhibiting a forkhead transcription factor. Cell 1999;96:857–868.
184. Jin Z, Dicker DT, El-Deiry WS. Enhanced sensitivity of G1 arrested human cancer cells suggests a novel therapeutic strategy using a combination of simvastatin and TRAIL. Cell Cycle 2002;1:82–89.

185. Fulda S, Debatin KM. Sensitization for tumor necrosis factor-related apoptosis-inducing ligand-induced apoptosis by the chemopreventive agent resveratrol. Cancer Res 2004;64:337–346.
186. Keane MM, Ettenberg SA, Nau MM, Russell EK, Lipkowitz S. Chemotherapy augments TRAIL-induced apoptosis in breast cell lines. Cancer Res 1999;59:734–741.
187. Nagane M, Pan G, Weddle JJ, Dixit VM, Cavenee WK, Huang HJ. Increased death receptor 5 expression by chemotherapeutic agents in human gliomas causes synergistic cytotoxicity with tumor necrosis factor-related apoptosis-inducing ligand in vitro and in vivo. Cancer Res 2000;60:847–853.
188. Mizutani Y, Nakao M, Ogawa O, Yoshida O, Bonavida B, Miki T. Enhanced sensitivity of bladder cancer cells to tumor necrosis factor related apoptosis inducing ligand mediated apoptosis by cisplatin and carboplatin. J Urol 2001;165:263–270.
189. An J, Sun YP, Adams J, Fisher M, Belldegrun A, Rettig MB. Drug interactions between the proteasome inhibitor bortezomib and cytotoxic chemotherapy, tumor necrosis factor (TNF) alpha, and TNF-related apoptosis-inducing ligand in prostate cancer. Clin Cancer Res 2003;9:4537–4545.
190. Kim DM, Koo SY, Jeon K, et al. Rapid induction of apoptosis by combination of flavopiridol and tumor necrosis factor (TNF)-alpha or TNF-related apoptosis-inducing ligand in human cancer cell lines. Cancer Res 2003;63:621–626.
191. Inoue H, Shiraki K, Ohmori S, et al. Histone deacetylase inhibitors sensitize human colonic adenocarcinoma cell lines to TNF-related apoptosis inducing ligand-mediated apoptosis. Int J Mol Med 2002;9:521–525.
192. Rosato RR, Almenara JA, Dai Y, Grant S. Simultaneous activation of the intrinsic and extrinsic pathways by histone deacetylase (HDAC) inhibitors and tumor necrosis factor-related apoptosis-inducing ligand (TRAIL) synergistically induces mitochondrial damage and apoptosis in human leukemia cells. Mol Cancer Ther 2003;2:1273–1284.
193. Sayers TJ, Brooks AD, Koh CY, et al. The proteasome inhibitor PS-341 sensitizes neoplastic cells to TRAIL-mediated apoptosis by reducing levels of c-FLIP. Blood 2003;102:303–310.
194. Johnson TR, Stone K, Nikrad M, et al. The proteasome inhibitor PS-341 overcomes TRAIL resistance in Bax and caspase 9-negative or Bcl-xL overexpressing cells. Oncogene 2003;22:4953–4963.
195. Fan Z, Shang BY, Lu Y, Chou JL, Mendelsohn J. Reciprocal changes in p27(Kip1) and p21(Cip1) in growth inhibition mediated by blockade or overstimulation of epidermal growth factor receptors. Clin Cancer Res 1997;3:1943–1948.
196. Janicke RU, Sprengart ML, Wati MR, Porter AG. Caspase-3 is required for DNA fragmentation and morphological changes associated with apoptosis. J Biol Chem 1998;273:9357–9360.
197. Kurokawa H, Nishio K, Fukumoto H, Tomonari A, Suzuki T, Saijo N. Alteration of caspase-3 (CPP32/Yama/apopain) in wild-type MCF-7, breast cancer cells. Oncol Rep 1999;6:33–37.
198. Soung YH, Lee JW, Kim HS, et al. Inactivating mutations of CASPASE-7 gene in human cancers. Oncogene 2003;22:8048–8052.
199. Soengas MS, Capodieci P, Polsky D, et al. Inactivation of the apoptosis effector Apaf-1 in malignant melanoma. Nature 2001;409:207–211.
200. Wolf BB, Schuler M, Li W, et al. Defective cytochrome c-dependent caspase activation in ovarian cancer cell lines due to diminished or absent apoptotic protease activating factor-1 activity. J Biol Chem 2001;276:34,244–34,251.
201. Weil M, Jacobson MD, Coles HS, et al. Constitutive expression of the machinery for programmed cell death. J Cell Biol 1996;133:1053–1059.
202. Pegoraro L, Palumbo A, Erikson J, et al. A 14;18 and an 8;14 chromosome translocation in a cell line derived from an acute B-cell leukemia. Proc Natl Acad Sci USA 1984;81:7166–7170.
203. McDonnell TJ, Troncoso P, Brisbay SM, et al. Expression of the protooncogene bcl-2 in the prostate and its association with emergence of androgen-independent prostate cancer. Cancer Res 1992;52:6940–6944.
204. Charpin C, Garcia S, Bouvier C, et al. Automated and quantitative immunocytochemical assays of Bcl-2 protein in breast carcinomas. Br J Cancer 1997;76:340–346.
205. Buchholz TA, Davis DW, McConkey DJ, et al. Chemotherapy-induced apoptosis and Bcl-2 levels correlate with breast cancer response to chemotherapy. Cancer J 2003;9:33–41.
206. Bush JA, Li G. The role of Bcl-2 family members in the progression of cutaneous melanoma. Clin Exp Metastasis 2003;20:531–539.
207. Termuhlen PM, Sweeney-Gotsch BM, Berman RS, et al. Increased apoptosis in metastatic human colonic adenocarcinomas. Cancer Biol Ther 2002;1:58–63.

208. Agui T, McConkey DJ, Tanigawa N. Comparative study of various biological parameters, including expression of survivin, between primary and metastatic human colonic adenocarcinomas. Anticancer Res 2002;22:1769–1776.
209. Rampino N, Yamamoto H, Ionov Y, et al. Somatic frameshift mutations in the BAX gene in colon cancers of the microsatellite mutator phenotype. Science 1997;275:967–969.
210. Ionov Y, Yamamoto H, Krajewski S, Reed JC, Perucho M. Mutational inactivation of the proapoptotic gene BAX confers selective advantage during tumor clonal evolution. Proc Natl Acad Sci USA 2000;97:10,872–10,877.
211. Ouyang H, Furukawa T, Abe T, Kato Y, Horii A. The BAX gene, the promoter of apoptosis, is mutated in genetically unstable cancers of the colorectum, stomach, and endometrium. Clin Cancer Res 1998;4:1071–1074.
212. Yamamoto H, Sawai H, Perucho M. Frameshift somatic mutations in gastrointestinal cancer of the microsatellite mutator phenotype. Cancer Res 1997;57:4420–4426.
213. Kondo S, Shinomura Y, Miyazaki Y, et al. Mutations of the bak gene in human gastric and colorectal cancers. Cancer Res 2000;60:4328–4330.
214. Altieri DC. Survivin, versatile modulation of cell division and apoptosis in cancer. Oncogene 2003;22:8581–8589.
215. Davis DW, Buchholz TA, Hess KR, Sahin AA, Valero V, McConkey DJ. Automated quantification of apoptosis after neoadjuvant chemotherapy for breast cancer: early assessment predicts clinical response. Clin Cancer Res 2003;9:955–960.
216. Boehm T, Folkman J, Browder T, O'Reilly MS. Antiangiogenic therapy of experimental cancer does not induce acquired drug resistance. Nature 1997;390:404–407.
217. Shaheen RM, Davis DW, Liu W, et al. Antiangiogenic therapy targeting the tyrosine kinase receptor for vascular endothelial growth factor receptor inhibits the growth of colon cancer liver metastasis and induces tumor and endothelial cell apoptosis. Cancer Res 1999;59:5412–5416.
218. Bruns CJ, Harbison MT, Davis DW, et al. Epidermal growth factor receptor blockade with C225 plus gemcitabine results in regression of human pancreatic carcinoma growing orthotopically in nude mice by antiangiogenic mechanisms. Clin Cancer Res 2000;6:1936–1948.
219. Inoue K, Slaton JW, Davis DW, et al. Treatment of human metastatic transitional cell carcinoma of the bladder in a murine model with the anti-vascular endothelial growth factor receptor monoclonal antibody DC101 and paclitaxel. Clin Cancer Res 2000;6:2635–2643.
220. Davis DW, McConkey DJ, Abbruzzese JL, Herbst RS. Surrogate markers in antiangiogenesis clinical trials. Br J Cancer 2003;89:8–14.
221. Herbst RS, Hess KR, Tran HT, et al. Phase I Study of recombinant human endostatin in patients with advanced solid tumors. J Clin Oncol 2002;20:3792–3803.
222. Herbst RS, Mullani NA, Davis DW, et al. Development of biologic markers of response and assessment of antiangiogenic activity in a clinical trial of human recombinant endostatin. J Clin Oncol 2002;20:3804–3814.
223. Davis DW, Shen Y, Mullani NA, et al. Quantitative analysis of biomarkers defines an optimal biological dose for recombinant human endostatin in primary human tumors. Clin Cancer Res 2004;10:33-42.
224. Blankenberg F, Mari C, Strauss HW. Imaging cell death in vivo. Q J Nucl Med 2003;47:337–348.
225. Blankenberg FG, Katsikis PD, Tait JF, et al. In vivo detection and imaging of phosphatidylserine expression during programmed cell death. Proc Natl Acad Sci USA 1998;95:6349–6354.
226. Meade TJ, Taylor AK, Bull SR. New magnetic resonance contrast agents as biochemical reporters. Curr Opin Neurobiol 2003;13:597–602.

3 Structures of TNF Receptors and Their Interactions With Ligands

Sarah G. Hymowitz, PhD,
and Abraham M. de Vos, PhD

SUMMARY

The tumor necrosis factor receptors (TNFRs), in conjunction with their ligands, influence many important biological processes, including activation of apoptosis, modulation of the immune system, and regulation of developmental pathways in some tissue types. Some TNFRs positively regulate cell growth, whereas others initiate apoptotic pathways upon stimulation by ligand *(1)*. These contradictory biological activities are determined to some extent by differences in the intracellular domains of these receptors. In particular, a subfamily of TNFRs, termed the *death receptors*, including TNFR1, Fas, death receptor (DR)3, DR4, DR5, DR6, EDAR, and p75^{NGFR}, all contain an intracellular death domain, and many but not all of these receptors activate apoptotic pathways. None of the other members of the TNFR family identified to date contain recognizable intracellular domains, and instead present binding sites for interactions with TNF receptor-associated factors (TRAFs) and other adaptor proteins.

The death receptors are functionally distinguished by their ability to trigger the assembly of the death-inducing signaling complex (DISC), leading to initiation of the apoptotic cascade upon stimulation by ligand. However, the primary function of at least three of the death receptors—DR3, EDAR and p75^{NTR}—does not appear to be induction of apoptosis. DR3 is a receptor for a T-cell co-stimulator *(2)*. EDAR is involved in ectodermal development and signals through a novel death domain containing adaptor protein, but has not been observed to initiate DISC formation *(3,4)*. p75^{NTR} is not known to interact with a TNF ligand (TNFL), but instead binds to the neurotrophins, which are members of the cystine-knot family of growth factors. The complex between NGF and p75^{NTR} stimulates apoptosis, whereas the higher affinity ternary complex formed by p75^{NTR}, trkA, and NGF initiates nonapoptotic activities *(5)*.

From: *Cancer Drug Discovery and Development: Death Receptors in Cancer Therapy*
Edited by: W. S. El-Deiry © Humana Press Inc., Totowa, NJ

Whereas the intracellular consequences of signaling by the death receptors and their ligands can be considerably different from that by the other TNFRs, their extracellular domains (ECDs) and cognate ligands share some structural similarities. Structural information about the death receptors is based on the structures of the LTα–TNFR1 complex *(6)*, of TNFR1 by itself *(7)*, of herpes virus entry mediator (HveA, also called HVEM *[8]*), and of the Apo2L/TRAIL–DR5 complex *(9–11)*. These structures show that the ECD of the death receptors as well as those of other TNFR family members contain several (typically 2 to 4) cysteine-rich pseudo-repeats, which form elongated structures composed of loops tethered together by disulfide bridges. These receptors bind at the monomer-monomer interfaces of their trimeric ligands to form a complex consisting of three copies of the receptor and one trimeric ligand *(6,12,13)* (Figs. 1, 2). Recently, distant members of the TNFR family have been discovered that are much smaller and are composed of a single (BCMA, TWEAKR) *(14,15)* or partial cysteine-rich extracellular domain (CRD) (BR3) *(16,17)*.

The ligands for both the death receptors and the other TNFRs are members of the TNF family. The ligands have been more thoroughly structurally characterized than the receptors. The structure of TNF was the first to be determined and has been supplemented by the structures of several other family members in the last decade. These structures show that TNFLs are homotrimeric globular proteins with distant structural homology to viral capsid proteins as well as to the complement protein C1q and to the NC1 domain of collagen X *(18–20)* (Fig. 3). This review will focus on the structures of the TNFLs, the TNFRs, and their interactions.

LIGANDS

Overall Structure

The sequence similarity among TNFLs varies from nondetectable to as high as 28% between Apo2L/TRAIL (Apo2 ligand or TNF-related apoptosis-inducing ligand) and RANKL. TNFLs are type II membrane proteins containing an amino-terminal cytoplasmic motif, a transmembrane (TM) domain, a linker region of varying length, and a C-terminal TNF domain of approx 150 amino acids. TNFLs can have additional functional motifs such as a putative collagen-like stalk, seen in the sequence of EDA, or proteolytic sites between the TM and the TNF domain in some ligands, which allows for shedding of a soluble ligand from the cell surface. Several of the TNFLs have truncated features. For example, LTα has a cryptic signal sequence and OX40L lacks a linker region, such that the TNF domain follows the TM almost immediately.

Regardless of these differences, the TNFLs are united by sharing the same basic fold. Seven members of the TNF family have been structurally characterized (TNF-α *[18,21]*, LTα *[22]*, CD40L *[23]*, Apo2L/TRAIL *[24,25]*, BAFF *[26,27,28]*, murine *[29]* and human RANKL *[30]*, and EDA [SGH, unpublished data]). Elucidation of the structure of TNF-α (also called TNF or TNFSF2) in 1992 revealed a jelly-roll monomer fold that is conserved in the structure of all TNFLs determined to date (Fig. 3). The monomer is formed by two beta sheets, one consisting of strands A'AHCF, the other of strands B'BGDE. These monomers homotrimerize with the A'AHCF sheet mostly buried and the B'BGDE sheet mostly exposed. The shape of the trimer is roughly pyramidal with the N- and C-termini protruding from the wide part of the pyramid, the tip of the pyramid being formed by the CD and EF loops. Changes in the shape and size of these loops can make

A

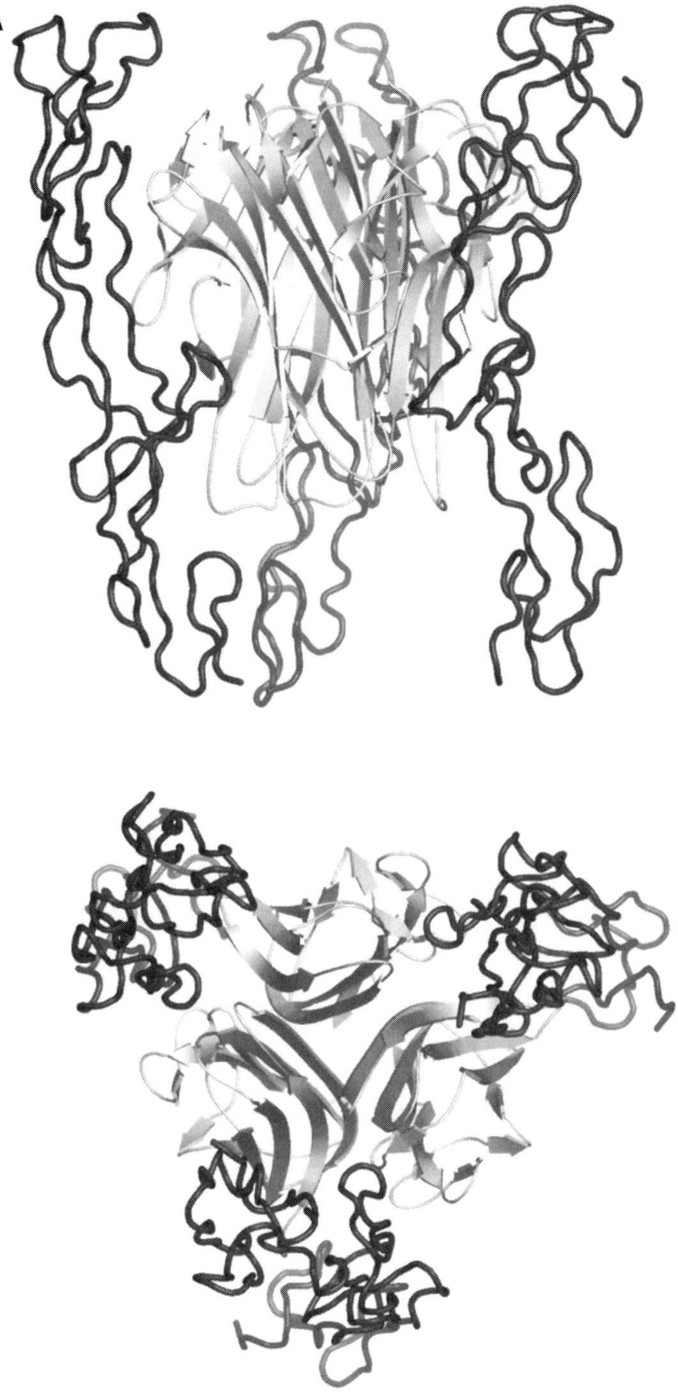

B

Fig. 1. The LTα–TNFR1 complex *(6)*. The LTα trimer is drawn as ribbon rendering in gray, and the Cα trace of the three copies of TNFR1 are colored black. (**A**) Side view. In this orientation, the membrane of the receptor-containing cell is at the bottom of the figure. (**B**) View up the threefold axis of the complex, perpendicular to A.

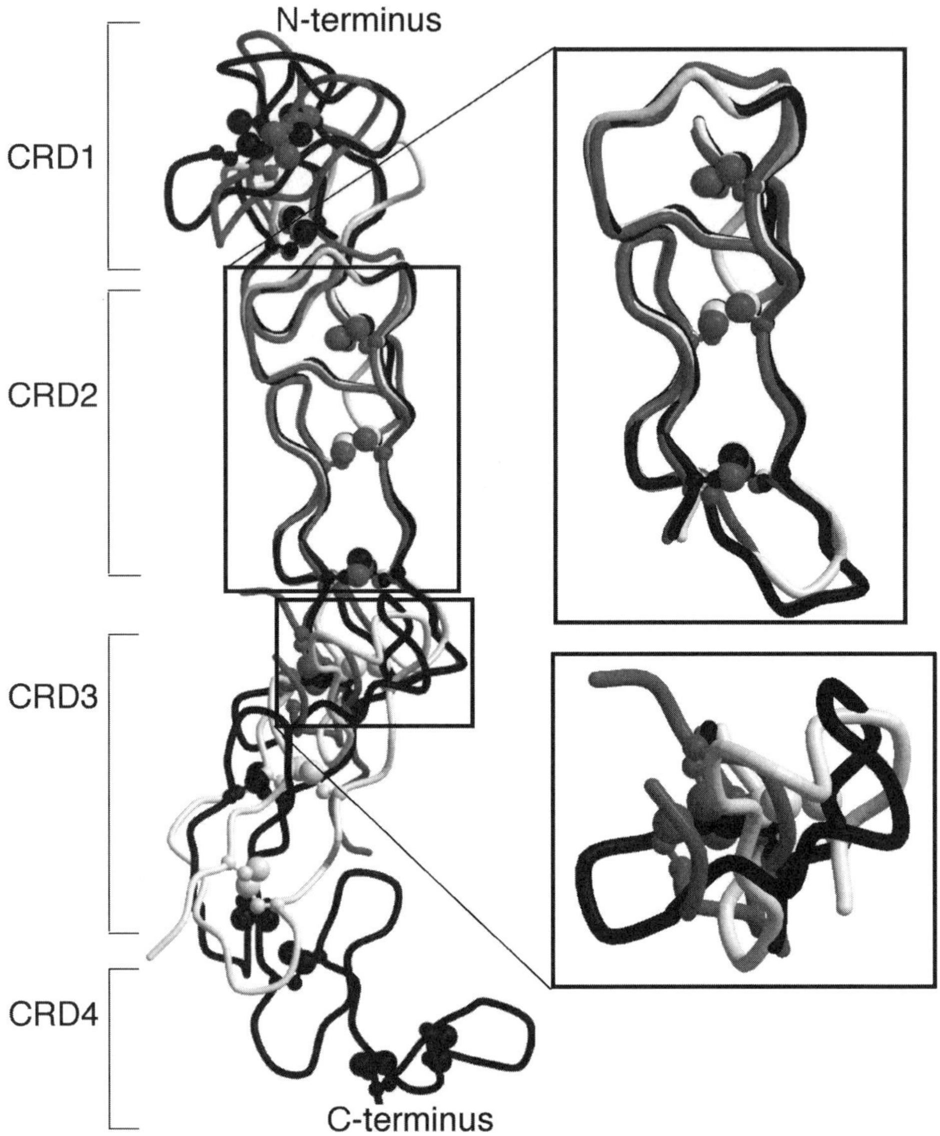

Fig. 2. Superposition of the Cα traces of the ECD of DR5 *(9)*, HveA *(8)*, and TNFR1 *(48)*. DR5 is colored white, HveA is gray, and TNFR1 is black. Disulfide linkages are shown as ball-and-stick representation. The receptors were superimposed based on the Cα atoms of the structurally equivalent residues in CRD2. Insets show the structurally conserved CRD2 and the very divergent first loop in CRD3.

some members (especially EDA) appear less pyramidal. Based on sequence similarity, all TNFLs are expected to have the same core β-structure, although length of the beta strands, the shape and size of the connecting loops, the location and number of disulfide bridges, as well as the presence or absence of metal-binding sites vary considerably among the family members (Figs. 3, 4).

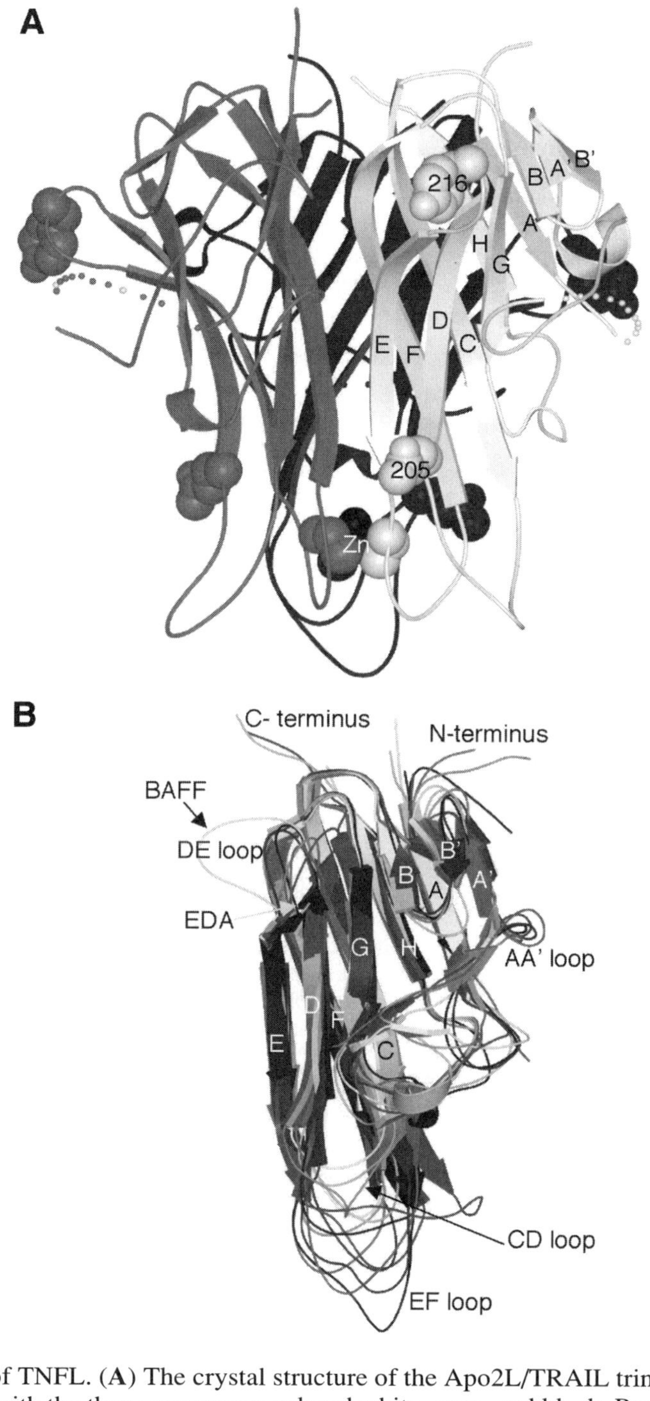

Fig. 3. Structure of TNFL. (**A**) The crystal structure of the Apo2L/TRAIL trimer *(9)* drawn as a ribbon rendering with the three monomers colored white, gray, and black. Residues 132–143 of Apo2L/TRAIL are disordered and shown as small balls. The zinc-binding site, including the three symmetry-related cysteines and a putative chloride ligand, are shown in close rendering, as are side chains of residues Tyr 216 and Gln 205, which are critical for bioactivity and form the center of the two receptor binding patches *(9,24)*. (**B**) Ribbon rendering of a superposition of monomers from crystal structures of BAFF *(26)*, EDA (SGH unpublished data), CD40L *(28)*, Apo2L/TRAIL *(9)*, RANKL *(30)*, LTα *(6)*, and TNF *(21)*, colored from white to dark gray, respectively, showing the conservation of the core β-strands and the variation in loop conformation.

```
                                                                 A                                        A'
         TNF KPVAHVVAN. .......... .....PQAEG QLQWLNRRAN .ALLAN.GVE
        FasL RKVAHLTGK. .......... ....SNSRSM PLEWEDT... YGIVLLSGVK
 Apo2L/TRAIL RVAAHITGTR GRSNTLSSPN SKNEKALGRK INSWESSRSG HSFLSN..LH
       CD40L QIAAHVISE. .......... ...ASSKTTS VLQWAEK..G YYTMSNNLVT
        BAFF QDCLQLIAD. ........SE TPTIQKGSYT FVPWLL.... .SFKRGSALE
      EDA-A2 PAVVHLQGQ. ......GSAI QVKNDLSGGV LNDWSR.... .ITMNPKVFK

             B'   B          C                        D
                                                  *
         TNF LRD..NQLVV PSEGLYLIYS QVLFKGQGC. ...PSTHVLL THTISRIAVS
        FasL YKK..GGLVI NETGLYFVYS KVYFRGQSC. .....NNLPL SHKVYMRNSK
 Apo2L/TRAIL LRN..GELVI HEKGFYYIYS QTYFRFQEEI KENTKNDKQM VQYIYKYT.S
       CD40L LENG.KQLTV KRQGLYYIYA QVTFCSNR.. ..EASSQAPF IASLCLKSPG
        BAFF EKE..NKILV KETGYFFIYG QVLYTDK... ......TYAM GHLIQRKKVH
      EDA-A2 LHPRSGELEV LVDGTYFIYS QVYYINFTD. ........FA SYEVVVD...

                         E                             F
             *
         TNF Y....QTKVN LLSAIKSPCQ RETPEGAEAK PWYEPIYLGG VFQLEKGDRL
        FasL Y....PQDLV MMEGKMMSYC TT......GQ MWARSSYLGA VFNLTSADHL
 Apo2L/TRAIL Y....PDPIL LMKSARNSCW S.....KDAE YGLYSIYQGG IFELKENDRI
       CD40L RF.....ERI LLRAANTHSS .......AKP CGQQSIHLGG VFELQPGASV
        BAFF VFGDELSLVT LFRCIQNMPE T......... LPNNSCYSAG IAKLEEGDEL
      EDA-A2 .......EKP FLQCTRS.IE T.......GK TNYNTCYTAG VCLLKARQKI

             G                    H
         TNF SAEINR.PDY LLFAESGQVY FGIIAL....
        FasL YVNVSE.LSL VNFE.ESQTF FGLYKL....
 Apo2L/TRAIL FVSVTN.EHL IDMD.HEASF FGAFLVG...
       CD40L FVNVTD.PSQ VSHG.TGFTS FGLLKL....
        BAFF QLAIPRENAQ ISLD.GDVTF FGALKLL...
      EDA-A2 AVKMVHADIS INMS.KHTTF FGAIRLGEAP
```

Fig. 4. Alignment of the TNF domain of four conventional ligands (TNFα, FasL, Apo2L/TRAIL, CD40L) and two divergent ligands (BAFF and EDA), showing the conservation of the β-strands and the range in size of the intervening loops. Cysteine residues are underlined with a solid line. Residues which have been identified by mutagenesis as important for receptor binding are boxed *(24,61,39)*. Apo2L/TRAIL residues that bury at least 50% of their accessible surface area upon binding receptor are shaded gray *(9)*. The residues either observed or predicted to be at the center of the two receptor binding sites in ligands that bind multi-domain receptors are marked with an asterisk (*).

Conserved Features

The conserved features of the TNFLs that are easiest to identify in sequence alignments include the tryptophan residue forming part of the hydrophobic core of the monomer, which is present at the end of the AA' loop in almost all human TNFLs known to date (the exception being OX40L), the BC loop, and the long C strand. Of the structurally characterized ligands, TNF-α, LTα, CD40L, and RANKL are relatively conventional ligands with well conserved strands and significant variation confined to the EF, CD, and

AA' loops as well as the presence and location of disulfide linkages. With the exception of the novel zinc-binding site and a long but poorly ordered AA' loop, Apo2L/TRAIL also belongs with the conventional ligands. Sequence analysis suggests that structurally, TL1A, LIGHT, and FasL are likely to closely resemble these ligands. Due to their sequence homology, this subgroup of ligands is expected to have structurally similar receptor binding sites (Figs. 3, 4).

In contrast, EDA (SGH, unpublished data) and BAFF *(26–28)* are more divergent. EDA is more globular than other TNFLs due to short EF and CD loops combined with a long but well ordered AA' loop. The combination of a very short DE loop and the divergent C-terminal portion of the AA' loop suggests that EDA may interact with receptors slightly differently than the more conventional ligands. BAFF has a divergent sequence in the A strand as well as a very long DE loop, which mediates formation of an unusual supra-molecular assembly in some crystal forms of the ligand. Other TNFLs that may have more divergent structures include OX40L and GITRL. For instance, OX40L lacks the conserved tryptophan and is unusually small (approx 130 residues in the TNF domain), with very short CD, DE, and FG loops and very divergent A and H strands, whereas GITRL is predicted to be similarly compact with a possible disulfide involving the A strand.

Variable Features, Including Metal-Binding Sites

The locations of significant sequence and structural variation in the TNFLs include the A strand, the AA' loop, and the CD and EF loops. Although the A strand is well conserved structurally, its sequence is not, and it is followed by the very poorly conserved AA' loop, which varies in length and sequence throughout the family. These two features can make it difficult to determine the N-terminus of the TNF domain based on sequence analysis for some family members. This lack of N-terminal conservation was likely the reason that the full-length TL1A gene was cloned *(2)* several years after a sequence missing the A strand, TM, and signal sequence was described in the literature as VEGI/TL1 *(31,32)*.

Most of the ligands (CD40L, TNF-α, OX40L, BAFF, EDA, APRIL, TWEAK, LIGHT, CD27L, FASL) either have been predicted or have been shown to contain disulfide bridges, but some family members (including Apo2L/TRAIL, LTα, LTβ, RANKL, and 4-1BBL) do not contain disulfides. Even in disulfide-containing members, the location (and number) of the disulfide(s) can vary considerably. For instance, the structures of TNF-α *(18,21)* and CD40L *(23)* contain a disulfide connecting the CD and EF loops, which is also present in the sequencees of Fas, LIGHT, and VEGI. Both BAFF *(26–28)* and EDA (SGH, unpublished data) (Figs. 3, 4) contain a disulfide connecting the E and F strands, which is also expected to be present in TWEAK and APRIL, whereas OX40L is predicted to contain a disulfide in yet another location.

Other features which may stabilize the ligand structure also differ throughout the family. Both Apo2L/TRAIL *(9,23)* and BAFF *(26)* contain a metal-binding site at the tip of the trimer, as does the structurally homologous NC1 domain of collagen X *(20)*. In the case of Apo2L/TRAIL, a zinc-binding site formed by three cysteine residues, one from the EF loop of each monomer, together with an interior solvent molecule, has been shown to stabilize the trimer (Fig. 3A). Removing the zinc-binding site either by dialysis against chelating agents or by mutating the cysteines to other residues reduces Apo2L/TRAIL bioactivity and stability *(9,23,33)*. Similarly, BAFF binds two magnesium ions using residues from the E and F strands. Removing this site has been shown to have a detrimental effect on BAFF function *(26)*. From sequence alignments, no other TNFLs are expected to have a cysteine-containing metal-binding site like Apo2L/TRAIL. However, since neither of these metal-binding sites was suspected before the crystal structures of Apo2L/TRAIL and BAFF were determined, other TNFLs may yet be shown to contain cysteine-independent metal-binding sites.

Ligand Clustering and Activity of Soluble Ligands

Optimal biological activity of several of the ligands may depend on whether the ligand is membrane bound or soluble. Furthermore, aggregation of soluble ligands into larger oligomeric states (generally thought to be dimers or trimers of trimers) can also alter ligand activity. For instance, TNF-α has different (and antagonistic) biological effects when it is membrane bound vs soluble *(34,35)*. FasL has generally decreased apoptotic activity with concomitant loss of liver toxicity when soluble *(36,37)*. Soluble CD40L is unable to promote cell-cycle progression in B-cells but can prevent apoptosis *(38)*. It has been proposed that proteolytic processing sites N-terminal to the TNF domain in some ligands may represent an "off" switch. Release of soluble ligand may terminate biological activity. In contrast, release from the membrane seems to be required for full EDA activity, as mutations that alter the furin cleavage site result in impaired biological activity *(39)*.

Aggregation of soluble trimers can restore biological activity, suggesting that one consequence of being membrane bound is increased local concentration of ligand. For example, soluble FasL that has been crosslinked by antibodies can activate both apoptotic and c-JNK pathways *(36,40)*. Inappropriate ligand clustering can have unintended consequences due to overactivity. Soluble Apo2L/TRAIL may have adverse effects on normal tissue in aggregated states induced by removal of the bound zinc ion whereas it is nontoxic when soluble and trimeric *(41)*. Other ligands require both solubility and clustering for full activity. EDA has a collagen-like domain, which is believed to be important for optimal function and may facilitate formation of dimers or trimers of trimers. Mutations which affect this oligomeriztion domain but leave the TNFL domain intact result in the same phenotype as EDA deficiency or mutations in the TNFL domain *(39,42)*.

BAFF Assemblies

BAFF has been reported to have an unusual tendency to form very large supra-molecular assemblies in some circumstances. Liu et al. have shown that recombinant BAFF composed of residues 135–285 expressed in bacteria forms a spherical assembly of twenty trimers at or above physiological pH but not at lower pH. The molecular contacts stabilizing this assembly are formed almost exclusively by reciprocal interactions between the unusually long DE loops of the trimers *(27)*. Liu et al. also observed particles consistent with this assembly in the serum of mammalian cells overproducing soluble BAFF *(27)*. Longer BAFF constructs or constructs with different N-terminal sequences do not seem to form this assembly. For instance, glycosylated BAFF residues 136–285, with an N-terminal 14 residue myc, tag at pH 4.5 *(28)*; untagged BAFF, consisting of residues 134–285 at pH 6.0 *(26)*, or bacterially produced BAFF, with a longer N-terminal sequence (a GSHM tag followed by residues 82–285 *[43]*) at pH 7.0, all produce crystals with no evidence of supra-molecular assembly.

The functional importance of the assembly is also unclear. Liu et al. observed that mutant BAFF in which the DE loop has been replaced with a short glycine-rich linker retains full receptor affinity, but is impaired in cell-based biological activity assays, suggesting that the assembly may be important for full activity *(27)*. This result conflicts with data from Schneider et al. indicating that flag-tagged BAFF residues 136–285 exclusively form trimers but not higher-order oligomers (at pH 7.0) and appear fully active in cell-based assays *(44)*. Furthermore, crosslinking this form of BAFF using antiflag antibodies did not result in enhanced activity *(44)*. The homologous ligand APRIL, which shares receptors TACI and BCMA with BAFF, lacks the DE extension required for formation of the twenty-trimer oligomer and is not expected to form similar assemblies. Finally, the twenty-trimer assembly cannot fully form when BAFF is attached to the cell surface, since all of the N-termini would point inward to the center of the assembly and thus would be unable to connect to the transmembrane helix.

These observations do not eliminate the possibility that a smaller clustering of two or three BAFF trimers mediated by contacts using the DE loops could exist and be functional on the surface of the cell. Clustering of BAFF in this manner could affect bioactivity by increasing the local ligand concentration, producing apparent increases in receptor affinity as a result of avidity. Further characterization of larger BAFF assemblies, including a better understanding of the importance of the length and sequence of the N-terminal residues for assembly formation, determination of the K_d for super-molecular assembly to assess whether the assembly process is likely to occur at physiological concentrations of BAFF, and the resolution of the apparent discrepancy between the activity observed for the various constructs and variants of BAFF, will likely to be important for determining whether this assembly is physiologically relevant.

Formation of Heterotrimers

In general, TNFLs form homotrimers. LTβ is the exception to this rule *(45,46)*. It has been found exclusively in heterotrimers with LTα rather than as a homotrimeric protein. There have also been reports that heterotrimers of APRIL and BAFF have been detected in the serum of patients with autoimmune diseases *(47)*. Some of the less well characterized TNFLs may also have this propensity. Since the receptor binding sites are located at the monomer-monomer interfaces of the ligands, heterotrimers would present three distinct receptor binding surfaces. Since residues forming the monomer-monomer interfaces are some of the most conserved parts of TNFL sequences and structures, more heterotrimers may be observed as the family is studied more closely.

RECEPTORS

Overview

Most TNFRs are type I transmembrane proteins with an N-terminal signal sequence followed by the CRD, a transmembrane helix and a C-terminal intracellular segment. However, some of the family members, including BCMA, TACI, BR3, and XEDAR, are type III transmembrane proteins without a signal sequence. The TNFRs are even more divergent than the ligands and have very low pairwise sequence identity. This divergence is a consequence of a nonglobular fold composed of cysteine-rich pseudorepeats, which are not constrained by the packing requirements of a hydrophobic core but

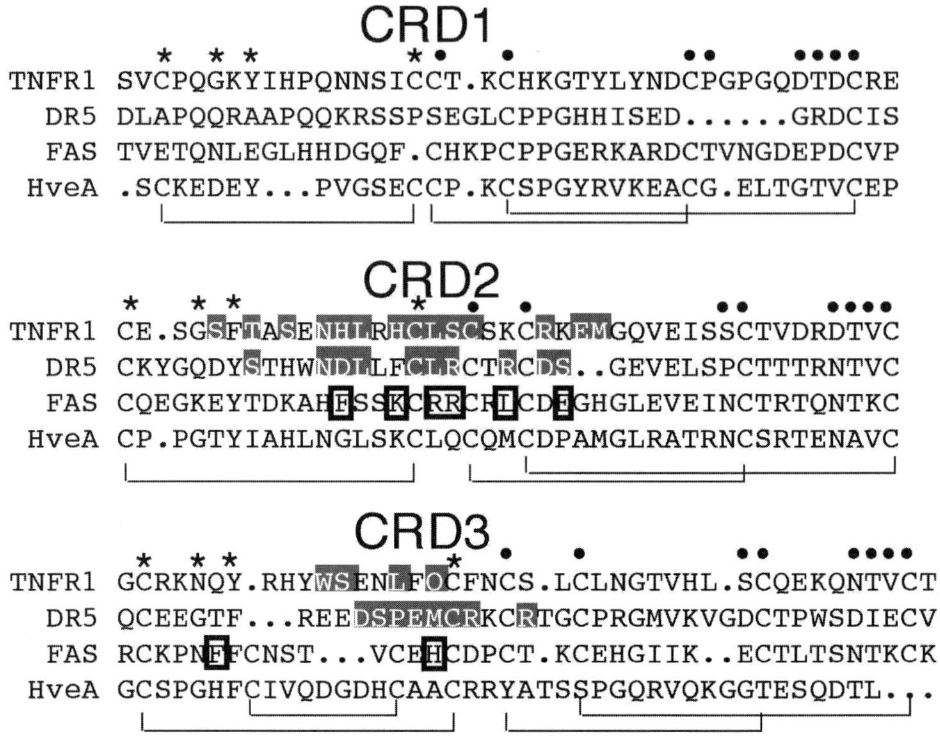

Fig. 5. CRD structure and sequence alignment of selected TNFRs (TNFR1, DR5, FAS, HveA). Disulfide connectivity is indicated. Residues that bury at least 50% of their accessible surface area upon binding ligand are shaded gray *(6,9)*. Residues that have been identified by mutagenesis as important for binding are boxed *(52,53,62,24)*. Positions that are part of the A1 consensus motif of Cys1-x_2-Gly-x-Tyr(or Phe)-$x_{4\text{-}9}$-Cys2 are indicated with an asterisk (*) *(13)*. Positions that are part of the B2 consensus motif of Cys1-x_2-Cys2-$x_?$-Cys3-Thr-$x_{2\text{-}5}$-Asn-Thr-Val-Cys4 are indicated with a bullet (•) *(13)*.

instead are stabilized by a large number of disulfides. Unfortunately, the TNFRs are less well structurally characterized than the ligands. Structures of four receptors have been determined: TNFR1 *(6,7,48)*, DR5 *(9–11)*, HveA *(8)*, and BR3 *(43)*. These structures indicate that tandem CRD-containing receptors have several common features, whereas the smaller receptors (BR3, BCMA, TWEAKR) are more divergent.

CRD Substructure

A typical CRD contains approx 40 residues with 6 cystines connected in a 1-2, 3-5, 4-6 pattern of disulfide linkages (Figs. 2, 5). Different connectivity has been observed in the fourth CRD of TNFR1 *(7)* and is postulated to exist in other TNFRs. However, not all CRDs have these sequence motifs. DR5 has only a partial CRD1 with one disulfide corresponding to the 4-6 disulfide of a typical CRD. EDAR is predicted to be missing the 3-5 disulfide in CRD2, and both XEDAR and EDAR lack the 4-6 disulfide in CRD3. Several of the TNFRs, including HveA, CD40, DR3, and Fas, are predicted to have an extra disulfide in the first loop of CRD3 (the A1 module in TNFR1 and DR5, below). This disulfide is observed in the crystal structure of HveA *(8)* and serves as a structural model for all TNFRs containing this motif (Figs. 2, 5).

Structural and sequence analysis of the CRD motif has allowed further subdivision into modules *(12,13)* such that each typical CRD can be described as a being composed of an A1 and a B2 module. The A1 nomenclature indicates a structural unit containing one disulfide whereas the B2 indicates two disulfides connected in a 1-3, 2-4 bonding topology (the 3-5, 4-6 disulfide of a typical CRD). These modules are defined by sequence conservation. In an A1 module, glycine is frequently the third residue following the first cysteine, with a hydrophobic residue later in the sequence that packs against the following disulfide (Figs. 2, 5). Other modules have been proposed based on sequence analysis. Consideration of modules in this manner, although cumbersome, can facilitate identification and alignment of CRDs from sequence data. The structure of BR3 *(43)* reveals that this divergent receptor is essentially an A1 module containing a β-hairpin receptor interaction loop that has been stabilized with an additional noncanonical disulfide.

Preligand Assembly Via the PLAD

Several TNFR family members have been shown to be preoligomerized by FRET, co-immunoprecipitation, and FACS analysis *(49,50)*. This activity seems to be dependent on a portion of the N-terminal CRD, termed the *preligand assembly domain* (PLAD). Although other receptor families have also been shown to be maintained in a quiescent form in the absence of ligand, this mode of regulation had not been expected for TNFRs. However, further biophysical characterization of the PLAD is necessary before it can be determined whether this is a widespread feature of TNFR regulation. For instance, the K_d for the receptor-receptor interaction, neither for recombinant protein or at the surface of the cell membrane, has not been reported, nor has it been established whether PLAD function corresponds to any conserved structural or sequence features in the TNFRs.

LIGAND–RECEPTOR COMPLEXES

LTα–TNFR1 Reveals the Basic Interaction Motif

Our understanding of the formation of TNFL–TNFR complexes has largely been derived from the structure of the LTα homotrimer (also called LT, TNFSF1, or TNF-β) bound to the ECD of TNFR1 (Fig. 1). This structure revealed that TNFLs bind their receptors in an arrangement of three receptors per trimeric ligand, with each elongated receptor nestled at the three monomer-monomer interfaces of the trimer *(6)*. Determination of the structure of Apo2L/TRAIL bound to DR5 by several groups confirmed that this binding mode is conserved for other multidomain TNFRs and showed that the structurally equivalent loops in other TNFRs are similar *(9–11)*. In particular, CRD2 and the first loop of CRD3 mediate most of the contacts to the ligand in both the LTα–TNFR1 and Apo2L/TRAIL–DR5 complexes. This is consistent with the observation that CRD2 is the best conserved feature in TNFR1, HveA, and DR5. The first loop of CRD2 makes interactions with hydrophobic residues in the DE loop and with the C-terminal portion of the AA' loop. The first loop of CRD3 makes contacts near the tip of the pyramidal ligand, interacting with residues from the D, E, C, and F strands from adjacent monomers (Figs. 1, 4, 5). In one of the three independently determined structures of Apo2L/TRAIL bound to DR5, an additional contact was postulated between a very poorly ordered C-terminal portion of the AA' loop and DR5 *(11)*; however, this is not likely to be physiologically relevant. Modeling studies of other receptor–ligand pairs including Fas *(51,52)*, CD40 *(53)*, and EDAR (*54*, SGH unpublished data) suggest that these receptors also interact with their receptors in a similar fashion, which is likely conserved in the interactions of all multi-CRD TNFRs with their ligands

In both the LTα–TNFR1 and Apo2L/TRAIL–DR5 complexes, the spacing of the C-termini of the receptors as they enter the cell form an almost equilateral triangle with sides of approx 50 Å (Fig. 1). These dimensions are consistent with the observation that the receptor binding sites on the cytosolic adaptor proteins, the TRAFs *(55)*, which interact either directly or indirectly with the intracellular domains of many TNFRs, also form a triangle with sides of approx 50 Å. This similarity in geometry suggests that this spacing is likely physiologically relevant and may be required for signaling.

More divergent, single domain TNFRs are not expected to make all of the same binding interactions seen in the complexes between multidomain TNFRs and their ligands, but should retain the overall features such as binding at monomer-monomer interfaces and the geometry of the signaling complex. For instance, BR3, which contains only a partial CRD, has a very small focused binding epitope with sequences from one loop in the receptor containing most of the binding energy *(43,56)*. The recently determined solution structure of BR3 and the crystal structure of a complex between BAFF and a peptide derived from BR3 reveal that BR3 is essentially an elaborate A1 module and binds in the same location on the ligand as the A1 module of CRD3 from TNFR1 or DR5 *(43,56)*. In contrast to the large (>2000 $Å^2$) and relatively flat interfaces seen in the LTα–TNFR1 and Apo2L/TRAIL–DR5 complexes, the core BAFF–BR3 interaction consists of a salt bridge between a conserved aspartate in BR3 and an arginine residue in BAFF together with a leucine from BR3 filling a tight hydrophobic cavity on BAFF. No similar knob-and-hole interaction is seen in the LTα–TNFR1 or Apo2L/TRAIL–DR5 complexes. Whether TWEAKR *(15)*, which contains only a single CRD, binds TWEAK in a similar fashion as BR3 interacting with BAFF remains to be seen.

Determinants of Ligand–Receptor Specificity

TNFL–TNFR interactions are highly specific, with observed dissociation constants generally in the low n*M* or even p*M* range, although some interactions such as those of BAFF with its receptors, are only in the 50–100 n*M* range *(1,49,54)*. Various mechanisms have been proposed that lead to receptor specificity. Hymowitz et al. proposed that the interactions made by CRD3 of the receptors are likely to contribute more to specificity than the interactions made by CRD2, since the CRD3 loop is more diverse in length, chemical composition, and structure than CRD2 *(9)* (Fig. 5). This proposal is consistent with the observation that the EDA splice variants EDA-A1 and EDA-A2 differ by two amino acids in a region which likely interacts with CRD3 of their respective receptors *(39,42)*.

Mongkolsapaya et al. noted that the position of CRD3 relative to the rest of the receptor differs considerably between TNFR1 and DR5, and proposed that this may be a means of achieving specificity *(10)*. However, independent structures of Apo2L/TRAIL with DR5 showed that the orientation of CRD3 can differ considerably even within the same complex and is therefore inherently variable. Finally, Cha et al. suggested that the conformation of the AA' loop may influence specificity *(11)*.

As more structures and further biochemical characterization takes place, it seems likely that one mechanism alone is not enough to explain receptor specificity across the family. For instance, BAFF interacts intimately with a very focused part of the receptor

(43), while the multidomain receptors make more extensive contact with their ligands *(6,9–11)*. Finally, splice variations as seen in the discrimination between EDA-A1 and EDA-A2 for EDAR and XEDAR, respectively, may represent another evolutionary approach to achieving specificity between TNFRs and their ligands *(42,54)*.

Formation of Multireceptor Complexes

Several ligands bind more than one receptor. For instance, Apo2L/TRAIL has two signaling and at least two decoy receptors, whereas FasL interacts with both Fas and DcR3. There is no apparent structural reason why hetero-receptor complexes could not form on the surface of cells; for example, Apo2L/TRAIL has been reported to simultaneously interact with DR5 and DR4 *(57)*. The propensity for these interactions to occur in vivo may depend on receptor sequestration or on the selective expression of receptors on various cell types rather than active discrimination by either the ligands or the receptors.

FUNCTIONAL DETERMINANTS OF TNFR–TNFL INTERACTIONS

Ligand Mutagenesis

Mutagenesis experiments have been carried out in several systems. Due to the differences in assay format and reagent preparation, it is impossible to quantitatively compare these results. Qualitatively, these studies identify similar portions of different ligands as important for receptor binding. For Apo2L/TRAIL, two residues, Q205 and Y216, at the center of the two receptor binding patches, have been identified by activity assays as well as direct binding experiments as the most important residues for receptor interactions. Mutations of either of these residues to alanine impairs bioactivity by several hundred fold and results in at least a 10-fold reduction in receptor affinity as determined by surface plasmon resonance (Biacore) measurements using recombinant protein *(24)*. Mutation of the analogous residues (P206 and Y218) in FasL shows similar results *(58)*, supporting the assertion that FasL interacts with Fas in the same manner as Apo2L/TRAIL with DR5 or LTα with TNFR1, using two-site CRD2- and CRD3-mediated binding. Mutational analysis of CD40L *(59)* and LTα *(60)* is also consistent with two areas of the monomer-monomer interface forming the receptor-binding site (Fig. 4).

For EDA, disease-causing mutations have been mapped to the same area of the ligand surface as Q205 in Apo2L/TRAIL. Recombinant protein containing some of these naturally occurring mutations (for instance, Y343C or T378M) has been produced and shown to have impaired receptor binding *(39)*. Other surface mutations in EDA map to a second surface patch on EDA, which is not expected to interact with receptor.

Receptor Mutagenesis

Both Fas and CD40 have been studied by receptor mutagenesis (Fig. 5). Serine scanning of Fas identified residues in CRD2 and CRD3 that resulted in decreased binding affinity when mutated to serine in the context of recombinant Fas–Ig fusions *(61,62)*. Similar serine scanning experiments in CD40 have identified residues in CRD2 as well as the beginning of CRD3 that are important for receptor binding *(59)*. Chimeras between Fas and TNFR1 are also consistent with the expectation that CRD2 and CRD3 mediate all significant ligand contacts. Although all Fas CRDs were required for full receptor function, chimeric receptors containing CRD1 of TNFR1 with CRD2 and 3 of Fas retained significant activity and FasL specificity *(63)*. All of these results are consistent with the binding modes seen in the crystal structures of the complex between Apo2L/TRAIL with DR5 as well as LTα with TNFR1 being typical for most members of the TNFR–TNFL families.

Construction of Homology Models

The availability of crystal structures of several TNFLs facilitates the construction of homology models of family members that thus far have proved resistant to structure determination. These models can be very useful for determining potential residues to mutate in order to identify the receptor binding sites *(52,54)*. However, although most homology models are generally correct about strand location and disulfide formation, they can be misleading about the most interesting aspects of the ligands in that they miss the features that make each ligand distinct, such as the presence of metal-binding sites or unusual loop conformations, which may influence ligand stability or receptor specificity.

The situation for homology modeling the receptors is not as good. In general, the homology models constructed of the receptors are less reliable than models of the ligands, due the greater degree of structural and sequence variation between the family members, their nonglobular fold, and the lack of extensive regular secondary structure. Additionally, there is a paucity of templates available as starting points, since many fewer receptors than ligands have been structurally characterized *(64)*. Experimental determination of further receptor structures as well as of more complexes between receptors and divergent ligands is therefore highly desirable.

MISSING FAMILY MEMBERS

There is reason to believe that there are more TNFLs and TNFRs yet to be cloned. Several receptors (DR6, TROY, RELT) lack ligands. Intriguingly, TROY and RELT share significant sequence homology to EDAR and XEDAR *(65–67)*. In particular, TROY is 50% homologous to XEDAR, suggesting than another EDA-A2-like ligand is likely to exist. Additionally, although all known ligands have been shown to interact with at least one receptor, many ligands bind to more than one receptor, and more receptors may yet be found for some of the ligands. In particular, small receptors without intracellular death domains or with only a single or partial CRD may have been missed by conventional sequence- and structure-based searches of genomic databases.

CONCLUSION

This is an exciting time in the study of the structure and function of not just the death receptors but of all TNFLs and receptors. Whereas most of the basic structural motifs have likely been determined, the structures of more divergent complexes and identification of novel ligands and receptors remains a promising area of investigation, likely to reveal novel structural features and interactions. In addition, the structural aspects of regulation of receptors and ligand activity by oligomerization remains an area of much interest.

NOTE ADDED IN PROOF

The structure of EDA referred to SGH, unpublished data, has been published *(68)*. Structures of the BAFF-BR3 and BAFF-BCMA complexes have also been published *(69,70)* and agree well with the data presented in ref. *43*.

REFERENCES

1. Locksely RM, Killeen N, Lenardo MJ. The TNF and TNF receptor superfamilies: integrating mammalian biology. Cell 2001;104:487–501.
2. Mignone T-S, Zhang J, Luo X, et al. TL1A is a TNF-like ligand for DR3 and TR6/DcR3 and functions as a T cell co-stimulator. Immunity 2002;16:479–492.
3. Headon DJ, Emmal SA, Ferguson BM, et al. Gene defect in ectodermal dysplasia implicates a death domain adapter in development. Nature 2001;414:913–916.
4. Yan M, Zhang Z, Brady JR, Schilbach S, Fairbrother WJ, Dixit VM. Indentification of a novel death domain-containing adaptor molecule for ectodysplasin-A receptor that is mutated in *crinkled* mice. Curr Biol 2002;12:1–20.
5. Wiesmann C, de Vos AM. Nerve growth factor: structure and function. Cell Mol Life Sci 2001;58:748–759.
6. Banner DW, D'Arcy A, Janes W, et al. Crystal structure of the soluble human 55 kd TNF receptor–human TNFβ complex: implications for TNF receptor activation. Cell 1993;73:431–445.
7. Naismith JH, Devine TQ, Brandhuber BJ Sprang SR. Crystallographic evidence for dimerization of unliganded tumor necrosis factor receptor. J Biol Chem 1995;270:13,303–13,307.
8. Carfi A, Willis SH, Whitback JC, et al. Herpes simplex virus glycoprotein D bound to the human receptor HveA. Mol Cell 2001;8:169–179.
9. Hymowitz SG, Christinger HW, Fuh G, et al. Triggering cell death: the crystal structure of Apo2L/TRAIL in a complex with death receptor 5. Mol Cell 1999;4:563–571.
10. Mongkolsapaya J, Grimes JM, Chen J, et al. The structure of the TRAIL-DR5 complex reveals mechanisms conferring specificity in apoptotic initiation. Nat Struc Biol 1999;6:1048–1053.
11. Cha S-S, Sung B-J, Kim Y-A, et al. Crystal structure of TRAIL-DR5 complex identifies a critical role of the unique frame insertion in conferring recognition specificity. J Biol Chem 2000;275:31,171–31,177.
12. Bazan JF. Emerging families of cytokines and receptors. Curr Biol 1993;3:603–606.
13. Naismith JH, Sprang SR. Modularity in the TNF-receptor family. TIBS 1998;23:74–79.
14. Madry C, Laabi Y, Callebaut I, et al. The characterization of the murine BCMA gene defines it as a new member of the tumor necrosis factor receptor family. Int Immunol 1998;10:1693–1702.
15. Wiley SR, Cassiano L, Lofton T, et al. A novel TNF receptor family member binds TWEAK and is implicated in angiogenesis. Immunity 2001;15:837–846.
16. Thompson JS, Bixler SA, Qian F, et al. BAFF-R, a newly identified TNF receptor that specifically interacts with BAFF. Science 2001;293:2108–2111.
17. Yan M, Brady JR, Chan B, et al. Indentification of a novel receptor for B lymphocyte stimulator that is mutated in a mouse strain with severe B cell deficiency. Curr Biol 2001;11:1547–1552.
18. Jones EY, Stuart DI, Walker NPC. Structure of tumour necrosis factor. Nature 1989;338:225–228.
19. Shapiro L, Scherer PE. The crystal structure of a complement-1q family protein suggests an evolutionary link to the tumor necrosis factor. Curr Biol 1998;8:335–338.
20. Bogin O, Kvansakul M, Rom E, Singer J, Yayon A, Hohenester E. Insight into Schmid metaphyseal chondrodysplasia from the crystal structure of the collagen X NC1 domain trimer. Structure 2002;10:165–173.
21. Eck MJ, Sprang SR. The structure of tumor necrosis factor-α at 2.6 Å resolution. J Biol Chem 1989;264:17,595–17,605.
22. Eck MJ, Ultsch M, Rinderknecht E, de Vos AM, Sprang SR. The structure of human lymphotoxin (tumor necrosis factor-β) at 1.9-Å resolution. J Biol Chem 1992;267:2119–2122.
23. Karpusas M, Hsu Y-M, Wang J-H, et al. 2 Å crystal structure of an extracellular fragment of human CD40 ligand. Structure 1995;3:1031–1039.
24. Hymowitz SG, O'Connell MP, Ultsch MH, et al. A unique zinc-binding site revealed by a high-resolution x-ray structure of homotrimeric Apo2L/TRAIL. Biochem 2000;39:633–640.

25. Cha S-S, Kim M-S, Choi YH, et al. 2.8 Å resolution crystal structure of human TRAIL, a cytokine with selective anitumor activity. Immunity 1999;11:253–261.
26. Oren DC, Li Y, Volovik Y, et al. Structural basis of BLyS receptor recognition. Nat Struc Biol 2002;9: 288–292.
27. Liu Y, Xu L, Opalka N, Kappier J, Shu H-B, Zhang G. Crystal structure of stall-1 reveals a virus-like assembly of TNF family ligands. Cell 2002;108:383–394.
28. Karpusas M, Cachero TG, Qian F, et al. Crystal structure of extracellular human BAFF, a TNF family member that stimulates B lymphocytes. J Mol Biol 2002;315:1145–1154.
29. Ito S, Wakabayashi k, Ubukata O, Hayashi S, Okada F, Hata T. Crystal structure of the extracellular domain of mouse RANK ligand at 2.2-Å resolution. J Biol Chem 2002;277:6631–6636.
30. Lam J, Nelson CA, Ross FP, Tietelbaum SL, Fremont DH. Crystal structure of the TRANCE/RANKL cytokine reveals determinants of receptor-ligand specificity. J Clin Invest 2001;108:971–979.
31. Yue T, Ni J, Romanic AM, et al. TL1, a novel tumor necrosis factor-like cytokine, induces apoptosis in endothelial cells. J Biol Chem 1999;274:1479–1486.
32. Zhai Y, Ni J, Jian GW, et al. VEGI, a novel cytokine of the tumor necrosis factor family, is an angiogenesis inhibitor that suppresses growth of colon carcinomas in vivo. FASEB J 1999;13:181–189.
33. Bodmer J-L, Meier P, Tschopp J, Schneider P. Cysteine 230 is essential for the structure and activity of the cytotoxic ligand TRAIL. J Biol Chem 2000; 275: 20,632–20,637.
34. Grell M, Douni E, Wajant H, et al. The transmembrane form of tumor necrosis factor is the prime activating ligand of the 80 kDa tumor necrosis factor receptor. Cell 1995;83:793–802.
35. Krippner-Heidenreich A, Tübing F, Bryde S, Willi S, Zimmermann G, Scheurich P. Control of receptor-induced signaling complex formation by the kinetics of ligand/receptor interaction. J Biol Chem 2002;277:44,155–44,163.
36. Schneider P, Holler N, Bodmer J-L, et al. Conversion of membrane-bound Fas (CD95) ligand to its soluble form is associated with downregulation of its proapoptotic activity and loss of liver toxicity. J Exp Med 1998;187:1205–1213.
37. Huang DCS, Hahne M, Schroeter M, et al. Activation of Fas by FasL induces apoptosis by a mechanism that cannot be blocked by Bcl-2 or Bcl-xL. Proc Natl Acad Sci USA 1999;96:14,871–14,876.
38. Pound JD, Challa A, Holder MJ, et al. Minimal cross-linking and epitope requirements for CD40-dependent suppression of apoptosis contrast with those for promotion of the cell cycle and homotypic adhesions in human B cells. Int Immunol 1999;11:11–20.
39. Schneider P, Street SL, Gaide O, et al. Mutations leading to X-linked hypohidrotic ectodermal dysplasia affect three major functional domains in the tumor necrosis factor family member ectodysplasin-A. J Biol Chem 2001;276:18,819–18,827.
40. Villunger A, Huang DCS, Holler N, Tschopp J, Strasser A. Fas ligand-induced c-jun kinase activation in lymphoid cells requires extensive receptor aggregation but is independent of DAXX, and fas-mediated cell death does not involve DAXX, RIP or RAIDD. J Immunol 2000;165:1337–1343.
41. Lawrence D, Shahrokh Z, Marsters S, et al. Differential hepatocyte toxicity of recombinant Apo2L/TRAIL versions. Nat Med 2001;7:383–385.
42. Bayés M, Hartung AJ, Ezer S, et al. The anihidrotic ectodermal dysplasia gene (EDA) undergoes alternative splicing and encodes ecotdyplasin-A with deletion mutations in collagenous repeats. Hum Mol Genet 1998;7:1661–1669.
43. Gordon NC, Pan B, Hymowitz SG, et al. BAFF/BLyS receptor 3 comprises a minimal TNF receptor-like module that encodes a highly focused ligand-binding site. Biochemistry 2003;42(20):5977–5983.
44. Schneider P, MacKay F, Steiner V, et al. BAFF, a novel ligand of the tumor necrosis factor family, stimulates B cell growth. J Exp Med 1999;189:1747–1756.
45. Browning JL, Androlewicz MJ, Ware CF. Lymphotoxin and an associated 33-kDa glycoprotein are expressed on the surface of an activated human T cell hybridoma. J Immunol 1991 147:1230–1237.
46. Browning JL, Miatkowski K, Griffiths DA, et al. Preparation and characterization of soluble recombinant heterotrimeric complexes of human lymphotoxins α and β. J Biol Chem 1996;271:8618–8626.
47. Roschke V, Sosnovtseva S, Ward CD, et al. BLyS and APRIL form biologically active heterotrimers that are expressed in patients with systematic immune-based rheumatic diseases. J. Immunol 2002;169: 4314–4321.
48. Naismith JH, Devine TQ, Kohno T, Sprang SR. Structures of the extracellular domain of type I tumor necrosis factor receptor. Structure 1996;4:1251–1262.

49. Papoff G, Hausler P, Eramo A, et al. Identification and characterization of a ligand-independent oligomerization domain in the extracellular region of the CD95 death receptor. J Biol Chem 1999;274: 38,241–38,250.
50. Chan FK-M, Chun HJ, Zheng L, Siegel RM, Bui KL, Lenardo MJ. A domain in TNF receptors that mediates ligand-independent receptor assembly and signaling. Science 2000;288:2351–2354.
51. Bajorath J. Identification of the ligand binding site in Fas (CD95) and analysis of the Fas-ligand interactions. Proteins: Struc Func Genet 1999;35:475–482.
52. Peitsch MC, Tschopp J. Comparative molecular modeling of the Fas-ligand and other members of the TNF family. Mol Immun 1995;32:762–772.
53. Bajorath J, Marken JS, Chalupny NJ, et al. Analysis of gp39/CD40 interactions using molecular models and site-directed mutagenesis. Biochem1995;34:9884–9892.
54. Yan M, Wang L-C, Hymowitz SG, et al. Two-amino acid molecular switch in an epithelial morphogen that regulates binding to two distinct receptors. Science 2000;290:523–527.
55. Park YC, Burkitt V, Villa AR, Tong L, Wu Hao. Structural basis for self-association and receptor recognition of human TRAF2. Nature 1999;398:533–538.
56. Kayagaki N, Yan M, Seshasayee D, et al. BAFF/BLyS receptor 3 binds the B cell survival factor BAFF ligand through a discrete surface loop and promotes processing of NF-κB2. Immunity 2002;10:515–524.
57. Scheider P, Thome M, Burns K, et al. TRAIL receptors 1 (DR4) and 2 (DR5) signal FADD-dependent apoptosis and activate NF-κB. Immunity 1997;7:831–836.
58. Schneider P. Bodmer J-L, Holler N., et al. Characterization of the Fas (Apo-1, CD95)-Fas ligand interaction. J Biol Chem 1997;272:18,827–18,833.
59. Bajorath J, Chalupny NJ, Marken JS, et al. Identification of residues on CD40 and its ligand which are critical for the receptor-ligand interaction. Biochem 1995;34:1833–1844.
60. Goh C, Loh C-S, Porter AG. Aspartic acid 50 and tyrosine 108 are essential for receptor binding and cytotoxic activity of tumour necrosis factor beta (lymphotoxin). Prot Engin 1991;4:785–791.
61. Starling GC, Bajorath J, Emswiler J, Ledbetter JA, Aruffo A, Kiener PA. Identification of amino acid residues important for ligand binding to Fas. J Exp Med 1997;185:1487–1492.
62. Startling GC, Kiener PA, Aruffo A, Bajorath J. Analysis of the ligand binding site in Fas (CD95) by site-directed mutagenesis and comparison with TNFR and CD40. Biochem 1998;37:3723–3726.
63. Orlinick JR, Vaishnaw A, Elkon KB, Chao MV. Requirement of cysteine-rich repeats of the fas receptor for binding by the Fas ligand. J Biol Chem 1997;272:28,889–28,894.
64. Bodmer J-L, Schneider P, Tschopp J. The molecular architecture of the TNF superfamily. TIBS 2002;27:19–26.
65. Kojima T, Morikawa Y, Copelan NG, et al. TROY, a newly identified member of the tumor necrosis factor receptor superfamily, exhibits a homology with Edar and is expressed in embryonic skin and hair follicles. J Biol Chem 2000;275:20,742–20,747.
66. Eby MT, Jasmin AJ, Kumar A, Sharma K, Chaudhary PM. TAJ, a novel member of the tumor necrosis factor receptor family, activates the c-Jun N-terminal kinase pathway and mediates caspase-independent cell death. J Biol Chem 2000;275:15,336–15,342.
67. Sica GL, Zhu G, Tamada K, Liu D, Ni J, Chen L. RELT, a new member of the tumor necrosis factor receptor superfamily is selectively expressed in hematopoietic tissues and activates transcription factor NF-κB. Blood 2001;97:2702–2707.
68. Hymowitz SG, Compaan DM, Yan M, et al. The crystal structures of EDA-A1 and EDA-A2: splice variants with distant receptor specificity. Structure 2003;11:1513–1520.
69. Liu Y, Hong X, Kappler J, et al. Ligand-receptor binding revealed by the TNF family member TALL-1. Nature 2003;423:49–56.
70. Kim HM, Yu KS, Lee ME, et al. Crystal sturcture of the BAFF-BAFF-R complex and its implications for receptor activation. Nat Struc Biol 2003;10:342–348.

4 Death Receptor Signaling in Embryonic Ectodermal Development

Preet M. Chaudhary, MD, PhD

SUMMARY

The ectodermal dysplasias (EDs) are a heterogeneous group of genetic disorders which are identified by the absent or deficient function of at least two derivatives of ectoderm (e.g., skin, nails, sweat glands, or teeth) *(1)*. More than 150 different types of EDs have been identified, and the combined incidence of these disorders may be as high as 7 per 10,000 births. However, a large number of cases go undetected due to the relatively mild phenotype and the apparent ability of the affected individuals to cover up their disease by application of cosmetics, wigs, or dentures. Although Charles Darwin wrote one of the earliest descriptions of an ED involving "the toothless men of Sind" *(2)*, the diagnosis of these disorders may be extremely difficult, partly because there can be many different permutations of ectodermal defects. EDs have been broadly classified into two major subgroups based on the absence or presence of sweat gland function—hidrotic ectodermal dysplasia (or Clouston syndrome) and hypohidrotic ectodermal dysplasias (HEDs). Recent studies suggest an important role of signaling via the tumor necrosis factor receptor (TNFR) family in the pathogenesis of hypohidrotic ectodermal dysplasias, and that will be the focus of this discussion.

HYPOHIDROTIC ECTODERMAL DYSPLASIAS

HEDs are characterized by the triad of signs consisting of sparse hair, abnormal or missing teeth, and inability to sweat *(3)*. Many individuals with hypohidrotic ectodermal dysplasias also have characteristic facial abnormalities, including prominent forehead, saddle nose, unusually thick lips, and/or large chin *(3)*. The skin on most parts of the body may be abnormally thin, dry, soft, and hypopigmented. Four mouse mutants (*Tabby, downless, Sleek,* and *crinkled*) have phenotypes similar to patients with HEDs and represent the mouse equivalents of human disorders. HEDs can be transmitted either as an X-linked disorder, designated *ED1*, or morphologically indistinguishable autosomal dominant or recessive conditions in both humans and mouse *(3)*.

From: *Cancer Drug Discovery and Development: Death Receptors in Cancer Therapy*
Edited by: W. S. El-Deiry © Humana Press Inc., Totowa, NJ

ROLE OF ECTODYSPLASIN A IN THE PATHOGENESIS OF X-LINKED HYPOHIDROTIC ECTODERMAL DYSPLASIA (ED1)

Darwin's "toothless men of Sind" suffered from *ED1*, which is also the most common form of HED. In 1996, an international group of scientists used positional cloning to isolate the gene responsible for *ED1* and designated it EDA *(4)*. However, the transcript identified in the original study was a truncated spliced variant, and the true identity of EDA was not revealed until the molecular cloning of the gene responsible for the *Tabby* mutation in mice, which is the counterpart of human *ED1 (5,6)*. Sequence analysis of the protein encoded by the *Tabby* gene, which was named ectodysplasin (EDA), revealed it to be a novel ligand of the TNF superfamily *(7)*. Like the majority of the ligands of the TNF family, EDA is a type II membrane protein, and possesses a TNF homology domain at its COOH terminal (Fig. 1). However, EDA also possesses a unique glycine-rich collagenous domain, which is composed of three subdomains (Fig. 1). EDA is proteolytically processed into a soluble molecule by cleavage at Arg^{159}, which lies within a furin consensus cleavage site *(8–10)*. Analysis of mutations in families with X-linked ectodermal dysplasia has revealed that the three domains of EDA described above (collagenous domain, TNF homology domain, and furin cleavage site) play essential yet distinct roles in its biological activity. Mutations in the collagenous domain inhibit EDA multimerization, those in TNF homology domain prevent its binding to the receptor, while those in the consensus furin recognition site prevent its proteolytic cleavage *(8–12)*. Several alternatively spliced transcripts of EDA have been identified *(5,7,12)*. Two of these transcripts, EDA-A1 and EDA-A2, which differ from each other by only two amino acids in the TNF homology domain, bind to two different receptors and appear to have distinct biological activities *(13)*.

ROLE OF EDAR IN THE PATHOGENESIS OF AUTOSOMAL FORMS OF HEDS

As discussed above, *downless, sleek*, and *crinkled* mice have phenotypes similar to *Tabby* and represent the counterparts of autosomal forms of human HEDs. While the genetic defect in *downless* and *crinkled* mice is autosomal recessive, *sleek* represents an autosomal dominant mutation at the *downless* locus. The candidate gene at the *downless* locus was isolated using positional cloning, and was found to encode a novel receptor of the TNFR family *(14)*. This gene was supposed to code for the receptor for ectodysplasin A, termed EDAR (ectodermal dysplasia receptor) *(14)*. Mutations in *dl* were found in both the autosomal recessive (downless^{Jackson}, dl^{J}) and autosomal dominant (downless^{sleek}, Dl^{slk}) forms of disease. Subsequently, mutations in the human homolog of *dl* were found in three HED families displaying recessive inheritance and in two with dominant inheritance *(15)*. Three independent research groups found that EDAR was physically associated with the EDA-A1 isoform, which established EDAR and EDA-A1 as a receptor-ligand pair and explained the identical phenotype of the mutations in the respective genes *(10,13,16)*.

Structural analysis of EDAR has revealed it to be a type I transmembrane protein that bears significant sequence homology to an orphan TNF family receptor termed TAJ (also known as TNRFSF19 and TROY), in its extracellular ligand binding domain *(17,18)*. This homology is due to the presence of cysteine-rich pseudorepeats, a hallmark of the

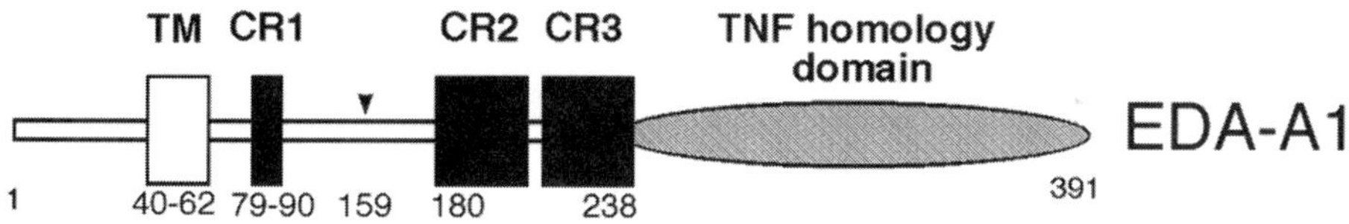

Fig. 1. A schematic representation of human EDA-A1 protein. The position of the furin cleavage site at Arg^{159} is marked with an arrowhead. The EDA-A2 isoform is identical to EDA-A1 except for two-residue (Glu^{308} and Val^{309}) deletion in the TNF homology domain. TM, transmembrane domain; CR, collagenous repeat domain.

TNFR family (Fig. 2) *(14,15)*. The cytoplasmic region of EDAR contains a domain with modest homology to the death domain (DD) present in the p75 nerve growth factor receptor, and only a weak homology to the death domain present in the classical death receptors such as Fas and TNFR1 (Fig. 3) *(14,15)*. Accordingly, EDAR does not interact with the death domain adaptor proteins FADD and TRADD *(16)*. Nevertheless, the death domain of EDAR was shown to play a critical role in EDAR signaling, since point mutations within this domain or its deletion (as in Dl^{slk}) were found to be associated with HED *(14,15)*.

SIGNAL TRANSDUCTION VIA EDA-A1/EDAR

Signal transduction via the TNFR family members has been shown to lead to cellular proliferation, differentiation, activation, or programmed cell death, depending upon cellular context, nature of the receptor, and the stimulus *(19)*. Signaling via these receptors is initiated upon ligand-induced receptor trimerization, which results in the recruitment of cytosolic adaptor proteins to their cytoplasmic domains *(19)*. These adaptor proteins can be broadly classified into two main categories: death domain-containing proteins (e.g., TRADD, FADD, and RIP) and TNF receptor-associated factors (TRAFs) *(19)*. Most members of the TNFR family lack a death domain and interact directly with the TRAFs. In contrast, signaling via the death domain-containing receptors is initiated upon the recruitment of the death adaptors, which subsequently leads to the activation of two main signaling pathways—a kinase cascade leading to NF-κB and JNK activation, and a caspase cascade leading to cell death *(19)*.

Activation of the NF-κB Pathway by EDA-A1/EDAR Interaction

As EDAR also possesses a death domain, its ability to activate the above signaling pathways was tested. Transient transfection of EDAR strongly activated the NF-κB pathway, and this activity was significantly impaired in mutants that lacked the death domain *(13,16,20)*. Furthermore, a R420Q ($Arg^{420} \rightarrow Gln^{420}$) mutation in the death domain of EDAR, which was discovered in a family with an autosomal dominant form of HED, led to a severe loss of NF-κB activity. In contrast, an EDAR construct with an E379K mutation, which is seen in the autosomal recessive $dl^{Jackson}$ mice, retained nearly 60% activity of the wild-type protein *(13,16)*. Taken together, the above results suggested that impaired ability to activate the NF-κB pathway via EDAR may play a key role in the pathogenesis of HED.

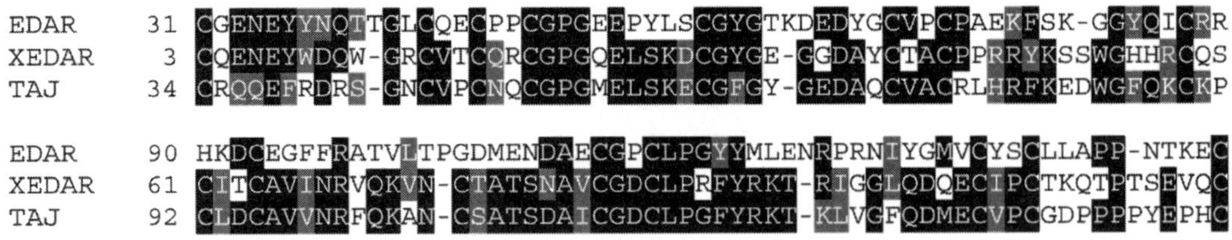
EDAR 31 CGENEYYNQTTGLCQECPPCGPGEEPYLSCGYGTKDEDYGCVPCPAEKFSK-GGYQICRR
XEDAR 3 CQENEYWDQW-GRCVTCQRCGPGQELSKDCGYGE-GGDAYCTACPPRRYKSSWGHHRCQS
TAJ 34 CRQQEFRDRS-GNCVPCNQCGPGMELSKECGFGY-GEDAQCVACRLHRFKEDWGFQKCKP
EDAR 90 HKDCEGFFRATVLTPGDMENDAECGPCLPGYYMLENRPRNIYGMVCYSCLLAPP-NTKEC
XEDAR 61 CITCAVINRVQKVN-CTATSNAVCGDCLPRFYRKT-RIGGLQDQECIPCTKQTPTSEVQC
TAJ 92 CLDCAVVNRFQKAN-CSATSDAICGDCLPGFYRKT-KLVGFQDMECVPCGDPPPPYEPHC

Fig. 2. Sequence alignment of the extracellular domain of human EDAR, XEDAR, and TAJ receptors. Identical amino acids are shaded dark and homologous residues are shaded gray.

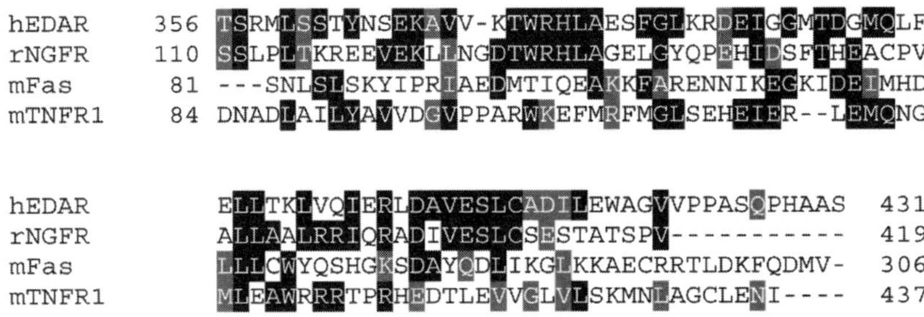

Fig. 3. Sequence alignment of the death domain of human EDAR, rat nerve growth factor receptor, mouse Fas, and mouse TNFR1 receptors. Identical amino acids are shaded dark and homologous residues are shaded gray.

As discussed above, although EDAR possesses a death domain, it does not interact with FADD or TRADD *(16)*. Further characterization of EDAR signaling revealed that EDAR-induced NF-κB could not be blocked by a dominant negative mutant of TRAF2 *(16)*, an adaptor that has been shown to play a key role in NF-κB activation via various TNF family receptors. The above results suggested that EDAR employs a novel adaptor protein in the proximal aspect of its signal transduction pathway *(16)*.

The molecular mechanism of EDAR signaling and the role of its death domain in this process were clarified by the cloning of the gene responsible for the *crinkled* phenotype by two different groups *(21,22)*. One of the groups used a positional cloning approach to isolate a novel adaptor protein with a death domain from the human chromosome 1q42.3-43 region, which is syntenic to the *cr* region on mouse chromosome 13 *(21)*. This adaptor protein, designated EDAR-associated death domain (EDARADD), contained a COOH-terminal death domain that is most homologous to the death domain of MyD88, a signaling intermediate in the Toll/interleukin receptor pathway. EDARADD was independently cloned as *crinkled* (*CR*) by Yan et al., who searched the mouse genomic database to identify a novel death domain containing exon in the *cr* locus and subsequently used this information to clone both human and mouse cDNAs *(22)*. EDARADD was found to associate with the cytoplasmic domain of EDAR in GST-pull-down and coimmunoprecipitation assays, and this interaction was dependent on the presence of their respective death domains *(21)*. In addition to its interaction with EDAR, EDARADD was also shown to self-associate, and this interaction was also dependent on its death domain. EDARADD was shown to interact with TRAF1, -2, and -3 via its amino-terminal domain *(21)*. This domain contains the consensus TRAF-binding sequence Pro-X-Gln-X-Thr, and a deletion mutant lacking this consensus sequence (EDARADDΔ34–40) lost the ability to interact with TRAFs *(21)*. A weak interaction between EDARADD/*CR* and TRAF5 and -6 was detected as well *(22)*. Finally, a GST fusion protein containing the cytoplasmic domain of EDAR was shown to recruit TRAF2 in the presence of EDARADD when all three proteins were overexpressed in 293T cells *(22)*.

Transient transfection of EDARADD in 293T cells led to robust NF-κB activation, and this activity was absent in its deletion mutants that lacked the entire N-terminal domain but contained an intact death domain *(21,22)*. Interestingly, removal of only the TRAF-binding motif (amino acids 34–40) had little effect on EDARADD-induced NF-κB activation, suggesting that a region outside this motif is important for this activity *(21)*. The N-terminal deletion mutants of EDARADD not only failed to activate NF-κB but also blocked EDAR-induced NF-κB activation in a dominant-negative fashion, presumably by blocking the recruitment of the wild-type protein to the aggregated receptor complex *(21,22)*.

The involvement of EDARADD in EDAR-induced NF-κB was supported by the discovery of a missense mutation (E142K) in the death domain of EDARADD in a family with autosomal recessive HED *(21)*. This mutation modestly reduced EDARADD self-association and significantly reduced its interaction with EDAR *(21)*. The E142K mutant demonstrated impaired ability to activate NF-κB upon transient transfection in 293T cells, presumably reflecting its diminished ability to self-aggregate *(21)*.

Taken together, the above studies provide strong molecular and genetic evidence in support of the hypothesis that EDARADD is a key signaling intermediate in EDAR-induced NF-κB activation. However, it remains to be seen whether EDARADD uses TRAF2 for NF-κB activation. For example, although interaction between the EDAR cytoplasmic domain (expressed as a GST fusion protein) and TRAF2 required cotransfection of EDARADD in one study *(22)*, we have previously demonstrated that full-length EDAR can recruit TRAF1, -2, and -3 even without the overexpression of EDARADD *(16)*. Furthermore, a COOH-terminal deletion mutant of EDAR, which completely lacks the death domain and cannot interact with EDARADD, was as effective as the wild-type protein in recruiting TRAFs, suggesting that the TRAF-interacting domain lies outside the death domain *(16)*. The above result also argued against the possibility that the observed interactions between EDAR and TRAFs were due to the presence of endogenously expressed EDARADD. Other arguments against a key role of TRAF2 in EDAR signaling include the lack of effect of dominant-negative TRAF2 on EDAR-induced NF-κB activation *(16)* and the lack of effect of removal of the TRAF2-binding motif on EDARADD-induced NF-κB activation *(21)*. However, almost all the above studies involved GST pull-down or overexpression-based coimmunoprecipitation assays, and the final resolution of this question awaits the demonstration of recruitment of endogenously expressed TRAFs to EDAR in a ligand-dependent fashion.

Although the involvement of TRAFs in EDAR signaling stills need confirmation, there is molecular and genetic evidence supporting the involvement of the IκB kinase (IKK) complex in this process. The IKK complex is a multisubunit signalsome complex that consists of two catalytic subunits, IKK1/IKKα and IKK2/IKKβ, and a regulatory subunit called NEMO/IKKγ *(23)*. The IKK complex phosphorylates IκBα protein, an inhibitory protein that sequesters the NF-κB subunits in the cytoplasm. IKK complex-induced phosphorylation of IκBα leads to its ubiquitination and subsequent proteasome-mediated degradation *(23)*. Once IκBα is degraded, the NF-κB subunits are free to migrate to the nucleus and turn on the transcription of their target genes.

The involvement of the IKK complex in EDAR signaling was suggested by studies using kinase-inactive mutants of IKK1 and IKK2, which could block EDAR-induced NF-κB activation in a dominant-negative fashion *(16)*. Genetic proof of the involvement of the IKK complex in EDAR signaling was provided by the discovery of mutations in NEMO/IKKγ in several families with HED and immunodeficiency *(24–26)*. In addition, a deletion mutant of NEMO has been shown to block EDAR-induced NF-κB activation in a dominant-negative fashion *(25)*.

Other Signaling Pathways Activated by EDAR

Although NF-κB is the predominant pathway activated by EDAR, it is also known to activate the JNK pathway *(16)*. However, JNK activation via EDAR was relatively weak as compared to other members of the TNFR *(16)*. Transient transfection of EDAR in 293T, 293EBNA, and MCF7 cells also led to cellular rounding, detachment, and ultimately cell death *(16)*. However, EDAR-induced cell death was not accompanied by caspase activation and could not be blocked by caspase inhibitors *(16)*.

SIGNAL TRANSDUCTION VIA XEDAR

As discussed previously, EDA-A1 and EDA-A2 are two alternatively spliced isoforms of ectodysplasin A that differ from each other by two amino acids in the TNF homology domain. While EDA-A1 binds to EDAR, EDA-A2 was shown to bind to an EDAR homolog located on the X-chromosome, designated XEDAR *(13)*. Two alternatively spliced isoforms of XEDAR, designated XEDAR-L (for long) and XEDAR-s (for short), have been described; these differ from each other by 21 amino acids in the juxta-membrane region of the cytoplasmic domain *(27)*. Unlike the majority of the other receptors of its family, XEDAR is a type III membrane protein that bears significant sequence homology to EDAR and TAJ in its extracellular domain (Fig. 2) *(13)*. Unlike EDAR, the cytoplasmic domain of XEDAR lacks a death domain. Nevertheless, XEDAR is a strong activator of the NF-κB pathway *(13,27)*, and this activity has been mapped to the amino acid regions 249–254 and 273–281 of XEDAR-L isoform, with the latter region accounting for most of this activity *(27)*. Interestingly, the region between amino acid residues 249 and 254 contains the sequence PTQES, which is homologous to the consensus binding motif PXQXT/S for TRAF2, -3, and -5 *(28,29)*. On the other hand, the region between 273 and 281 contains the sequence PIECTE, which is homologous to the consensus binding motif PXEXXaromatic/acidic for TRAF6 *(30)*. Consistent with the results of deletion mutagenesis, a mutant containing a glutamine to lysine change at amino acid 253 (E253K), showed a marginal loss of NF-κB activity, whereas a similar mutant at position 277 (E277K) showed a more significant loss *(27)*. Finally, a double mutant, EE253/277KK (EE/KK), demonstrated almost a complete lack of NF-κB activity, confirming the importance of the two regions in NF-κB activation *(27)*.

Coimmunoprecipitation studies have revealed the recruitment of TRAF3 and TRAF6 to XEDAR in an EDA-A2-dependent fashion *(27)*. In contrast, no interaction between XEDAR and TRAF2 was observed *(27)*. The involvement of TRAF3 and -6 in XEDAR-induced NF-κB activation was also supported by the ability of dominant-negative mutants of these proteins to block EDA-A2-induced NF-κB activation in a dominant-negative fashion *(27)*. The involvement of TRAF6 in XEDAR signaling is also supported by the presence of hypohidrotic ectodermal dysplasia in *Traf-6–/–* animals *(31)*. These animals show focal alopecia behind the ears, alopecia of the tail, a distinctive kink near the tip of their tail, and lack of sweat gland development, features also seen in Ta, dl, and cr mice. While EDAR and XEDAR use distinct proximal adaptor proteins, both depend on the IKK distally for activating the NF-κB pathway *(27)*. Therefore, defects in ectodermal differentiation seen in patients with mutations in NEMO/IKKγ *(25)* might be due to inhibition of signaling via both these receptors.

As discussed above, EDAR is a relatively weak activator of the JNK pathway. XEDAR differs in this respect from EDAR, and strongly stimulates JNK activity in an EDA-A2-dependent fashion *(27)*. Similar to the situation with NF-κB, JNK activation via XEDAR is dependent on its interaction with TRAF3 and -6. ASK1 is believed to be the intermediate kinase in XEDAR-induced JNK activation *(27)*. XEDAR is also known to activate the ERK pathway *(30)*. Finally, we have recently discovered that XEDAR can also induce apoptosis (unpublished observation).

The involvement of XEDAR in ectodermal differentiation is supported by the recent discovery of a mutation in this gene in a patient with HED *(32)* and the phenotype of *Traf 6–/–* animals *(31)*. Interestingly, transgenic expression of EDA-A1 isoform in male Tabby mice was recently shown to rescue development of several skin appendages, with near complete restoration of hair growth, dermal ridges, sweat glands, and molars *(33)*. However, while the number of hair follicles in the transgenic mice was the same as in wild-type animals, a block in the development of follicles and associated glands was noted in some of the transgenic animals *(33)*. The above study suggests that while EDA-A2-mediated XEDAR signaling may not be absolutely essential for skin appendage formation, it may be required for appropriate timing and completeness of this process *(33)*. Consistent with the above hypothesis, EDAR and XEDAR are expressed in a distinctive temporal and spatial pattern during embryonic development in mice *(13)*. For example, expression of EDAR is seen as early as d 14 in the basal cells of developing epidermis with elevated focal expression in placodes, while XEDAR expression is not expressed at this stage *(13)*. However, both receptors are highly expressed in maturing hair follicles by embryonic d 16–17, and their expression is confined to hair follicles by postnatal day *(13)*. Similarly, while EDA-A1 is expressed in both developing epidermis and hair follicles, expression of EDA-A2 appears later and is confined to hair follicles *(13)*.

SIGNAL TRANSDUCTION VIA TAJ/TROY

TAJ/TROY is the third TNF family receptor with preferential expression during embryonic development and ectodermal derivatives *(17,18)*. The human TAJ cDNA encodes for a type I membrane protein of 423 amino acids with an N-terminal signal peptide and a single transmembrane domain *(17,18)*. Although the extracellular domain of TAJ bears significant sequence homology to EDAR, it possesses a unique cytoplasmic domain with no sequence homology to any known protein *(17,18)*. In addition to its full-length isoform, two alternatively spliced isoforms of mouse TAJ have been described *(17)*. One of these clones lacks a transmembrane region and, therefore, may represent a soluble receptor, while the second clone possesses a transmembrane region and a short cytoplasmic tail, and may represent a decoy receptor *(17)*. Similar soluble and decoy receptors have been isolated for other members of the TNFR family and have been shown to block signaling through the full-length receptors in a dominant-negative fashion.

During mouse development, TAJ is highly expressed beginning on embryonic d 11. Interestingly, expression of TAJ/TROY during embryogenesis is mainly limited to the epithelium. Thus, high-level expression was detected in the neuroepithelium in the frontal and lateral lobes of the brain, and in the epithelium of skin and hair follicles, tongue, stomach, cochlea, conjunctiva, and lungs *(18)*. TAJ expression is also seen in the ossification centers in the mandible and maxilla (our unpublished observations). The above results suggest that TAJ may be involved in craniofacial development and ectodermal differentiation. In adult human tissues, major expression of TAJ is seen in prostate gland, brain, heart, and lungs *(17,18)*. The TAJ/TROY gene has been mapped to the central region of the mouse chromosome 14 *(18)*. Interestingly, the genetic defect in *waved coat* (*Wc*) mice, which present with abnormalities in skin and hair, have been mapped to the same region *(18)*. It remains to be seen whether the genetic defect in *Wc* mice involves TAJ/TROY.

Activation of the NF-κB pathway by TAJ/TROY is controversial. While we have reported the inability of TAJ to activate the NF-κB pathway *(17)*, Kojima et al. reported NF-κB activation upon transient transfection of TROY in 293T cells *(18)*. Unfortunately, the TAJ ligand is yet to be cloned and, therefore, the physiological significance of the NF-κB activation upon overexpression of the receptor is not clear. Unlike the NF-κB pathway, TAJ is a strong activator of the JNK pathway, and this activity cannot be blocked by dominant-negative mutants of ASK1 *(17)*. Thus, although both XEDAR and TAJ activate the JNK pathway, they appear to utilize different signaling intermediates. Finally, like the situation with EDAR, transient transfection-based overexpression of TAJ is known to induce cellular rounding detachment and cell death, and this process is independent of the activation of the caspase cascade *(17)*. Consistent with the above results and lack of a death domain in its cytoplasmic region, TAJ does not interact with TRADD or FADD *(17)*. However, TAJ is known to coimmunoprecipitate with TRAF1, -2, and -3 upon overexpression in 293T cells *(17)*. Again, the physiological relevance of these interactions and TAJ-induced cell death awaits the isolation of its ligand.

CONCLUSION

The members of the TNF family and their receptors have been known to play a central role in the regulation of cellular proliferation, activation, and programmed cell death *(34)*. The recent discovery of mutations in ligands and receptors of this family in patients with ectodermal dysplasias has led to an increased appreciation of the role of this family in the regulation of embryonic development and epithelial morphogenesis *(4,12,25,35)*. Abnormalities in developmentally regulated genes have been implicated in several human malignancies. It remains to be seen whether dysregulated expression and/or activity of EDAR and its homologs similarly play a role in the pathogenesis of human carcinomas and whether their death-inducing ability can be exploited for cancer treatment.

ACKNOWLEDGMENT

This work was supported by grants from the March of Dimes Foundation, Children's Cancer Fund, and the Department of Defense Breast Cancer Research Program (DAMD17-02-1-590), which is managed by the U.S. Army Medical Research and Materiel Command.

REFERENCES:

1. Freire-Maia N, Pinheiro M. Ectodermal dysplasias: a clinical and genetic study. Alan R. Liss, New York: 1984.
2. Darwin C. The variation of animals and plants under domestication. Vol. II. John Murray, London: 1875:319.
3. Pinheiro M, Freire-Maia N. Ectodermal dysplasias: a clinical classification and a causal review. Am J Med Genet 1994;53:153–162.
4. Kere J, Srivastava AK, Montonen O, et al. X-linked anhidrotic (hypohidrotic) ectodermal dysplasia is caused by mutation in a novel transmembrane protein. Nat Genet 1996;13:409–416.
5. Srivastava AK, Pispa J, Hartung AJ, et al. The Tabby phenotype is caused by mutation in a mouse homologue of the EDA gene that reveals novel mouse and human exons and encodes a protein (ectodysplasin-A) with collagenous domains. Proc Natl Acad Sci USA 1997;94:13,069–13,074.
6. Ferguson BM, Brockdorff N, Formstone E, Ngyuen T, Kronmiller JE, Zonana J. Cloning of Tabby, the murine homolog of the human EDA gene: evidence for a membrane-associated protein with a short collagenous domain. Hum Mol Genet 1997;6:1589–1594.
7. Mikkola ML, Pispa J, Pekkanen M, et al. Ectodysplasin, a protein required for epithelial morphogenesis, is a novel TNF homologue and promotes cell-matrix adhesion. Mechanisms of Development 1999;88:133–146.
8. Chen Y, Molloy SS, Thomas L, et al. Mutations within a furin consensus sequence block proteolytic release of ectodysplasin-A and cause X-linked hypohidrotic ectodermal dysplasia. Proc Natl Acad Sci USA 2001;98:7218–7223.
9. Schneider P, Street SL, Gaide O, et al. Mutations leading to X-linked hypohidrotic ectodermal dysplasia affect three major functional domains in the tumor necrosis factor family member ectodysplasin-A. J Biol Chem 2001;276:18,819–18,827.
10. Elomaa O, Pulkkinen K, Hannelius U, Mikkola M, Saarialho-Kere U, Kere J. Ectodysplasin is released by proteolytic shedding and binds to the EDAR protein. Hum Mol Gen 2001; 10:953–962.
11. Monreal AW, Zonana J, Ferguson B. Identification of a new splice form of the EDA1 gene permits detection of nearly all X-linked hypohidrotic ectodermal dysplasia mutations.[erratum appears in Am J Hum Genet 1998 Oct;63(4):1253–1255]. Am J Hum Gen 1998;63:380–389.
12. Bayes M, Hartung AJ, Ezer S, et al. The anhidrotic ectodermal dysplasia gene (EDA) undergoes alternative splicing and encodes ectodysplasin-A with deletion mutations in collagenous repeats. Hum Mol Genet 1998;7:1661–1669.
13. Yan M, Wang LC, Hymowitz SG, et al. Two-amino acid molecular switch in an epithelial morphogen that regulates binding to two distinct receptors. Science 2000;290:523–527.
14. Headon DJ, Overbeek PA. Involvement of a novel Tnf receptor homologue in hair follicle induction. Nat Genet 1999;22:370–374.
15. Monreal AW, Ferguson BM, Headon DJ, Street SL, Overbeek PA, Zonana J. Mutations in the human homologue of mouse dl cause autosomal recessive and dominant hypohidrotic ectodermal dysplasia. Nat Genet 1999;22:366–369.
16. Kumar A, Eby MT, Sinha S, Jasmin A, Chaudhary PM. Ectodermal dysplasia receptor activates the nuclear factor kappa B, c-Jun N-terminal kinase and cell death pathways and binds to ectodysplasin A. J Biol Chem 2001;276:2668–2677.
17. Eby MT, Jasmin A, Kumar A, Sharma K, Chaudhary PM. TAJ, a novel member of the tumor necrosis factor receptor family, activates the c-Jun N-terminal kinase pathway and mediates caspase-independent cell death. J Biol Chem 2000;275:15,336–15,342.
18. Kojima T, Morikawa Y, Copeland NG, et al. TROY, a newly identified member of the tumor necrosis factor receptor superfamily, exhibits a homology with Edar and is expressed in embryonic skin and hair follicles. J Biol Chem 2000;275:20,742–20,747.

19. Aggarwal BB. Tumour necrosis factors receptor associated signalling molecules and their role in activation of apoptosis, JNK and NF-kappaB. Ann Rheum Dis 2000;59 Suppl 1:i6–i16.
20. Koppinen P, Pispa J, Laurikkala J, Thesleff I, Mikkola ML. Signaling and subcellular localization of the TNF receptor Edar. Exp Cell Res 2001;269:180–192.
21. Headon DJ, Emmal SA, Ferguson BM, et al. Gene defect in ectodermal dysplasia implicates a death domain adapter in development. Nature 2001;414:913–916.
22. Yan M, Zhang Z, Brady JR, Schilbach S, Fairbrother WJ, Dixit VM. Identification of a novel death domain-containing adaptor molecule for ectodysplasin-A receptor that is mutated in *crinkled* mice. Curr Biol 2002;12:409–413.
23. Israel A. The IKK complex: an integrator of all signals that activate NF-kappaB? Trends Cell Biol 2000;10:129–133.
24. Zonana J, Elder ME, Schneider LC, et al. A novel X-linked disorder of immune deficiency and hypohidrotic ectodermal dysplasia is allelic to incontinentia pigmenti and due to mutations in IKK-gamma (NEMO). Am J Hum Genet 2000;67:1555–1562.
25. Doffinger R, Smahi A, Bessia C, et al. X-linked anhidrotic ectodermal dysplasia with immunodeficiency is caused by impaired NF-kappaB signaling. Nat Genet 2001;27:277–285.
26. Dupuis-Girod S, Corradini N, Hadj-Rabia S, et al. Osteopetrosis, lymphedema, anhidrotic ectodermal dysplasia, and immunodeficiency in a boy and incontinentia pigmenti in his mother. Pediatrics 2002;109:e97.
27. Sinha SK, Zachariah S, Quinones HI, Shindo M, Chaudhary PM. Role of TRAF3 and -6 in the activation of the NF-kappa B and JNK pathways by X-linked ectodermal dysplasia receptor. J Biol Chem 2002;277:44,953–44,961.
28. Ye H, Park YC, Kreishman M, Kieff E, Wu H. The structural basis for the recognition of diverse receptor sequences by TRAF2. Mol Cell 1999;4:321–330.
29. Qian Y, Zhao Z, Jiang Z, Li X. Role of NFkappa B activator Act1 in CD40-mediated signaling in epithelial cells. Proc Natl Acad Sci USA 2002;99:9386–9391.
30. Ye H, Arron JR, Lamothe B, et al. Distinct molecular mechanism for initiating TRAF6 signalling. Nature 2002;418:443–447.
31. Naito A, Yoshida H, Nishioka E, et al. TRAF6-deficient mice display hypohidrotic ectodermal dysplasia. Proc Natl Acad Sci USA 2002;99:8766–8771.
32. Smahi A, Courtois G, Rabia SH, et al. The NF-kappaB signalling pathway in human diseases: from incontinentia pigmenti to ectodermal dysplasias and immune-deficiency syndromes. Hum Mol Genet 2002;11:2371–2375.
33. Srivastava AK, Durmowicz MC, Hartung AJ, et al. Ectodysplasin-A1 is sufficient to rescue both hair growth and sweat glands in Tabby mice. Hum Mol Genet 2001;10:2973–2981.
34. Locksley RM, Killeen N, Lenardo MJ. The TNF and TNF receptor superfamilies: integrating mammalian biology. Cell 2001;104:487–501.
35. Munoz F, Lestringant G, Sybert V, et al. Definitive evidence for an autosomal recessive form of hypohidrotic ectodermal dysplasia clinically indistinguishable from the more common X-linked disorder. Am J Hum Genet 1997;61:94–100.

5 Adaptor Proteins in Death Receptor Signaling

Nien-Jung Chen, PhD
and Wen-Chen Yeh, MD, PhD

SUMMARY

Signal transduction induced by death receptors belonging to the tumor necrosis factor receptor (TNFR) superfamily has been an area of intensive research for the past several years. The major advances arising from these studies have been the characterization of critical signal-transducing adaptor molecules and the delineation of parallel but opposing signaling pathways, some inducing apoptosis and others promoting cell survival. An imbalance in favor of either apoptosis or cell survival can have disastrous pathological consequences, including cancer, autoimmunity, or immune deficiency. Many adaptor proteins have been reported in the literature to be involved in death receptor signaling. In this chapter, we will focus on molecules whose functions have been investigated by multiple approaches, particularly gene targeting in mice and ex vivo biochemical studies. By validating or clarifying the function of each adaptor, we hope to construct a blueprint of the various signaling channels triggered by death receptors, providing a foundation for further scientific investigations and practical therapeutic designs.

INTRODUCTION

Cancer biologists and oncologists have struggled for years to devise ways of eradicating cancer cells while sparing normal ones. One breakthrough that has emerged during the past decade has been the investigation of the molecular mechanisms of apoptosis *(1)*. Apoptosis is a critical physiological process that is subject to intricate regulation. Indeed, many cancers arise from the dysregulation of apoptotic or antiapoptotic signals, and such dysregulation is often attributable to mutation or altered expression of specific molecules *(1,2)*. The elucidation of the nature of the individual signaling proteins in pathways leading to apoptosis or antiapoptosis has become a central issue in cancer biology as well as in tissue development and immune system regulation.

From: *Cancer Drug Discovery and Development: Death Receptors in Cancer Therapy*
Edited by: W. S. El-Deiry © Humana Press Inc., Totowa, NJ

Some of the most important apoptotic signaling pathways are those induced by engagement of the death receptors (DRs). The death receptors are a subset of ligand-specific cell-surface receptors belonging to the TNFR superfamily, and are characterized by the presence of a motif called the death domain (DD) in their cytoplasmic tails *(3)*. It is these death domains that confer the ability to induce apoptosis on the death receptors. Apoptosis is triggered when the death receptors are engaged by specific death factors, ligands such as Fas ligand (FasL) *(4)*, TNF *(5,6)*, TNF-like molecule 1A (TL1A) *(7)*, and TNF-related apoptosis-inducing ligand (TRAIL) *(8)*. The death factors are not only toxic to many transformed cell types in vitro but also play important roles in the regulation of immune responses. The physiological and clinical relevance of the death receptor family thus makes its study very compelling. Over the past 8 yr, the apoptosis signaling pathways induced by stimulation of various death receptors, including TNFR1 *(9,10)*, Fas (CD95) *(11,12)*, the TRAIL receptors (DR4 and DR5) *(13–16)*, DR3 *(17)*, and DR6 *(18)*, have come under intense investigation.

There are two basic models of death receptor-induced apoptosis signaling cascades: one exemplified by the engagement of Fas and the other by the engagement of TNFR1 (Fig. 1). In the first two sections of this chapter, we will discuss the adaptor proteins that are involved in Fas and TNFR1 signaling. We start with an overview of each model system and move to a detailed description of validated and putative functions of selected adaptors. A special emphasis will be placed on information gained from studies of gene-targeted "knockout mice." In the third section, we will discuss signaling pathways triggered by other death receptors that share features with our model systems but also contain some unique adaptor proteins. In the final section, we will discuss perspectives on questions in death receptor signaling that remain to be answered and on the knowledge that can potentially be garnered from studies of new adaptor proteins.

STIMULATION OF FAS TRIGGERS A "SUPERHIGHWAY" APOPTOTIC SIGNAL

Engagement of Fas triggers a swift and efficient apoptotic signal. The first event following the binding of the death factor FasL to Fas is the direct recruitment of Fas-associated death domain protein (FADD) *(19,20)* to the cytoplasmic tail of Fas. As we shall see in the following sections, FADD is the common adaptor protein upon which almost all death receptor signaling pathways converge *(21)* (Fig. 1). FADD binds to Fas through the interaction of their homologous death domains, an event that unmasks the N-terminal death-effector domain (DED) of FADD. The DED allows FADD to then recruit caspase-8 (also called FLICE) *(22,23)* to the growing complex of proteins, which is now called the "death-inducing signaling complex" (DISC) *(24)*. The interaction of the DISC with caspase-8 activates the latter, possibly by auto-proteolytic processing *(25)*, and activated caspase-8 in turn triggers the caspase cascade. Caspase-8 either directly activates execution caspases *(26)*, or cleaves Bid (BH3 interacting domain death agonist) which leads to activation of the mitochondrial apoptotic pathway *(27)*. The involvement of FLICE-associated huge protein (FLASH) *(28)*, a protein that binds to and activates caspase-8, will be discussed in another chapter of this book. One of the controls of apoptotic signaling takes effect at the level of caspase-8. Recruitment of caspase-8 to the DISC can be inhibited by cellular FLICE-inhibitory protein (c-FLIP) *(29)*, a protein that plays a crucial role in keeping Fas-mediated apoptosis in check.

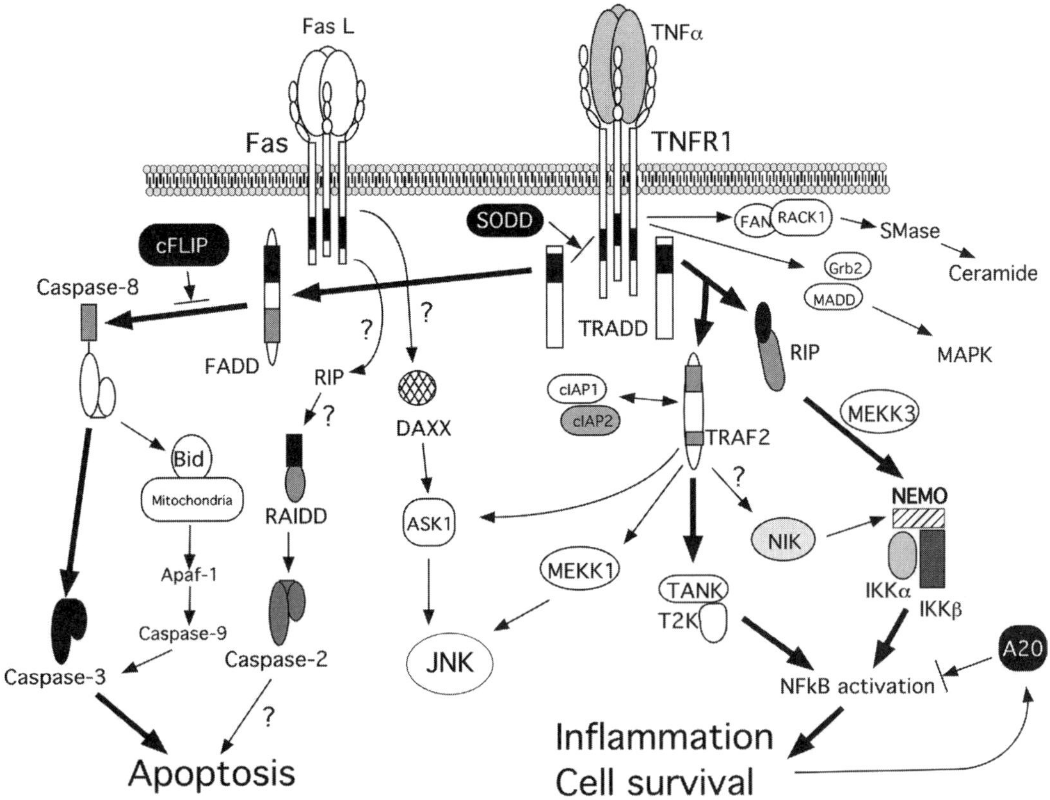

Fig. 1. Signaling pathways modulated by Fas (left) and TNFR1 (right).

Several other molecules have been implicated in minor pathways of death receptor-mediated apoptosis. It has recently been proposed that an alternative apoptotic pathway can be triggered by Fas via direct recruitment of death domain-associated protein (DAXX) *(30)*. DAXX activates apoptosis signal-regulated kinase 1 (ASK1) which in turn activates the downstream c-Jun N-terminal kinase (JNK) pathway *(31)*. Others have reported that Fas engagement may trigger necrosis in a process that requires the recruitment of receptor-interacting protein (RIP) *(32)* and FADD *(33)*. Finally, association of RIP with RIP-associated ICH-1/CED-3-homologous protein (RAIDD) *(34,35)* followed by recruitment of caspase-2 has been implicated in death receptor-induced apoptotic signaling. In the following sub-sections, we will discuss most of the adaptor proteins mentioned above with the exception of RIP (which will be discussed in the section headed "Signaling by TNFR1 Triggers Both Apoptotic and Antiapoptotic Pathways").

FADD

The majority of genetic and biochemical studies addressing FADD function have provided evidence that this molecule is not only essential for Fas-mediated apoptosis but also plays a key role in almost all death receptor-induced apoptosis *(19–21)*. In addition, FADD is required for a recently described pathway of T-cell necrosis that is mediated by

Fas or TRAIL but is independent of caspase-8 *(33)*. Paradoxically, FADD is also required for embryonic cell survival, particularly at the stage of heart ventricular development *(36)*. The precise function of FADD in embryogenesis remains to be determined. At the cellular level, FADD-deficient T-cells exhibit a defect in T-cell receptor (TCR)-mediated proliferation and deregulation of the cell-cycle machinery *(37,38)*. The involvement of FADD in heart development and T-cell proliferation implies functions for this molecule in addition to its role as a common proapoptotic adaptor for death receptor signaling, and further suggests that death receptor functions may extend beyond inducing cell death.

Caspase-8 and c-FLIP

Caspase-8 is the key initiator caspase acting downstream of FADD during apoptosis induced by Fas and other death receptors *(22,23,39)*. Not surprisingly, caspase-8-deficient cells are highly resistant to Fas- and death receptor-mediated apoptosis. Interestingly, caspase-8-knockout mice die during embryogenesis and exhibit a heart defect similar to that observed in FADD-deficient embryos *(40)*. Caspase-8-deficient T-cells also show defects in TCR-mediated proliferation. However, unlike FADD-deficient T-cells, caspase-8-deficient T-cells have a normal cell cycle. Curiously, caspase-8-deficient T-cells stimulated via their TCRs fail to expand due to a paradoxical increase in cell death *(41)*.

The function of c-FLIP as an inhibitor of caspase-8 recruitment *(29)* led researchers to assume that c-FLIP-deficient mice would exhibit phenotypes opposite to those of FADD- or caspase-8-knockout mice. Indeed, cells lacking c-FLIP become highly sensitive to apoptosis induced by FasL as well as by other death factors such as TNF and TRAIL (V. Wong and W-C. Yeh, unpublished results). However, embryos lacking c-FLIP unexpectedly show a defect in heart development analogous to that in FADD- or caspase-8-knockouts *(42)*. The mystery is deepened by the observation that the developing heart tissues of FADD- or c-FLIP-deficient embryos show normal apoptosis in vivo. With respect to T lymphocytes, c-FLIP may play a role in responses to TCR engagement, since T-cells overexpressing c-FLIP show enhanced proliferation in response to TCR stimulation *(43)*. Taken together, these results imply that FADD, caspase-8 and c-FLIP function in the cytoplasm as a block and are involved in signaling pathways in addition to death receptor-mediated apoptosis. These interactions may be cooperative or antagonistic in nature, and may depend on other players present in each unique signaling context.

Bid

Bid is a proapoptotic Bcl-2 family member that is recruited and cleaved by caspase-8 *(44)*. Cleaved Bid then translocates to the mitochondria, where it mediates cytochrome c release and apoptotic changes *(27,45)*. Bid-deficient mice are resistant to the anti-Fas antibody-induced hepatocyte apoptosis that kills wild-type mice. However, a milder defect of FasL- or TNF-induced apoptosis has been observed in Bid-deficient thymocytes and mouse embryonic fibroblasts (MEF), suggesting that, depending on tissue type, death receptor-induced apoptosis may or may not depend on Bid *(46)*. Interestingly, Bid-deficient mice develop myeloid hyperplasia and chronic leukemia-like disorders, indicating that Bid and death receptor-mediated apoptosis are essential for maintaining myeloid cell homeostasis *(47)*.

DAXX, ASK1, RAIDD AND CASPASE-2

The functions of DAXX, ASK1, RAIDD, and caspase-2 in Fas- or death receptor-mediated apoptosis remain controversial. For example, DAXX is proapoptotic when overexpressed and triggers the activation of JNK via ASK1 *(30,31)*. However, gene targeting and RNAi knock-down experiments suggest that DAXX antagonizes antiapoptosis *(48,49)*. Like FADD, DAXX is essential for embryonic development. Genetic evidence has also shown that ASK1 is tightly linked to the activation of JNK mediated by TNF or endoplasmic reticulum (ER) stress *(31,50)*. However, a gene-targeting study has indicated that TNF-, but not Fas-, induced apoptosis requires the presence of ASK1 *(51)*. An interesting alternative to the FADD/caspase-8 pathway of death receptor-mediated apoptosis may be the recruitment by RIP of RAIDD and subsequently caspase-2 *(34,35)*. Whereas FADD and caspase-8 are essential for Fas-mediated apoptosis, the RIP–RAIDD–caspase-2 pathway may be relevant for apoptosis induced by engagement of other death receptors. Although there has been no report as yet on RAIDD-deficient mice, introduction of a dominant negative form of RAIDD fails to inhibit FasL-mediated cell death *(52)*. Furthermore, caspase-2-deficient cells do not exhibit a defect in either Fas- or TNF-mediated apoptosis *(53)*.

SIGNALING BY TNFR1 TRIGGERS BOTH APOPTOTIC AND ANTIAPOPTOTIC PATHWAYS

The TNFR1 signaling cascade is one of the best characterized receptor signaling systems. The effects of TNF are mediated by two cell-surface receptors, TNFR1 and TNFR2, but only TNFR1 contains a DD *(54)*. At the cellular level, TNF stimulation of TNFR1 activates either a cell suicide program or an antideath activity. As shown in Fig. 1, TNFR-associated death-domain protein (TRADD), an adaptor protein that binds directly to the DD of TNFR1, can transduce signals both for apoptosis and for NF-κB activation leading to cell survival *(55,56)*. For the apoptotic arm, the first event is the recruitment of FADD by TRADD through the interaction of their homologous death domains. Caspase-8 activation and downstream signaling events follow that are similar to those constituting the Fas-mediated cascade. The adaptors involved in TNFR1-mediated apoptotic signaling are thus essentially the same as those discussed in the previous section.

For the cell-survival arm of TNFR1 signaling, TRADD recruits TNFR-associated factor-2 (TRAF2) and RIP to the TNFR1 complex *(56–58)*. These molecules then trigger the recruitment of additional mediators that promote NF-κB activation. NF-κB is a key transcription factor whose activation can lead to cell survival. Mice lacking RelA (p65), a principal subunit of NF-κB, die during embryogenesis due to massive liver apoptosis *(59)*. NF-κB is normally held inactive in the cytoplasm by its association with the inhibitor protein IκB (inhibitor of NF-κB) *(60)*. To activate NF-κB, IκB must be removed via phosphorylation followed by ubiquitination and proteasomal degradation. Phosphorylation of IκB *(61)* is mediated primarily by the IκB kinase (IKK) complex containing the proteins IKKα, IKKβ *(62)* and NEMO (NF-κB essential modulator; also known as IKKγ) *(63)*. In response to TNF, RIP recruits NEMO and also interacts with MEKK-3, stimulating degradation of IκB *(64)*. Another study has suggested that TRAF2 may be involved in recruiting IKK *(65)*. In this section, we will discuss each of the adaptor proteins functioning in TNFR1-mediated NF-κB activation.

It is important to point out that the many signaling cascades co-existing in a cell have effects on each other, and that TNF-mediated NF-κB activation may also be regulated in part by the actions of protein kinase B (PKB/Akt) *(66)*, protein kinase Cζ (PKCζ) *(67)* and glycogen synthase kinase 3β (GSK3β) *(68)*. Although knockout animal models for these proteins are available, these molecules are not canonical adaptors, and their positions in the TNFR1 signaling cascade remain to be determined *(69,70)*. A discussion of these proteins is thus beyond the scope of this chapter.

TRAF2 is a central player in TNFR1-mediated antiapoptotic signaling. As well as its direct involvement in TNFR1-mediated NF-κB activation, TRAF2 can mediate TNF-induced activation of the JNK pathway. TRAF2 interacts with upstream mediators in this pathway such as the mitogen-activated protein kinase kinase kinase (MAP3K) family members ASK1 *(50)*, NF-κB-inducing kinase (NIK) *(71)*, and MEKK-3 *(64)*. Also associated with TRAF2 is the protein complex of TANK (TRAF family member associated NF-κB activator, also called I-TRAF) *(72)* and T2K (TRAF2-associated kinase, also called TBK1 or NAK) *(73,74)*. In addition, TRAF2 recruits cellular inhibitor of apoptosis protein 1 and 2 (cIAP1 and cIAP2) to TNFR1 *(75)*. The functions of the cIAPs in death receptor signaling remain to be resolved. Each of these adaptors is discussed in the following sections.

TNF is capable of triggering a plethora of cellular responses in addition to apoptosis and activation of NF-κB and JNK. For example, TNF stimulation leads to activation of ERK/MAPK, p38 MAPK, and sphinogomyelinase *(76,77)*, as well as ceramide production and the generation of reactive oxygen species. The molecular mechanisms underlying these events are largely unknown. Fittingly, there are several adaptor proteins that interact with TNFR1 but whose functions remain to be defined, including BRE, Grb2, MADD, FAN, PIP5K, and p60TRAK (for more detail, see review by MacEwan *[78]*). Some of these adaptors may have pathway-specific functions, as exemplified by the putative roles of Grb2 *(79)* and MADD *(80)* in the TNF-mediated MAPK pathway. Interaction of FAN (factor associated with neutral sphingomyelinase activation) with TNFR1 may lead to sphingomyelinase activation and also contribute to the induction of apoptosis *(77)*. Among these adaptors, FAN will be discussed further in this section since its function in TNF signaling has been extensively studied.

Adaptors are also involved in the regulation of TNF-induced signaling. For example, the TNFR1 signaling cascade is controlled by an auto-regulatory and feedback inhibition mechanism. The adaptor silencer of death domain (SODD) is thought to bind directly to TNFR1 and inhibit any accidental triggering of ligand-independent TNFR1 oligomerization *(81)*. In contrast, A20 is a protein induced by TNF-mediated NF-κB signaling that is recruited to the TNFR1 signaling complex by TRAF2 to inhibit further triggering of NF-κB activation *(82)*. These interesting regulatory mechanisms have been explored in knockout mice and will be discussed at the end of this section.

TRADD

No knockout studies have been reported for TRADD. However, given the complicated picture of TNFR1 signaling, it is unlikely that a deficiency of TRADD would abrogate the entire signaling cascade. Overexpression of TRADD activates both apoptotic and cell-survival signals *(55)*. It will be very intriguing to determine the effect of TRADD deficiency on the cell-death/survival decision triggered by TNF. TRADD (and FADD) are also involved in acid sphingomyelinase activation, an event that may contribute to TNF cytotoxicity *(83)*.

TRAF2

Overexpression studies have indicated that TRAF2 plays a critical role in transducing signals initiated by engagement of TNFR1 and several other TNFR superfamily members *(84)*. Biochemical examination of *TRAF2*$^{-/-}$ cells shows a severe reduction in TNF-mediated JNK activation. However, TRAF2 deficiency has only a mild effect on TNF-induced NF-κB activation, in that the kinetics of NF-κB activation are delayed and the intensity of NF-κB DNA-binding activity is mildly reduced in mutant MEF *(85)*. These results suggest that TRAF2-independent pathway(s) of TNF-induced NF-κB activation exist. As we will see in the following section, RIP plays a critical role in TRAF2-independent TNF-mediated NF-κB activation. Interestingly, TNF-induced NF-κB activation is normal in cells lacking TRAF5 *(86)*, a protein homologous to TRAF2. However, cells lacking both TRAF2 and TRAF5 show more severe impairment of NF-κB activation than TNF-stimulated *TRAF2*$^{-/-}$ cells *(87)*. This result suggests that TRAF2 and TRAF5 have redundant roles in TNF-stimulated NF-κB activation.

Roughly half of TRAF2-deficient animals die at E14.5 with massive liver apoptosis, a phenotype strikingly similar to that of mice with a severe impairment of NF-κB activation. Furthermore, TRAF2-deficient thymocytes, hematopoietic progenitors, and MEFs are highly sensitive to TNF-induced cell death. TRAF2-deficient mice that survive birth are runty, devoid of fat deposits, and have reduced muscle mass. Moribund mutant mice have elevated basal levels of serum TNF, and show depletion of thymocytes, B-cell precursors, and peripheral lymphocytes *(85)*. Intriguingly, *TRAF2*$^{-/-}$ *TNFR1*$^{-/-}$ and *TRAF2*$^{-/-}$*TNF*$^{-/-}$ mutants are viable and generally healthy, indicating that much of the pathology in *TRAF2*$^{-/-}$ mice is due to deregulated effects of TNF *(88)*. In addition, TRAF2-deficient macrophages are hypersensitive to TNF stimulation and produce copious quantities of inflammatory cytokines and mediators *(88)*. Although the molecular mechanism of this phenomenon remains to be delineated, it seems that TRAF2 may anchor the negative regulation of TNF signal transduction that appears to be exerted at later time points during TNF stimulation.

RIP

RIP is a death domain-containing adaptor protein. Originally identified by its interaction with Fas, RIP is also recruited to TNFR1 upon ligand stimulation and can interact with TNFR1, TRADD, and TRAF2 *(32,58)*. Analysis of RIP-deficient mice has shown that RIP plays a role in TNF-induced NF-κB activation. *RIP*$^{-/-}$ mice appear normal at birth but fail to thrive, dying at 1–3 d of age with extensive apoptosis in both lymphoid and adipose tissues *(89)*. Given the function of RIP in TNF-mediated NF-κB activation, it is interesting to note that RIP can be cleaved upon caspase-8 activation and that the cleavage of RIP blocks NF-κB activation *(90)*. RIP is dispensable for TNF-mediated JNK activation and apoptosis induction. However, a recent study has suggested that RIP is involved in necrotic death induced by TNF or TRAIL *(91)*. Although RIP is not required for the development of B-lymphocytes or the myeloid lineages, RIP appears to be involved in T-cell development, and RIP-deficient thymocytes are highly sensitive to TNF-induced cell death *(92)*. Interestingly, unlike *TRAF2*$^{-/-}$ mice, thymocyte apoptosis associated with

RIP deficiency is not rescued by the elimination of TNFR1, but is restored by an absence of TNFR2. TNFR2 has been implicated in the apoptosis of Jurkat T-cells induced by TNF. In this context, TNFR2 induces apoptosis only in the presence of RIP, but does not require RIP to signal for NF-κB activation *(92)*.

MAP3Ks

During the induction of cell survival by TNFR1 engagement, a number of MAP3K family members associate with TRAF2 or RIP (Fig. 1). The kinase NIK was initially proposed to be the downstream target of TRAF2 in mediating TNF-induced NF-κB *(71)*. However, NIK-deficient mice show a specific defect in LTβR signaling and lymph node development, and cells lacking NIK respond normally to TNF by activating NF-κB *(93)*. The kinase MEKK-1 has also been implicated in TNF-induced NF-κB activation *(94)*. In addition, MEKK-1 and ASK-1 have been reported to mediate TRAF2-triggered JNK activation. From studies of knockout mice, however, it seems that MEKK-1 is required for TNF-induced JNK activation only in embryonic stem cells but not in fibroblasts or T-cells *(95)*. ASK-1 is not required for early phase TNF-induced JNK activation, but *ASK-1*$^{-/-}$ cells exhibit a partial defect in sustained JNK activation *(51,96)*.

Recently, a new member of the MEKK family called MEKK-3 has been found to associate with RIP and can directly phosphorylate IKK, meaning that it could potentially play a role in downstream survival signaling *(64)*. Indeed, disruption of MEKK-3 severely impairs the activation of NF-κB induced by TNF, and *MEKK-3*$^{-/-}$ cells are highly sensitive to TNF-induced apoptosis. MEKK-3-deficient embryos die at E10.5-11 just as the fetal liver starts to develop *(97)*. MEKK-3 may promote NF-κB activation induced by proinflammatory cytokines by linking RIP to the IKK complex.

NEMO

NEMO-deficient mice display a phenotype of fetal liver apoptosis and embryonic lethality, consistent with an essential role for NEMO in signaling leading to NF-κB activation *(98)*. Like *RelA*$^{-/-}$ and *IKKβ*$^{-/-}$ cells *(59,99)*, *NEMO*$^{-/-}$ cells show an increased susceptibility to TNF-induced apoptosis. NEMO is an X-linked gene, and female *NEMO*$^{+/-}$ mice develop a self-limiting inflammatory skin disorder characterized by hyperkeratosis and increased apoptosis. This phenotype is presumably dependent on X-chromosome inactivation. Importantly, these symptoms are reminiscent of incontinentia pigmenti, an X-linked dominant hereditary disease in humans. Indeed, genetic studies of incontinentia pigmenti patients have revealed mutations in the NEMO gene and defects in NF-κB activation in the majority of cases *(100,101)*.

TANK and T2K

NF-κB activation can occur via signaling pathways that are independent of the IKK complex. T2K (also called TBK and NAK) *(73,74)* associates with TRAF2 through an intermediary adaptor protein called TANK *(72)*. T2K is a serine threonine kinase that is distantly related to IKKα and IKKβ. T2K phosphorylates serine 36 on the IκBα subunit of IκB, but does so only weakly, such that degradation of IκB is not triggered. Although no study of *TANK*$^{-/-}$ mice has been reported to date, T2K-deficient mice have been generated and analyzed. *T2K*$^{-/-}$ cells show normal IκB phosphorylation and degradation, normal NF-κB translocation into the nucleus, and normal NF-κB binding to target DNA sequences in response to TNF and interleukin-1. However, NF-κB transactivation activity is decreased in cells lacking T2K *(74)*. Consistent with the latter observation, *T2K*$^{-/-}$ mice show liver apoptosis and embryonic lethality similar to that in mice lacking RelA *(59,102)*, IKKβ *(99)*, or NEMO *(95)*. Furthermore, elimination of TNFR1 rescues T2K-deficient mice from embryonic lethality, and the double-knockout animals survive for extended periods with no gross abnormalities *(74)*.

cIAP proteins

cIAP1 and cIAP2 belong to a family of IAP proteins that generally inhibit apoptosis by interacting with caspases and blocking their enzymatic activities *(103)*. Although no knockout studies of cIAP1 and cIAP2 have been reported to date, deletion of XIAP, a close homolog of the cIAPs, causes no obvious defects in mice *(104)*. Interestingly, overexpression of XIAP or the baculoviral IAP homolog in T-cells results in altered T-cell homeostasis and resistance to apoptosis *(104)*. The effects of cIAP1 and cIAP2 on TNF-mediated apoptosis remain unclear. cIAP1 and cIAP2 can be recruited by TRAF2 to the receptor complex, and cIAP1 and cIAP2 contain RING domains. These observations have led to speculation that cIAP1 and cIAP2 may function as E3-ligase. Indeed, one study has suggested that cIAP2 may direct the ubiquitination of caspase-3 and caspase-7. However, a more recent study has shown that cIAP1, but not cIAP2, is involved in TRAF2 ubiquitination and degradation induced by TNFR2 signaling, and can thus potentiate TNF-induced apoptosis *(105,106)*.

FAN

FAN binds to TNFR1 through a cytoplasmic region that is distinct from the death domain and required for activation of neutral sphingomyelinase (N-Smase) and ceramide generation *(77)*. Indeed, FAN-deficient mice fail to activate N-Smase in response to TNF and demonstrate a defect in epidermal barrier repair. Interestingly, evidence from studies of FAN knockout mice and FAN-dominant negative mutants indicates that the FAN-dependent pathway may also play a role in TNF-mediated apoptosis *(107,108)*. Recently, RACK1 (receptor for activated C-kinase 1) was identified as a binding partner of FAN that is involved in TNF-mediated N-Smase activation *(109)*.

A20 and SODD

SODD *(81)* and A20 are adaptors that are thought to regulate TNFR1 signaling via distinct mechanisms. SODD-deficient mice display a mild enhancement of TNF responses. In vitro work has shown that SODD associates constitutively with TNFR1, perhaps preventing the recruitment of TRADD and other downstream signal transducers until the receptor is stimulated by ligand. These data suggest that SODD may function as a gatekeeper type of inhibitor. In contrast, A20 is a cytoplasmic zinc finger-containing protein whose expression is rapidly induced after TNF stimulation. Overexpression studies have shown that A20 interacts with both TRAF1 and TRAF2 and can inhibit both NF-κB activation and TNF-mediated cell death *(82,110)*. Studies of A20-deficient mice have demonstrated that A20 is a key negative regulator of TNF signaling. *A20*$^{-/-}$ mice are runty, develop severe multi-organ inflammation, and die prematurely. These mutant animals are also highly susceptible to sublethal doses of LPS or TNF. *A20*$^{-/-}$ cells exhibit prolonged NF-κB activation in response to TNF stimulation and are more sensitive to

TNF-induced apoptosis. A20 must physically bind to the TNFR signaling complex in order to quench the transduction of newly initiated signals *(111)*. A20 can interact with two other proteins, ABIN-1 and ABIN-2, which overexpression studies have shown can also inhibit NF-κB activation *(110,112,113)*. Further investigation of the physiological functions of these molecules will expand our understanding of mechanisms underlying the negative feedback regulation of TNF signaling.

ADAPTOR PROTEINS THAT TRANSDUCE SIGNALS INITIATED BY OTHER DEATH RECEPTORS

In this section, we discuss death receptors other than Fas and TNFR1 whose engagement induces apoptosis. DR3 *(17)* and DR6 *(18)* are capable of recruiting TRADD, whereas DR4 and DR5 (the TRAIL receptors) *(114)* appear to interact directly with FADD. Thereafter, signaling associated with DR3 and DR6 generally follows that described above for the TNFR1 and Fas models, respectively. We will focus on studies that emphasize the unique features of signaling induced by engagement of these death receptors. We will also discuss ectodermal dysplasia receptor (EDAR) *(115)* and nerve growth factor receptor (NGFR) *(116)*, receptors that contain death domains in their cytoplasmic tails but use signaling pathways that are distinct from the Fas and TNFR1 models.

DR3 Signaling

DR3 is highly homologous to TNFR1 and is preferentially expressed in lymphocytes *(17)*. Although Tweak/Apop3L has been reported to bind to DR3, more recent studies suggest that TL1A may be the physiological ligand for DR3. Based on overexpression experiments, engagement of DR3, like TNFR1, results in the recruitment of TRADD and the subsequent association of FADD, RIP, and TRAF2 with the signaling complex. Triggering of DR3 by TL1A can activate caspase-dependent apoptosis in an erythroleukemic cell line, and NF-κB activation in mitogen-activated primary T-cells *(7)*.

DR4 and DR5 Signaling

Five receptors (DR4, DR5, DcR1, DcR2, and OPG) have been reported to bind to TRAIL. Whereas all these receptors contain conserved extracellular domains that allow them to associate with TRAIL, only DR4 and DR5 also contain compact intracellular death domains that are capable of transducing signals *(114)*. Similar to Fas signaling, TRAIL signaling leading to apoptosis requires FADD and caspase-8 activation *(117–119)*. Overexpression of Bcl-2 or Bcl-xL delays, but does not inhibit, TRAIL-induced apoptosis. However, TRAIL-induced apoptosis is blocked by overexpression of XIAP, CrmA, or p35 *(120)*. A putative nucleotide-binding protein called death-associated protein 3 (DAP-3) *(121)*, which was initially identified by expression cloning, has been implicated in the regulation of apoptosis associated with DR4 and DR5 *(122)*. Yeast two-hybrid and immunoprecipitation studies have shown that DAP3 serves as an adaptor protein linking DR4 and DR5 (but not Fas) to FADD. Moreover, DAP3 binds to FADD in a GTP-dependent manner. Interestingly, overexpression of a dominant-negative mutant of DAP3 suppresses apoptosis induced by engagement of DR4, DR5, or Fas *(122)*.

DR6 Signaling

The DR6 signaling pathway remains a bit of a puzzle. DR6 is expressed in a number of tissues, including lymphoid organs, but the ligand(s) binding to DR6 remains to be identified. Ectopic expression of DR6 in mammalian cells induces apoptosis but also the activation of NF-κB and JNK *(18)*. Knockout studies have shown that DR6 is an important regulator of T- and B-lymphocyte homeostasis *(101,123)*, and that DR6 is required for JNK activation linked to T-helper cell differentiation *(124)*. DR6 is capable of recruiting TRADD, but not FADD, RIP, or RAIDD, to the DD *(18)*. It is unclear whether the intracellular domain of DR6 interacts with the members of TRAF family.

EDAR Signaling

EDAR plays a key role in the process of ectodermal differentiation. The biological ligand of EDAR is ectodysplasin A (EDA). Genetic mutations of EDAR in humans (anhydrotic ectodermal dysplasia) and in mice (*downless* mice) result in similar phenotypes, including sparse hair, abnormal or missing teeth, and an inability to sweat *(125)*. Engagement of EDAR leads to NF-κB and JNK activation and the triggering of a caspase-independent cell-death pathway. Unlike other death receptors, EDAR does not interact with TRADD or FADD; it can interact with NIK and TRAF family members. Activation of NF-κB by EDAR is NIK- and IKK-dependent *(115)*. Recently, a new death domain-containing adaptor called EDAR-associated death domain (EDARADD) was found to interact with the death domain of EDAR. A mutation of EDARADD has been identified in a natural mutant mouse strain called *crinkled*, and these animals share phenotypes with *downless* mice. In vitro, EDARADD interacts primarily with TRAF2 and to a lesser extent with TRAF5 and TRAF6. EDARADD is required for DR6-mediated NF-κB activation *(126)*.

NGFR Signaling

NGFR (or p75) is an intriguing neurotrophin receptor that induces apoptosis in certain cell types but appears to have a protective role in many others. The intracellular portion of NGFR contains a TRAF-binding domain and a death domain. TRAF6 has been shown to interact with NGFR, and is potentially important for NF-κB activation induced by NGFR engagement *(127)*. Apoptosis induced by NGFR is unique among death receptors in that it involves the activation of caspase-1, caspase-2, and caspase-3, but not caspase-8. Fittingly, the DD of NGFR does not appear to bind to TRADD or FADD. Recent studies have shown that proteins such as neurotrophin receptor interacting factor (NRIF) *(128)*, SC-1 (a zinc finger protein) *(129)*, and FAP-1 (Fas-associated phosphatase 1) *(130)* may bind to NGFR cytoplasmic domains. The functions of these potential signaling adaptors remain to be investigated.

PERSPECTIVES

Signal transduction via members of the death receptor family results in a delicate balance of cell death and survival. Mutations or environmental damage leading to excessive apoptosis or an abnormal survival advantage have been causally implicated in cancers, autoimmune disorders, graft-vs-host disease, and neurodegenerative diseases. Many of these serious disorders have also been linked to death receptor-mediated signaling. It is therefore possible that proper modulation of apoptotic and survival pathways could restore the critical balance of the cell life/death decision and reverse the progression of these diseases. To this end, understanding the signal transduction mechanisms underlying apoptosis and survival signaling is essential.

As we have described in this chapter, death receptors require the recruitment of various cytoplasmic adaptors for signal transduction. The key issue is to match the many adaptors identified as associating with death receptors, with their functional places in each signaling pathway. The combined efforts of many research laboratories have resulted in the thorough investigation of the physiological functions of several adaptors and their involvement in death receptor-mediated pathways. This knowledge may lead to the development of agents that can strategically interfere with adaptor function and thus death receptor signaling. For example, compounds that can specifically inhibit TNF-induced NF-κB activation by targeting RIP or TRAF2 may be useful for the treatment of certain types of cancers. On the other hand, there remain several interesting death receptor-mediated pathways whose signaling mechanisms are still poorly understood. Studies of novel adaptors using a combination of gene targeting and biochemical approaches will be very helpful in assigning specific functions to individual signaling proteins. It is hoped that increased knowledge of these pathways and their component molecules will eventually lead to still more targets for rational therapeutic strategies.

REFERENCES

1. Green DR, Evan GI. A matter of life and death. Cancer Cell 2002;1:19–30.
2. Hanahan D, Weinberg RA. The hallmarks of cancer. Cell 2000;100:57–70.
3. Tartaglia LA, Ayres TM, Wong GH, Goeddel DV. A novel domain within the 55 kd TNF receptor signals cell death. Cell 1993;74:845–853.
4. Suda T, Takahashi T, Golstein P, Nagata S. Molecular cloning and expression of the Fas ligand, a novel member of the tumor necrosis factor family. Cell 1993;75:1169–1178.
5. Carswell EA, Old LJ, Kassel RL, Green S, Fiore N, Williamson B. An endotoxin-induced serum factor that causes necrosis of tumors. Proc Natl Acad Sci U S A 1975;72:3666–3670.
6. Beutler B, Greenwald D, Hulmes JD, et al. Identity of tumour necrosis factor and the macrophage-secreted factor cachectin. Nature 1985;316:552–554.
7. Migone TS, Zhang J, Luo X, et al. TL1A is a TNF-like ligand for DR3 and TR6/DcR3 and functions as a T cell costimulator. Immunity 2002;16:479–492.
8. Wiley SR, Schooley K, Smolak PJ, et al. Identification and characterization of a new member of the TNF family that induces apoptosis. Immunity 1995;3:673–682.
9. Lewis M, Tartaglia LA, Lee A, et al. Cloning and expression of cDNAs for two distinct murine tumor necrosis factor receptors demonstrate one receptor is species specific. Proc Natl Acad Sci USA 1991;88:2830–2834.
10. Tartaglia LA, Weber RF, Figari IS, Reynolds C, Palladino MA, Jr., Goeddel DV. The two different receptors for tumor necrosis factor mediate distinct cellular responses. Proc Natl Acad Sci USA 1991;88:9292–9296.
11. Itoh N, Yonehara S, Ishii A, et al. The polypeptide encoded by the cDNA for human cell surface antigen Fas can mediate apoptosis. Cell 1991;66:233–243.
12. Oehm A, Behrmann I, Falk W, et al. Purification and molecular cloning of the APO-1 cell surface antigen, a member of the tumor necrosis factor/nerve growth factor receptor superfamily. Sequence identity with the Fas antigen. J Biol Chem 1992;267:10,709–10,715.
13. Pan G, O'Rourke K, Chinnaiyan AM, et al. The receptor for the cytotoxic ligand TRAIL. Science 1997;276:111–113.
14. Chaudhary PM, Eby M, Jasmin A, Bookwalter A, Murray J, Hood L. Death receptor 5, a new member of the TNFR family, and DR4 induce FADD-dependent apoptosis and activate the NF-kappaB pathway. Immunity 1997;7:821–830.

15. MacFarlane M, Ahmad M, Srinivasula SM, Fernandes-Alnemri T, Cohen GM, Alnemri ES. Identification and molecular cloning of two novel receptors for the cytotoxic ligand TRAIL. J Biol Chem 1997;272:25,417–25,420.
16. Walczak H, Degli-Esposti MA, Johnson RS, et al. TRAIL-R2: a novel apoptosis-mediating receptor for TRAIL. Embo J 1997;16:5386–5397.
17. Chinnaiyan AM, O'Rourke K, Yu GL, et al. Signal transduction by DR3, a death domain-containing receptor related to TNFR-1 and CD95. Science 1996;274:990–992.
18. Pan G, Bauer JH, Haridas V, et al. Identification and functional characterization of DR6, a novel death domain-containing TNF receptor. FEBS Lett 1998;431:351–356.
19. Chinnaiyan AM, O'Rourke K, Tewari M, Dixit VM. FADD, a novel death domain-containing protein, interacts with the death domain of Fas and initiates apoptosis. Cell 1995;81:505–512.
20. Boldin MP, Varfolomeev EE, Pancer Z, Mett IL, Camonis JH, Wallach D. A novel protein that interacts with the death domain of Fas/APO1 contains a sequence motif related to the death domain. J Biol Chem 1995;270:7795–7798.
21. Chinnaiyan AM, Tepper CG, Seldin MF, et al. FADD/MORT1 is a common mediator of CD95 (Fas/APO-1) and tumor necrosis factor receptor-induced apoptosis. J Biol Chem 1996;271:4961–4965.
22. Muzio M, Chinnaiyan AM, Kischkel FC, et al. FLICE, a novel FADD-homologous ICE/CED-3-like protease, is recruited to the CD95 (Fas/APO-1) death-inducing signaling complex. Cell 1996;85:817–827.
23. Boldin MP, Goncharov TM, Goltsev YV, Wallach D. Involvement of MACH, a novel MORT1/FADD-interacting protease, in Fas/APO-1- and TNF receptor-induced cell death. Cell 1996;85:803–815.
24. Kischkel FC, Hellbardt S, Behrmann I, et al. Cytotoxicity-dependent APO-1 (Fas/CD95)-associated proteins form a death-inducing signaling complex (DISC) with the receptor. Embo J 1995;14:5579–5588.
25. Medema JP, Scaffidi C, Kischkel FC, et al. FLICE is activated by association with the CD95 death-inducing signaling complex (DISC). Embo J 1997;16:2794–2804.
26. Srinivasula SM, Ahmad M, Fernandes-Alnemri T, Litwack G, Alnemri ES. Molecular ordering of the Fas-apoptotic pathway: the Fas/APO-1 protease Mch5 is a CrmA-inhibitable protease that activates multiple Ced-3/ICE-like cysteine proteases. Proc Natl Acad Sci USA 1996;93:14,486–14,491.
27. Li H, Zhu H, Xu CJ, Yuan J. Cleavage of BID by caspase 8 mediates the mitochondrial damage in the Fas pathway of apoptosis. Cell 1998;94:491–501.
28. Imai Y, Kimura T, Murakami A, Yajima N, Sakamaki K, Yonehara S. The CED-4-homologous protein FLASH is involved in Fas-mediated activation of caspase-8 during apoptosis. Nature 1999;398:777–785.
29. Irmler M, Thome M, Hahne M, et al. Inhibition of death receptor signals by cellular FLIP. Nature 1997;388:190–195.
30. Yang X, Khosravi-Far R, Chang HY, Baltimore D. Daxx, a novel Fas-binding protein that activates JNK and apoptosis. Cell 1997;89:1067–1076.
31. Chang HY, Nishitoh H, Yang X, Ichijo H, Baltimore D. Activation of apoptosis signal-regulating kinase 1 (ASK1) by the adapter protein Daxx. Science 1998;281:1860–1863.
32. Stanger BZ, Leder P, Lee TH, Kim E, Seed B. RIP: a novel protein containing a death domain that interacts with Fas/APO-1 (CD95) in yeast and causes cell death. Cell 1995;81:513–523.
33. Holler N, Zaru R, Micheau O, et al. Fas triggers an alternative, caspase-8-independent cell death pathway using the kinase RIP as effector molecule. Nat Immunol 2000;1:489–495.
34. Duan H, Dixit VM. RAIDD is a new "death" adaptor molecule. Nature 1997;385:86–89.
35. Ahmad M, Srinivasula SM, Wang L, et al. CRADD, a novel human apoptotic adaptor molecule for caspase-2, and FasL/tumor necrosis factor receptor-interacting protein RIP. Cancer Res 1997;57:615–619.
36. Yeh WC, Pompa JL, McCurrach ME, et al. FADD: essential for embryo development and signaling from some, but not all, inducers of apoptosis. Science 1998;279:1954–1958.
37. Zhang J, Cado D, Chen A, Kabra NH, Winoto A. Fas-mediated apoptosis and activation-induced T-cell proliferation are defective in mice lacking FADD/Mort1. Nature 1998;392:296–300.
38. Kabra NH, Kang C, Hsing LC, Zhang J, Winoto A. T cell-specific FADD-deficient mice: FADD is required for early T cell development. Proc Natl Acad Sci USA 2001;98:6307–6312.
39. Fernandes-Alnemri T, Armstrong RC, Krebs J, et al. In vitro activation of CPP32 and Mch3 by Mch4, a novel human apoptotic cysteine protease containing two FADD-like domains. Proc Natl Acad Sci USA 1996;93:7464–7469.
40. Varfolomeev EE, Schuchmann M, Luria V, et al. Targeted disruption of the mouse caspase 8 gene ablates cell death induction by the TNF receptors, Fas/Apo1, and DR3 and is lethal prenatally. Immunity 1998;9:267–276.

41. Salmena L, Lemmers B, Matysiak-Zablocki E, et al. Essential role for caspase 8 in T-cell homeostasis and T-cell mediated immunity. Genes Dev 2003;17(7):883–95.
42. Yeh WC, Itie A, Elia AJ, et al. Requirement for Casper (c-FLIP) in regulation of death receptor-induced apoptosis and embryonic development. Immunity 2000;12:633–642.
43. Chastagner P, Reddy J, Theze J. Lymphoadenopathy in IL-2-deficient mice: further characterization and overexpression of the antiapoptotic molecule cellular FLIP. J Immunol 2002;169:3644–3651.
44. Wang K, Yin XM, Chao DT, Milliman CL, Korsmeyer SJ. BID: a novel BH3 domain-only death agonist. Genes Dev 1996;10:2859–2869.
45. Luo X, Budihardjo I, Zou H, Slaughter C, Wang X. Bid, a Bcl2 interacting protein, mediates cytochrome c release from mitochondria in response to activation of cell surface death receptors. Cell 1998;94:481–490.
46. Yin XM, Wang K, Gross A, et al. Bid-deficient mice are resistant to Fas-induced hepatocellular apoptosis. Nature 1999;400:886–891.
47. Zinkel SS, Ong CC, Ferguson DO, et al. Proapoptotic BID is required for myeloid homeostasis and tumor suppression. Genes Dev 2003;17:229–239.
48. Michaelson JS, Bader D, Kuo F, Kozak C, Leder P. Loss of Daxx, a promiscuously interacting protein, results in extensive apoptosis in early mouse development. Genes Dev 1999;13:1918–1923.
49. Michaelson JS, Leder P. RNAi reveals anti-apoptotic and transcriptionally repressive activities of DAXX. J Cell Sci 2003;116:345–352.
50. Nishitoh H, Saitoh M, Mochida Y, et al. ASK1 is essential for JNK/SAPK activation by TRAF2. Mol Cell 1998;2:389–395.
51. Matsuzawa A, Nishitoh H, Tobiume K, Takeda K, Ichijo H. Physiological roles of ASK1-mediated signal transduction in oxidative stress- and endoplasmic reticulum stress-induced apoptosis: advanced findings from ASK1 knockout mice. Antioxid Redox Signal 2002;4:415–425.
52. Villunger A, Huang DC, Holler N, Tschopp J, Strasser A. Fas ligand-induced c-Jun kinase activation in lymphoid cells requires extensive receptor aggregation but is independent of DAXX, and Fas-mediated cell death does not involve DAXX, RIP, or RAIDD. J Immunol 2000;165:1337–1343.
53. Bergeron L, Perez GI, Macdonald G, et al. Defects in regulation of apoptosis in caspase-2-deficient mice. Genes Dev 1998;12:1304–1314.
54. Tartaglia LA, Goeddel DV. Two TNF receptors. Immunol Today 1992;13:151–153.
55. Hsu H, Xiong J, Goeddel DV. The TNF receptor 1-associated protein TRADD signals cell death and NF-kappa B activation. Cell 1995;81:495–504.
56. Hsu H, Shu HB, Pan MG, Goeddel DV. TRADD-TRAF2 and TRADD-FADD interactions define two distinct TNF receptor 1 signal transduction pathways. Cell 1996;84:299–308.
57. Rothe M, Wong SC, Henzel WJ, Goeddel DV. A novel family of putative signal transducers associated with the cytoplasmic domain of the 75 kDa tumor necrosis factor receptor. Cell 1994;78:681–692.
58. Hsu H, Huang J, Shu HB, Baichwal V, Goeddel DV. TNF-dependent recruitment of the protein kinase RIP to the TNF receptor-1 signaling complex. Immunity 1996;4:387–396.
59. Beg AA, Sha WC, Bronson RT, Ghosh S, Baltimore D. Embryonic lethality and liver degeneration in mice lacking the RelA component of NF-kappa B. Nature 1995;376:167–170.
60. Gilmore TD, Morin PJ. The I kappa B proteins: members of a multifunctional family. Trends Genet 1993;9:427–433.
61. Zandi E, Chen Y, Karin M. Direct phosphorylation of IkappaB by IKKalpha and IKKbeta: discrimination between free and NF-kappaB-bound substrate. Science 1998;281:1360–1363.
62. Mercurio F, Zhu H, Murray BW, et al. IKK-1 and IKK-2: cytokine-activated IkappaB kinases essential for NF-kappaB activation. Science 1997;278:860–866.
63. Yamaoka S, Courtois G, Bessia C, et al. Complementation cloning of NEMO, a component of the IkappaB kinase complex essential for NF-kappaB activation. Cell 1998;93:1231–1240.
64. Yang J, Lin Y, Guo Z, et al. The essential role of MEKK3 in TNF-induced NF-kappaB activation. Nat Immunol 2001;2:620–624.
65. Devin A, Lin Y, Yamaoka S, Li Z, Karin M, Liu Z. The alpha and beta subunits of IkappaB kinase (IKK) mediate TRAF2-dependent IKK recruitment to tumor necrosis factor (TNF) receptor 1 in response to TNF. Mol Cell Biol 2001;21:3986–3994.
66. Ozes ON, Mayo LD, Gustin JA, Pfeffer SR, Pfeffer LM, Donner DB. NF-kappaB activation by tumour necrosis factor requires the Akt serine-threonine kinase. Nature 1999;401:82–85.
67. Muller G, Ayoub M, Storz P, Rennecke J, Fabbro D, Pfizenmaier K. PKC zeta is a molecular switch in signal transduction of TNF-alpha, bifunctionally regulated by ceramide and arachidonic acid. Embo J 1995;14:1961–1969.

68. Kim JW, Lee JE, Kim MJ, Cho EG, Cho SG, Choi EJ. Glycogen synthase kinase 3b is a natural activator of mitogen-activated protein kinase/extracellular signal-regulated kinase kinase kinase 1 (MEKK1). J Biol Chem 2003;12:12.
69. Cho H, Thorvaldsen JL, Chu Q, Feng F, Birnbaum MJ. Akt1/PKBalpha is required for normal growth but dispensable for maintenance of glucose homeostasis in mice. J Biol Chem 2001;276:38,349–38,352.
70. Martin P, Duran A, Minguet S, et al. Role of zeta PKC in B-cell signaling and function. Embo J 2002;21:4049–4057.
71. Malinin NL, Boldin MP, Kovalenko AV, Wallach D. MAP3K-related kinase involved in NF-kappaB induction by TNF, CD95 and IL-1. Nature 1997;385:540–544.
72. Cheng G, Baltimore D. TANK, a co-inducer with TRAF2 of TNF- and CD 40L-mediated NF-kappaB activation. Genes Dev 1996;10:963–973.
73. Pomerantz JL, Baltimore D. NF-kappaB activation by a signaling complex containing TRAF2, TANK and TBK1, a novel IKK-related kinase. Embo J 1999; 18:6694–6704.
74. Bonnard M, Mirtsos C, Suzuki S, et al. Deficiency of T2K leads to apoptotic liver degeneration and impaired NF-kappaB-dependent gene transcription. Embo J 2000;19:4976–4985.
75. Rothe M, Pan MG, Henzel WJ, Ayres TM, Goeddel DV. The TNFR2-TRAF signaling complex contains two novel proteins related to baculoviral inhibitor of apoptosis proteins. Cell 1995;83:1243–1252.
76. Adam D, Adam-Klages S, Kronke M. Identification of p55 tumor necrosis factor receptor-associated proteins that couple to signaling pathways not initiated by the death domain. J Inflamm 1995;47:61–66.
77. Adam-Klages S, Adam D, Wiegmann K, et al. FAN, a novel WD-repeat protein, couples the p55 TNF-receptor to neutral sphingomyelinase. Cell 1996;86:937–947.
78. MacEwan DJ. TNF receptor subtype signalling: differences and cellular consequences. Cell Signal 2002;14:477–492.
79. Hildt E, Oess S. Identification of Grb2 as a novel binding partner of tumor necrosis factor (TNF) receptor I. J Exp Med 1999;189:1707–1714.
80. Schievella AR, Chen JH, Graham JR, Lin LL. MADD, a novel death domain protein that interacts with the type 1 tumor necrosis factor receptor and activates mitogen-activated protein kinase. J Biol Chem 1997;272:12,069–12,075.
81. Jiang Y, Woronicz JD, Liu W, Goeddel DV. Prevention of constitutive TNF receptor 1 signaling by silencer of death domains. Science 1999;283:543–546.
82. Song HY, Rothe M, Goeddel DV. The tumor necrosis factor-inducible zinc finger protein A20 interacts with TRAF1/TRAF2 and inhibits NF-kappaB activation. Proc Natl Acad Sci USA 1996;93:6721–6725.
83. Schwandner R, Wiegmann K, Bernardo K, Kreder D, Kronke M. TNF receptor death domain-associated proteins TRADD and FADD signal activation of acid sphingomyelinase. J Biol Chem 1998;273:5916–5922.
84. Rothe M, Sarma V, Dixit VM, Goeddel DV. TRAF2-mediated activation of NF-kappa B by TNF receptor 2 and CD40. Science 1995;269:1424–1427.
85. Yeh WC, Shahinian A, Speiser D, et al. Early lethality, functional NF-kappaB activation, and increased sensitivity to TNF-induced cell death in TRAF2-deficient mice. Immunity 1997;7:715–725.
86. Nakano H, Sakon S, Koseki H, et al. Targeted disruption of Traf5 gene causes defects in CD40- and CD27-mediated lymphocyte activation. Proc Natl Acad Sci USA 1999;96:9803–9808.
87. Tada K, Okazaki T, Sakon S, et al. Critical roles of TRAF2 and TRAF5 in tumor necrosis factor-induced NF-kappa B activation and protection from cell death. J Biol Chem 2001;276:36,530–36,534.
88. Nguyen LT, Duncan GS, Mirtsos C, et al. TRAF2 deficiency results in hyperactivity of certain TNFR1 signals and impairment of CD40-mediated responses. Immunity 1999;11:379–389.
89. Kelliher MA, Grimm S, Ishida Y, Kuo F, Stanger BZ, Leder P. The death domain kinase RIP mediates the TNF-induced NF-kappaB signal. Immunity 1998;8:297–303.
90. Lin Y, Devin A, Rodriguez Y, Liu ZG. Cleavage of the death domain kinase RIP by caspase-8 prompts TNF-induced apoptosis. Genes Dev 1999;13:2514–2526.
91. Lin Y, Devin A, Cook A, et al. The death domain kinase RIP is essential for TRAIL (Apo2L)-induced activation of IkappaB kinase and c-Jun N-terminal kinase. Mol Cell Biol 2000;20:6638–6645.
92. Cusson N, Oikemus S, Kilpatrick ED, Cunningham L, Kelliher M. The death domain kinase RIP protects thymocytes from tumor necrosis factor receptor type 2-induced cell death. J Exp Med 2002;196:15–26.
93. Xue Y, Wang X, Li Z, Gotoh N, Chapman D, Skolnik EY. Mesodermal patterning defect in mice lacking the Ste20 NCK interacting kinase (NIK). Development 2001;128:1559–1572.
94. Lee FS, Peters RT, Dang LC, Maniatis T. MEKK1 activates both IkappaB kinase alpha and IkappaB kinase beta. Proc Natl Acad Sci USA 1998;95:9319–9324.

95. Yujiri T, Ware M, Widmann C, et al. MEK kinase 1 gene disruption alters cell migration and c-Jun NH2-terminal kinase regulation but does not cause a measurable defect in NF-kappa B activation. Proc Natl Acad Sci USA 2000;97:7272–7277.
96. Tobiume K, Matsuzawa A, Takahashi T, et al. ASK1 is required for sustained activations of JNK/p38 MAP kinases and apoptosis. EMBO Rep 2001;2:222–228.
97. Yang J, Boerm M, McCarty M, et al. Mekk3 is essential for early embryonic cardiovascular development. Nat Genet 2000;24:309–313.
98. Rudolph D, Yeh WC, Wakeham A, et al. Severe liver degeneration and lack of NF-kappaB activation in NEMO/IKKgamma-deficient mice. Genes Dev 2000;14:854–862.
99. Li ZW, Chu W, Hu Y, et al. The IKKbeta subunit of IkappaB kinase (IKK) is essential for nuclear factor kappaB activation and prevention of apoptosis. J Exp Med 1999;189:1839–1845.
100. Makris C, Godfrey VL, Krahn-Senftleben G, et al. Female mice heterozygous for IKK gamma/NEMO deficiencies develop a dermatopathy similar to the human X-linked disorder incontinentia pigmenti. Mol Cell 2000;5:969–979.
101. Schmidt CS, Liu J, Zhang T, et al. Enhanced B cell expansion, survival, and humoral responses by targeting death receptor 6. J Exp Med 2003;197:51–62.
102. Alcamo E, Mizgerd JP, Horwitz BH, et al. Targeted mutation of TNF receptor I rescues the RelA-deficient mouse and reveals a critical role for NF-kappa B in leukocyte recruitment. J Immunol 2001;167:1592–1600.
103. Salvesen GS, Duckett CS. IAP proteins: blocking the road to death's door. Nat Rev Mol Cell Biol 2002;3:401–410.
104. Harlin H, Reffey SB, Duckett CS, Lindsten T, Thompson CB. Characterization of XIAP-deficient mice. Mol Cell Biol 2001;21:3604–3608.
105. Huang H, Joazeiro CA, Bonfoco E, Kamada S, Leverson JD, Hunter T. The inhibitor of apoptosis, cIAP2, functions as a ubiquitin-protein ligase and promotes in vitro monoubiquitination of caspases 3 and 7. J Biol Chem 2000;275:26,661–26,664.
106. Li X, Yang Y, Ashwell JD. TNF-RII and c-IAP1 mediate ubiquitination and degradation of TRAF2. Nature 2002;416:345–347.
107. Segui B, Cuvillier O, Adam-Klages S, et al. Involvement of FAN in TNF-induced apoptosis. J Clin Invest 2001;108:143–151.
108. Kreder D, Krut O, Adam-Klages S, et al. Impaired neutral sphingomyelinase activation and cutaneous barrier repair in FAN-deficient mice. Embo J 1999;18:2472–2479.
109. Tcherkasowa AE, Adam-Klages S, Kruse ML, et al. Interaction with factor associated with neutral sphingomyelinase activation, a WD motif-containing protein, identifies receptor for activated C-kinase 1 as a novel component of the signaling pathways of the p55 TNF receptor. J Immunol 2002;169: 5161–5170.
110. Heyninck K, De Valck D, Vanden Berghe W, et al. The zinc finger protein A20 inhibits TNF-induced NF-kappaB-dependent gene expression by interfering with an RIP- or TRAF2-mediated transactivation signal and directly binds to a novel NF-kappaB-inhibiting protein ABIN. J Cell Biol 1999;145:1471–1482.
111. Lee EG, Boone DL, Chai S, et al. Failure to regulate TNF-induced NF-kappaB and cell death responses in A20-deficient mice. Science 2000;289:2350–2354.
112. Van Huffel S, Delaei F, Heyninck K, De Valck D, Beyaert R. Identification of a novel A20-binding inhibitor of nuclear factor-kappa B activation termed ABIN-2. J Biol Chem 2001;276:30,216–30,223.
113. Heyninck K, Kreike MM, Beyaert R. Structure-function analysis of the A20-binding inhibitor of NF-kappaB activation, ABIN-1. FEBS Lett 2003;536:135–140.
114. Schneider P, Thome M, Burns K, et al. TRAIL receptors 1 (DR4) and 2 (DR5) signal FADD-dependent apoptosis and activate NF-kappaB. Immunity 1997;7:831–836.
115. Koppinen P, Pispa J, Laurikkala J, Thesleff I, Mikkola ML. Signaling and subcellular localization of the TNF receptor Edar. Exp Cell Res 2001;269:180–192.
116. Gruss HJ. Molecular, structural, and biological characteristics of the tumor necrosis factor ligand superfamily. Int J Clin Lab Res 1996;26:143–159.
117. Bodmer JL, Holler N, Reynard S, et al. TRAIL receptor-2 signals apoptosis through FADD and caspase-8. Nat Cell Biol 2000;2:241–243.
118. Kischkel FC, Lawrence DA, Chuntharapai A, Schow P, Kim KJ, Ashkenazi A. Apo2L/TRAIL-dependent recruitment of endogenous FADD and caspase-8 to death receptors 4 and 5. Immunity 2000;12:611–620.

119. Sprick MR, Weigand MA, Rieser E, et al. FADD/MORT1 and caspase-8 are recruited to TRAIL receptors 1 and 2 and are essential for apoptosis mediated by TRAIL receptor 2. Immunity 2000;12:599–609.
120. Suliman A, Lam A, Datta R, Srivastava RK. Intracellular mechanisms of TRAIL: apoptosis through mitochondrial-dependent and -independent pathways. Oncogene 2001;20:2122–2133.
121. Kissil JL, Cohen O, Raveh T, Kimchi A. Structure-function analysis of an evolutionary conserved protein, DAP3, which mediates TNF-alpha- and Fas-induced cell death. Embo J 1999;18:353–362.
122. Miyazaki T, Reed JC. A GTP-binding adapter protein couples TRAIL receptors to apoptosis-inducing proteins. Nat Immunol 2001;2:493–500.
123. Liu J, Na S, Glasebrook A, et al. Enhanced CD4+ T cell proliferation and Th2 cytokine production in DR6-deficient mice. Immunity 2001;15:23–34.
124. Zhao H, Yan M, Wang H, Erickson S, Grewal IS, Dixit VM. Impaired c-Jun amino terminal kinase activity and T cell differentiation in death receptor 6-deficient mice. J Exp Med 2001;194:1441–1448.
125. Headon DJ, Emmal SA, Ferguson BM, et al. Gene defect in ectodermal dysplasia implicates a death domain adapter in development. Nature 2001;414:913–916.
126. Yan M, Zhang Z, Brady JR, Schilbach S, Fairbrother WJ, Dixit VM. Identification of a novel death domain-containing adaptor molecule for ectodysplasin-A receptor that is mutated in crinkled mice. Curr Biol 2002;12:409–413.
127. Roux PP, Barker PA. Neurotrophin signaling through the p75 neurotrophin receptor. Prog Neurobiol 2002;67:203–233.
128. Casademunt E, Carter BD, Benzel I, Frade JM, Dechant G, Barde YA. The zinc finger protein NRIF interacts with the neurotrophin receptor p75(NTR) and participates in programmed cell death. Embo J 1999;18:6050–6061.
129. Chittka A, Chao MV. Identification of a zinc finger protein whose subcellular distribution is regulated by serum and nerve growth factor. Proc Natl Acad Sci USA 1999;96:10,705–10,710.
130. Irie S, Hachiya T, Rabizadeh S, et al. Functional interaction of Fas-associated phosphatase-1 (FAP-1) with p75(NTR) and their effect on NF-kappaB activation. FEBS Lett 1999;460:191–198.

6 Caspase Activation by the Extrinsic Pathway

Xiaolu Yang, PhD

CASPASES AND APOPTOSIS

Caspases As the Central Executioners of Apoptosis

Apoptosis, or programmed cell death, has been an area of extensive study since the early 1990s, largely due to its essential role in the development and maintenance of homeostasis and its implication in numerous diseases, ranging from cancer and autoimmunity to neurodegeneration and immunodeficiency *(1)*. To date, one of the most important insights into the molecular mechanism of apoptosis is the discovery that apoptosis is executed by a family of intracellular proteases known as caspases. Caspases are cysteine aspases, i.e., they use cysteine as the nucleophilic group in their active site to cleave proteins after aspartic acid residues. This discovery initially came a decade ago with the cloning of CED-3, a *Caenorhabditis elegans* gene required for developmental cell death. During the development of this small organism, 1090 somatic cells are generated, 131 of which are deleted by apoptosis *(2,3)*. Genetic analysis has revealed a core apoptotic program in *C. elegans* comprised of three genes: CED-3, CED-4, and CED-9, with the first two promoting apoptosis and the latter inhibiting it. Epistatic analysis has identified CED-3 as the most downstream component of this program, suggesting that the functions of CED-4 and CED-9 are to control CED-3 activity. CED-3 encodes a protein this is significantly similar to the only other caspase identified at that time, caspase-1, or interleukin(IL)-1β converting enzyme (ICE), which, as its name indicates, is responsible for processing pro-IL-1β to its mature form, a potent inflammatory cytokine *(4,5)*. This finding has placed caspases at the center of apoptosis study, leading to earnest efforts to identify additional caspases in a range of organisms and extensive investigation of their functions and regulation. Presently, fourteen caspases have been found in mammals, five in *Drosophila*, and three in *C. elegans*. A large number of studies using inhibitors of caspases (either small peptide inhibitors or protein inhibitors encoded by viruses) and cells and animals deficient in caspases have confirmed a critical role of some caspases in apoptosis *(6–8)*. However, other caspases appear to mainly function in nonapoptotic

From: *Cancer Drug Discovery and Development: Death Receptors in Cancer Therapy*
Edited by: W. S. El-Deiry © Humana Press Inc., Totowa, NJ

processes such as inflammation. Mammalian caspases are named according to the order in which they were identified *(9)*. The apoptosis caspases include caspase-2, -3, -6, -7, -8, -9, -10, and -12, and the inflammatory caspases are caspase-1, -4, -5, and -11 (Fig. 1).

Caspases are Highly Specific Proteases

The involvement of caspases in apoptosis signaling initially came as a surprise because, until then, intracellular proteases had been studied almost exclusively in the context of protein degradation, either for protein turnover or for antigen processing. However, with its propensities for self-amplification and for affecting a large number of proteins, and, perhaps more importantly, with its irreversibility, a proteolytic system seems to fit nicely with the terminal nature of dismantling cells. Caspases, unlike the proteases in the proteosome and endosome, are among the most specific proteases known. They do not degrade proteins. Rather, they specifically cleave proteins at highly selective sites often located in their inter-domain regions. This specificity is achieved in part through an almost absolute requirement for an Asp residue immediately NH_2-terminal to the cleaved bond (the P1 position) *(5)*. In addition, they show high preference for certain amino acid residues at the P2 through P4 positions. There are substantial differences in the substrate recognition sites of the various caspases, a feature likely reflecting their distinct roles in apoptosis and inflammation (*see* below) *(10)*. In contrast, there appears to be no preference for amino acid residues COOH-terminal to the cleavage bond (the P' position) *(5)*.

Caspases Cleave a Wide Range of Cellular Proteins to Dismantle Cells

With such high specificity, caspases not only inactivate some cellular proteins but also activate others, orchestrating the cellular events that lead to cell demise and qualifying them as signaling molecules. To date, over 100 caspase substrates have been identified, and the list is still growing. These substrates fall into several categories *(6,7)*. Caspase substrates include other pro- and antiapoptotic proteins. DNA laddering, a long-recognized biochemical hallmark of apoptosis, is due to intrachromosome cleavage, which is mainly carried out by caspase activated DNase (CAD)/DNA fragmentation factor (DFF)40. CAD is normally kept inactive by its inhibitor ICAD or DFF45 through direct protein-protein interaction. Cleavage of ICAD by caspase-3 at two sites abolishes this interaction and releases CAD, allowing it to translocate to the nucleus to cleave chromosomes *(11–13)*. The Bcl-2 family proteins, which regulate the release of mitochondrial apoptosis inducers, are also caspase substrates. For example, Bid, a BH3-only protein, is cleaved by caspase-8 in the cytosol, generating an active COOH-terminal fragment that translocates to the outer membrane of the mitochondria and promotes the release of cytochrome c. Apoptosis is accompanied by profound changes in the cytoskeleton, as the nucleus fragments, the cell body shrinks, and cells detach from the surrounding cell and basal membranes, eventually breaking down to membrane-bound apoptotic bodies. Cytoskeletal proteins and their regulatory factors are among prominent caspase substrates. Cleavage of the nuclear lamin, a scaffold protein associated with the nuclear envelope, contributes to nuclear fragmentation *(14,15)*. Caspases also cleave gelsolin, an actin-depolymerizing enzyme, and the ROCK1 kinase, a Rho effetor protein, generating constitutively active fragments of these proteins that cause membrane blebbing, a morphological characteristic of apoptotic cells *(16,17)*. Caspase substrates include a large number of signal transduction molecules, transcription factors, cell-cycle regulatory

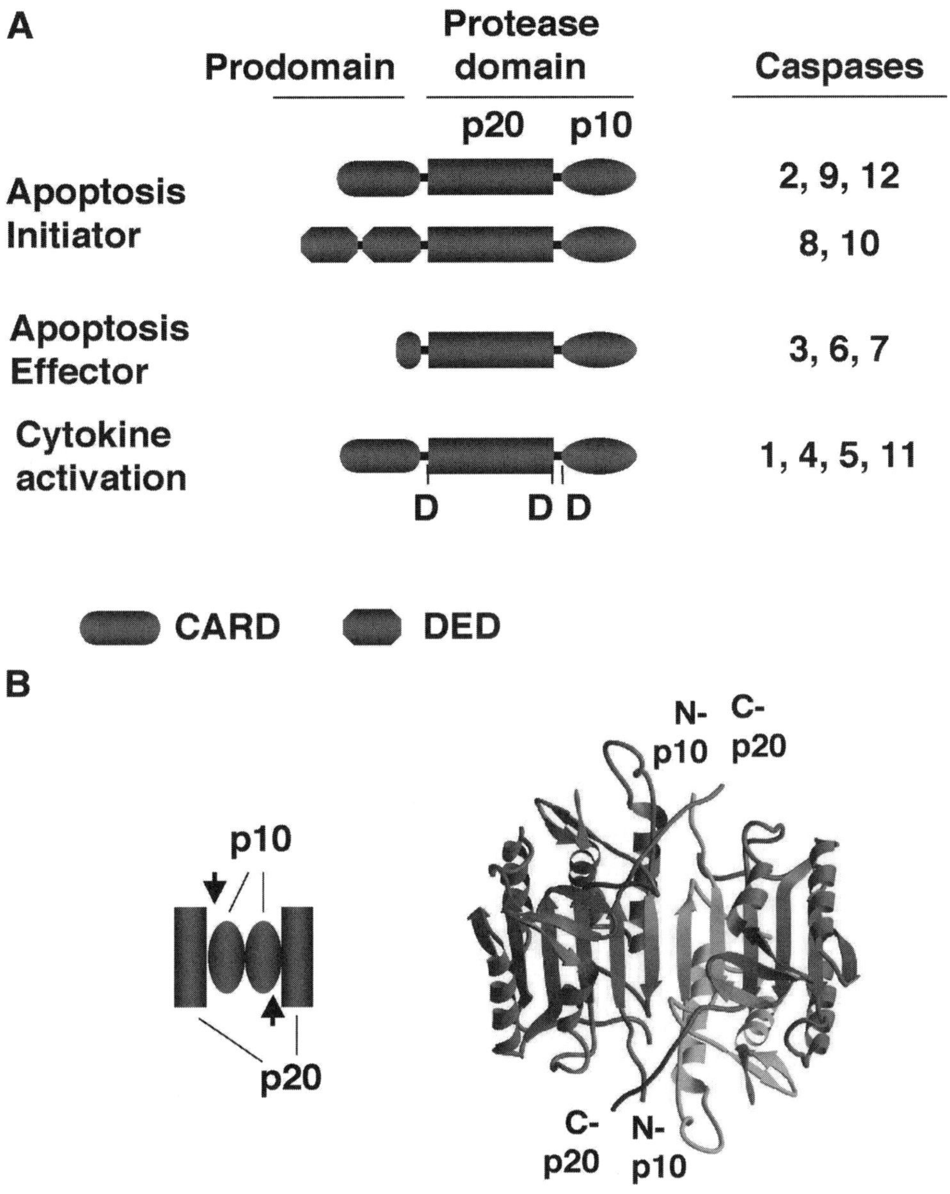

Fig. 1. Structure of mammalian caspases. (**A**) Primary structure of procaspases. All caspases are of human origin except caspase-11, whose human homolog is likely to be capase-5. A procaspase consists of a prodomain and the characteristic protease domain, which can be divided into the large (p20) and small (p10) subunits. The prodomain of apical caspases (apoptosis initiator and inflammatory caspases) contains distinct motifs such as death effector domain (DED) and caspase recruitment domain (CARD). The cleavage site aspartic acids (D) are indicated. For some procaspases, the region between p20 and p10 has two cleavage sites. (**B**) Structure of mature caspases. Left, a mature caspase is a tetramer comprising two p10s surrounded by two p20s with twofold rotational symmetry. Each unit is a p20:p10 heterodimer, which forms one active site (shown by arrow). Right, structure of active caspase-3 in complex with a peptide inhibitor Ac-DEVD-CHO *(27)*. The active sites are indicated by arrows. The N-termini of the p10 and C-termini of p20 are indicated.

proteins, and DNA metabolism proteins. The cleavage of these proteins serves a range of functions, such as shutting down cell survival and proliferative pathways, inactivating DNA-damage responses, and conserving energy that is needed for the execution of apoptosis. Finally, inappropriate cleavage by caspases is implicated in a range of diseases, notably neurodegenerative diseases. To date, eight inherited neurodegenerative diseases, including Huntington's disease and spinocerebellar ataxias, all of which are characterized by neuronal cell death in specific regions of the brain, are thought to be caused by aggregates formed by polyglutamine (PolyQ)-containing protein fragments *(18,19)*. Caspases can cleave and release the precursor proteins of the polyQ fragments, thus exacerbating the pathogenesis of these diseases *(20)*. In many cases, the function and consequence of the cleavage remain to be determined. Some substrates may merely be "innocent" bystanders due to the large amount of active caspases generated during apoptosis. It is also possible that individual cleavages may have only minor effects on the cell; however, taken together in large quantities, they ensure cell death, making the assessment of each individual cleavage difficult.

Caspase Structure

Apoptosis often occurs within a short time span and in most scenarios does not require the synthesis of new proteins. Consequently, caspases, and many of the other components of the apoptosis pathways, exist in virtually every healthy cell. As is the case of many proteases, caspases are synthesized as inactive precursors, or procaspases, which undergo proteolytic processing during apoptosis to generate the mature enzymes *(5,21)*. A procaspase is comprised of three domains: an NH_2-terminal prodomain of varying length (ranging from a dozen to over 100 amino acids), a middle large subunit of approx 180 amino acids (p20), and a COOH-terminal small subunit of approx 100 amino acids (p10). Relatively long prodomains typically contain distinct protein motifs of approx 80 amino acids, notably the death effector domain (DED) and the caspase recruitment domain (CARD), which facilitate homophilic protein-protein interactions during caspase activation (Fig. 1). These two domains as well as a third one that is also commonly found in apoptosis proteins, the death domain (DD), have similar three-dimensional structures *(22–24)*. The p20 and p10 subunits form the protease domain characteristic of all caspases. Based on the crystal structures of several caspases, an active caspase is a tetramer arranged in twofold rotational symmetry, with two small subunits in the center and two large subunits on the outside *(25–29)*. The functional unit is a p20:p10 heterodimer, which forms an active site consisting of amino acids from both subunits. The two dimers are held together through extensive hydrophobic and polar interactions along their interface, which is most likely required for the proper formation of the active site. To generate the individual p20 and p10 subunits, two cleavages need to occur (Fig. 1). However, for a few caspases, such as caspase-9 and most likely also caspase-2, only one cleavage event occurs that severs the link between the large and small subunits. In this case, the prodomain is still attached to the large subunit *(30–33)*. This pattern of processing may have important ramifications for the regulation of caspase activation (*see* below).

Caspase Cascade

Intriguingly, caspase processing occurs at aspartic acid residues, which conforms to the substrate recognition site of these proteases. Therefore, it is generally believed that a mature caspase can facilitate the maturation of its own as well as other procaspases. While this seems to be the case in some circumstances, recent studies have revealed that initiator caspases may not cleave their own precursors (*see* below). In a few well studied cases, the activation of procaspases occurs in a cascade. The first caspases to be activated are called initiator caspases, and include capase-8, -9, and -10. Initiator procaspases contain relatively long prodomains with distinct motifs. They are activated by distinct death stimuli in large protein complexes. Caspases 8 and 10 are recruited to the death-inducing signaling complex (DISC) formed at the intracellular tails of cell-surface death receptors, while caspase-9 becomes associated with a cytosolic complex, known as the apoptosome, in response to various intracellular death signals that trigger the release of cytocrome c from the mitochondria. Although there are several well documented cases in which initiator capases cleave noncaspase proteins, such as the cleavage of Bid by caspase-8, their major targets are downstream effector caspases, such as caspase-3, -6, and -7. The optimal substrate recognition sequences for initiator caspases are often present in effector caspases. Effector caspases represent the majority of active caspases during apoptosis *(34)*, and their activation ensures the amplification of lethal signaling from a small number of active initiator caspases. The optimal substrate recognition sequences for effector caspases are present in a wide range of cellular proteins, and effector caspases are responsible for the majority of cleavage events observed during apoptosis. For example, caspase-3 cleaves a large number of cellular proteins, including the above-mentioned ICAD, gelsolin, ROCK1, and PolyQ-containing proteins. Caspase-7 has similar enzymatic properties and tissue distribution to caspase-3, and is believed to be able to replace caspase-3 when the latter is absent, providing a redundant mechanism to ensure the effective execution of apoptosis. In contrast, the substrates for caspase-6 are limited in number, although one important example is nuclear lamin, the nuclear envelope scaffold protein *(14)*. The substrate specificity of caspase-6 is distinct from that of caspase-3 and -7, and is more like that of the initiator caspases *(10)*. It is possible that this caspase may have an additional role beyond that as an effector caspase. For example, caspase-6 may function as an intermediate between initiator caspases and caspase-3 and -7.

While the existence of a caspase cascade has been well established for some initiator caspases, including caspase-8 and -9, it is not clear that this is the case for other initiator caspases such as caspase-2 *(35,36)*. Although early studies have revealed that caspase-2 is processed in multiple scenarios of apoptosis *(31,33)*, mice deficient in caspase-2 develop normally and show minimal defects in apoptosis *(37)*. Given the similarity in overall structure of caspase-2 and -9, it is possible that a compensatory mechanism involving caspase-9 comes into play in these mice. This possibility is bolstered by a recent study using caspase-2-specific small interference RNA (siRNA), which works over a time span perhaps too short to activate a compensatory mechanism. This study showed an essential role for caspase-2 in genotoxic drug-induced apoptosis *(38)*, and, together with other studies, placed caspase-2 functioning upstream of the mitochondrial pathway *(38–40)*. In this regard, caspase-2 is similar to caspase-8 in that they both can engage the mitochondrial pathway for the amplification of caspase activation. Nevertheless, caspase-2 has a substrate specificity distinct from that of caspase-8 and -9, and it does not seem to activate effector caspases directly. The lack of a cascade amplification event prior to the activation of the mitochondrial apoptosis pathway may force the apoptotic signals generated by caspase-2 to be transmitted to the mitochondria, allowing for multiple levels of regulation before it can cause irreversible damage. The regulation of caspase-2 activation is currently unknown.

The massive destructive power of caspases and the universal existence of their precursors inside cells demand tight regulation to avoid unwanted death. The mechanism that controls caspase activation has to strictly prevent accidental activation while at the same time allowing for rapid and efficient activation when needed. Caspase activation, particularly that of the initiator caspases, is thus intricately modulated by a large number of pro- and antiapoptotic proteins. To date, two apoptosis pathways leading to caspase activation have been extensively studied: the extrinsic and intrinsic pathways. The extrinsic pathway is engaged by a group of plasma membrane receptors known as death receptors. Upon activation by their ligands, these receptors form the DISC complex, where caspase-8 and, in the case of human cells, caspase-10, are processed. The intrinsic pathway, on the other hand, is initiated by various intracellular stimuli, such as developmental lineage information, oncogenic transformation, and severe DNA damage caused by radiation and certain therapeutic drugs. These signals converge on mitochondria and cause them to release, among several apoptotic inducers, cytochrome c, which binds to caspase-activating factor-1 (Apaf-1), leading to the recruitment and activation of caspase-9. After the cleavage between the large and small subunits, no further processing of caspase-9 occurs. This product can thus stay with Apaf-1 through its interaction mediated by its prodomain. Interestingly, Apaf-1-bound caspase-9 is markedly more active than the free form, suggesting that caspase-9 and Apaf-1 function as a holoenzyme *(41)*. Following activation, both caspase-8 and caspase-9 process and activate effector caspase-3, -6, and -7.

DEATH RECEPTORS AND THE FORMATION OF THE CASPASE-ACTIVATING COMPLEX

Death Receptors

Death receptors form a subgroup in the tumor necrosis factor receptor (TNFR)/nerve growth factor receptor (NGFR) superfamily and include CD95 (Fas/APO-1), type I TNF receptor (TNFRI), death receptor (DR) 3 (APO-3/TRAMP), DR4 (TNF-related apoptosis inducing ligand or TRAIL receptor 1, TRAIL-R1), DR5 (TRAIL-R2/KILLER), and DR6 *(42)*. Members of this family share characteristic cysteine-rich repeats in their extracellular domains but have distinct cytoplasmic tails. However, all of the death receptors contain a homophilic protein–protein interaction motif, the death domain, in their intracellular region. Death receptor-mediated apoptosis plays various cellular roles, particularly in the immune system. For example, CD95-mediated apoptosis is important in maintaining immune tolerance in peripheral tissues and downregulating immune responses at the end of infection. Cytotoxic T-lymphocytes also use this kind of apoptosis for killing virus-infected cells. In addition, CD95-mediated apoptosis has been implicated in the protection of immune privileged sites, such as the eyes and testis, against harmful inflammatory responses, as well as in the evasion of tumor cells from the immune system. In the latter two cases, the CD95 ligand is thought to induce apoptosis in nearby lymphocytes, thereby preventing the opportunity for an immune response *(43,44)*. The role of TNF-mediated apoptosis is less clear. TNF is a potent proinflammatory cytokine that orchestrates the acute inflammatory response to Gram-negative bacteria and other infectious microbes *(45)*. It does so mainly by activating transcription factors, such as nuclear factor-κB (NF-κB) and activation factor-1 (AP-1). TNF can induce apoptosis in vitro in a range of cells, particularly tumor cells. However, it often requires the addition of transcription or translation inhibitors, such as actinomycin D or cycloheximide, for effective killing. TRAIL can kill a wide range of tumor cells while sparing most normal cells by engaging two receptors, DR4 and DR5 *(46–48)*. This observation has generated a lot of interest in TRAIL as a potential cancer therapeutic agent. The physiological function of TRAIL is not well understood. The ligand for DR6 is not known and its cellular function remains unclear, although it appears to affect T-cell differentiation *(49)*.

CD95 is the best-characterized death receptor in terms of its apoptosis function. Consequently, the activation of caspases by CD95 has been extensively studied as a paradigm for apoptosis signaling in mammalian cells. The activation of initiator caspases by TRAIL receptors is thought to be similar to that by CD95, in that both occur in the membrane-associated DISC complex comprising the same set of proteins. On the contrary, caspase-8 appears to be activated in a cytosolic complex during TNFRI-mediated apoptosis.

Components and Assembly of the CD95 and TRAIL DISC Complexes

The CD95 DISC complex contains several proteins: FADD (Fas-associated death domain, also known as MORT), caspase-8 (MACH/FLICE), caspase-10 (Mch4/FLICE-2), and a caspase-8/10-like protein called cellular FLICE-inhibitory protein (c-FLIP) (also known as Casper, MRIT, CLARP, CASH, I-FLICE, FLAME, and Usurpin). FADD was identified using the intracellular tail of CD95 as bait in yeast two-hybrid screens *(50,51)*. It is a bipartite adapter protein with a COOH-terminal death domain, which mediates its interaction with the CD95 death domain, and an NH_2-terminal DED. The presence of FADD in the DISC complex was subsequently confirmed through biochemical analysis *(52)*. Caspase-8 was independently identified using FADD as bait in a yeast two-hybrid screen and through mass spectrometry analysis of the DISC *(53–55)*. Caspase-8 contains two tandem DEDs in its prodomain, which bind to the FADD DED. Although a large number of splicing variants have been cloned for caspase-8, only two isoforms are predominantly expressed in cells, caspase-8a (p55) and caspase-8b (p53), with the former having extra amino acids in the linker region between the large subunit and prodomain *(56)*. During apoptosis, both isoforms are recruited to the DISC, where they are processed. It is not clear how the expression of these two alternative splicing forms is regulated, nor whether they play different roles in caspase-8 activation.

Caspase-10 and c-FLIP were originally identified through homology cloning and database searching, because they both contain tandem DEDs and share high sequence similarity to caspase-8 *(57–65)*. Their existence in the DISC complex has been subsequently confirmed by biochemical analysis *(66–69)*. Caspase-10 is mainly present in three isoforms—caspase-10a (p55), caspase-10c (p31), and caspase-10d (p59)—with the d isoform having a longer large subunit than the a isoform and the c isoform missing the majority of the protease domain *(67)*. All of these isoforms are recruited to the DISC complex, where the a and d isoforms undergo proteolytic processing during CD95- or TRAIL-induced apoptosis. c-FLIP is the cellular homolog of viral FLIP, an apoptotic inhibitor that is structurally similar to the prodomains of caspase-8 and -10 and contains two tandem DED repeats. It is found in two splicing variants *(62)*. The short form, c-$FLIP_S$, is most similar to v-FLIP and has two DEDs. The long form, c-$FLIP_L$, has a domain highly homologous to the caspase-8 and -10 protease domains in addition to the tandem DED repeats, and is thus similar to caspase-8 and -10 throughout its length. Notably, several amino acids critical for the formation of the active site of caspase-8 and -10, including the requisite cysteine, are missing in c-$FLIP_L$. Human caspase-8, caspase-10, and c-FLIP reside in the same chromosome region, and mice have caspase-8 and c-$FLIP_L$ but not caspase-10, suggesting that caspase-10 and possibly also c-$FLIP_L$ arose from gene duplication events.

The three-dimensional structure of the CD95 ligand is believed to be similar to that of TNF, a homotrimer that binds to three molecules of the TNFRI *(45)*. Thus, each DISC complex should theoretically contain three molecules each of CD95 and FADD, and the same number of caspase-8/caspase-10/c-FLIP molecules in various combinations. Intriguingly, CD95 and TNFRI preform homotrimers on the plasma membrane before binding to their ligands or agonistic antibodies *(70,71)*. CD95 mutants have been identified in human patients that retain this ability but cannot bind to the CD95 ligand and thus interfere with CD95 signaling. It is not clear what prevents these preformed receptor trimers from recruiting intracellular signaling molecules, nor is it clear how binding of the ligands or agonistic antibodies promotes the assembly of the DISC complex. It is conceivable that the intracellular domain of CD95 undergoes a conformational change, which may generate high-affinity binding sites to FADD. Recruitment of FADD to the receptor may in turn create strong binding sites for caspase-8, caspase-10, and c-FLIP. In this regard, it is noted that the FADD DED shows high cytotoxicity when overexpressed in cells compared to the full-length protein, suggesting that this domain may normally be masked by its intra-molecular association with the death domain *(51)*. In addition, the presence of two DEDs on procaspase-8/-10 and c-FLIP may enable their association with each other to prevent binding to the FADD DED in healthy cells. The exposure of the FADD DED upon recruitment to the DISC may abstract one of the two DEDs of procaspase-8, procaspase-10, and c-FLIP. However, this scenario is likely too simplistic, as the assembly of the DISC during CD95-mediated apoptosis appears to be a highly dynamic process involving at least four steps *(72)*. First, the receptor forms a microcomplex. Next, FADD is recruited to the complex in an actin-dependent manner. Third, a large receptor cluster forms in a manner that is enhanced by caspase-8 found in the DISC. Finally, the DISC complex is internalized via an endosomal pathway. Thus, FADD and possibly also procaspase-8 appear to be actively transported from the cytosol to the receptor, where they in turn contribute to the further assembly of the DISC complex and its eventual internalization.

Because three tandem DED-containing proteins—caspase-8, caspase-10, and c-FLIP—are recruited to the DISC by FADD, DISC complexes may vary in their content. c-FLIP and caspase-8 have been shown to co-exist in the same DISC complex *(69)*. However, it is not clear whether this is the case for caspase-8 and caspase-10 or for caspase-10 and c-$FLIP_L$. In addition, caspase-8 and c-$FLIP_L$ are expressed at markedly different levels in the cell, with nearly 100 times more caspase-8 than c-$FLIP_L$ *(68,69)*. This ratio seems to be fairly consistent across various cell lines, suggesting the existence of a "counting" mechanism, although the nature of this mechanism is far from clear. Furthermore, the recruitment of these two proteins to the DISC is quite different, with c-$FLIP_L$ being recruited much more efficiently than caspase-8, even though it is expressed at a much lower level *(68)*. This difference appears to play an important function in regulating CD95-mediated apoptosis (*see* below), although the underlying mechanism for this difference is not understood. To date, the expression level of procaspase-10 and its recruitment to the DISC has not been quantitatively compared to caspase-8 and c-FLIP$_L$.

The DISC complex formed in response to the engagement of the two TRAIL receptors, DR4 and DR5, is very similar to the CD95 DISC. For example, although initial analyses using overexpressed proteins suggested otherwise, recent studies have confirmed the existence of FADD in the endogenous TRAIL DISC *(73)*. In addition, like the CD95 DISC, the TRAIL DISC contains caspase-8 and caspase-10 *(67,73)*.

Two Types of CD95 Apoptotic Cells

A survey of various tumor cell lines revealed two different types of cells in terms of their response to CD95-mediated apoptosis. Although both cell types are sensitive to killing by CD95, they employ distinct intracellular pathways for caspase activation *(74)*. In type I cells, the DISC complex is readily formed and a large amount of active caspase-8 is generated, which then goes on to effectively cleave effector caspases. In these cells, the mitochondrial pathway plays little if any role in apoptosis induction, and overexpression of the antiapoptotic members of the Bcl-2 family of proteins, such as Bcl-2 and Bcl-X$_L$, does not prevent apoptosis. In contrast, in the type II cells, DISC is poorly formed, and consequently, only a small amount of active caspase-8 is generated. The mitochondrial pathway is activated in these cells to amplify the apoptosis signal. This is achieved in part through the cleavage of BID by caspase-8, generating a truncated BID (tBID) that translocates from the cytosol to the outer membrane of the mitochondria, where it acts together with Bax and Bak to release cytochrome c *(75,76)*. It is believed that BID oligomerizes Bax and Bak, two proapoptotic members of the Bcl-2 family of proteins, to form a large channel on the outer membrane. This channel releases cytochrome c, which resides in the inter-membrane space, into the cytosol *(77)*. The release of cytochrome c facilitates the formation of the apoptosome, which activates caspase-9 *(32)*. Thus, because of its mitochondrial dependence, CD95-mediated apoptosis is partially inhibited in type II cells by the overexpression of Bcl-2 or Bcl-X$_L$.

Evidence suggests that type I and type II tumor cells most likely have normal counterparts in vivo. For example, thymocytes and hepatocytes are both sensitive to CD95-induced apoptosis. However, the lack of BID or the overexpression of Bcl-2 renders hepatocytes partially resistant to killing by CD95 but has no effect on thymocytes, similar to the type II and type I cells, respectively *(78–80)*. The mechanism underlying the differential formation of the DISC complex in these two types of cells is currently not understood.

An Intracellular Complex for Caspase Activation During TNF-Induced Apoptosis

TNF has pleiotropic functions in the regulation of inflammation, cell proliferation, differentiation, and apoptosis. Unlike CD95 and the TRAIL receptors, TNF-RI directly binds to the death domain-containing adapter TRADD, as opposed to FADD *(81)*, although TRADD has been shown to interact with FADD *(82)*. The TRADD-FADD connection was originally thought to recruit procaspase-8 and -10 to the TNFRI complex. However, a recent study showed that upon binding to TNF, TNFRI formed a complex that contains TRADD and other signaling proteins but not FADD, procaspase-8, or procaspase-10 *(83)*. The TNF-RI complex actives NF-κB. Notably, a cytosolic complex is subsequently formed comprising TRADD, FADD, and procaspase-8 and -10, whereby the caspases are activated *(83)*. The separation of this cytosolic complex from the proximal receptor complex may enable differential regulation of the multiple signals originated from TNFRI.

MECHANISM AND REGULATION OF CASPASE ACTIVATION BY DEATH RECEPTORS

Activation of Procaspase-8 in the DISC Complex

Given the critical role of initiator caspases in the induction of apoptosis, understanding their activation mechanism is central to our understanding of apoptosis. Caspase-8 plays a central role in death receptor-mediated apoptosis, as cells deficient in caspase-8 are largely resistant to killing by the CD95 ligand (CD95L), TRAIL, and TNF *(84,85)*. During activation, procaspase-8 undergoes two cleavage events to generate a large and small subunit, which tetramerize to form active caspase-8. All of the components of caspase-8—including the separate large and small subunits, the prodomain, and the processing intermediate lacking the small subunit—are found in the DISC, indicating that both cleavage events occur there *(54,55,86)*. Mature caspase-8 is then released into the cytosol, where it activates downstream caspases. It has been shown that a caspase-8 processing mutant that cannot be released into the cytosol also loses its ability to kill cells *(87)*. To prevent the unprocessed protease domain from being released, the two cleavage events need to proceed in a defined order, with the large and small subunits being separated first, followed by the separation of the large subunit from the prodomain, which links procaspase-8 to the DISC. Thus, any model for caspase-8 activation in the DISC needs to account not only for the generation of the two mature caspase-8 subunits, but also for the order of the processing events. It is also helpful to consider what the enzymes and the substrates may be during caspase processing.

The finding that caspase-8 is recruited to the DISC upon aggregation of CD95 by its cognate ligand or agonistic antibodies led to the hypothesis that procaspases are activated by oligomerization. Using a heterologous oligomerization system, it has been shown that oligomerization of procaspase-8 leads to its self-processing in vitro *(88)*. In addition, oligomerization of procaspase-8 enhances its cell death activity in vivo *(87–90)*. Furthermore, in an experiment where the CD95 extracellular region was fused to the caspase-8 protease domain, thereby bypassing the intermediary signaling proteins in the DISC, the fusion protein induced apoptosis in an anti-CD95 antibody-dependent manner *(88)*. These results indicate that oligomerization triggers auto-proteolytic processing of procaspase-8. Subsequent studies have shown that caspase-1, -2, -9, -10, -11, and the *C. elegans* caspase CED-3 are all activated by oligomerization, establishing oligomerization as a general mechanism for the activation of apical caspases, including both apoptosis initiator caspases and inflammatory caspases *(30,68,88,91–95)*. This finding is critical in providing a common molecular framework for the functions of various pro- and antiapoptotic proteins. For example, the function of CED-4, the activator of CED-3, is to oligomerize CED-3, while CED-9, the apoptosis inhibitor in *C. elegans*, is to inhibit CED-4 oligomerization *(91)*. Thus, CED-4 oligomerization is a unifying mechanism for the various components of the *C. elegans* apoptosis pathway. Similarly, in a manner dependent on cytochrome c and dATP, mammalian Apaf-1 forms homo-oligomers, which in turn aggregate procaspase-9, leading to its activation *(91–93,96,97)*.

How does oligomerization lead to procaspase activation? A well established paradigm for oligomerization-induced signal transduction is that mediated by receptor tyrosine kinases, in which ligand-mediated dimerization of these kinases facilitates cross-phosphorylation among the individual kinase molecules *(98)*. Previously, it was proposed that, similar to receptor tyrosine kinases, individual caspases in close proximity cleave one another (the close-proximity model) *(99)*. Indeed, an early study suggested that a nonprocessible caspase-8 mutant possessed weak enzymatic activity, rending support for this model *(89)*. Since then, however, new evidence has contradicted this model. Most notable is the finding that c-FLIP$_L$, the proteolytically inactive caspase-8 homolog found in the DISC, enhances rather than inhibits caspase-8 activation upon heterodimerization with caspase-8 (*see* below).

Additional studies have shown that procaspase-8 gains significant activity upon oligomerization prior to processing *(100–102)*. This has been confirmed not only in vitro for recombinant nonprocessible caspase-8 mutants *(100–102)*, but also in vivo for procaspase-8 in the DISC complex *(100)*. This activity requires the stable association of the unprocessed protease domains in a manner similar to the association of the processed protease domains in a mature caspase; the same residues that participate in the interaction along the interface of the two p20:p10 heterodimers of a mature caspase are also required for the association of the protease domains in procaspase-8 *(100)*. Interestingly, when recombinant nonprocessible caspase-8 mutants were expressed in bacteria, a small portion of the proteins formed stable dimers, which may explain the above-mentioned enzyme activity thought to have originated from an individual precursor molecule *(101,102)*. Therefore, individual procaspase-8 molecules most likely do not possess any significant activity. The first step during caspase-8 activation appears to be the formation of a procaspase-8 dimeric intermediate that is structurally similar to a mature caspase and is proteolytically active. There is, however, at least one major difference between this intermediate and mature caspase-8 (*see* below).

Theoretically, the substrate for the active procaspase-8 dimer could be either monomeric procaspase-8 or another dimer. The former seems to be reasonable, given that there may be up to three procaspase-8 molecules present in every DISC complex. However, in actuality, the preferred substrate is another dimeric procaspase-8 molecule, which has been shown by using a heterologous dimerization system *(100)*. The ability of the paired procaspase-8 molecules to serve as substrate required the stable association of their protease domains, and mutants that were defective in this association were resistant to cleavage *(100)*. This is intriguing because the cleavage sites were intact in these mutants, thus suggesting that these sites may not become accessible in the individual precursor molecules until after the two protease domains associate. Therefore, procaspase-8 is likely activated by an interdimer cleavage mechanism. This mechanism provides a remarkably simple way to achieve safe and efficient caspase activation. It is safe because only the dimerized procaspases and not the individual procaspases possess significant protease activity. Furthermore, if a procaspase-8 dimer is randomly formed, another dimer must be nearby in order to initiate the irreversible process of caspase cleavage, further decreasing the chance of accidental activation. The interdimer cleavage mechanism is efficient because oligomeric complexes are formed during apoptosis. The presence of multiple procaspase-8 dimers in this complex effectively creates an environment where an active enzyme and its optimal substrate are in close proximity, facilitating caspase processing. Consistent with this mechanism, higher orders of death receptor oligomerization are often required for the effective induction of apoptosis *(52,103)*. Proper alignment of these procaspase dimers may be required for optimal cleavage. In this regard, it is interesting to speculate that the function of the third individual procaspase-8 molecule in one DISC is to pair with a similar individual procaspase-8 molecule in another DISC to properly arrange these complexes. Notably, the caspase-9-activating apoptosome complex is a heptamer of Apaf-1, which recruits the same number of procaspase-9 molecules *(104)*.

There are at least two possible explanations that would ensure that the large and small subunits of procspase-8 separate before the large subunit and the prodomain. First, a procaspase dimer may perform both cleavage events, but the second cleavage site may not be accessible to the enzyme until after the large and small subunits are separated (the sequential accessibility model). Alternatively, the second cleavage site may not be recognized by the active procaspase dimer. Instead, it may be cleaved only by the intermediate generated from the first cleavage (the sequential activity model). Evidence suggests that the sequential accessibility model is most likely correct. It has been shown that a nonprocessible caspase-8 mutant can cleave a nonmutant precursor at both sites. In addition, when a heterologous thrombin cleavage site was introduced between the large and small subunits, cleavage of the large subunit and the prodomain occurred only after the large and small subunits were severed by thrombin *(100)* (Fig. 2).

The activation of procaspase-8 involves a shift in substrate specificities. Although procaspase-8 dimers can readily cleave one another, they cannot cleave caspase-3. Mature caspase-8, on the other hand, can cleave caspase-3 well but cannot process procaspase-8, even when procaspase-8 is dimerized *(100)*. Consequently, inhibitors of mature caspase-8 may not affect the activity of procaspase-8 dimers, and vice versa. For example, crmA, a sepin caspase inhibitor specific for mature caspase-1 and -8, does not inhibit the activation of procaspase-8, indicating that it selectively targets mature caspase-8 *(100)*. Contrary to the popular notion that caspase activation is always a self-amplifying process, these results indicate that the activation of initiator procaspases may not feed back on itself and may therefore be limited in amplitude. This property of initiator caspase activation could play a critical cellular function. For example, accumulating evidence has indicated that caspase-8 is required for the activation and proliferation of lymphocytes. This function of caspase-8 would not be possible if the activation of caspase-8 necessarily led to massive caspase activation. The linearity of procaspase-8 activation may allow the generation of only small amounts of active caspase-8, which may cleave certain cellular proteins to promote cell proliferation. Another interesting possibility is that the active procaspase-8 dimer may be responsible for the prolife ability of caspase-8 in lymphocytes. This possibility is supported by the observation that caspase-8-deficient mice show defects in lymphocyte proliferation *(105,106)*, but mice expressing the crmA transgene do not *(107)*. As enzymes, caspases provide attractive targets for therapeutic intervention. The different enzymatic characteristics of procaspases and mature caspases should be further examined with regard to their roles in cell proliferation and apoptosis. This could lead to the design of specific inhibitors that could better modulate cell life and death.

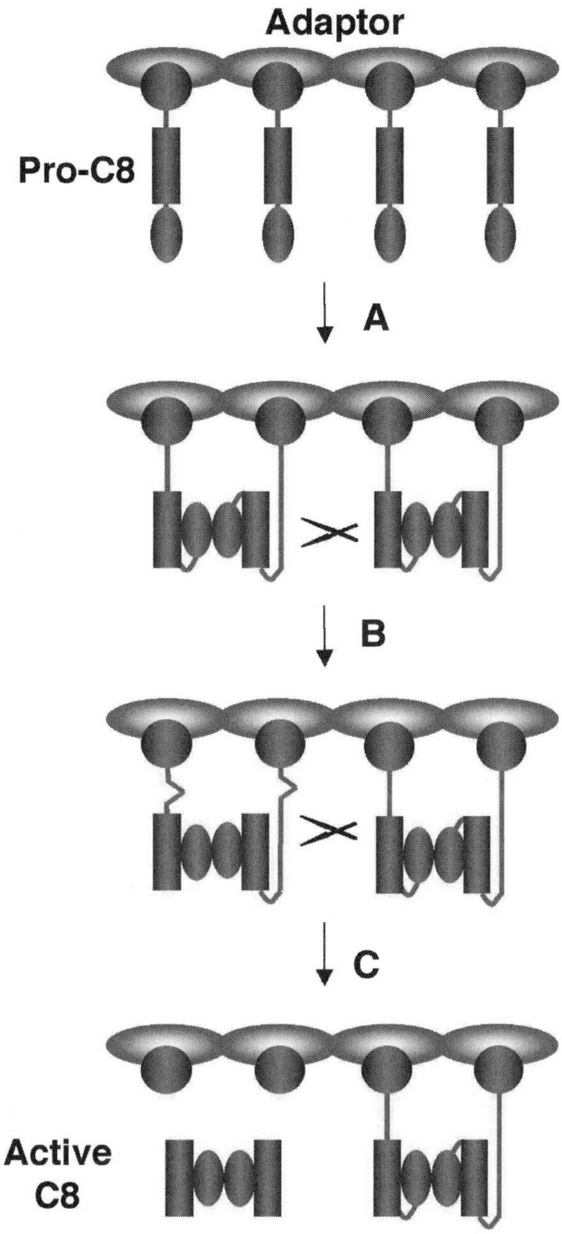

Fig. 2. An interdimer cleavage mechanism for procaspase-8 activation. Upon oligomerization, procaspase-8 molecules form multiple dimers (**A**). These dimers are not only enzymatically active but also are more susceptible to cleavage than individual procaspases, leading to their cross-processing (**B**). The first cleavage occurs between the large and small subunits, which induces a conformational change in the region between the prodomain and large subunit, allowing this region to be cleaved by another procaspase-8 dimer (**C**). The resulting mature caspase-8 then leaves the DISC complex to active effector caspases. The different enzymatic characteristics of active procaspase-8 and mature caspase-8 prevent a positive feedback loop for the activation of procaspase-8.

Activation of Caspase-10

The activation mechanism of procaspase-10 is similar to that of procaspase-8. For example, procaspase-10 can be induced to undergo self-processing upon oligomerization *(30,94)*. In addition, activation of both procaspase-8 and -10 is enhanced by c-FLIP$_L$. During CD95 ligand- and TRAIL-induced apoptosis, procaspase-10 is recruited to the DISC complex, where it becomes activated in a similar manner as procaspase-8 *(66–68)*. However, the recruitment of procaspase-8 and -10 to and their activation in the DISC appears to be independent of each other *(66,67)*. Despite understanding its activation mechanism, the function of procaspase-10 in apoptosis is not well defined. Mice do not have caspase-10. In humans, missense mutations in procaspase-10 have been found in two patients with autoimmune and lymphoproliferative syndrome (ALPS), which manifests as a defect in CD95-induced cell death *(108)*. These procaspase-10 mutants have decreased protease activity. However, one mutation has been identified as a common polymorphism in the Danish population *(109)*. Transient overexpression of caspase-10 in caspase-8-deficient cells has been shown to restore apoptosis sensitivity *(66,94)*, but this was not the case when exogenous caspase-10 was stably expressed in the same cells to levels comparable to that found in wild-type cells *(67)*. Although no clear picture has emerged to explain the function of caspase-10, several studies have shown that unlike caspase-8, caspase-10 is frequently mutated in certain tumors, suggesting a tumor suppression function for this caspase *(66,110–112)*. Consistent with this hypothesis, caspase-8 and -10 appear to recognize different substrates *(94,113)*.

Dual Regulation of Caspase-8 Activation by c-FLIP$_L$

c-FLIP has been independently identified by eight different groups, and consequently, it probably has more aliases than any other apoptosis protein *(58–65)*. But that is not the only thing that makes c-FLIP unique. While c-FLIP$_S$ is generally believed to be an apoptosis inhibitor, the role of c-FLIP$_L$ in apoptosis was a matter of controversy for years *(109,114)*. c-FLIP$_S$, like viral FLIP, contains tandem DEDs. It therefore can compete with tandem DED-containing caspases, caspase-8 and -10, for binding to FADD *(115)*. Although the same logic may apply to c-FLIP$_L$, the presence of a domain highly similar to the protease domains of procaspase-8 and -10 makes the matter more complex. Originally, c-FLIP$_L$ was reported to be an antiapoptotic protein by some initial studies *(62–65)*, a proapoptotic protein by others *(58–60)*, and as both (dependent on the cell type) by one study *(61)*, all of which employed either stable or transient overexpression of exogenous c-FLIP$_L$. The proapoptotic function of c-FLIP$_L$ was observed only upon transient overexpression, and in that case was dependent on its protease-like domain. In addition, a survey of a panel of different cell lines failed to identify a single cell in which c-FLIP$_L$ is not part of the DISC regardless of the CD95 apoptosis sensitivity *(69)*. Subsequent generation and analysis of c-FLIP-deficient mice (which lack both c-FLIP$_L$ and c-FLIP$_S$) did not solve this controversy *(116)*. The mice died between embryonic day 10.5 and 11.5 of a failure in heart formation and extreme hemorrhaging, which was strikingly similar to caspase-8- and FADD-deficient mice, suggesting that c-FLIP$_L$, like FADD, is an activator and not an inhibitor of caspase-8. On the other hand, embryonic fibroblasts (MEFs) derived from these mice showed enhanced sensitivity towards CD95-induced apoptosis, supporting the notion that c-FLIP$_L$ is an inhibitor of apoptosis.

These seemingly contradictory results have been reconciled at least in part by a recent study *(68)*. The role of c-FLIP$_L$ is directly related to the above-mentioned finding that a procaspase-8 dimer, rather than individual procaspases, is the active unit during procaspase-8 activation. This mechanism does not require both dimeric partners to have an active site. In fact, a proteolytically inactive mutant of procaspase-8 did not significantly inhibit the activation of the wild-type protein upon their dimerization *(100)*. Remarkably, c-FLIP$_L$ has intrinsic activity that promotes procaspase-8 activation; the c-FLIP$_L$ protease-like domain strongly induces protease activity in the procaspase-8 protease domain when heterodimerized with it. This has been shown both in vitro using recombinant proteins and in the endogenous DISC complex obtained from cells that inducibly or stably express exogenous c-FLIP$_L$ at various levels *(68,117)*. The interaction between the c-FLIP$_L$ protease-like domain and the procaspase-8 protease domain is much stronger than the homophilic interaction of the procaspase-8 protease domains, thereby suggesting that c-FLIP$_L$ may effectively help procaspase-8 to gain enzymatic activity. In addition, c-FLIP$_L$ enhances the auto-processing of procaspase-10 but not of procaspase-9, which acts in the mitochondrial pathway *(68)*. Thus, in many cells where it is expressed at low levels, c-FLIP$_L$ specifically enhances procaspase-8 (and likely procaspase-10) activation. Consistently, expression of c-FLIP$_L$ in these cells at physiologically relevant levels stimulates CD95-induced apoptosis, whereas a decrease in c-FLIP$_L$ expression attenuates apoptosis. This may also be the case during development, where c-FLIP$_L$ could be critical in the activation of procaspase-8, and thus may explain why the same developmental defects are seen in c-FLIP$_L$- and caspase-8-deficient mice. At high levels of expression, c-FLIP$_L$ behaves like c-FLIP$_S$ and blocks procaspase-8 recruitment to the DISC through competing for binding to FADD (Fig. 3). However, at extremely high levels of expression achievable by transient overexpression, c-FLIP$_L$ may complex with endogenous procaspase-8 outside the DISC and induce apoptosis, which may explain the initial reports on its proapoptotic activity. Upregulation of c-FLIP$_L$ may occur during certain physiological or pathological conditions. For example, c-FLIP$_L$ is highly expressed in several melanoma cell lines, which is thought to contribute to the resistance of these cells to CD95-induced apoptosis *(62)*. This may also be the case in MEF cells, which could explain why the lack of c-FLIP$_L$ in MEFs leads to enhanced apoptosis sensitivity *(116)*. Alternatively, because c-FLIP-deficient cells lack both isoforms, the enhanced apoptosis sensitivity may be due to the absence of the apoptosis inhibitor c-FLIP$_S$. These possibilities remain to be determined.

Although the expression level of c-FLIP$_L$ is only about one percent of that of caspase-8 in many cells, it has a profound effect on CD95-mediated apoptosis. Quantitative analysis of the levels of c-FLIP$_L$ in the DISC over time revealed that c-FLIP$_L$ is much more effectively recruited to the DISC than caspase-8 at the initial stage of apoptosis. Consequently, its level in the DISC reaches one-sixth of that of caspase-8 *(68)*. This ratio in the DISC is still relatively low, which may be for a good reason. In the DISC, c-FLIP$_L$ is rapidly processed by caspase-8. This cleavage contributes to the activation of caspase-8, most likely due to the stabilization of the caspase-8:c-FLIP$_L$ dimer by this cleavage *(68)*. However, there is an important difference between the cleavage of caspase-8 and that of c-FLIP$_L$: the prodomain of c-FLIP$_L$ is not separated from its large subunit. Therefore, c-FLIP$_L$ may not leave the DISC complex. Consequently, although having a small amount of c-FLIP$_L$ in the DISC is beneficial for the generation of highly active procaspase-

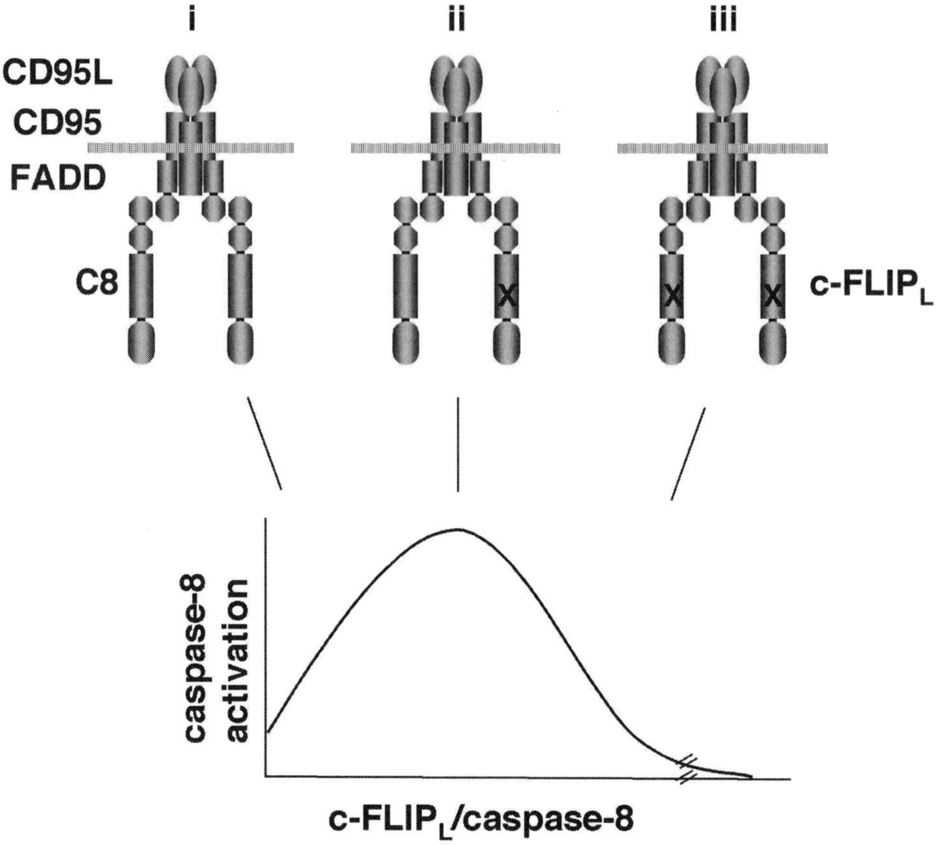

Fig. 3. Dual function of c-FLIP$_L$ in procaspase-8 activation in the DISC. Homo-oligomerization of procaspase-8 in the DISC can lead to its activation in the absence of c-FLIP$_L$(i). However, at low levels of expression, c-FLIP$_L$ potently enhances procaspase-8 activation by hetero-dimerizing with procaspase-8 and inducing caspase activity in the zymogen (ii). This may be the scenario in most cells and during development. At high expression levels, which may occur under certain physiological and pathological conditions, c-FLIP$_L$ inhibits procaspase-8 activation, likely by both competing with procaspase-8 for binding to the DISC and preventing the release of processed caspase-8 subunits (iii).

8 molecules, modest to high amounts of c-FLIP$_L$ may hinder the release of the mature caspase-8 molecules that associate with it. Thus, higher levels of c-FLIP$_L$ may inhibit apoptosis by inhibiting both the recruitment of procaspase-8 to the DISC and the release of mature caspase-8.

Unlike the other DISC components such as FADD and caspase-8, c-FLIP$_L$ is a relatively unstable protein whose expression level is highly regulated. For example, both the MAP kinase pathway and NF-κB upregulate c-FLIP$_L$ *(118,119)*. Therefore, c-FLIP$_L$ may represent a focal point for regulating death receptor-induced apoptosis. Additionally, c-FLIP$_L$ and c-FLIP$_S$ appear to be differentially regulated. c-FLIP$_S$, but not c-FLIP$_L$, is upregulated upon the stimulation of T-cells through either the T-cell receptor or the CD28 co-stimulatory receptor *(120,121)*. Modulation of the levels of c-FLIP$_L$ and c-FLIP$_S$ may provide an effective way to adjust cellular sensitivity toward death receptor-induced apoptosis.

ACKNOWLEDGMENTS

I thank R. Stratt for scientific editing of the manuscript. The research in my lab is supported by the National Institutes of Health. I am a scholar of the Leukemia & Lymphoma Society of America.

REFERENCES

1. Thompson CB. Apoptosis in the pathogenesis and treatment of disease. Science 1995;267:1456–1462.
2. Metzstein MM, Stanfield GM, Horvitz HR. Genetics of programmed cell death in *C. elegans*: past, present and future. Trends Genet 1998;14:410–416.
3. Liu QA, Hengartner MO. The molecular mechanism of programmed cell death in *C. elegans*. Ann N Y Acad Sci 1999;887:92–104.
4. Yuan J, Shaham S, Ledoux HM, Horvitz HR. The C. elegans cell death gene ced-3 encodes a protein similar to mammalian interleukin-b-converting enzyme. Cell 1993;75:641–652.
5. Thornberry NA, Bull HG, Calaycay JR, et al. A novel heterodimeric cysteine protease is required for interleukin-1 beta processing in monocytes. Nature 1992;356:768–774.
6. Chang HY, Yang X. Proteases for Cell Suicide: Functions and regulation of caspases. Microbiol Mol Biol Rev 2000;64:821–846.
7. Degterev A, Boyce M, Yuan J. A decade of caspases. Oncogene 2003;22:8543–8567.
8. Nicholson DW. Caspase structure, proteolytic substrates, and function during apoptotic cell death. Cell Death Differ 1999;6:1028–1042.
9. Alnemri ES, Livingston DJ, Nicholson DW, et al. Human ICE/CED-3 protease nomenclature. Cell 1996;87:171.
10. Thornberry NA, Rano TA, Peterson EP, et al. A combinatorial approach defines specificities of members of the caspase family and granzyme B. Functional relationships established for key mediators of apoptosis. J Biol Chem 1997;272:17,907–17,911.
11. Liu X, Li P, Widlak P, et al. The 40-kDa subunit of DNA fragmentation factor induces DNA fragmentation and chromatin condensation during apoptosis. Proc Natl Acad Sci USA 1998;95:8461–8466.
12. Liu X, Zou H, Slaughter C, Wang X. DFF, a heterodimeric protein that functions downstream of caspase-3 to trigger DNA fragmentation and apoptosis. Cell 1997;89:175–184.
13. Enari M, Sakahira H, Yokoyama H, Okawa K, Iwamatsu A, Nagata S. A caspase-activated DNase that degrades DNA during apoptosis, and its inhibitor ICAD. Nature 1998;391:43–50.
14. Lazebnik YA, Takahashi A, Moir RD, et al. Studies of the lamin proteinase reveal multiple parallel biochemical pathways during apoptotic execution. Proc Natl Acad Sci USA 1995;92:9042–9046.
15. Takahashi A, Alnemri ES, Lazebnik YA, et al. Cleavage of lamin A by Mch2 alpha but not CPP32: multiple interleukin 1 beta-converting enzyme-related proteases with distinct substrate recognition properties are active in apoptosis. Proc Natl Acad Sci USA 1996;93:8395–8400.
16. Kothakota S, Azuma T, Reinhard C, et al. Caspase-3-generated fragment of gelsolin: effector of morphological change in apoptosis. Science 1997;278:294–298.
17. Coleman ML, Sahai EA, Yeo M, Bosch M, Dewar A, Olson MF. Membrane blebbing during apoptosis results from caspase-mediated activation of ROCK I. Nat Cell Biol 2001;3:339–345.
18. Martin JB. Molecular basis of the neurodegenerative disorders. New Engl J Med 1999;340:1970–1980.
19. Yuan J, Yankner BA. Apoptosis in the nervous system. Nature 2000;407:802–809.
20. Goldberg YP, Nicholson DW, Rasper DM, et al. Cleavage of huntingtin by apopain, a proapoptotic cysteine protease, is modulated by the polyglutamine tract. Nat Genet 1996;13:442–429.
21. Nicholson DW, Ali A, Thornberry NA, et al. Identification and inhibition of the ICE/CED-3 protease necessary for mammalian apoptosis. Nature 1995;376:37–43.
22. Huang B, Eberstadt M, Olejniczak ET, Meadows RP, Fesik SW. NMR structure and mutagenesis of the Fas (APO-1/CD95) death domain. Nature 1996;384:638–641.
23. Eberstadt M, Huang B, Chen Z, et al. NMR structure and mutagenesis of the FADD (Mort1) death-effector domain. Nature 1998;392:941–945.
24. Chou JJ, Matsuo H, Duan H, Wagner G. Solution structure of the RAIDD CARD and model for CARD/CARD interaction in caspase-2 and caspase-9 recruitment. Cell 1998;94:171–180.
25. Wilson KP, Black JA, Thomson JA, et al. Structure and mechanism of interleukin-1 beta converting enzyme. Nature 1994;370:270–275.

26. Walker NP, Talanian RV, Brady KD, et al. Crystal structure of the cysteine protease interleukin-1 beta-converting enzyme: a (p20/p10)2 homodimer. Cell 1994;78:343–352.
27. Rotonda J, Nicholson DW, Fazil KM, et al. The three-dimensional structure of apopain/CPP32, a key mediator of apoptosis. Nat Struct Biol 1996;3:619–625.
28. Blanchard H, Kodandapani L, Mittl PR, et al. The three-dimensional structure of caspase-8: an initiator enzyme in apoptosis. Structure Fold Des 1999;7:1125–1133.
29. Watt W, Koeplinger KA, Mildner AM, Heinrikson RL, Tomasselli AG, Watenpaugh KD. The atomic-resolution structure of human caspase-8, a key activator of apoptosis. Structure Fold Des 1999;7:1135–1143.
30. Chang DW, Ditsworth D, Liu H, Srinivasula SM, Alnemri ES, Yang X. Oligomerization is a general mechanism for the activation of apoptosis initiator and inflammatory procaspases. J Biol Chem 2003;278:16,466–16,469.
31. Li H, Bergeron L, Cryns V, et al. Activation of caspase-2 in apoptosis. J Biol Chem 1997;272:21,010–21,017.
32. Li P, Nijhawan D, Budihardjo I, et al. Cytochrome c and dATP-dependent formation of Apaf-1/caspase-9 complex initiates an apoptotic protease cascade. Cell 1997;91:479–489.
33. Harvey NL, Butt AJ, Kumar S. Functional activation of Nedd2/ICH-1 (caspase-2) is an early process in apoptosis. J Biol Chem 1997;272:13,134–13,139.
34. Faleiro L, Kobayashi R, Fearnhead H, Lazebnik Y. Multiple species of CPP32 and Mch2 are the major active caspases present in apoptotic cells. EMBO J 1997;16:2271–2281.
35. Wang L, Miura M, Bergeron L, Zhu H, Yuan J. Ich-1, an Ice/ced-3-related gene, encodes both positive and negative regulators of programmed cell death. Cell 1994;78:739–750.
36. Kumar S, Kinoshita M, Noda M, Copeland NG, Jenkins NA. Induction of apoptosis by the mouse Nedd2 gene, which encodes a protein similar to the product of the *Caenorhabditis elegans* cell death gene ced-3 and the mammalian IL-1 beta-converting enzyme. Genes Dev 1994;8:1613–1626.
37. Bergeron L, Perez GI, Macdonald G, et al. Defects in regulation of apoptosis in caspase-2-deficient mice. Genes Dev 1998;12:1304–1314.
38. Lassus P, Opitz-Araya X, Lazebnik Y. Requirement for caspase-2 in stress-induced apoptosis before mitochondrial permeabilization. Science 2002;297:1352–1354.
39. Guo Y, Srinivasula SM, Druilhe A, Fernandes-Alnemri T, Alnemri ES. Caspase-2 induces apoptosis by releasing proapoptotic proteins from mitochondria. J Biol Chem 2002;277:13,430–13,437.
40. Paroni G, Henderson C, Schneider C, Brancolini C. Caspase-2 can trigger cytochrome C release and apoptosis from the nucleus. J Biol Chem 2002;277:15,147–15,161.
41. Rodriguez J, Lazebnik Y. Caspase-9 and APAF-1 form an active holoenzyme. Genes Dev 1999;13: 3179–184.
42. Ashkenazi A, Dixit VM. Death receptors: signaling and modulation. Science 1998;281:1305–1308.
43. Nagata S. Fas ligand-induced apoptosis. Annu Rev Genet 1999;33:29–55.
44. Krammer PH. CD95's deadly mission in the immune system. Nature 2000;407:789–795.
45. Locksley RM, Killeen N, Lenardo MJ. The TNF and TNF receptor superfamilies: integrating mammalian biology. Cell 2001;104:487–501.
46. Sheridan JP, Marsters SA, Pitti RM, et al. Control of TRAIL-induced apoptosis by a family of signaling and decoy receptors [see comments]. Science 1997;277:818–821.
47. Pan G, Ni J, Wei YF, Yu G, Gentz R, Dixit VM. An antagonist decoy receptor and a death domain-containing receptor for TRAIL [see comments]. Science 1997;277:815–818.
48. Ashkenazi A, Pai RC, Fong S, et al. Safety and antitumor activity of recombinant soluble Apo2 ligand. J Clin Invest 1999;104:155–162.
49. Liu J, Na S, Glasebrook A, et al. Enhanced CD4+ T cell proliferation and Th2 cytokine production in DR6-deficient mice. Immunity 2001;15:23–34.
50. Boldin MP, Varfolomev EE, Pancer Z, Mett IL, Camonis JH, Wallach D. A novel protein that interacts with the death domain of Fas/APO1 contains a sequence motif related to the death domain. J Biol Chem 1995;270:7795–7798.
51. Chinnaiyan AM, O'Rourke K, Tewari M, Dixit VM. FADD, a novel death domain-containing protein, interacts with the death domain of Fas and initiates apoptosis. Cell 1995;81:505–512.
52. Kischkel FC, Hellbardt SH, Behrmann I, et al. Cytotoxicity-dependent APO-1 (Fas/CD-95)-associated proteins form a death-inducing signaling complex (DISC) with the receptor. EMBO J. 1995;14: 5579–5588.
53. Boldin MP, Goncharov TM, Goltsev YV, Wallach D. Involvement of MACH, a novel MORT1/FADD interacting protease, in Fas/APO-1 and TNF receptor-induced cell death. Cell 1996;85:803–815.

54. Muzio M, Chinnaiyan AM, Kischkel FC, et al. FLICE, a novel FADD-homologous ICE/CED-3 like protease, is recruited to the CD95 (Fas/Apo1) death inducing signal complex. Cell 1996;85:817–827.
55. Medema JP, Scaffidi C, Kischkel FC, et al. FLICE is activated by association with the CD95 death-inducing signaling complex (DISC). Embo J 1997;16:2794–2804.
56. Scaffidi C, Medema JP, Krammer PH, Peter ME. FLICE is predominantly expressed as two functionally active isoforms, caspase-8/a and caspase-8/b. J Biol Chem 1997;272:26,953–26,958.
57. Fernandes-Alnemri T, Armstrong RC, Krebs J, et al. In vitro activation of CPP32 and Mch3 by Mch4, a novel human apoptotic cysteine protease containing two FADD-like domains. Proc Natl Acad Sci USA 1996;93:7464–7469.
58. Shu HB, Halpin DR, Goeddel DV. Casper is a FADD- and caspase-related inducer of apoptosis. Immunity 1997;6:751–763.
59. Han D, Chaudhary PM, Wright ME, et al. MRIT, a novel death-effector domain-containing protein, interacts with caspases and BclXL and initiates cell death. Proc Natl Acad Sci USA 1997;94:11,333–11,338.
60. Inohara N, Koseki T, Hu Y, Chen S, Nunez G. CLARP, a death effector domain-containing protein interacts with caspase-8 and regulates apoptosis. Proc Natl Acad Sci USA 1997;94:10,717–10,722.
61. Goltsev YV, Kovalenko AV, Arnold E, Varfolomeev EE, Brodianskii VM, Wallach D. CASH, a novel caspase homologue with death effector domains. J Biol Chem 1997;272:19,641–19,644.
62. Irmler M, Thome M, Hahne M, et al. Inhibition of death receptor signals by cellular FLIP. Nature 1997;388:190–195.
63. Hu S, Vincenz C, Ni J, Gentz R, Dixi VM. I-FLICE, a novel inhibitor of tumor necrosis factor receptor-1- and CD-95-induced apoptosis. J Biol Chem 1997;272:17,255–17,257.
64. Srinivasula SM, Ahmad M, Ottilie S, et al. FLAME-1, a novel FADD-like anti-apoptotic molecule that regulates Fas/TNFR1-induced apoptosis. J Biol Chem 1997;272:18,542–18,545.
65. Rasper DM, Vaillancourt JP, Hadano S, et al. Cell death attenuation by 'Usurpin', a mammalian DED-caspase homologue that precludes caspase-8 recruitment and activation by the CD-95 (Fas, APO-1) receptor complex. Cell Death Differ 1998;5:271–288.
66. Kischkel FC, Lawrence DA, Tinel A, et al. Death receptor recruitment of endogenous caspase-10 and apoptosis initiation in the absence of caspase-8. J Biol Chem 2001;276:46,639–46,646.
67. Sprick MR, Rieser E, Stahl H, Grosse-Wilde A, Weigand MA, Walczak H. Caspase-10 is recruited to and activated at the native TRAIL and CD95 death-inducing signalling complexes in a FADD-dependent manner but can not functionally substitute caspase-8. Embo J 2002;21:4520–4530.
68. Chang DW, Xing Z, Pan Y, et al. c-FLIP(L) is a dual function regulator for caspase-8 activation and CD95-mediated apoptosis. Embo J 2002;21:3704–3714.
69. Scaffidi C, Schmitz I, Krammer PH, Peter ME. The role of c-FLIP in modulation of CD95-induced apoptosis. J Biol Chem 1999;274:1541–1548.
70. Chan FK, Chun HJ, Zheng L, Siegel RM, Bui KL, Lenardo MJ. A domain in TNF receptors that mediates ligand-independent receptor assembly and signaling [see comments]. Science 2000;288:2351–2354.
71. Siegel RM, Frederiksen JK, Zacharias DA, et al. Fas preassociation required for apoptosis signaling and dominant inhibition by pathogenic mutations [see comments]. Science 2000;288:2354–2357.
72. Algeciras-Schimnich A, Shen L, Barnhart BC, Murmann AE, Burkhardt JK, Peter ME. Molecular ordering of the initial signaling events of CD95. Mol Cell Biol 2002;22:207–220.
73. Kischkel FC, Lawrence DA, Chuntharapai A, Schow P, Kim KJ, Ashkenazi A. Apo2L/TRAIL-dependent recruitment of endogenous FADD and caspase-8 to death receptors 4 and 5. Immunity 2000;12:611–620.
74. Scaffidi C, Fulda S, Srinivasan A, et al. Two CD95 (APO-1/Fas) signaling pathways. Embo J 1998;17:1675–1687.
75. Li H, Zhu H, Xu C, Yuan J. Cleavage of BID by caspase-8 mediates the mitochondrial damage in the Fas pathway of apoptosis. Cell 1998;94:491–501.
76. Luo X, Budihardjo I, Zou H, Slaughter C, Wang X. BID, a Bcl-2 interacting protein, mediates cytochrome c release from mitochondria in response to activation of cell surface death receptors. Cell 1998;94:481–490.
77. Korsmeyer SJ, Wei MC, Saito M, Weiler S, Oh KJ, Schlesinger PH. Pro-apoptotic cascade activates BID, which oligomerizes BAK or BAX into pores that result in the release of cytochrome c. Cell Death Differ 2000;7:1166–1173.
78. Rodriguez I, Matsuura K, Khatib K, Reed JC, Nagata S, Vassalli P. A bcl-2 transgene expressed in hepatocytes protects mice from fulminant liver destruction but not from rapid death induced by anti-Fas antibody injection. J Exp Med 1996;183:1031–1036.

79. Strasser A, Harris AW, Huang DC, Krammer PH, Cory S. Bcl-2 and Fas/APO-1 regulate distinct pathways to lymphocyte apoptosis. EMBO J. 1995;14:6136–6147.
80. Yin XM, Wang K, Gross A, et al. Bid-deficient mice are resistant to Fas-induced hepatocellular apoptosis. Nature 1999;400:886–891.
81. Hsu H, Xiong J, Goeddel DV. The TNF receptor 1-associated protein TRADD signals cell death and NF-kB activation. Cell 1995;81:495–504.
82. Hsu H, Shu H-B, Pan M-G, Goeddel DV. TRADD-TRAF2 and TRADD-FADD interactions define two distinct TNF receptor 1 signal transduction pathways. Cell 1996;84:299–308.
83. Micheau O, Tschopp J. Induction of TNF receptor I-mediated apoptosis via two sequential signaling complexes. Cell 2003;114:181–190.
84. Juo P, Kuo CJ, Yuan J, Blenis J. Essential requirement for caspase-8/FLICE in the initiation of the Fas-induced apoptotic cascade. Curr Biol 1998;8:1001–1008.
85. Varfolomeev EE, Schuchmann M, Luria V, et al. Targeted disruption of the mouse caspase 8 gene ablates cell death induction by the TNF receptors, Fas/Apo1, and DR3 and is lethal prenatally. Immunity 1998;9:267–276.
86. Lavrik I, Krueger A, Schmitz I, et al. The active caspase-8 heterotetramer is formed at the CD95 DISC. Cell Death Differ 2003;10:144–145.
87. Martin DA, Siegel RM, Zheng L, Lenardo MJ. Membrane oligomerization and cleavage activates the caspase-8 (FLICE/MACHalpha1) death signal. J Biol Chem 1998;273:4345–4349.
88. Yang X, Chang HY, Baltimore D. Autoproteolytic activation of pro-caspases by oligomerization. Mol Cell 1998;1:319–325.
89. Muzio M, Stockwell BR, Stennicke HR, Salvesen GS, Dixit VM. An induced proximity model of caspase-8 activation. J Biol Chem 1998;273:2926–2930.
90. MacCorkle RA, Freeman KW, Spencer DM. Synthetic activation of caspases: artificial death switches. Proc Natl Acad Sci USA 1998;95:3655–3660.
91. Yang X, Chang HY, Baltimore D. Essential role of CED-4 oligomerization in CED-3 activation and apoptosis. Science 1998;281:1355–1357.
92. Srinivasula SM, Ahmad M, Fernandes-Alnemri T, Alnemri ES. Autoactivation of procaspase-9 by Apaf-1-mediated oligomerization. Mol Cell 1998;1:949–957.
93. Hu Y, Ding L, Spencer DM, Nunez G. WD-40 repeat region regulates Apaf-1 self-association and procaspase-9 activation. J Biol Chem 1998;273:33,489–33,494.
94. Wang J, Chun HJ, Wong W, Spencer DM, Lenardo MJ. Caspase-10 is an initiator caspase in death receptor signaling. Proc Natl Acad Sci USA 2001;98:13,884–13,888.
95. Colussi PA, Harvey NL, Kumar S. Prodomain-dependent nuclear localization of the caspase-2 (Nedd2) precursor. A novel function for a caspase prodomain. J Biol Chem 1998;273:24,535–24,542.
96. Zou H, Li Y, Liu X, Wang X. An APAF-1.cytochrome c multimeric complex is a functional apoptosome that activates procaspase-9. J Biol Chem 1999;274:11,549–11,556.
97. Jiang X, Wang X. Cytochrome c promotes caspase-9 activation by inducing nucleotide binding to Apaf-1. J Biol Chem 2000;275:31,199–31,203.
98. Schlessinger J. Cell signaling by receptor tyrosine kinases. Cell 2000;103:211–225.
99. Salvesen GS, Dixit VM. Caspase activation: the induced-proximity model. Proc Natl Acad Sci USA 1999;96:10,964–10,967.
100. Chang DW, Xing Z, Capacio VL, Peter ME, Yang X. Interdimer processing mechanism of procaspase-8 activation. Embo J 2003;22:4132–4142.
101. Boatright KM, Renatus M, Scott FL, et al. A unified model for apical caspase activation. Mol Cell 2003;11:529–541.
102. Donepudi M, Sweeney AM, Briand C, Grutter MG. Insights into the regulatory mechanism for caspase-8 activation. Mol Cell 2003;11:543–549.
103. Holler N, Tardivel A, Kovacsovics-Bankowski M, et al. Two adjacent trimeric fas ligands are required for fas signaling and formation of a death-inducing signaling complex. Mol Cell Biol 2003;23:1428–440.
104. Acehan D, Jiang X, Morgan DG, Heuser JE, Wang X, Akey CW. Three-dimensional structure of the apoptosome: implications for assembly, procaspase-9 binding, and activation. Mol Cell 2002;9:423–432.
105. Chun HJ, Zheng L, Ahmad M, et al. Pleiotropic defects in lymphocyte activation caused by caspase-8 mutations lead to human immunodeficiency. Nature 2002;419:395–399.
106. Salmena L, Lemmers B, Hakem A, et al. Essential role for caspase 8 in T-cell homeostasis and T-cell-mediated immunity. Genes Dev 2003;17:883–895.

107. Smith KG, Strasser A, Vaux DL. CrmA expression in T lymphocytes of transgenic mice inhibits CD95 (Fas/APO-1)-transduced apoptosis, but does not cause lymphadenopathy or autoimmune disease. Embo J 1996;15:5167–5176.
108. Wang J, Zheng L, Lobito A, et al. Inherited human caspase 10 mutations underlie defective lymphocyte and dendritic cell apoptosis in autoimmune lymphoproliferative syndrome type II. Cell 1999;98:47–58.
109. Barnhart BC, Lee JC, Alappat EC, Peter ME. The death effector domain protein family. Oncogene 2003;22:8634–8644.
110. Park WS, Lee JH, Shin MS, et al. Inactivating mutations of the caspase-10 gene in gastric cancer. Oncogene 2002;21:2919–2925.
111. Shin MS, Kim HS, Lee SH, et al. Alterations of Fas-pathway genes associated with nodal metastasis in non-small cell lung cancer. Oncogene 2002;21:4129–4136.
112. Shin MS, Kim HS, Kang CS, et al. Inactivating mutations of CASP10 gene in non-Hodgkin lymphomas. Blood 2002;99:4094–4099.
113. Kang JJ, Schaber MD, Srinivasula SM, et al. Cascades of mammalian caspase activation in the yeast *Saccharomyces cerevisiae*. J Biol Chem 1999;274:3189–3198.
114. Krueger A, Baumann S, Krammer PH, Kirchhoff S. FLICE-inhibitory proteins: regulators of death receptor-mediated apoptosis. Mol Cell Biol 2001;21:8247–8254.
115. Krueger A, Schmitz I, Baumann S, Krammer PH, Kirchhoff S. Cellular FLICE-inhibitory protein splice variants inhibit different steps of caspase-8 activation at the CD95 death-inducing signaling complex. J Biol Chem 2001;276:20,633–20,640.
116. Yeh WC, Itie A, Elia AJ, et al. Requirement for Casper (c-FLIP) in regulation of death receptor-induced apoptosis and embryonic development. Immunity 2000;12:633–642.
117. Micheau O, Thome M, Schneider P, et al. The long form of FLIP is an activator of caspase-8 at the Fas death-inducing signaling complex. J Biol Chem 2002;277:45,162–45,171.
118. Micheau O, Lens S, Gaide O, Alevizopoulos K, Tschopp J. NF-kappaB signals induce the expression of c-FLIP. Mol Cell Biol 2001;21:5299–5305.
119. Kreuz S, Siegmund D, Scheurich P, Wajant H. NF-kappaB inducers upregulate cFLIP, a cycloheximide-sensitive inhibitor of death receptor signaling. Mol Cell Biol 2001;21:3964–3973.
120. Kirchhoff S, Muller WW, Krueger A, Schmitz I, Krammer PH. TCR-mediated up-regulation of c-FLIPshort correlates with resistance toward CD95-mediated apoptosis by blocking death-inducing signaling complex activity. J Immunol 2000;165:6293–6300.
121. Kirchhoff S, Muller WW, Li-Weber M, Krammer PH. Up-regulation of c-FLIPshort and reduction of activation-induced cell death in CD28-costimulated human T cells. Eur J Immunol 2000;30:2765–2774.

7 Death Signaling and Therapeutic Applications of TRAIL

Mi-Hyang Kim and Dai-Wu Seol, PhD

SUMMARY

Apoptosis is a biological process that plays a pivotal role in the development and homeostasis of multicellular organisms *(1–3)*. Aberrations of this process can be detrimental to organisms. Excessive apoptosis causes damage to normal tissues in certain autoimmune disorders; however, a failure of apoptosis allows cells to grow unlimitedly, resulting in neoplasia. A wide variety of molecules have been identified to induce apoptosis. Among these molecules, ligand-type cytokine molecules including the tumor necrosis factor (TNF) family members have been best characterized. The TNF family members most extensively characterized for death signaling and structure include TNF-α, Fas ligand (FasL), and TNF-related apoptosis-inducing ligand (TRAIL).

TRAIL, also known as Apo2L, has been identified by a homology search of an expressed sequence tag database with a highly conserved sequence motif characteristic for the TNF family members *(4,5)*. The open reading frame encodes 281 amino acids for human TRAIL and 291 amino acids for mouse TRAIL *(4)*. TRAIL is primarily expressed as a type II membrane protein in which the carboxyl terminus of the receptor-binding domain protrudes extacellularly. As reported for TNF-α and FasL, TRAIL can also be cleaved from the cell membrane by metalloproteases to yield a soluble and biologically active form *(6)*. Structural studies have demonstrated that biologically active soluble TRAIL forms a homotrimer *(7,8)*. The homotrimeric structure of TRAIL is stabilized by a cysteine residue at position 230 that coordinates with a divalent zinc ion *(8,9)*. The depletion of the zinc ion or a mutation of the cysteine residue to alanine or glycine abrogated functional activity of TRAIL protein *(9,10)*, indicating that the trimeric structure of TRAIL is critical for biological activity.

TRAIL has been identified to bind five different receptor molecules, such as death receptor (DR)4, DR5, decoy receptor (DcR)1, DcR2 (Table 1), and osteoprotegerin (OPG). These receptor molecules, members of the TNF receptor (TNFR) family, are type I transmembrane polypeptides with two to five cysteine-rich domains at the extracellular

From: *Cancer Drug Discovery and Development: Death Receptors in Cancer Therapy*
Edited by: W. S. El-Deiry © Humana Press Inc., Totowa, NJ

Table 1
TRAIL Receptors

Receptors	TRAIL-R1	TRAIL-R2	TRAIL-R3	TRAIL-R4	Osteoprotegrin
Other name	DR4	DR5	DcR1	DcR2	OPG
		TRICK2	TRID	TRUNDD	
		Killer	LIT		

region. DR4 and DR5 are intact functional TRAIL receptors that contain a cytoplasmic death domain and transmit the apoptosis-inducing activity of TRAIL across the cell membrane *(11–14)*. In contrast, the three other receptors do not have a functional death domain. Thus, they may act as decoy receptors, probably by competing with DR4 or DR5 for TRAIL. The decoy receptor DcR1 is a glycosylphosphatidylinositol (GPI)-linked membrane molecule and acts as an antagonizing receptor for TRAIL *(12–16)*. The decoy receptor DcR2 contains a truncated death domain and is unable to elicit an apoptotic response upon stimulation by TRAIL *(17–19)*. Similar to DcR1, overexpression of DcR2 blocks the function of DR4 and DR5 by competing with DR4 or DR5 for TRAIL. TRAIL has also been shown to interact with OPG, a soluble protein that regulates osteoclastogenesis by competing with receptor activator of NF-κB (RANK) for RANK ligand (RANKL) *(20)*. However, TRAIL has been shown to have a much weaker affinity for OPG *(21)*; therefore, it is unclear whether or not OPG can efficiently act as a decoy receptor for TRAIL under physiological conditions. Except for OPG, the genes of the other four TRAIL receptors are tightly clustered on human chromosome 8q21-22 *(16)*, suggesting that they have evolved by gene duplication.

Although TRAIL is a TNF family member protein, it has some notable differences from other family member proteins. Unlike other members of TNF family, whose expression is restricted to some cells and tissues such as activated T-cells, natural killer (NK) cells, and immune-privileged sites, TRAIL is widely expressed in many cell types and tissues *(4)*. Expression of TRAIL receptors closely parallels that of TRAIL *(11–14)*, suggesting that most tissues and cell types are potential targets for TRAIL.

TRAIL has a unique selectivity for triggering apoptosis in tumor cells *(22–24)* and may be less active against normal cells. Hence, in contrast to FasL or agonistic Fas antibody, which induce fulminant massive liver damage *(25,26)* when introduced systemically, TRAIL does not exhibit any undesirable cytotoxicity in mice *(23)* and nonhuman primates *(22,24)*. Human immunodeficiency virus (HIV)-1-infected T-cells were also shown to be more susceptible to TRAIL than uninfected T-cells *(27)*. Recent results demonstrated that TRAIL knockout mice are more susceptible to experimental and spontaneous tumorigenesis and metastasis *(28)*. These mice were also observed to be defective in thymocyte apoptosis and impaired in negative selection of thymocytes. As a result of defective thymocyte apoptosis, TRAIL-deficient mice showed accelerated experimental autoimmune diseases such as collagen-induced arthritis and streptozotocin-induced diabetes *(29)*. Recent studies have also shown that TRAIL is an active NK cell-mediated blocker of tumor metastasis *(30)*. These features have focused considerable attention on TRAIL as an important cellular factor of natural defense mechanisms and as a potential therapeutic to treat human cancers and acquired immunodeficiency syndrome (AIDS).

DEATH SIGNALING TRIGGERED BY TRAIL

The exact sequence of the signaling events triggered by TRAIL is not fully understood. Nevertheless, it has been well known that caspase activation is a critical step to transmit TRAIL-initiated proapoptotic signals, and the activation of the executioner caspases, such as caspase-3 and -7, are pivotal to accomplish TRAIL-induced apoptosis. Based on their structural features, caspases can be divided into at least two groups: initial caspases (caspase-8, -9, and -10), with a long prodomain, and executioner caspases (caspase-3, -6, and -7), with a short prodomain. In the activation process, especially in death receptor-mediated apoptosis, each group of caspases is activated by different mechanisms. Initial caspases are activated by noncaspase cellular factors such as Fas-associated death domain (FADD) *(31,32)* and Apaf-1 *(33)*, and executioner caspases are activated by upstream active caspases *(33)*.

Biologically active trimeric TRAIL protein activates TRAIL receptors (Fig. 1) via trimerization *(7,8)*. Similar to other TNF family receptors, stimulation of the death domain-containing TRAIL receptors DR4 or DR5 recruits cellular adaptor protein FADD through interaction of the death domains on each molecule *(31,32)*. Recently, the GTP-binding adaptor protein death-associated protein-3 (DAP3), originally found as a mediator of interferon-γ-induced apoptosis, has been identified as an additional adaptor protein for DR4 and DR5 *(34)*. DAP3 has been shown to bind to the death domain of DR4 and DR5 and the death effector domain of FADD, presumably linking activation of DR4 and DR5 to FADD. However, recent studies have demonstrated that DAP3 is a ribosomal protein localized to the mitochondrial matrix, and DAP3 does not interact with FADD as long as subcellular compartments remain intact *(35,36)*. Therefore, the involvement of DAP3 in TRAIL receptor-mediated apoptotic signaling is uncertain. Numerous studies have demonstrated a critical role of FADD in TRAIL-induced apoptosis; therefore, the recruitment of FADD to activated DR4 or DR5 is considered to be an initial step for DR4- and DR5-mediated signaling cascades. FADD, which is also crucially involved in apoptotic signaling for other death receptors such as Fas and TNFR1, recruits procasepase-8 *(31,32)* and procaspase-10 *(37,38)*, forming a death-inducing signaling complex (DISC). The recruited procaspase-8 and procaspase-10 molecules undergo autopro-teolytic activation by induced proximity *(39,40)*. Despite identification of procaspase-10 as a component of DISC, the involvement of caspase-10 in initial death signaling activated by stimulated TRAIL receptors is unclear. Several studies suggest a minor role of caspase-10 in initial events of the caspase cascade *(37,41)*. A better understanding of subcellular localization and expression levels of caspase-10 is important to analyze its functional role in death receptor-mediated signaling cascades.

Once activated, caspase-8 initiates caspase signaling leading to cleavage of many cellular components (Fig. 1). Proapoptotic signals following activation of caspase-8 are known to transmit through at least two pathways *(42,43)*. One proapoptotic signal pathway, termed *mitochondria-independent pathway*, involves direct activation of executioner caspases (caspase-3 and -7) by caspase-8. Another proapoptotic signal pathway, termed *mitochondria-dependent pathway*, employs mitochondrial events to activate the executioner caspases. The mitochondria-dependent pathway is initiated by Bid, a Bcl-2 family member. After cleavage of Bid by caspase-8, truncated Bid (tBid) translocates to the mitochondria and induces cytochrome c release into the cytoplasm *(42,44)*. The cytoplasmic cytochrome c binds to Apaf-1 and participates in caspase-9 activation *(33)*.

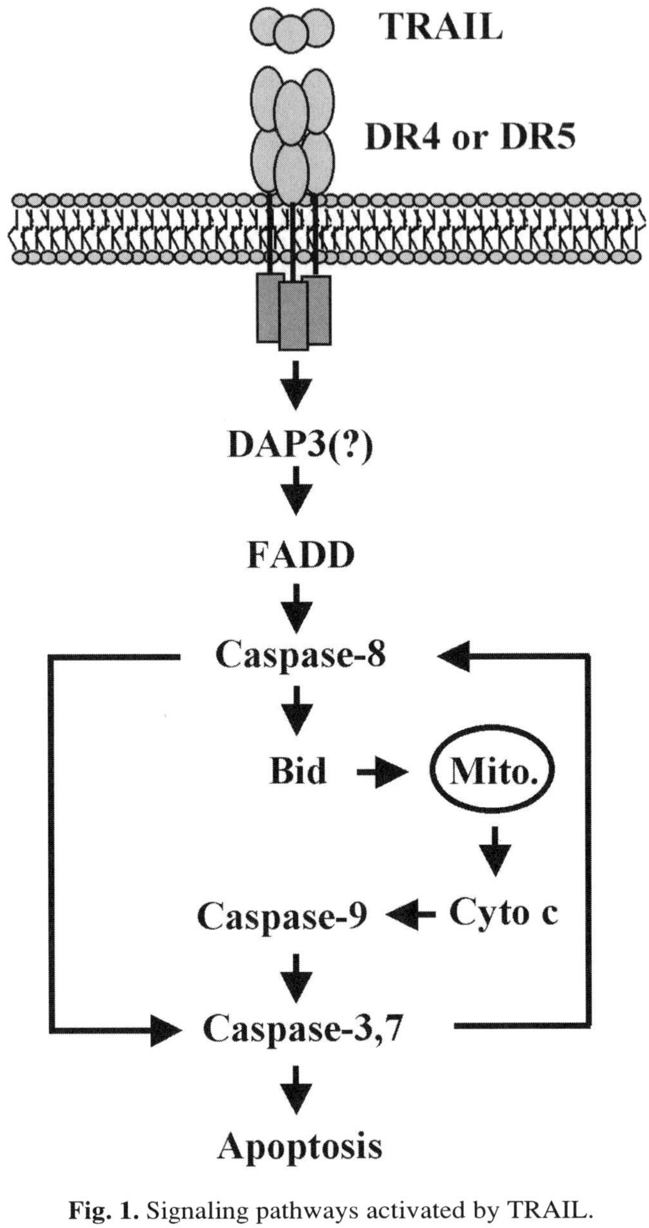

Fig. 1. Signaling pathways activated by TRAIL.

The activated caspase-9 is then able to activate executioner caspases *(33)*. Thus, activation of executioner caspases is the point that mitochondria-dependent and -independent proapoptotic signal pathways meet. In most cell types, the mitochondria-dependent signaling pathway is required for efficient induction of apoptosis despite the existence of a mitochondria-independent signal pathway. The mitochondrial events also include the release of Smac/DIABLO *(45,46)*, apoptosis-inducing factor (AIF) *(47)* and other propapoptotic factors *(48,49)* from the mitochondria. The release of Smac/DIABLO from mitochondria appears to be induced by tBid and occurs simultaneously with cytochrome c release. Once activated, executioner caspases liberate a DNase termed CAD (caspase-activated DNase) by cleaving an inhibitor of CAD (ICAD/DFF-45) *(50–52)*. CAD activation leads to DNA degradation, a hallmark event in apoptosis. Activation of executioner caspases also leads to cleavage of numerous cytosolic, cytoskeletal, and nuclear proteins

There are two types of cells, termed type I and type II cells, depending on their response to stimulation by death ligands. In type I cells, stimulation of TRAIL receptors activates caspase-8 to an extent that is sufficient to activate an adequate amount of executioner caspases and induce apoptosis *(53,54)*. Since mitochondria-independent direct activation of executioner caspases by caspase-8 plays a major role in this cell type, high expression levels of death domain-containing TRAIL receptors and caspase-8 are important for induction of apoptosis. In type II cells, caspase-8 activation is limited and only sufficient to cleave Bid. Generation of tBid triggers the mitochondrial events leading to activation of the mitochondria-dependent proapoptotic signal pathway. Postmitochondrial activation of executioner caspases leads to activation of initial caspase such as caspase-8, forming a proapoptotic amplification loop, which results in effective induction of apoptosis.

REGULATION OF SUSCEPTIBILITY TO TRAIL-INDUCED APOPTOSIS

Regulation of TRAIL-induced apoptosis occurs at multiple points and involves a battery of molecules and signals. Expression and subcellular localization of major signaling factors, including receptor molecules, affect the TRAIL susceptibility of the cell. Antiapoptotic molecules and other factors can regulate TRAIL-induced apoptosis by affecting the activity of proapoptotic factors involved in the signaling cascades. Diverse extracellular cell survival signals also influence TRAIL susceptibility of cells by modulating many cellular factors involved in TRAIL signaling.

The expression levels of the factors involved in TRAIL-triggered death signaling may influence signal strength generated by stimulated TRAIL receptors. Early studies suggested that the expression levels of decoy receptor DcR1 and DcR2 might be critical in TRAIL-induced selective induction of apoptosis in tumor cells because the levels of these decoy receptors were higher in normal cells than in tumor cells *(12,13,15,18)*. In experimental settings, overexpression of decoy receptors protected TRAIL-sensitive cells from TRAIL-induced apoptosis. However, subsequent studies, including more cell types derived from tumor and normal tissues, did not show a solid correlation between the expression levels of decoy receptors and TRAIL susceptibility *(55–57)*. These results suggest that physiological levels of decoy receptors may not be sufficient to inhibit TRAIL-induced apoptosis. Nevertheless, these decoy receptors may contribute to TRAIL resistance under certain physiologic or pathologic conditions, since these conditions regulate the expression levels and subcellular localization of these decoy receptors *(58)*.

Expression and mutations of death domain-containing TRAIL receptors DR4 and DR5 can influence TRAIL susceptibility *(59,60)*. DNA-damaging agents, such as chemotherapeutic agents and ionizing radiation, have been shown to upregulate DR5 expression in both a p53-dependent and -independent manner *(61,62)*. However, these DNA-damaging agents also upregulate TRAIL decoy receptors DcR1 and DcR2 *(63,64)*, which may abrogate the augmented susceptibility due to the increased expression of DR4 and DR5. Since numerous DNA-damaging agents have been shown to sensitize cells to TRAIL, whether or not TRAIL sensitization by DNA-damaging agents requires upregulation of DR5 is unclear. A mutation of the DR5 gene in head and neck cancer tissues truncates its death domain, converting it to a decoy receptor-like molecule and resulting in loss of TRAIL-induced apoptosis induction *(60)*. Similarly, a homozygous deletion of the death domain region in the DR4 gene has been identified in a nasopharyngeal carcinoma cell line and associated with TRAIL resistance in this cell line *(59)*.

In addition to receptor molecules, many cytosolic factors involved in TRAIL signaling also modulate TRAIL-induced apoptosis. In accordance with an essential role in death signaling, the adaptor molecule FADD regulates the TRAIL susceptibility of a cell *(31,37,65)*. A FADD-deficient cell line failed to recruit procaspase-8 to the activated TRAIL receptors, resulting in complete resistance to TRAIL-induced apoptosis. Similarly, mouse embryonic fibroblasts derived from FADD knockout mouse were also resistant to apoptosis induced by DR4 and DR5 overexpression.

Caspase-8, another component of DISC, plays a critical role in TRAIL death signaling. Caspase-8-deficient cells were shown to be resistant to TRAIL-induced apoptosis *(41,66)*. In childhood neuroblastoma, the gene for caspase-8 was found to be frequently silenced through DNA methylation and gene deletion *(67–71)*. Cell lines established from the neuroblastoma tissues were resistant to apoptosis induced by TRAIL. Cellular FLICE-inhibitory protein (c-FLIP), structurally related to procaspase-8 but lacking an active site for proteolytic action, inhibits TRAIL-induced apoptosis *(72,73)* by competing with procaspase-8 for FADD, preventing the formation of a functional DISC. High expression of c-FLIP has been observed in many cancer cells that are resistant to TRAIL *(55,74,75)*, suggesting that the expression levels of c-FLIP may be an important determinant in controlling the susceptibility of tumor cells to TRAIL. The level of c-FLIP is regulated by the transcription factor NF-κB *(76–78)*, an antiapoptotic factor that upregulates antiapoptotic genes.

Cell survival factor Akt has been shown to inhibit TRAIL-induced apoptosis. Receptor ligation by platelet-derived growth factor (PDGF) *(79)* and insulin-like growth factor (IGF)-1 *(80)* activates Akt following PI-3K activation. Akt is a protein kinase with targets including proapoptotic factors Bad *(79)* and caspase-9 *(81)* as well as a forkhead transcription factor FKHR *(82–85)*. Activation of Akt by phosphorylation leads to phosphorylation of its downstream targets. Phosphorylation of Bad and caspase-9 attenuates their proapoptotic activity *(79,81)*, ablating the propagation of downstream proapoptotic signaling cascades. Phosphorylation of the FKHR prevents translocation of FKHR to the nucleus and results in a blockade of target gene transcription *(82–85)*. However, the detailed mechanism by which FKHR regulates apoptosis has not yet been determined, including the identity of the target genes regulated by FKHR. A human prostate cancer cell line with constitutive activation of Akt is almost completely resistant to TRAIL *(86,87)*, indicating that Akt may play a critical role in normal cell physiology, tumorigenensis, and apoptosis.

The protein kinase C (PKC) family of serine-threonine kinases is activated by diverse stimuli and participates in many cellular processes, such as cell growth, differentiation, and apoptosis. Different isoforms of PKC act as negative regulators of TRAIL-induced apoptosis *(88)*. A dominant-negative form of PKC sensitized TRAIL-resistant glioma cells to TRAIL, and reintroduction of PKC to TRAIL-sensitive cells resulted in the reduction of apoptosis induced by TRAIL *(88,89)*. Furthermore, inhibition of PKC activity restored sensitivity in TRAIL-resistant glioma cells. Thus, diverse cell-survival stimuli activating Akt and PKC may negatively regulate TRAIL-induced apoptosis.

The deficiency of Bax, a proapoptotic Bcl-2 family member, also results in significant reduction of apoptosis induced by TRAIL *(90–93)*. Treatment of Bax-deficient cells with TRAIL induced the formation of a functional DISC and led to caspase-8 activation and Bid cleavage. However, mitochondrial events involving the release of mitochondrial factors, such as cytochrome c and Smac/DIABLO, were impaired in Bax-deficient cells. The impaired mitochondrial events prevented postmitochondrial proapoptotic events, including caspase-9 activation. Although the studies using Bax-deficient cells have shown that Bax plays a critical role in the release of mitochondrial factors, another available line of evidence indicates that Bax requires Bak, another Bcl-2 family member, to act as a gateway for the tBid-induced release of mitochondrial factors *(94)*. Cells lacking both Bax and Bak, but not the cells lacking only one of these components, are completely resistant to tBid-induced cytochrome c release and apoptosis.

Antiapoptotic Bcl-2 family members such as Bcl-2 and Bcl-x_L have been shown to inhibit apoptosis mediated by various death receptors. Overexpression of these proteins prevents the release of mitochondrial factors by interacting with proapoptotic Bax and Bad and attenuating their proapoptotic functions *(95)*. Overexpression of Bcl-2 and/or Bcl-x_L protects various TRAIL-sensitive cells from TRAIL-induced apoptosis *(96–100)*. Upregulation of Bcl-2 and Bcl-x_L is also controlled by many extracellular cell-survival stimuli including growth factors *(101,102)* and hypoxia *(103)*.

Inhibitor of apoptosis protein (IAP) family members including c-IAP1, c-IAP2, X chromosome-linked IAP (XIAP), and Survivin are potent inhibitors of caspases *(104–110)*. These proteins exert their inhibitory activity by interacting with caspases, specifically caspase-9, -3, and -7 but not caspase-8. Smac/DIABLO interacts with IAP family members, antagonizing their inhibitory activity and releasing the bound IAPs from caspases *(45,111–115)*. Caspases free of IAPs are more susceptible to proteolytic cleavage and activation from upstream signals. As shown by caspase inhibitors, IAP family proteins block TRAIL-induced apoptosis. The protein levels of the family members are regulated by diverse signals, including self-regulation by an intrinsic ubiquitin protein ligase activity *(116,117)*. This intrinsic ligase activity has also been shown to regulate the levels of other proteins such as caspase-3 and Smac/DIABLO. Downregulation or inactivation of IAPs induced spontaneous apoptosis and resulted in augmentation of apoptosis induced by TRAIL *(118,119)*.

THERAPEUTIC APPLICATIONS OF TRAIL

TRAIL has been shown to be a potent inducer of apoptosis in a wide variety of tumor cell lines in vitro and cancer xenograft animal models in vivo. Despite its efficacy, TRAIL did not show any detectable toxic side effects in safety tests using animals such as mice *(23)*, monkeys *(22)*, and chimpanzees *(24)*. Administration of soluble recombinant TRAIL protein induced selective apoptosis in grafted tumor cells and improved survival in mice bearing solid tumors without detectable damage to normal tissues.

In addition to administration of soluble recombinant TRAIL protein, gene therapy approaches have also produced promising results *(120–124)*. Adenoviral vectors encoding the full-length human TRAIL gene induced apoptosis in many tumor cell lines in vitro. Intratumoral delivery of the TRAIL gene to the grafted tumor tissues in animal models led to apoptotic cell death and suppression of tumor growth. The transfer of the TRAIL gene induced apoptosis of target cells via direct activation of TRAIL receptors. Interestingly, apoptosis is also increased in TRAIL-negative cells located in close proximity to TRAIL-transfected cells. Although the biochemical mechanism of this phenomenon, termed the *bystander effect (124)*, is unclear, this result suggests that apoptosis induced by the full-length TRAIL gene can sequentially propagate to neighboring cells to an extent. A gene therapy approach using a proliferation-specific promoter that drives the full-length TRAIL gene has not shown any cytotoxic effects in hepatocytes *(125)*. Instead, this approach selectively induced apoptosis in the established tumors in an animal model.

In addition to suppression of primary tumors, TRAIL also appears to participate in the suppression of metastasis. In human mammary carcinoma cells, nonanchored tumor cells were shown to be more susceptible to TRAIL than anchored cells *(126)*. Furthermore, TRAIL has been found to play an important role in liver NK cell-mediated suppression of tumor metastasis *(127)*. Blockade of TRAIL action using a neutralizing antibody against TRAIL significantly increased experimental liver metastases of TRAIL-sensitive tumor cells.

Recent studies suggest that TRAIL may also be effective for autoimmune diseases including rheumatoid arthritis. Chronic blockade of TRAIL by a soluble DR5 receptor exacerbated autoimmune arthritis in mice *(128)*. TRAIL blockade in vivo resulted in profound hyperproliferation of synovial cells and arthritogenic lymphocytes. The blockade of TRAIL action also led to the production of inflammatory cytokines and autoantibodies. TRAIL was shown to inhibit DNA synthesis and prevent cell-cycle progression of lymphocytes. In accordance with these observations, TRAIL-deficient mice showed accelerated experimental autoimmune diseases such as collagen-induced arthritis and streptozotocin-induced diabetes *(29)*. The TRAIL-deficient mice turned out to be defective in thymocyte apoptosis and impaired in deletion of autoreactive T-cells, which may result in increase susceptibility to autoimmune disorders. Thus, delivery of TRAIL protein or the gene by a gene therapy approach may become a therapeutic tool to treat such autoimmune diseases as reumatoid arthritis and diabetes.

From a clinical point of view, one of the most important issues in drug development is safety. Numerous studies have demonstrated stringent selectivity of TRAIL to tumor cells but not to normal and nontransformed cells. However, recent reports challenge this established apoptotic selectivity of TRAIL to tumors, demonstrating effective induction of apoptosis in cultured normal human hepatocytes *(129)* and brain cells *(130)*. These observations suggested possible occurrence of severe damage in normal tissues and organs in clinical trials. Reevaluation of these results, however, revealed that the toxicity observed in cultured normal human hepatocytes is associated with the preparation and version of the recombinant TRAIL protein *(131,132)*. The soluble recombinant TRAIL with a histidine-tag or a leucine-zipper at its amino terminus has been shown to induce apoptosis in cultured normal human hepatocytes and keratinocytes. In sharp contrast, a non-histidine-tagged soluble form of TRAIL did not show any cytotoxic activity in cultured normal human hepatocytes or keratinocytes. Despite no cytotoxicity for normal cells, this non-histidine-tagged soluble TRAIL showed increased apoptotic activity against tumor cells. Mice, monkeys, and chimpanzees tolerated non-histidine-tagged TRAIL and showed no adverse reactions *(22,24)*. The non-histidine-tagged TRAIL effectively suppressed tumor xenografts in mice. Thus, this non-histidine-tagged TRAIL is believed to be safe and more appropriate for use in clinical trials; however, the structural difference between these TRAIL proteins is not fully known. The non-histidine-tagged TRAIL is mostly trimeric and contains more zinc ions than histidine-tagged TRAIL, which is a mixture of dimeric and trimeric proteins *(10,131)*. The leucine zipper-fused TRAIL is a homogeneous trimer *(23)* and believed to be structurally similar to non-histidine-tagged TRAIL. The toxicity to normal cells, however, is remarkably different for each version. Detailed understanding of structural differences between these molecules and identification of major receptors for each version of TRAIL protein will spur the development of TRAIL as an anticancer therapy. Nonetheless, these results indicate that TRAIL has a great potential to be developed as a promising anticancer drug that effectively restricts primary tumors as well as metastatic cancers. Furthermore, TRAIL may be applied in the therapy of autoimmune diseases. There is great interest to see whether clinical trials will produce positive results for human cancers as in animal models.

The distribution of TRAIL receptors in tissues suggests a wider scope of targets than TNF-α and FasL in apoptosis. Although TRAIL is a potent apoptosis inducer without damaging normal tissues in vivo, TRAIL alone has limited apoptotic capacity in some cancer cell lines *(22)*; however, combination therapies with TRAIL and chemotherapeutic agents may produce better efficacy than individual therapies in cancer treatment. Many chemotherapeutic agents are known to cause toxic side effects at an effective dose. If a low dose of a chemotherapeutic agent can sensitize cells to TRAIL-induced apoptosis (especially against TRAIL-resistant cancers), this combination therapy would be superior to TRAIL alone. Numerous chemotherapeutic agents have demonstrated augmentation of TRAIL-induced apoptosis in vitro and in vivo *(61,91,133–135)*. This augmentation of activity has been attributed to the inhibition of the antiapoptotic pathway, the activation of the proapoptotic pathway including the induction of the p53 pathway, or a combination of both. For example, doxorubicin increased death domain-containing TRAIL receptors in a p53-dependent manner *(61,136)* and significantly augmented TRAIL-induced apoptosis. Doxorubicin treatment also resulted in synergistic cytotoxicity and apoptosis for multiple myeloma cells that are resistant to TRAIL alone *(137)*. However, in many cases the molecular basis of the synergistic action of chemotherapeutic agents for TRAIL is poorly understood. Chemotherapeutic agents also directly damage mitochondria *(138,139)*, leading to activation of mitochondria-dependent proapoptotic signal pathways. Despite the significance of the proapoptotic mitochondrial events, the detailed mechanisms activated by and cellular targets for chemotherapeutic agents are largely unknown. In addition to chemotherapeutic agents, a Smac/DIABLO antagonizing peptide for IAPs has also showed a potent sensitization activity for TRAIL-induced apoptosis *(118,119)*. In an animal tumor model for brain cancer, this peptide molecule significantly promoted TRAIL-induced apoptosis. The combination of this antagonizing peptide and TRAIL eradicated established tumors without inducing detectable adverse side effects *(118)*. It would be interesting to test whether combinations of TRAIL and enhancers such as chemotherapeutic agents and Smac/DIABLO peptide can be applied to nontransformed normal cells including synovial cells in arthritis.

PERSPECTIVES

Accumulated experimental evidence supports the conclusion that TRAIL selectively induces apoptosis in tumors without damaging normal tissues. However, safety issues related to the different versions of TRAIL proteins have not yet been completely resolved. Although the non-histidine-tagged version of TRAIL looks safe for clinical use, further clarification of structure versus potential toxicity to normal cells is needed.

For the past few years, most of the TRAIL research has been focused on proapoptotic activity of TRAIL. Thus, the normal physiological functions of TRAIL are poorly understood. Recent studies using TRAIL knockout mice and an animal model for chronic blockade of TRAIL function have shed light on the role of TRAIL in normal physiology. A better understanding on the physiological role of TRAIL will broaden the possible therapeutic applications of the molecule.

Despite advancement in understanding of TRAIL action, little is known about TRAIL-triggered death signaling. In particular, modulation of TRAIL death signaling under conditions of continuous challenge with extracelluar cell-survival stimuli is poorly understood. Many extracelluar cell-survival stimuli have been shown to play an important role in apoptosis, since under normal cell physiology, apoptosis is counterbalanced with cell survival. Identification of signal pathways and cellular factors involved in cell-survival signaling will provide information for the potential targets to be specifically blocked, thereby enhancing TRAIL activity in therapeutic applications.

Understanding of the mechanisms by which chemotherapeutic agents act and sensitize TRAIL-induced apoptosis will provide various combination therapies using TRAIL. Although numerous chemotherapeutic agents have shown death augmentation in TRAIL-induced apoptosis in vitro and in vivo, toxicity testing of the combinations in cultured normal human cells has not been intensively performed. These tests would reduce the concerns raised in clinical trials and provide better combination therapies that have higher efficacy and less toxicity than individual therapies.

TRAIL has a great potential to be developed as a promising new drug for cancers and autoimmune diseases. Even though there is a concern for toxic side effects, clinical trials using TRAIL should move forward. The benefits of TRAIL can only be proven through clinical trials.

REFERENCES

1. Ashkenazi A, Dixit VM. Death receptors: signaling and modulation. Science 1998;281:1305–1308.
2. Nagata S. Apoptosis by death factor. Cell 1997;88:355–3365.
3. Salvesen GS, Dixit VM. Caspases: intracellular signaling by proteolysis. Cell 1997;91:443–446.
4. Wiley SR, Schooley K, Smolak PJ, et al. Identification and characterization of a new member of the TNF family that induces apoptosis. Immunity 1995;3:673–682.
5. Pitti RM, Marsters SA, Ruppert S, Donahue CJ, Moore A, Ashkenazi A. Induction of apoptosis by Apo-2 ligand, a new member of the tumor necrosis factor cytokine family. J Biol Chem 1996;271:12,687–12,690.
6. Liabakk NB, Sundan A, Torp S, Aukrust P, Froland SS, Espevik T. Development, characterization and use of monoclonal antibodies against sTRAIL: measurement of sTRAIL by ELISA. J Immunol Methods 2002;259:119–128.
7. Cha SS, Kim MS, Choi YH, et al. 2.8 A resolution crystal structure of human TRAIL, a cytokine with selective antitumor activity. Immunity 1999;11:253–261.
8. Hymowitz SG, Christinger HW, Fuh G, et al. Triggering cell death: the crystal structure of Apo2L/TRAIL in a complex with death receptor 5. Mol Cell 1999;4:563–571.
9. Hymowitz SG, O'Connell MP, Ultsch MH, et al. A unique zinc-binding site revealed by a high-resolution X-ray structure of homotrimeric Apo2L/TRAIL. Biochemistry 2000;39:633–640.

10. Seol DW, Billiar TR. Cysteine 230 modulates tumor necrosis factor-related apoptosis-inducing ligand activity. Cancer Res 2000;60:3152–3154.
11. Pan G, O'Rourke K, Chinnaiyan AM, et al. The receptor for the cytotoxic ligand TRAIL. Science 1997;276:111–113.
12. Pan G, Ni J, Wei YF, Yu G, Gentz R, Dixit VM. An antagonist decoy receptor and a death domain-containing receptor for TRAIL. Science 1997;277:815–818.
13. Sheridan JP, Marsters SA, Pitti RM, et al. Control of TRAIL-induced apoptosis by a family of signaling and decoy receptors. Science 1997;277:818–821.
14. MacFarlane M, Ahmad M, Srinivasula SM, Fernandes-Alnemri T, Cohen GM, Alnemri ES. Identification and molecular cloning of two novel receptors for the cytotoxic ligand TRAIL. J Biol Chem 1997;272:25,417–25,420.
15. Mongkolsapaya J, Cowper AE, Xu XN, et al. Lymphocyte inhibitor of TRAIL (TNF-related apoptosis-inducing ligand): a new receptor protecting lymphocytes from the death ligand TRAIL. J Immunol 1998;160:3–6.
16. Degli-Esposti MA, Smolak PJ, Walczak H, et al. Cloning and characterization of TRAIL-R3, a novel member of the emerging TRAIL receptor family. J Exp Med 1997;186:1165–1170.
17. Pan G, Ni J, Yu G, Wei YF, Dixit VM. TRUNDD, a new member of the TRAIL receptor family that antagonizes TRAIL signalling. FEBS Lett 1998;424:41–45.
18. Marsters SA, Sheridan JP, Pitti RM, et al. A novel receptor for Apo2L/TRAIL contains a truncated death domain. Curr Biol 1997;7:1003–1006.
19. Degli-Esposti MA, Dougall WC, Smolak PJ, Waugh JY, Smith CA, Goodwin RG. The novel receptor TRAIL-R4 induces NF-kappaB and protects against TRAIL-mediated apoptosis, yet retains an incomplete death domain. Immunity 1997;7:813–820.
20. Emery JG, McDonnell P, Burke MB, et al. Osteoprotegerin is a receptor for the cytotoxic ligand TRAIL. J Biol Chem 1998;273:14363–4367.
21. Truneh A, Sharma S, Silverman C, et al. Temperature-sensitive differential affinity of TRAIL for its receptors. DR5 is the highest affinity receptor. J Biol Chem 2000;275:23,319–23,325.
22. Ashkenazi A, Pai RC, Fong S, et al. Safety and antitumor activity of recombinant soluble Apo2 ligand. J Clin Invest 1999;104:155–162.
23. Walczak H, Miller RE, Ariail K, et al. Tumoricidal activity of tumor necrosis factor-related apoptosis-inducing ligand in vivo. Nat Med 1999;5:157–163.
24. Kelley SK, Harris LA, Xie D, et al. Preclinical studies to predict the disposition of Apo2L/tumor necrosis factor- apoptosis-inducing ligand in humans: characterization of in vivo efficacy, pharmacokinetics, and safety. J Pharmacol Exp Ther 2001;299:31–38.
25. Ogasawara J, Watanabe-Fukunaga R, Adachi M, et al. Lethal effect of the anti-Fas antibody in mice. Nature 1993;364:806–809.
26. Galle PR, Hofmann WJ, Walczak H, et al. Involvement of the CD95 (APO-1/Fas) receptor and ligand in liver damage. J Exp Med 1995;182:1223–1230.
27. Jeremias I, Herr I, Boehler T, Debatin KM. TRAIL/Apo-2-ligand-induced apoptosis in human T cells. Eur J Immunol 1998;28:143–152.
28. Cretney E, Takeda K, Yagita H, Glaccum M, Peschon JJ, Smyth MJ. Increased susceptibility to tumor initiation and metastasis in TNF-related apoptosis-inducing ligand-deficient mice. J Immunol 2002;168:1356–1361.
29. Lamhamedi-Cherradi SE, Zheng SJ, Maguschak KA, Peschon J, Chen YH. Defective thymocyte apoptosis and accelerated autoimmune diseases in TRAIL(–/–) mice. Nat Immunol 2003;4:255–260.
30. Takeda K, Smyth MJ, Cretney E, et al. Critical role for tumor necrosis factor-related apoptosis-inducing ligand in immune surveillance against tumor development. J Exp Med 2002;195:161–169.
31. Sprick MR, Weigand MA, Rieser E, et al. FADD/MORT1 and caspase-8 are recruited to TRAIL receptors 1 and 2 and are essential for apoptosis mediated by TRAIL receptor 2. Immunity 2000;12:599–609.
32. Kischkel FC, Lawrence DA, Chuntharapai A, Schow P, Kim KJ, Ashkenazi A. Apo2L/TRAIL-dependent recruitment of endogenous FADD and caspase-8 to death receptors 4 and 5. Immunity 2000;12:611–620.
33. Li P, Nijhawan D, Budihardjo I, et al. Cytochrome c and dATP-dependent formation of Apaf-1/caspase-9 complex initiates an apoptotic protease cascade. Cell 1997;91:479–489.
34. Miyazaki T, Reed JC. A GTP-binding adapter protein couples TRAIL receptors to apoptosis-inducing proteins. Nat Immunol 2001;2:493–500.
35. Berger T, Kretzler M. Interaction of DAP3 and FADD only after cellular disruption. Nat Immunol 2002;3:3–5.

36. Berger T, Kretzler M. TRAIL-induced apoptosis is independent of the mitochondrial apoptosis mediator DAP3. Biochem Biophys Res Commun 2002;297:880–884.
37. Sprick MR, Rieser E, Stahl H, Grosse-Wilde A, Weigand MA, Walczak H. Caspase-10 is recruited to and activated at the native TRAIL and CD95 death-inducing signalling complexes in a FADD-dependent manner but can not functionally substitute caspase-8. Embo J 2002;21:4520–4530.
38. Kischkel FC, Lawrence DA, Tinel A, et al. Death receptor recruitment of endogenous caspase-10 and apoptosis initiation in the absence of caspase-8. J Biol Chem 2001;276:46,639–46,646.
39. Muzio M, Stockwell BR, Stennicke HR, Salvesen GS, Dixit VM. An induced proximity model for caspase-8 activation. J Biol Chem 1998;273:2926–2930.
40. Salvesen GS, Dixit VM. Caspase activation: the induced-proximity model. Proc Natl Acad Sci USA 1999;96:10,964–10,967.
41. Seol DW, Li J, Seol MH, Park SY, Talanian RV, Billiar TR. Signaling events triggered by tumor necrosis factor-related apoptosis-inducing ligand (TRAIL): caspase-8 is required for TRAIL-induced apoptosis. Cancer Res 2001;61:1138–1143.
42. Li H, Zhu H, Xu CJ, Yuan J. Cleavage of BID by caspase 8 mediates the mitochondrial damage in the Fas pathway of apoptosis. Cell 1998;94:491–501.
43. Gross A, Yin XM, Wang K, et al. Caspase cleaved BID targets mitochondria and is required for cytochrome c release, while BCL-XL prevents this release but not tumor necrosis factor-R1/Fas death. J Biol Chem 1999;274:1156–1163.
44. Luo X, Budihardjo I, Zou H, Slaughter C, Wang X. Bid, a Bcl2 interacting protein, mediates cytochrome c release from mitochondria in response to activation of cell surface death receptors. Cell 1998;94:481–490.
45. Verhagen AM, Ekert PG, Pakusch M, et al. Identification of DIABLO, a mammalian protein that promotes apoptosis by binding to and antagonizing IAP proteins. Cell 2000;102:43–53.
46. Du C, Fang M, Li Y, Li L, Wang X. Smac, a mitochondrial protein that promotes cytochrome c-dependent caspase activation by eliminating IAP inhibition. Cell 2000;102:33–42.
47. Susin SA, Lorenzo HK, Zamzami N, et al. Molecular characterization of mitochondrial apoptosis-inducing factor. Nature 1999;397:441–446.
48. Li LY, Luo X, Wang X. Endonuclease G is an apoptotic DNase when released from mitochondria. Nature 2001;412:95–99.
49. Susin SA, Lorenzo HK, Zamzami N, et al. Mitochondrial release of caspase-2 and -9 during the apoptotic process. J Exp Med 1999;189:381–394.
50. Enari M, Sakahira H, Yokoyama H, Okawa K, Iwamatsu A, Nagata S. A caspase-activated DNase that degrades DNA during apoptosis, and its inhibitor ICAD. Nature 1998;391:43–50.
51. Sakahira H, Enari M, Nagata S. Cleavage of CAD inhibitor in CAD activation and DNA degradation during apoptosis. Nature 1998;391:96–99.
52. Liu X, Li P, Widlak P, et al. The 40-kDa subunit of DNA fragmentation factor induces DNA fragmentation and chromatin condensation during apoptosis. Proc Natl Acad Sci USA 1998;95:8461–8466.
53. Scaffidi C, Fulda S, Srinivasan A, et al. Two CD95 (APO-1/Fas) signaling pathways. Embo J 1998;17:1675–1687.
54. Ozoren N, El-Deiry WS. Defining characteristics of Types I and II apoptotic cells in response to TRAIL. Neoplasia 2002;4:551–557.
55. Zhang XD, Franco A, Myers K, Gray C, Nguyen T, Hersey P. Relation of TNF-related apoptosis-inducing ligand (TRAIL) receptor and FLICE-inhibitory protein expression to TRAIL-induced apoptosis of melanoma. Cancer Res 1999;59:2747–2753.
56. Griffith TS, Rauch CT, Smolak PJ, et al. Functional analysis of TRAIL receptors using monoclonal antibodies. J Immunol 1999;162:2597–2605.
57. Leverkus M, Neumann M, Mengling T, et al. Regulation of tumor necrosis factor-related apoptosis-inducing ligand sensitivity in primary and transformed human keratinocytes. Cancer Res 2000;60:553–559.
58. Zhang XD, Franco AV, Nguyen T, Gray CP, Hersey P. Differential localization and regulation of death and decoy receptors for TNF-related apoptosis-inducing ligand (TRAIL) in human melanoma cells. J Immunol 2000;164:3961–3970.
59. Ozoren N, Fisher MJ, Kim K, et al. Homozygous deletion of the death receptor DR4 gene in a nasopharyngeal cancer cell line is associated with TRAIL resistance. Int J Oncol 2000;16:917–925.
60. Pai SI, Wu GS, Ozoren N, et al. Rare loss-of-function mutation of a death receptor gene in head and neck cancer. Cancer Res 1998;58:3513–3518.
61. Wu GS, Burns TF, McDonald ER, 3rd, et al. KILLER/DR5 is a DNA damage-inducible p53-regulated death receptor gene. Nat Genet 1997;17:141–143.

62. Sheikh MS, Burns TF, Huang Y, et al. p53-dependent and -independent regulation of the death receptor KILLER/DR5 gene expression in response to genotoxic stress and tumor necrosis factor alpha. Cancer Res 1998;58:1593–1598.
63. Sheikh MS, Huang Y, Fernandez-Salas EA, et al. The antiapoptotic decoy receptor TRID/TRAIL-R3 is a p53-regulated DNA damage-inducible gene that is overexpressed in primary tumors of the gastrointestinal tract. Oncogene 1999;18:4153–4159.
64. Meng RD, McDonald ER, 3rd, Sheikh MS, Fornace AJ, Jr., El-Deiry WS. The TRAIL decoy receptor TRUNDD (DcR2, TRAIL-R4) is induced by adenovirus-p53 overexpression and can delay TRAIL-, p53-, and KILLER/DR5-dependent colon cancer apoptosis. Mol Ther 2000;1:130–144.
65. Kuang AA, Diehl GE, Zhang J, Winoto A. FADD is required for DR4- and DR5-mediated apoptosis: lack of TRAIL-induced apoptosis in FADD-deficient mouse embryonic fibroblasts. J Biol Chem 2000;275:25,065–25,068.
66. Kim IK, Chung CW, Woo HN, Hong GS, Nagata S, Jung YK. Reconstitution of caspase-8 sensitizes JB6 cells to TRAIL. Biochem Biophys Res Commun 2000;277:311–316.
67. Teitz T, Wei T, Valentine MB, et al. Caspase 8 is deleted or silenced preferentially in childhood neuroblastomas with amplification of MYCN. Nat Med 2000;6:529–535.
68. Hopkins-Donaldson S, Bodmer JL, Bourloud KB, Brognara CB, Tschopp J, Gross N. Loss of caspase-8 expression in highly malignant human neuroblastoma cells correlates with resistance to tumor necrosis factor-related apoptosis-inducing ligand-induced apoptosis. Cancer Res 2000;60:4315–4319.
69. Grotzer MA, Eggert A, Zuzak TJ, et al. Resistance to TRAIL-induced apoptosis in primitive neuroectodermal brain tumor cells correlates with a loss of caspase-8 expression. Oncogene 2000;19:4604–4610.
70. Eggert A, Grotzer MA, Zuzak TJ, Wiewrodt BR, Ikegaki N, Brodeur GM. Resistance to TRAIL-induced apoptosis in neuroblastoma cells correlates with a loss of caspase-8 expression. Med Pediatr Oncol 2000;35:603–607.
71. Eggert A, Grotzer MA, Zuzak TJ, et al. Resistance to tumor necrosis factor-related apoptosis-inducing ligand (TRAIL)-induced apoptosis in neuroblastoma cells correlates with a loss of caspase-8 expression. Cancer Res 2001;61:1314–1319.
72. Kim Y, Suh N, Sporn M, Reed JC. An inducible pathway for degradation of FLIP protein sensitizes tumor cells to TRAIL-induced apoptosis. J Biol Chem 2002;277:22,320–22,329.
73. Xiao C, Yang BF, Asadi N, Beguinot F, Hao C. Tumor necrosis factor-related apoptosis-inducing ligand-induced death-inducing signaling complex and its modulation by c-FLIP and PED/PEA-15 in glioma cells. J Biol Chem 2002;277:25,020–25,025.
74. Bullani RR, Huard B, Viard-Leveugle I, et al. Selective expression of FLIP in malignant melanocytic skin lesions. J Invest Dermatol 2001;117:360–364.
75. Olsson A, Diaz T, Aguilar-Santelises M, et al. Sensitization to TRAIL-induced apoptosis and modulation of FLICE-inhibitory protein in B chronic lymphocytic leukemia by actinomycin D. Leukemia 2001;15:1868–1877.
76. Kreuz S, Siegmund D, Scheurich P, Wajant H. NF-kappaB inducers upregulate cFLIP, a cycloheximide-sensitive inhibitor of death receptor signaling. Mol Cell Biol 2001;21:3964–3973.
77. Micheau O, Lens S, Gaide O, Alevizopoulos K, Tschopp J. NF-kappaB signals induce the expression of c-FLIP. Mol Cell Biol 2001;21:5299–5305.
78. Wu Xiao C, Asselin E, Tsang BK. Nuclear factor kappaB-mediated induction of FLICE-like inhibitory protein prevents tumor necrosis factor alpha-induced apoptosis in rat granulosa cells. Biol Reprod 2002;67:436–441.
79. Datta SR, Dudek H, Tao X, et al. Akt phosphorylation of BAD couples survival signals to the cell-intrinsic death machinery. Cell 1997;91:231–241.
80. Dudek H, Datta SR, Franke TF, et al. Regulation of neuronal survival by the serine-threonine protein kinase Akt. Science 1997;275:661–665.
81. Cardone MH, Roy N, Stennicke HR, et al. Regulation of cell death protease caspase-9 by phosphorylation. Science 1998;282:1318–1321.
82. Brunet A, Bonni A, Zigmond MJ, et al. Akt promotes cell survival by phosphorylating and inhibiting a Forkhead transcription factor. Cell 1999;96:857–868.
83. Tang ED, Nunez G, Barr FG, Guan KL. Negative regulation of the Forkhead transcription factor FKHR by Akt. J Biol Chem 1999;274:16,741–16,746.

84. Kashii Y, Uchida M, Kirito K, et al. A member of Forkhead family transcription factor, FKHRL1, is one of the downstream molecules of phosphatidylinositol 3-kinase-Akt activation pathway in erythropoietin signal transduction. Blood 2000;96:941–949.
85. Nakamura N, Ramaswamy S, Vazquez F, Signoretti S, Loda M, Sellers WR. Forkhead transcription factors are critical effectors of cell death and cell cycle arrest downstream of PTEN. Mol Cell Biol 2000;20:8969–8982.
86. Nesterov A, Lu X, Johnson M, Miller GJ, Ivashchenko Y, Kraft AS. Elevated AKT activity protects the prostate cancer cell line LNCaP from TRAIL-induced apoptosis. J Biol Chem 2001;276:10,767–10,774.
87. Chen X, Thakkar H, Tyan F, et al. Constitutively active Akt is an important regulator of TRAIL sensitivity in prostate cancer. Oncogene 2001;20:6073–6083.
88. Shinohara H, Kayagaki N, Yagita H, et al. A protective role of PKCepsilon against TNF-related apoptosis-inducing ligand (TRAIL)-induced apoptosis in glioma cells. Biochem Biophys Res Commun 2001;284:1162–1167.
89. Sarker M, Ruiz-Ruiz C, Lopez-Rivas A. Activation of protein kinase C inhibits TRAIL-induced caspases activation, mitochondrial events and apoptosis in a human leukemic T cell line. Cell Death Differ 2001;8:172–181.
90. Deng Y, Lin Y, Wu X. TRAIL-induced apoptosis requires Bax-dependent mitochondrial release of Smac/DIABLO. Genes Dev 2002;16:33–45.
91. LeBlanc H, Lawrence D, Varfolomeev E, et al. Tumor-cell resistance to death receptor—induced apoptosis through mutational inactivation of the proapoptotic Bcl-2 homolog Bax. Nat Med 2002;8:274–281.
92. Ravi R, Bedi A. Requirement of BAX for TRAIL/Apo2L-induced apoptosis of colorectal cancers: synergism with sulindac-mediated inhibition of Bcl-x(L). Cancer Res 2002;62:1583–1587.
93. He Q, Luo X, Huang Y, Sheikh MS. Apo2L/TRAIL differentially modulates the apoptotic effects of sulindac and a COX-2 selective non-steroidal anti-inflammatory agent in Bax-deficient cells. Oncogene 2002;21:6032–6040.
94. Wei MC, Zong WX, Cheng EH, et al. Proapoptotic BAX and BAK: a requisite gateway to mitochondrial dysfunction and death. Science 2001;292:727–730.
95. Yang E, Zha J, Jockel J, Boise LH, Thompson CB, Korsmeyer SJ. Bad, a heterodimeric partner for Bcl-XL and Bcl-2, displaces Bax and promotes cell death. Cell 1995;80:285–291.
96. Lamothe B, Aggarwal BB. Ectopic expression of Bcl-2 and Bcl-xL inhibits apoptosis induced by TNF-related apoptosis-inducing ligand (TRAIL) through suppression of caspases-8, 7, and 3 and BID cleavage in human acute myelogenous leukemia cell line HL-60. J Interferon Cytokine Res 2002;22:269–279.
97. Sun SY, Yue P, Zhou JY, et al. Overexpression of BCL2 blocks TNF-related apoptosis-inducing ligand (TRAIL)-induced apoptosis in human lung cancer cells. Biochem Biophys Res Commun 2001;280: 788–797.
98. Munshi A, Pappas G, Honda T, et al. TRAIL (APO-2L) induces apoptosis in human prostate cancer cells that is inhibitable by Bcl-2. Oncogene 2001;20:3757–3765.
99. Fulda S, Meyer E, Debatin KM. Inhibition of TRAIL-induced apoptosis by Bcl-2 overexpression. Oncogene 2002;21:2283–2294.
100. Rokhlin OW, Guseva N, Tagiyev A, Knudson CM, Cohen MB. Bcl-2 oncoprotein protects the human prostatic carcinoma cell line PC3 from TRAIL-mediated apoptosis. Oncogene 2001;20:2836–2843.
101. Pugazhenthi S, Miller E, Sable C, et al. Insulin-like growth factor-I induces bcl-2 promoter through the transcription factor cAMP-response element-binding protein. J Biol Chem 1999;274:27,529–27,535.
102. Pugazhenthi S, Nesterova A, Sable C, et al. Akt/protein kinase B up-regulates Bcl-2 expression through cAMP-response element-binding protein. J Biol Chem 2000;275:10,761–10,766.
103. Park SY, Billiar TR, Seol DW. Hypoxia inhibition of apoptosis induced by tumor necrosis factor-related apoptosis-inducing ligand (TRAIL). Biochem Biophys Res Commun 2002;291:150–153.
104. Suzuki Y, Nakabayashi Y, Nakata K, Reed JC, Takahashi R. X-linked inhibitor of apoptosis protein (XIAP) inhibits caspase-3 and -7 in distinct modes. J Biol Chem 2001;276:27,058–27,063.
105. Deveraux QL, Roy N, Stennicke HR, et al. IAPs block apoptotic events induced by caspase-8 and cytochrome c by direct inhibition of distinct caspases. Embo J 1998;17:2215–2223.
106. Silke J, Ekert PG, Day CL, et al. Direct inhibition of caspase 3 is dispensable for the anti-apoptotic activity of XIAP. Embo J 2001;20:3114–3123.
107. Huang Y, Park YC, Rich RL, Segal D, Myszka DG, Wu H. Structural basis of caspase inhibition by XIAP: differential roles of the linker versus the BIR domain. Cell 2001;104:781–790.

108. Riedl SJ, Renatus M, Schwarzenbacher R, et al. Structural basis for the inhibition of caspase-3 by XIAP. Cell 2001;104:791–800.
109. Bratton SB, Walker G, Srinivasula SM, et al. Recruitment, activation and retention of caspases-9 and -3 by Apaf-1 apoptosome and associated XIAP complexes. Embo J 2001;20:998–1009.
110. Chai J, Shiozaki E, Srinivasula SM, et al. Structural basis of caspase-7 inhibition by XIAP. Cell 2001;104:769–780.
111. Liu Z, Sun C, Olejniczak ET, et al. Structural basis for binding of Smac/DIABLO to the XIAP BIR3 domain. Nature 2000;408:1004–1008.
112. Wu G, Chai J, Suber TL, et al. Structural basis of IAP recognition by Smac/DIABLO. Nature 2000;408:1008–1012.
113. Srinivasula SM, Hegde R, Saleh A, et al. A conserved XIAP-interaction motif in caspase-9 and Smac/DIABLO regulates caspase activity and apoptosis. Nature 2001;410:112–116.
114. Srinivasula SM, Datta P, Fan XJ, Fernandes-Alnemri T, Huang Z, Alnemri ES. Molecular determinants of the caspase-promoting activity of Smac/DIABLO and its role in the death receptor pathway. J Biol Chem 2000;275:36,152–36,157.
115. Ekert PG, Silke J, Hawkins CJ, Verhagen AM, Vaux DL. DIABLO promotes apoptosis by removing MIHA/XIAP from processed caspase 9. J Cell Biol 2001;152:483–490.
116. Yang Y, Fang S, Jensen JP, Weissman AM, Ashwell JD. Ubiquitin protein ligase activity of IAPs and their degradation in proteasomes in response to apoptotic stimuli. Science 2000;288:874–877.
117. Suzuki Y, Nakabayashi Y, Takahashi R. Ubiquitin-protein ligase activity of X-linked inhibitor of apoptosis protein promotes proteasomal degradation of caspase-3 and enhances its anti-apoptotic effect in Fas-induced cell death. Proc Natl Acad Sci USA 2001;98:8662–8667.
118. Fulda S, Wick W, Weller M, Debatin KM. Smac agonists sensitize for Apo2L/TRAIL- or anticancer drug-induced apoptosis and induce regression of malignant glioma in vivo. Nat Med 2002;8:808–815.
119. Guo F, Nimmanapalli R, Paranawithana S, et al. Ectopic overexpression of second mitochondria-derived activator of caspases (Smac/DIABLO) or cotreatment with N-terminus of Smac/DIABLO peptide potentiates epothilone B derivative-(BMS 247550) and Apo-2L/TRAIL-induced apoptosis. Blood 2002;99:3419–3426.
120. Griffith TS, Anderson RD, Davidson BL, Williams RD, Ratliff TL. Adenoviral-mediated transfer of the TNF-related apoptosis-inducing ligand/Apo-2 ligand gene induces tumor cell apoptosis. J Immunol 2000;165:2886–2894.
121. Lee J, Hampl M, Albert P, Fine HA. Antitumor activity and prolonged expression from a TRAIL-expressing adenoviral vector. Neoplasia 2002;4:312–323.
122. Voelkel-Johnson C, King DL, Norris JS. Resistance of prostate cancer cells to soluble TNF-related apoptosis-inducing ligand (TRAIL/Apo2L) can be overcome by doxorubicin or adenoviral delivery of full-length TRAIL. Cancer Gene Ther 2002;9:164–172.
123. Griffith TS, Broghammer EL. Suppression of tumor growth following intralesional therapy with TRAIL recombinant adenovirus. Mol Ther 2001;4:257–266.
124. Kagawa S, He C, Gu J, et al. Antitumor activity and bystander effects of the tumor necrosis factor-related apoptosis-inducing ligand (TRAIL) gene. Cancer Res 2001;61:3330–3338.
125. Lin T, Gu J, Zhang L, et al. Targeted expression of green fluorescent protein/tumor necrosis factor-related apoptosis-inducing ligand fusion protein from human telomerase reverse transcriptase promoter elicits antitumor activity without toxic effects on primary human hepatocytes. Cancer Res 2002;62:3620–3625.
126. Goldberg GS, Jin Z, Ichikawa H, et al. Global effects of anchorage on gene expression during mammary carcinoma cell growth reveal role of tumor necrosis factor-related apoptosis-inducing ligand in anoikis. Cancer Res 2001;61:1334–1337.
127. Takeda K, Hayakawa Y, Smyth MJ, et al. Involvement of tumor necrosis factor-related apoptosis-inducing ligand in surveillance of tumor metastasis by liver natural killer cells. Nat Med 2001;7:94–100.
128. Song K, Chen Y, Goke R, et al. Tumor necrosis factor-related apoptosis-inducing ligand (TRAIL) is an inhibitor of autoimmune inflammation and cell cycle progression. J Exp Med 2000;191:1095–1104.
129. Jo M, Kim TH, Seol DW, et al. Apoptosis induced in normal human hepatocytes by tumor necrosis factor-related apoptosis-inducing ligand. Nat Med 2000;6:564–567.
130. Nitsch R, Bechmann I, Deisz RA, et al. Human brain-cell death induced by tumour-necrosis-factor-related apoptosis-inducing ligand (TRAIL). Lancet 2000;356:827–828.
131. Lawrence D, Shahrokh Z, Marsters S, et al. Differential hepatocyte toxicity of recombinant Apo2L/TRAIL versions. Nat Med 2001;7:383–385.

132. Qin J, Chaturvedi V, Bonish B, Nickoloff BJ. Avoiding premature apoptosis of normal epidermal cells. Nat Med 2001;7:385–386.
133. Gliniak B, Le T. Tumor necrosis factor-related apoptosis-inducing ligand's antitumor activity in vivo is enhanced by the chemotherapeutic agent CPT-11. Cancer Res 1999;59:6153–6158.
134. Wu XX, Kakehi Y, Mizutani Y, et al. Doxorubicin enhances TRAIL-induced apoptosis in prostate cancer. Int J Oncol 2002;20:949–954.
135. Wu XX, Kakehi Y, Mizutani Y, et al. Enhancement of TRAIL/Apo2L-mediated apoptosis by adriamycin through inducing DR4 and DR5 in renal cell carcinoma cells. Int J Cancer 2003;104:409–417.
136. Guan B, Yue P, Clayman GL, Sun SY. Evidence that the death receptor DR4 is a DNA damage-inducible, p53-regulated gene. J Cell Physiol 2001;188:98–105.
137. Jazirehi AR, Ng CP, Gan XH, Schiller G, Bonavida B. Adriamycin sensitizes the adriamycin-resistant 8226/Dox40 human multiple myeloma cells to Apo2L/tumor necrosis factor-related apoptosis-inducing ligand-mediated (TRAIL) apoptosis. Clin Cancer Res 2001;7:3874–3883.
138. Ahlemeyer B, Klumpp S, Krieglstein J. Release of cytochrome c into the extracellular space contributes to neuronal apoptosis induced by staurosporine. Brain Res 2002;934:107–116.
139. Robertson JD, Gogvadze V, Zhivotovsky B, Orrenius S. Distinct pathways for stimulation of cytochrome c release by etoposide. J Biol Chem 2000;275:32,438–32,443.

8 Death Receptor Mutations

Sug Hyung Lee, MD, PhD,
Nam Jin Yoo, MD, PhD,
and Jung Young Lee, MD, PhD,

SUMMARY

It is generally believed that human cancers may arise as the result of an accumulation of mutations in genes and subsequent clonal selection of variant progeny with increasingly aggressive behaviors. Also, among the remarkable advances in our understanding in cancer biology is the realization that apoptosis has a profound effect on the malignant phenotypes. Along with these, compelling evidence indicates that somatic mutations in the genes encoding apoptosis-related proteins contribute to either development or progression of human cancers. In this chapter, we present an overview of the death receptor pathway and its dysregulation in cancers. We then review the current knowledge of death receptor mutations that have been detected in humans.

INTRODUCTION

Programmed cell death through apoptosis plays a fundamental role in a variety of physiological processes, and its deregulation contributes to many diseases, including autoimmunity, cancer, acquisition of drug resistance in tumors, stroke, progression of some degenerative diseases, and acquired immunodeficiency syndrome (AIDS) *(1–4)*. Apoptosis is an active cell-suicide process executed by a cascade of molecular events involving a number of membrane receptors and cytoplasmic proteins *(1–4)*. Although many pathways for activating caspases may exist, only two, the intrinsic pathway and the extrinsic pathway, have been demonstrated in detail *(3)*. The extrinsic pathway can be induced by members of the tumor necrosis factor (TNF) receptor family, such as TNF receptor 1 (TNFR1) and Fas *(5–7)*. These proteins recruit adaptor proteins, including FADD, to their cytosolic death domains, which then bind caspases-8 and -10 *(8–12)*. The intrinsic pathway can be induced by release of cytochrome c from mitochondria *(13–15)*. In the cytosol, cytochrome c binds and activates apaf-1, allowing it to bind and activate caspase-9 *(14,15)*. Active initiator caspases of the extrinsic pathway (caspases-8 and -10)

From: *Cancer Drug Discovery and Development: Death Receptors in Cancer Therapy*
Edited by: W. S. El-Deiry © Humana Press Inc., Totowa, NJ

and the intrinsic pathway (caspase-9) have been shown to directly cleave and activate the effector protease, caspase-3 *(16,17)*. Also, though commonly viewed as separate pathways and capable of functioning independently, cross-talk can occur between these pathways at multiple levels, depending on the repertoire of apoptosis-modulating proteins expressed *(18–21)*.

APOPTOSIS AND CANCER

Several lines of evidence indicate that tumorigenesis is a multistep process and that these steps reflect genetic alterations that drive the progressive transformation of normal cells into malignant phenotypes *(22)*. The genomes of tumor cells are invariably altered at multiple sites, having suffered disruption through lesions as subtle as point mutations and as obvious as changes in chromosome complement *(23)*. In the multistep tumorigenesis model, mutations in key cellular genes produce a series of acquired capabilities that allow the developing cancer cell to grow unchecked in the absence of growth-stimulating signals, while overcoming growth-inhibitory signals and host immune responses *(22–25)*. They also allow the tumor to replicate indefinitely, maintain an oxygen and nutrient supply, and invade adjacent and distant tissues *(26–29)*. Finally, the ability of cells to evade apoptosis is also an essential hallmark of cancer *(22,30,31)*.

Since the discovery of *bcl-2* as an oncogene that promotes cell survival, it has been widely acknowledged that antiapoptotic genetic lesions are necessary for tumors to arise *(32,33)*. Clonal expansion and tumor growth are the results of the deregulation of intrinsic proliferation (cell division) and cell death (apoptosis). The evidence is mounting, from studies in mouse models and cultured cells, as well as from descriptive analyses of tumor tissues along the multistep carcinogenesis *(22,23)*. Enhanced cell survival is needed at several steps during tumorigenesis: deregulated oncogene expression not only leads to accelerated proliferation, but concomitantly induces apoptosis, which needs to be suppressed for the transformed cell to survive and multiply *(34)*. The tumor cells can persist in a hostile environment. For example, sufficient nutrition for every tumor cell becomes restricted; starvation of tumor cells from cytokines usually leads to apoptotic cell death *(26,27)*. Finally, defective apoptosis facilitates metastasis *(22)*. To metastasize, a tumor cell must acquire the ability to survive in the bloodstream and invade a foreign tissue. Normally, this process is prevented by the propensity of epithelial cells to die in suspension, or in the absence of appropriate tissue survival. During metastasis, cancer cells can ignore restraining signals from neighbors and survive detachment from the extracellular matrix *(29)*. Hence, loss of apoptosis can impact tumor development, progression, and metastasis. Loss of apoptosis is also a significant impediment to anticancer therapy. It is now well established that anticancer agents induce apoptosis, and the disruption of apoptotic machineries reduces treatment sensitivity *(35)*. The mutations that favored tumor development dampen the response to chemotherapy, and treatment might select more refractory clones.

DEATH RECEPTORS

Cell surface death receptors transmit an apoptosis signal on binding of a specific death ligand *(2)*. The best known family of death receptors is represented by tumor necrosis factor receptors (TNFRs), Fas (CD95, Apo-1), and TNF-related apoptosis-inducing ligand receptors (TRAIL-Rs) *(36-41)*. The receptors' ligands comprise another related family that includes TNF, CD95 ligand (FasL/CD95L), and TRAIL *(2)*. Each of the ligands is synthesized as a membrane-associated protein and shares a characteristic 150-amino-acid region towards the C-terminus by which each ligand interacts with its cognate receptor *(2)*. For the most part, these ligands exist as trimeric or multimeric membrane-bound proteins that may function to induce receptor aggregation.

The Fas-FasL system has been recognized as a major pathway for the induction of apoptosis in cells and tissues *(1,2)*. Fas is a member of the death receptor subfamily of the TNFR superfamily *(37–39)*. Ligation of Fas by either agonistic antibody or by its natural ligand transmits a death signal to the target cells, potentially triggering apoptosis. Fas has three cystein-rich extracellular domains and an intracellular death domain (DD) essential for signaling *(37–39)*.

The death domain, a name deriving from its ability to recruit downstream effectors that can induce apoptosis, is present in the cytoplasmic tail of all death receptors *(1)*. The death domain is a protein interaction module consisting of a compact bundle of six α-helices *(42)*. Death domains bind each other, probably forming oligomers of unknown stoichiometry. Stimulation of Fas results in aggregation of its intracellular death domain, leading to the recruitment of two key signaling proteins that, together with the receptor, form the death-inducing signaling complex (DISC) *(43)*. FADD/MORT-1 *(8)* couples through its C-terminal death domain to crosslinked Fas receptors and recruits caspase-8 *(9)* through its N-terminal death effector domain (DED) to the DISC. Caspase-10 (Mch4/FLICE2) is a caspase homologous to caspase-8 and is present as an inactive proenzyme, comprising a prodomain that contains two DEDs to allow caspase-10 to interact with the DED of FADD and a catalytic protease domain that can be further processed to give a large and a small subunit *(44)*. The local aggregation of the procaspases-8 and -10 is sufficient to allow autoprocessing or transprocessing to produce active caspases-8 and -10, which can subsequently activate downstream executioners, such as caspases 3 and 7 *(44)*.

Five receptors have been identified for TRAIL, including two apoptosis-inducing receptors (death receptor 4/TRAIL-R1 and DR5/TRICK-2/TRAIL-R2/KILLER-DR7), two decoy receptors (DcRs) (TRID/DcR1 and TRUNDD/DcR2), and osteo-progeterin. TRAIL induces apoptosis through DR4 and DR5 requiring FADD, caspase-8 and caspase-10, just like CD95-mediated cell killing *(45)*.

DEATH RECEPTOR MUTATIONS

Fas, DR5, and DR4 are widely expressed in normal and neoplastic cells *(46,47)*, but the expression of these proteins does not necessarily predict susceptibility to killing *(48,49)*. This can reflect the presence of inhibiting mechanisms of death receptor-mediated apoptosis. Fas-mediated apoptosis can be blocked by several mechanisms, including the production of soluble Fas *(50)*, the lack of cell-surface Fas expression *(51–53)*, the overexpression of inhibitory proteins in signal transduction pathways such as Fas-associated phosphatase-1 *(54)* and FLICE- inhibitory protein (FLIP) *(55)*, and the mutation of the primary structure of Fas *(56–65)*. TRAIL-induced apoptosis can be blocked by several mechanisms, including the expression of decoy receptors for TRAIL *(10)*, the loss of TRAIL receptor expression *(5)*, the overexpression of inhibitory proteins in signal transduction pathways such as FLIP *(7)*, and the mutation of the primary structure of DR4 and DR5 *(11)*.

Germline Mutation of Death Receptors

The consequences of naturally occurring mutants of Fas/FasL have been well demonstrated in both mice and humans. *lpr* and *gld* are mutations in mice of Fas and FasL, respectively *(56,66)*. Because the Fas/FasL system is involved in the apoptotic process that occurs during cell muturation, *lpr* and *gld* mutations result in the development of lymphadenopathy and autoimmune diseases in the mice *(67)*. To date, two *lpr* mutations are known: *lpr* and lpr^{cg}. The mouse *Fas* gene consists of over 70kb, and is split by 9 exons *(56)*. The restriction mapping of the *Fas* gene from lpr mice has revealed the insertion of an early transposable element (ETn) of 5.4 kb in intron 2. The ETn is a mouse endogenous retrovirus, of which about 1,000 copies can be found in the mouse genome. The ETn has long terminal repeat (LTR) sequences at both the 5' and 3' termini. This LTR sequence contains a polyadenylation signal, and transcription terminates at this area. Furthermore, insertion of ETn into an intron of a mammalian expression vector reduced the expression efficiency in mammalian cells. These data indicate that the *lpr* mice have a defect in the expression of Fas due to insertion of ETn in intron 2. Unlike the *lpr* mice, lpr^{cg} mice express full-length Fas mRNA as abundantly as wild-type mice *(56)*. However, the Fas mRNA carries a point mutation (T to A) in the death domain. This mutation results in an amino acid change, from isoleucine to asparagine, and abolishes the ability of Fas to transduce the cell-death signal to cells.

The autoimmune lymphoproliferative syndrome (ALPS; sometimes called the Canale–Smith syndrome) arises in early childhood and can have fatal complications *(44,51–67)*. It is associated with prominent nonmalignant lymphadenopathy, hepatosplenomegaly, and autoimmune manifestations. Underlying ALPS are heritable mutations in genes that regulate lymphocyte survival by triggering programmed death of lymphocytes, or apoptosis. By far, the most common form of ALPS is that associated with heterozygous Fas mutations (ALPS type Ia) *(51–67)*; ALPS is inherited in an autosomal dominant fashion. The region of the *Fas* gene most often mutated is the death domain. These mutations are predicted to result in early termination (frameshift insertions and deletions; amino acid changes to stop codons) or in single amino-acid substitutions (missense mutations) that disrupt the three-dimensional structure of the death domain. Patients with mutations of the *FasL (67)* or *caspase-10 (44)* gene are referred to as ALPS type Ib or II patients, respectively, whereas the remaining patients with the same symptoms but without identified mutations in genes involved in the induction of apoptosis are diagnosed as having ALPS type III *(44)*.

Interestingly, the *lpr* mice have been reported to have spontaneous development of plasmacytoid tumors *(69)*, and some ALPS patients have been reported to have malignancies *(59,60)*, including multiple tumor development in one patient *(59)*. Although it is not clear whether the tumors that occurred in ALPS patients arose as a result of *Fas* mutations, it is conceivable that *Fas* mutation might have influences on tumor development in these patients.

Somatic Mutation of Fas Gene

The key role of the Fas system in negative growth regulation has been studied mostly within the immune system, and the germline inactivation of the Fas system exhibits phenotypic abnormalities mainly in the lymphoid system *(2)*. Thus, mutational analyses of the *Fas* gene have been focused on hematopoietic tumors. However, there is mounting evidence that disruption of the Fas system frequently occurs in nonlymphoid malignancies as well *(48,50–52)*, and *Fas* gene mutations have been reported both in hematopoietic and nonhematopoietic tumors *(62–65,70–80)*. Mutational analysis of the *Fas* gene was performed in a number of human cancers. *Fas* mutation occurred in 0–65% of hematopoietic malignancies and 0–28% of nonhematopoietic malignancies (Table 1).

The dominant negative effect of monoallelic mutations within the death domain is likely attributable to the trimerization of the Fas receptor on the cell surface. The death domain is a highly conserved region that is required and sufficient for the transduction of the death signal *(37–39)*. Given the functional importance of this region, it is not surprising that approx 60% of somatic mutations in lymphoid or solid tumors involve this region.

Fas Mutations in Hematopoietic Tumors

The somatic mutation of *Fas* was first reported in multiple myelomas *(62)*. Multiple myelomas harbor *Fas* mutations at a frequency of 10% (5/48). All of the mutations identified were located in the death domain of the Fas antigen. Two separate individuals demonstrated an identical mutation at a site previously shown to be mutated in the congenital autoimmune syndrome ALPS. One patient exhibited a point mutation at a site only two amino acids removed from the documented lesion of the *lpr^{cg}* mouse. In childhood T-lineage acute lymphoblastic leukemias, two *Fas* mutations were observed in exon 3 and the AP-2-binding region of the promotor *(63)*. The mutation in exon 3 caused a 68Pro → 68Leu change, which resulted in decreased Fas-mediated apoptosis. By contrast, no Fas mutations could be detected in childhood B-lineage acute lymphoblastic leukemias *(81)*, although most of the leukemias were resistant to Fas-mediated apoptosis. Adult T-cell leukemia (ATL) is an aggressive neoplasm of activated T-lymphocytes, and human T-lymphotropic virus type I (HTLV-I) was found to be the causative virus of this tumor *(82)*. Tamiya et al. *(64)* reported that one Fas-negative ATL showed two types of aberrant transcripts: one had a 5-bp deletion and a 1-bp insertion in exon 2, and the other transcript lacked exon 4. These mutations caused the premature termination of both alleles, resulting in the loss of expression of surface Fas antigen. Also, analysis of 35 Fas-positive ATL cells revealed a mutation that lacked exon 4 *(64)*.

Lymphoma is another type of hematopoietic malignancy that has been reported to have *Fas* mutations. Grønbæk et al. *(65)* analyzed 150 cases of non-Hodgkin's lymphoma (NHL), and identified 16 tumors (11%) with *Fas* gene mutations. *Fas* mutations were identified in 3 (60%) MALT-type lymphomas, 9 (21%) diffuse large B-cell lymphomas, 2 (6%) follicle center-cell lymphomas, 1 (50%) anaplastic large-cell lymphoma, and 1 unusual case of B-cell chronic lymphocytic leukemia. They observed that missense mutations within the death domain of the receptor were associated with retention of the wild-type allele, indicating a dominant-negative mechanism, whereas missense mutations outside the death domain were associated with allelic loss. Of note, 10 of 13 evaluable patients with the *Fas* mutations showed features suggestive of autoimmune disease, suggesting a link between *Fas* mutation, cancer, and autoimmunity. Another suggestive commonality between *Fas* mutation, cancer, and autoimmunity is observed in thyroid lymphoma *(72)*, which is supposed to arise from active lymphoid cells formed in the preceding autoimmune chronic lymphocytic thyroiditis. Mutations of the *Fas* gene were detected in 3 (27.3%) of 11 cases of autoimmune chronic lymphocytic thyroiditis and 17

Table 1
Summary of the Somatic Mutations of *Fas* Gene in Human Cancers

Type of human cancers	*Frequency*	*Reference*
Multiple myeloma	5/48 (10.4%)	*62*
Childhood T-lineage leukemia	2/81 (2.5%)	*63*
Childhood B-lineage leukemia	0/32 (0%)	*81*
Adult T-cell leukemia	2/47 (4.3%)	*64*
Non-Hodgkin's lymphoma	16/150 (10.6%)	*65*
Hodgkin's lymphoma	2/10 (20%)	*75*
Mycosis fungoides	6/44 (13.6%)	*71*
Thyroid lymphoma	17/26 (65.4%)	*72*
Cutaneous T-cell lymphoma	13/22 (59%)	*73*
Nasal NK/T-cell lymphoma	7/14 (50%)	*74*
Large granular lymphocyte leukemia	0/11 (0%)	*85*
Marginal zone B-cell lymphomas	0/27 (0%)	*86*
Malignant melanoma	3/44 (6.8%)	*76*
NSCLC	5/65 (7.7%)	*77*
Bladder transitional cell carcinoma	12/43 (28%)	*78*
Gastric cancer	5/43 (11.6%)	*79*
Gastric cancer	2/20 (10%)	*87*
Colon cancer	2/20 (10%)	*87*
Colon cancer	0/24 (0%)	*93*
Burn scar-related SCC	3/21 (14.3%)	*80*
Conventional cutaneous SCC	0/50 (0%)	*80*
Breast cancer	0/58 (0%)	*89*
Hepatocellular carcinoma	0/50 (0%)	*90*
Hepatoblastoma	0/23 (0%)	*91*
Ovary cancer	0/8 (0%)	*92*
Glioblastoma multiforme	0/23 (0%)	*95*

Abbreviations: SCC, squamous cell carcinoma; NSCLC, non-small-cell lung cancer.

(65.4%) of 26 of thyroid lymphoma. Of note, all of the mutations involve the alteration of exon 9 that encodes the death domain. *Fas* mutations have also been detected in T-cell lymphoma, including cutaneous T-cell lymphoma *(74)*, mycosis fungoides *(72)*, and the nasal natural killer (NK)/T-cell lymphoma *(74)*. Doorn et al. *(73)* analyzed cutaneous T-cell lymphomas, a group of clinically heterogeneous malignancies of mature skin-homing T–cells, and identified a novel mutation of the *Fas* gene that displays retention of intron 5 in 13 of 22 patients (59%). Two of these 13 tumors were found to have additional missense mutations. Dereure et al. *(71)* described the presence of six point mutations of the coding sequence of the *Fas* gene in 6 of 44 patients (13%) with mycosis fungoides, a cutaneous T-cell lymphoma. Nasal NK/T-cell lymphoma (NKTCL) is a clinical condition of lethal midline granuloma that shows necrotic, granulomatous lesions in the upper respiratory tract, especially in the nasal cavity. Takakuwa et al. *(74)* reported mutations of the *Fas* gene in 7 (50%) of 14 NKTCLs which comprised four frameshift, two missense, and one silent mutations. All of the mutations involved the alteration of exon 9.

Hodgkin and Reed–Sternberg (H/RS) cells in classical Hodgkin's disease (HD) are thought to be derived from preapoptotic germinal center B-cells *(83)*. Single micromanipulated H/RS cells from 10 cases of HD were analyzed for somatic mutations within the *CD95* gene, and two cases displayed *Fas* mutation within the 5' region in one case and within exon 9 in another case *(75)*.

In contrast to the aforementioned reports of *Fas* mutations, some reports described the negative correlation between hematologic tumor pathogenesis and death receptor mutations. Rozenfeld-Granot et al. *(84)* screened somatic mutation at the death domains of *Fas, FADD, TNFR, TRADD,* and *RIP*, in the promoter region of *Fas* and in the protease domain of *caspase-10*, in a larger variety of hematological malignancies (31 chronic lymphocytic leukemias, 28 chronic myelogenous leukemias, 8 essential thrombocythemias, 6 acute lymphocytic leukemias, 6 acute myeloblastic leukemias, 3 hairy-cell leukemias, 3 Burkitt's lymphomas, 3 polycythemia veras, 2 myelofibroses, and 2 chronic myelomonocytic leukemias), but could not find any mutations in any of the malignancies. Also, no mutation could be detected in marginal zone B-cell lymphomas and large granular lymphocyte lymphoma *(85,86)*.

Fas Mutations in Nonhematopoietic Tumors

Fas mutations in nonhematopoietic tumors have been detected in non-small-cell lung cancers (NSCLC) *(77)*, malignant melanomas *(76)*, transitional cell carcinomas of the urinary bladder *(78)*, gastric carcinomas *(79,87)*, colon carcinomas *(87)*, burn scar-related squamous cell carcinomas *(80)*, and testicular germ-cell tumors *(88)*, while no *Fas* mutations have been detected in breast carcinomas *(89)*, hepatocellular carcinomas *(90)*, hepatoblastomas *(91)*, ovarian cancers *(92)*, and colon cancers *(93)*. Lee et al. and Shin et al. at the same laboratory have reported the majority of these mutations *(77–80,90,91)*. They analyzed the allelic status of the *Fas* gene as well as *Fas* mutations by using intragenic polymorphic markers.

In the NSCLCs, five tumors (7.7%) were found to have *Fas* mutations, which were all missense mutations *(77)*. Four of the five mutations identified were located in the cytoplasmic region (death domain) and one mutation was located in the transmembrane domain. In the cutaneous malignant melanomas, three tumors (6.8%) were found to have *Fas* mutations, which were all missense variants and identified in the death domain *(76)*. A particularly high incidence of *Fas* mutations was detected in bladder cancer (28%) *(78)*. Ten of the 12 identified mutations were located in the death domain and 8 of these 10 mutations showed an identical G to A transition at bp 993 (codon 251), indicating a potential mutation hotspot in bladder cancers. Burn scar-related squamous cell carcinoma, a skin tumor that is more aggressive and carries a poorer prognosis than conventional cutaneous squamous cell carcinoma, was reported to have a *Fas* mutation, whereas conventional cutaneous squamous cell carcinoma was not *(80)*. Microsatellite mutator phenotype (MMP) plays an important role in developing gastrointestinal cancer *(94)*. In the coding region of *Fas* (codons 133–135), there is a mononucleotide track (TTTTTTT). In the gastric and colon cancers with MMP, 10% of the cancers showed mutations in this repeat *(87)*.

The incidence of *Fas* mutation in nonhematopoietic tumors seems to be tissue-type specific. In the reports that analyzed *Fas* mutations in hepatocellular carcinomas *(90)*, hepatoblastomas *(91)*, breast carcinomas *(89)*, ovary carcinomas *(92)*, colon carcinomas

(93), glioblastoma multiformes *(95)*, and conventional squamous cell carcinomas *(80)*, the investigators could not detect any *Fas* mutations.

Mutations of TRAIL Receptor Genes

Mutational analyses of TRAIL receptors have been performed less widely in human cancers than analyses of *Fas*. Mutations of the death domain-containing receptors *TRAIL-R1* and *TRAIL-R2* have been found in different human cancers (Table 2) *(96–101)*. *TRAIL-R2* mutation was observed in 5% of head and neck cancer *(96)*, 10.6% of NSCLC *(97)*, 7% of gastric adenocarcinoma *(99)*, 1% of hepatocellular carcinoma *(101)*, 5.1% of non-Hodgkin's lymphoma *(100)*, and 11.7% of metastatic breast cancers *(98)*. Of note, all *TRAIL-R2* mutations were detected only in the death domain sequences of these genes, except for one in the splice site. The vast majority of mutations consisted of missense alterations; the remaining ones consisted of nonsense, splice-site, and silent mutations. By contrast, *TRAIL-R2* mutation was not detected in colorectal cancers *(102)*, breast cancers *(103)*, and NSCLC *(104)* by other researchers. A site-directed mutagenesis strategy and functional analysis of *TRAIL-R2* mutations derived from NSCLC *(105)*, breast cancer *(98)*, gastric adenocarcinoma *(99)*, and head/neck cancer *(96)* provided novel insights into the functional significance of specific structural determinants within the death domain of TRAIL-R2. It has been shown that death domain mutations displayed divergent phenotypes. *TRAIL-R2* mutation appears to be involved in the pathogenesis of breast cancers. A mutational analysis of the death domain of *TRAIL-R2* in breast cancer in a Korean population revealed mutations in tumors with metastasis to regional lymph nodes *(98)*. No mutations have been identified in any of the node-negative tumors. Transfection studies showed loss of apoptotic function in these mutants.

TRAIL-R1 mutation has been analyzed in several tumors, including breast cancer *(98)* and non-Hodgkin's lymphoma *(100)*. A mutational analysis of the death domain of *TRAIL-R1* in non-Hodgkin's lymphoma revealed mutations in two tumors (1.7%) *(100)*. The same research group also detected *TRAIL-R1* mutations in 8.8% of tumors with metastasis to regional lymph nodes *(98)*. In these two studies, analysis of *TRAIL-R1* mutation was performed only in the death domain. Seitz et al. analyzed the death domain of *TRAIL-R1* for the detection of mutations in breast cancers, but they did not detect any *(103)*. They also screened for *TRAIL-R2* and *TRAIL-R4* mutations in the same series of breast cancers, but they did not find any *(103)*. Next, they analyzed individuals from breast cancer families for the detection of *TRAIL-R2* germline mutations *(103)*. One alteration has been found in the Kozak consensus motif at position –4 with respect to the translation initiation AUG. Pai et al. *(96)* also found a germline *TRAIL-R2* mutation in a head/neck cancer, and observed loss of growth-suppressive function in the cell lines overexpressed with the tumor-derived *TRAIL-R2* mutant. In summary, it appears that TRAIL receptor mutation occurs occasionally in sporadic tumors as well as in familial tumors, and that it may contribute to cancer development and progression.

Death Receptors as Tumor Suppressor Genes

The development of human tumors results from clonal expansion of genetically modified cells that have acquired selective growth advantage through accumulated alterations of proto-oncogenes and tumor suppressor genes *(23)*. Inactivation of tumor suppressor gene is frequently accompanied by loss of portions of the chromosome on which the

Table 2
Summary of Mutations of *TRAIL-R1* and *TRAIL-R2* Genes in Cancers

Gene	*Type of human cancers*	*Frequency*	*References*
TRAIL-R1	Non-Hodgkin's lymphoma	2/117 (1.7%)	*100*
TRAIL-R1	Breast cancer	3/57 (5.3%)	*98*
TRAIL-R1	Breast cancer	0/115 (0%)	*103*
TRAIL-R2	Head/neck cancer	2/60 (3.3%)	*96*
TRAIL-R2	NSCLC	11/104 (10.6%)	*97*
TRAIL-R2	Non-Hodgkin's lymphoma	6/117 (5.1%)	*100*
TRAIL-R2	Breast cancer	4/57 (7.0%)	*98*
TRAIL-R2	Breast cancer	0/115 (0%)	*103*
TRAIL-R2	Gastric cancer	3/43 (7.0%)	*99*
TRAIL-R2	Hepatocellular carcinoma	1/100 (1%)	*101*
TRAIL-R2	Colon cancer	0/41 (0%)	*102*
TRAIL-R4	Breast cancer	0/115 (0%)	*103*

Abbreviation: NSCLC, non-small-cell lung cancer.

tumor suppressor gene resides *(23)*. Deletions and rearrangements of chromosome 10q24, where the *Fas* gene resides, have been reported in many types of human tumors, raising the possibility of the presence of tumor suppressor genes in this region *(106)*. *TRAIL-R1, -R2, -R3* and *-R4* genes are mapped to chromosome 8p21-22 *(93)*, suggesting that all of these genes have arisen by tandem duplication. Such duplications may reflect the relative instability of the chromosomal region. Allelic losses of chromosome 8p21-22 have been reported as a frequent event in several cancers *(106)*. These data strongly indicate that chromosome 8p21-22 may harbor one or more tumor suppressor genes, and suggest that *TRAIL-R2* gene might be one of the candidate tumor suppressor genes in this region. Because inaction of death receptors might result in deficient apoptotic signaling, *TRAIL-receptor* genes and the *Fas* gene are candidate tumor suppressor genes in these regions.

Many of the studies on mutational analysis of death receptors analyzed the allelic status of these genes, as well as their mutational status. Using the intragenic polymorphisms in the *Fas* gene, Lee et al. and Shin et al. have found loss of heterozygosity (LOH) with a range from 27 to 35% according to the tumor type *(76–78)*. The LOH in the tumors with *Fas* mutation was detected in 38 to 100% according to the tumor type *(76–78)*. Regarding *TRAIL-receptor* genes, LOH was observed in from 23 to 65%, and LOH in the tumors with *TRAIL-receptor* mutations was detected in 75 to 90% *(97,98,100)*. Higher incidence of the LOHs of *Fas* and *TRAIL receptor* genes in the tumors with the mutations indicates that these genes might be tumor suppressor genes in these loci. Also, the presence of LOH of *Fas* and *TRAIL receptor* genes in the tumors without the mutations suggests that there may be other tumor suppressor genes, such as DMBT1 in 10q25-26, in these loci *(107)*. The authenticity of a tumor suppressor gene is most clearly established by the identification of inactivating germline mutations that segregate with tumor predisposition, coupled with the identification of somatic mutations inactivating the wild-type allele in cancers arising from a germline mutation. At the current stage, the data may not be sufficient to call the death receptors tumor suppressor genes; the death receptor genes should be considered most appropriately as candidate tumor suppressor genes until additional data are available.

CONCLUSIONS

Mutations in apoptosis genes contribute to the pathogenesis of human tumors. The examples of mutated death receptor genes result in reduced apoptosis. However, mutation is only one mechanism of apoptosis dysregulation. Alterations in the expression of apoptosis genes in tumor cells, by known or still unknown mechanisms, may also be involved in the pathogenesis of diseases. The identification of alterations in death receptor genes contributes to the understanding of the function of the molecules involved, offers novel molecular tools for diagnosis, and reveals potential targets for therapeutic intervention.

REFERENCES

1. Reed JC. Mechanisms of apoptosis. Am J Pathol 2000;157:1415–1430.
2. Nagata S. Apoptosis by death factor. Cell 1997;88:355–365.
3. Thompson CB. Apoptosis in the pathogenesis and treatment of disease. Science 1995;267:1456–1462.
4. Kerr JF, Wyllie AH, Currie AR. Apoptosis: a basic biological phenomenon with wide-ranging implications in tissue kinetics. Br J Cancer 1972;26:239–257.
5. Salvesen GS, Dixit VM. Caspases: intracellular signaling by proteolysis. Cell 1997; 91:443–446.
6. Wallach D, Varfolomeev EE, Malinin NL, Goltsev YV, Kovalenko AV, Boldin MP. Tumor necrosis factor receptor and Fas signaling mechanisms. Annu Rev Immunol 1999;17:331–367.
7. Yuan J. Transducing signals of life and death. Curr Opin Cell Biol 1997;9:247–251.
8. Chinnaiyan AM, O'Rourke K, Tewari M, Dixit VM. FADD, a novel death domain-containing protein, interacts with the death domain of Fas and initiates apoptosis. Cell 1995;81:505–512.
9. Boldin MP, Varfolomeev EE, Pancer Z, Mett IL, Camonis JH, Wallach D. A novel protein that interacts with the death domain of Fas/APO1 contains a sequence motif related to the death domain. J Biol Chem 1995;270:7795–7798.
10. Muzio M, Chinnaiyan AM, Kischkel FC, et al. FLICE, a novel FADD-homologous ICE/CED-3-like protease, is recruited to the CD95 (Fas/APO-1) death-inducing signaling complex. Cell 1996;85:817–827.
11. Boldin MP, Goncharov TM, Goltsev YV, Wallach D. Involvement of MACH, a novel MORT1/FADD-interacting protease, in Fas/APO-1- and TNF receptor-induced cell death. Cell 1996;85:803–815.
12. Vincenz C, Dixit VM. Fas-associated death domain protein interleukin-1beta-converting enzyme 2 (FLICE2), an ICE/Ced-3 homologue, is proximally involved in CD95- and p55-mediated death signaling. J Biol Chem 1997;272:6578–6583.
13. Zou H, Henzel WJ, Liu X, Lutschg A, Wang X. Apaf-1, a human protein homologous to *C. elegans* CED-4, participates in cytochrome c-dependent activation of caspase-3. Cell 1997;90:405–413.
14. Zou H, Li Y, Liu X, Wang X. An APAF-1 cytochrome c multimeric complex is a functional apoptosome that activates procaspase-9. J Biol Chem 1999;274:11,549–11,556.
15. Saleh A, Srinivasula S, Acharya S, Fishel R, Alnemri E. Cytochrome c and dATP-mediated oligomerization of Apaf-1 is a prerequisite for procaspase-9 activation. J Biol Chem 1999;274:17,941–17,945.
16. Stennicke HR, Jurgensmeier JM, Shin H, et al. Pro-caspase-3 is a major physiologic target of caspase-8. J Biol Chem 1998; 273:27,084–27,090.
17. Slee EA, Harte MT, Kluck RM, et al. Ordering the cytochrome c-initiated caspase cascade: hierarchical activation of caspases-2, -3, -6, -7, -8, and -10 in a caspase-9-dependent manner. J Cell Biol 1999;144:281–292.
18. Li H, Zhu H, Xu C, Yuan J: Cleavage of BID by caspase 8 mediates the mitochondrial damage in the Fas pathway of apoptosis. Cell 1998, 94:491–501.
19. Luo X, Budihardjo I, Zou H, Slaughter C, Wang X. Bid, a Bcl2 interacting protein, mediates cytochrome c release from mitochondria in response to activation of cell surface death receptors. Cell 1998,94:481–490.
20. Du C, Fang M, Li Y, Li L, Wang X. Smac, a mitochondrial protein that promotes cytochrome c-dependent caspase activation by eliminating IAP inhibition. Cell 2000;102:33–42.

21. Guo F, Nimmanapalli R, Paranawithana S, et al. Ectopic overexpression of second mitochondria-derived activator of caspases (Smac/DIABLO) or cotreatment with N-terminus of Smac/DIABLO peptide potentiates epothilone B derivative-(BMS 247550) and Apo-2L/TRAIL-induced apoptosis. Blood 2002;99:3419–3426.
22. Hanahan D, Weinberg RA. The hallmarks of cancer. Cell 2000;100:57–70.
23. Kinzler KW, Vogelstein B. Lessons from hereditary colorectal cancer. Cell 1996;87: 159–170.
24. Giancotti FG, Ruoslahti E. Integrin signaling. Science 1996;285:1028–1032.
25. Weinberg RA. The retinoblastoma protein and cell cycle control. Cell 1995;81,323–330.
26. Bouck N, Stellmach V, Hsu SC. How tumors become angiogenic. Adv Cancer Res 1996;69:135–174.
27. Hanahan D, Folkman J. Patterns and emerging mechanisms of the angiogenic switch during tumorigenesis. Cell 1996;86:353–364.
28. Christofori G, Semb H. The role of the cell-adhesion molecule E-cadherin as a tumour-suppressor gene. Trends Biochem Sci 1999;24:73–76.
29. Sporn MB. The war on cancer. Lancet 1996;347:1377–1381.
30. Evan G., Littlewood T. A matter of life and cell death. Science 1998;281:1317–1322.
31. Ishizaki Y, Cheng L, Mudge AW, Raff MC. Programmed cell death by default in embryonic cells, fibroblasts, and cancer cells. Mol Biol Cell 1995;6:1443–1458.
32. McDonnell TJ, Deane N, Platt FM, et al. bcl-2-immunoglobulin transgenic mice demonstrate extended B cell survival and follicular lymphoproliferation. Cell 1989;57:79–88.
33. Tsujimoto Y, Cossman J, Jaffe E, Croce C. Involvement of the Bcl-2 gene in human follicular lymphoma. Science 1985;228:1440–1443.
34. Hueber AO, Zornig M, Lyon D, Suda T, Nagata S, Evan G.I. Requirement for the CD95 receptor-ligand pathway in c-Myc-induced apoptosis. Science 1997;278: 1305–1309.
35. Johnstone RW, Ruefli AA, Lowe SW. Apoptosis: a link between cancer genetics and chemotherapy. Cell 2002;108:153–164.
36. Hsu H, Xiong J, Goeddel DV. The TNF receptor 1-associated protein TRADD signals cell death and NF-κB activation. Cell 1995;81:495–504.
37. Itoh N, Yonehara S, Ishii A, et al. The polypeptide encoded by the cDNA for human cell surface antigen Fas can mediate apoptosis. Cell 1991;66:233–243.
38. Trauth BC, Klas C, Peters AMJ, et al. Monoclonal antibody-mediated tumor regression by induction of apoptosis. Science 1989;245:301–305.
39. Yonehara S, Ishii A, Yonehara M. A cell-killing monoclonal antibody (anti-Fas) to a cell surface antigen co-downregulated with the receptor of tumor necrosis factor. J Exp Med 1989;169:1747–1756.
40. Wiley SR, Schooley K, Smolak PJ, et al. Identification and characterization of a new member of the TNF family that induces apoptosis. Immunity 1995;3:673–682.
41. Degli-Esposti M. To die or not to die—the quest of the TRAIL receptors. J Leukoc Biol 1999;65:535–542.
42. Huang B, Eberstadt M, Olejniczak ET, Meadows RP, Fesik SW. NMR structure and mutagenesis of the Fas (APO-1/CD95) death domain. Nature 1996;384:638–641.
43. Kischkel FC, Lawrence DA, Chuntharapai A, Schow P, Kim KJ, Ashkenazi A. Apo2L/TRAIL-dependent recruitment of endogenous FADD and caspase-8 to death receptors 4 and 5. Immunity 2000;12:611–620.
44. Wang J, Zheng L, Lobito A, et al. Inherited human caspase 10 mutations underlie defective lymphocyte and dendritic cell apoptosis in autoimmune lymphoproliferative syndrome type II. Cell 1999;98:47–58.
45. Bodmer JL, Holler N, Reynard S, et al. TRAIL receptor-2 signals apoptosis through FADD and caspase-8. Nature Cell Biol 2000;2:241–243.
46. Leithäser F, Dhein J, Mechtersheimer G, et al. Constitutive and induced expression of APO-1, a new member of the new growth factor/tumor necrosis receptor superfamily, in normal and neoplastic cells. Lab Invest 1993;69:415–429.
47. MacFarlane M, Ahmad M, Srinivasula SM, Fernades-Alnemri T, Cohen G.M, Alnemri ES. Identification and molecular cloning of two novel receptors for the cytotoxic ligand TRAIL. J Biol Chem 1997;272:25,417–25,420.
48. Owen-Schaub LB, Radinsky R, Kruzel E, Berry K, Yonehara S. Anti-Fas on nonhematopoietic tumors: levels of Fas/APO-1 and bcl-2 are not predictive of biological responses. Cancer Res 1994;54:1580–1586.
49. Sheridan JP, Marsters SA, Pitti RM, et al. Control of TRAIL-induced apoptosis by a family of signaling and decoy receptors. Science 1997;277:818–821.
50. Natoli G, Ianni A, Costanzo A, et al. Resistance to Fas-mediated apoptosis in human hepatoma cells. Oncogene 1995; 11:1157–1164.

51. Hughes SJ, Nambu Y, Soldes OS, et al. Fas/APO-1 (CD95) is not translocated to the cell membrane in esophageal adenocarcinomas. Cancer Res 1997;57:5571–5578.
52. Nambu Y, Hughes SJ, Rehemtula A, Hamstra D, Orringer MB, Beer DG. Lack of cell surface Fas/APO-1 expression in pulmonary adenocarcinomas. J Clin Invest 1998;101:1102–1110.
53. Bennett M, Macdonald K, Chan S-W, Luzio JP, Simari R, Weissberg P. Cell surface trafficking of Fas: a rapid mechanism of p53-mediated apoptosis. Science 1998; 282:290–293.
54. Sato T, Irie S, Kituda S, Reed JC. FAP-1: a protein tyrosine phosphatase that associates with Fas. Science 1995;268:411–415.
55. Irmler M, Thome M, Hahne M, et al. Inhibition of death receptor signals by cellular FLIP. Nature 1997;388:190–195.
56. Watanabe-Fukunaga R, Brannan CI, Copeland NG, Jenkins NA, Nagata S. Lymphoproliferation disorder in mice explained by defects in Fas antigen that mediates apoptosis. Nature 1992;356:314–317.
57. Fisher GH, Rosenberg FJ, Straus SE, et al. Dominant interfering Fas gene mutations impair apoptosis in a human autoimmune lymphoproliferative syndrome. Cell 1995;81:935–946.
58. Rieux-Laucat F, Le Deist F, Hivroz C, et al. Mutations in Fas associated with human lymphoproliferative syndrome and autoimmunity. Science 1995;268:1347–1349.
59. Drappa J, Vaishnaw AK, Sullivan KE, Chu JL, Elkon KB. Fas gene mutations in the Canale-Smith syndrome, an inherited lymphoproliferative disorder associated with autoimmunity. N Engl J Med 1996;335:1643–1649.
60. Bettinardi A, Brugnoni B, Quiros-Roldan E, et al. Missense mutations in the Fas gene resulting in autoimmune lymphoproliferative syndrome: a molecular and immunological analysis. Blood 1997;89:902–909.
61. Infante AJ, Britton HA, DeNapoli T, et al. The clinical spectrum in a large kindred with autoimmune lymphoproliferative syndrome caused by a Fas mutation that impairs lymphocyte apoptosis. J Pediatr 1998;133:629–633.
62. Landowsky TH, Qu N, Buyuksal I, Painter JS, Dalton WS. Mutations in the Fas antigen in patients with multiple myeloma. Blood 1997;90:4266–4270.
63. Beltinger C, Kurz E, Bohler T, Schrappe M, Ludwig WD, Debatin KM. CD 95 (APO-1/Fas) mutations in childhood T-lineage acute lymphoblastic leukemia. Blood 1998;91:3943–3951.
64. Tamiya S, Etoh KI, Suzushima H, Takatsuki K, Matsuoka M. Mutation of CD 95 (Fas/APO-1) gene in adult T-cell leukemia cells. Blood 1998;91:3935–3942.
65. Grønbæk K, Straten PT, Ralfkiaer E, et al. Somatic Fas mutations in non-Hodgkin's lymphoma: association with extranodal disease and autoimmunity. Blood 1998; 92:3018–3024.
66. Takahashi T, Tanaka M, Brannan CI, et al. Generalized lymphoproliferative disease in mice, caused by a point mutation in the Fas ligand. Cell 1994;76,969–976.
67. Nagata S, Suda T. Fas and Fas ligand: lpr and gld mutations. Immunol Today 1995;16:39–43.
68. Wu J, Wilson J, He J, Xiang L, Schur PH, Mountz JD. Fas ligand mutation in a patient with systemic lupus erythematosus and lymphoproliferative disease. J Clin Invest. 1996;98:1107–1113.
69. Davidson WF, Giese T, Fredrickson TN. Spontaneous development of plasmacytoid tumors in mice with defective Fas-Fas ligand interactions. J Exp Med 1998, 187:1825–1838.
70. Maeda T, Yamada Y, Moriuchi R, et al. Fas gene mutation in the progression of adult T cell leukemia. J Exp Med;189:1063–1071.
71. Dereure O, Levi E, Vonderheid EC, Kadin ME. Infrequent Fas mutations but no Bax or p53 mutations in early mycosis fungoides: a possible mechanism for the accumulation of malignant T lymphocytes in the skin. J Invest Dermatol 2002;118:949–956.
72. Takakuwa T, Dong Z, Takayama H, Matsuzuka F, Nagata S, Aozasa K. Frequent mutations of Fas gene in thyroid lymphoma. Frequent mutations of Fas gene in thyroid lymphoma. Cancer Res 2001;61:1382–1385.
73. van Doorn R, Dijkman R, Vermeer MH, Starink TM, Willemze R, Tensen CP. A novel splice variant of the Fas gene in patients with cutaneous T-cell lymphoma. Cancer Res 2002;62:5389–5392.
74. Takakuwa T, Dong Z, Nakatsuka S, et al. Frequent mutations of Fas gene in nasal NK/T cell lymphoma. Oncogene 2002;21:4702–4705.
75. Muschen M, Re D, Brauninger A, et al. Somatic mutations of the CD95 gene in Hodgkin and Reed-Sternberg cells. Cancer Res 2000;60:5640–5643.
76. Shin MS, Park WS, Kim SY, et al. Alterations of Fas (Apo-1/CD95) gene in cutaneous malignant melanoma. Am J Pathol 1999;154:1785–1791.

77. Lee SH, Shin MS, Park WS, et al. Alterations of Fas (Apo-1/CD95) gene in non-small cell lung cancer. Oncogene 1999;18:3754–3760.
78. Lee SH, Shin MS, Park WS, et al. Alterations of Fas (APO-1/CD95) gene in transitional cell carcinomas of urinary bladder. Cancer Res 1999;59:3068–3072.
79. Park WS, Oh RR, Kim YS, et al. Somatic mutations in the death domain of the Fas (Apo-1/CD95) gene in gastric cancer. J Pathol 2001;193:162–168.
80. Lee SH, Shin MS, Kim HS, et al. Somatic mutations of Fas (Apo-1/CD95) gene in cutaneous squamous cell carcinoma arising from a burn scar. J Invest Dermatol 2000;114:122–126.
81. Beltinger C, Bohler T, Karawajew L, Ludwig WD, Schrappe M, Debatin KM. Mutation analysis of CD95 (APO-1/Fas) in childhood B-lineage acute lymphoblastic leukaemia. Br J Haematol 1998;102:722–728.
82. Wong-Staal F, Gallo RC. Human T-lymphotropic retroviruses. Nature 1985;317:395–403.
83. Kuppers R, Rajewsky K. The origin of Hodgkin and Reed/Sternberg cells in Hodgkin's disease. Annu Rev Immunol 1998;16:471–493.
84. Rozenfeld-Granot G, Toren A, Amariglio N, Brok-Simoni F, Rechavi G. Mutation analysis of the FAS and TNFR apoptotic cascade genes in hematological malignancies. Exp Hematol 2001;29:228–233.
85. Lamy T, Liu JH, Landowski TH, Dalton WS, Loughran TP Jr. Dysregulation of CD95/CD95 ligand-apoptotic pathway in CD3(+) large granular lymphocyte leukemia. Blood 1998;92:4771–4777.
86. Bertoni F, Conconi A, Luminari S, et al. Lack of CD95/FAS gene somatic mutations in extranodal, nodal and splenic marginal zone B cell lymphomas. Leukemia 2000;14:446–448.
87. Yamamoto H, Gil J, Schwartz S Jr, Perucho M. Frameshift mutations in Fas, Apaf-1, and Bcl-10 in gastro-intestinal cancer of the microsatellite mutator phenotype. Cell Death Differ 2000;7:238–239.
88. Takayama H, Takakuwa T, Tsujimoto Y, et al. Frequent Fas gene mutations in testicular germ cell tumors. Am J Pathol 2002;161:635–641.
89. Muschen M, Re D, Betz B, et al. Resistance to CD95-mediated apoptosis in breast cancer is not due to somatic mutation of the CD95 gene. Int J Cancer 2001;92:309–310.
90. Lee SH, Shin MS, Lee HS, et al. Expression of Fas and Fas-related molecules in human hepatocellular carcinoma. Hum Pathol 2001;32:250–256. 91. Lee SH, Shin MS, Lee JY, et al. In vivo expression of soluble Fas and FAP-1: possible mechanisms of Fas resistance in human hepatoblastomas. J Pathol 1999;188:207–212.
92. Bertoni F, Conconi A, Carobbio S, et al. Analysis of Fas/CD95 gene somatic mutations in ovarian cancer cell lines. Int J Cancer 2000;86:450.
93. Abdel-Rahman W, Arends M, Morris R, Ramadan M, Wyllie A. Death pathway genes Fas (Apo-1/CD95) and Bik (Nbk) show no mutations in colorectal carcinomas. Cell Death Differ 1999;6:387–388.
94. Fearon ER, Vogelstein B. A genetic model for colorectal tumorigenesis. Cell 1990;61:759–767.
95. Fults D, Pedone CA, Thompson GE, et al. Microsatellite deletion mapping on chromosome 10q and mutation analysis of MMAC1, FAS, and MXI1 in human glioblastoma multiforme. Int J Oncol 1998;12:905–910.
96. Pai SI, Wu GS, Ozoren N, et al. Rare loss-of-function mutation of a death receptor gene in head and neck cancer. Cancer Res 1998;58:3513–3518.
97. Lee SH, Shin MS, Kim HS, et al. Alterations of the DR5/TRAIL receptor 2 gene in non-small cell lung cancers. Cancer Res 1999;59:5683–5686.
98. Shin MS, Kim HS, Lee SH, et al. Mutations of tumor necrosis factor-related apoptosis-inducing ligand receptor 1 (TRAIL-R1) and receptor 2 (TRAIL-R2) genes in metastatic breast cancers. Cancer Res 2001;61:4942–4946.
99. Park WS, Lee JH, Shin MS, et al. Inactivating mutations of KILLER/DR5 gene in gastric cancers. Gastroenterology. 2001;121:1219–1225.
100. Lee SH, Shin MS, Kim HS, et al. Somatic mutations of TRAIL-receptor 1 and TRAIL-receptor 2 genes in non-Hodgkin's lymphoma. Oncogene 2001;20:399–403.
101. Jeng YM, Hsu HC. Mutation of the DR5/TRAIL receptor 2 gene is infrequent in hepatocellular carcinoma. Cancer Lett 2002;181:205–208.
102. Arai T, Akiyama Y, Okabe S, Saito K, Iwai T, Yuasa Y. Genomic organization and mutation analyses of the DR5/TRAIL receptor 2 gene in colorectal carcinomas. Cancer Lett 1998;133:197–204.
103. Seitz S, Wassmuth P, Fischer J, et al. Mutation analysis and mRNA expression of trail-receptors in human breast cancer. Int J Cancer 2002;102:117–128.
104. Wu WG, Soria JC, Wang L, Kemp BL, Mao L. TRAIL-R2 is not correlated with p53 status and is rarely mutated in non-small cell lung cancer. Anticancer Res 2000;20:4525–4529.

105. McDonald ER 3rd, Chui PC, Martelli PF, Dicker DT, El-Deiry WS. Death domain mutagenesis of KILLER/DR5 reveals residues critical for apoptotic signaling. J Biol Chem 2001;276:14,939–14,945.
106. Mitelman F, Mertens F, Johansson B. A breakpoint map of recurrent chromosomal rearrangements in human neoplasia. Nature Genet 1997;15:417–474.
107. Mollenhauer J, Wiemann S, Scheurlen W, et al. DMBT1, a new member of the SRCR superfamily, on chromosome 10q25.3-26.1 is deleted in malignant brain tumours. Nat Genet 1997;17:32–39.

9 Regulation of Death Receptors

Udo Kontny, MD *and Heinrich Kovar,* PhD

SUMMARY

Apoptotic cell death mediated through activation of death receptors is essential in the regulation of tissue homeostasis in development and differentiation. The expression of the members of the death receptor family is tightly regulated and varies among tissues. Dysregulation of death receptor expression is implicated in the pathogenesis of various diseases, including cancer, autoimmune disorders, neurodegenerative diseases, and infections. In this chapter we will focus on the stimuli and mechanisms that regulate the expression of death receptors.

TNF RECEPTORS

For tumor necrosis factor (TNF)-α, two different receptors, designated as TNF receptor 1 (TNFR1, also known as TNFR p55, CD120a) and TNF receptor 2 (TNFR2, also known as TNFR p75, CD120b) have been described *(1)*. Both receptors have been shown to mediate apoptosis *(2)*. Whereas TNFR1 is constitutively expressed on all nucleated cells, the expression of TNFR2 is primarily restricted to hematopoietic cells *(3)*. The relative ratio of TNFR1 and -R2 varies in different cells. It has been shown that myeloid progenitors downregulate the expression of TNFR1 as they differentiate into mature monocytes *(4)*. TNF receptor expression on the cell surface is regulated by three different mechanisms: (1) regulation of receptor synthesis; (2) shedding of receptors; and (3) internalization of receptors.

The TNF Receptor Promoters

The TNFR1 gene promoter resembles that of housekeeping genes lacking canonical TATA and CAAT box motifs with multiple start points for transcription *(5)*. Though a consensus sequence for NF-κB has been described, there is no clear evidence that TNFR1 is regulated by this transcription factor. The promoter of TNFR2 contains consensus

From: *Cancer Drug Discovery and Development: Death Receptors in Cancer Therapy*
Edited by: W. S. El-Deiry © Humana Press Inc., Totowa, NJ

elements for transcription factors involved in T-cell development and activation, such as T-cell factor 1, Ikaros, AP-1, CK-2, interleukin (IL)-6 receptor E, ISRE, GAS, NF-κB, and SP-1 *(3,6)*. The mRNA expression of TNFR2 is upregulated by various cytokines, such as TNF-α, IL-1β, IL-10, and bFGF *(7,8)*. TNFR2 mRNA is downregulated by interferon (IFN)γ *(8)*. Following T-cell activation, the expression of TNFR1 is increased, whereas TNFR2 expression is decreased *(9)*.

Regulation of TNF Receptor Expression by Shedding and Internalization

Shedding of TNFR has been shown to antagonize the effect of TNF-α *(10,11)*. However, when soluble TNFR (sTNFR) concentrations are low, they can increase TNF activity by stabilizing the death-inducing factor prolonging its availability to bind to membrane-bound TNFR. Shedding of TNFR1 and -R2 is mediated by the action of a metalloproteinase, probably identical to the TNF-α-converting enzyme (TACE) *(12)*. Its activity is stimulated by hydrogen peroxide and nitric oxide *(13,14)*. Injurious agents are known to induce shedding of TNFR1 from endothelial cells *(15)*. Also, IL-4 has been demonstrated to induce shedding of both TNFR1 and TNFR2 from cultured monocytes *(16)*. The production of sTNFR2 is increased after stimulation of cells with TNF-α, lipopolysaccharide (LPS), or IL-10 *(8,17)*. In contrast, dexamethasone suppresses the release of sTNFR1 and -R2 from human monocytes *(18)*. Internalization of the TNFR1 is observed after stimulating monocytes with LPS or TNF-α *(19)*.

TNF Receptor Expression and Disease

Increased expression of membrane-bound and soluble TNFR2 is seen in various autoimmune disorders, such as rheumatoid arthritis and Crohn's disease, and plays a pivotal role in the pathogenesis of these disorders *(20,21)*. Also, increased levels of sTNFR are observed in patients with malignancies including acute myelogenous leukaemia, non-Hodgkin's lymphoma, and breast cancer *(22–24)*.

THE CD95 RECEPTOR

The human CD95 antigen (also known as APO-1, Fas) is constitutively expressed in a wide range of hematopoietic and nonhematopoietic cells, and with particular abundance in the thymus, liver, and kidney *(25)*.

The CD95 Promoter

The human CD95 gene is a single-copy gene comprising nine exons and eight introns *(26,27)*. The 5' flanking sequence is GC rich (61%), with a high number of CpG dinucleotides between –590 and –1, and lacks conventional TATA and CAAT boxes *(28)*, properties characteristic of housekeeping genes *(29)*. The promoter sequence contains consensus binding sites for the transcription factors Sp1, AP-1, AP-2, Ets, GF-1, EBP20, *c-myb*, CREB, GAF, NF-κB, NF-AT, NF-Y, and NF-IL6 *(26,27,30)*. Rudert et al. identified a silencer region between nucleotide positions –1035 and –1008, and a strong enhancer region between –1007 and –964 *(31)*. The transcription factors YB-1, Purα, and Purβ were shown to bind to the silencer region and produce varying levels of transcriptional repression *(32)*. An enhancer element containing recognition motifs for GA-binding protein (GABP) and AP-1 resides between nucleotide positions –862 and –682 *(33)*. Regulation of CD95 expression has been described for a wide range of stimuli.

Upregulation of CD95 in T-Cell Activation

When T-cells get activated, CD95 mRNA is upregulated and cells gradually become sensitive to CD95L-mediated apoptosis *(34)*. In a first step, signaling through the TCR/CD3 complex activates the src family tyrosine kinases p56 lck and p59lyn, and the protein-tyrosine kinases ZAP-70 and Syk *(35)*. These kinases trigger three major pathways: (1) phospholipase Cγ1 → Ca2+ → calcineurin → NF-AT; (2) phosphatidylinositol (PI) 3-kinase → protein kinase (Akt) → S6 kinase; and (3) the Ras/Rac → mitogen-activated protein (MAP) kinase pathway. The MAP kinase pathways consist of three parallel signaling cascades, including the ERK1/2 MAP kinase cascade, the JNK/SAPK cascade, and the p38 MAP kinase cascade. Several targets of MAP kinase have been identified, including c-Jun and c-Fos, components of the transcription factor AP-1. Binding of both AP-1 and GABP to the upstream enhancer element has been shown to be required for initiating CD95 transcription after T-cell activation *(33)*. In addition, a composite binding site for Sp1 and NF-κB transcription factors at positions –295 to –286 is critical for T-cell activation-driven upregulation of CD95 *(36)*.

Regulation of CD95 in Viral Infections

Infection with influenza virus or HIV augments the production of CD95 at the mRNA level *(30,37)*. This may be due to a virus-stimulated increase of NF-IL6 (nuclear factor for interleukin 6 expression) binding to the 5' end of the human CD95 gene, containing eight copies of the NF-IL6 binding motif. NF-IL6 activation is likely to involve posttranslational modification, since no increase in NF-IL6 abundancy was observed after viral infection.

CD95 Expression After Genotoxic Stress

Chemotherapeutic drugs and irradiation stimulate upregulation of CD95 in many cell types *(38)*. The increase in CD95 mRNA has been shown to be p53-dependent by various groups *(39–42)*. After exposure to DNA-damaging agents, p53 protein gets stabilized, resulting in elevated steady-state levels *(43)*. Wild-type p53 protein governs cellular activity by regulating downstream genes that control various cellular pathways, including cell-cycle arrest and apoptosis *(44,45)*. A p53-responsive element is present in the first intron of the CD95 gene. Three additional putative p53 binding elements are contained 5' to the gene *(40)*. When the p53-binding intronic region was placed in conjunction with the CD95 promoter in a reporter plasmid, transcriptional activity was strongly induced by wild-type p53. Interestingly, in contrast to bax, another p53-regulated proapoptotic gene, the human CD95 p53-response element is still activated by the discriminatory p53 mutants Pro-175 and Ala-143 *(46)*. Different genotoxic treatments cause different phosphorylations of p53. Whereas both irradiation and the chemotherapeutic drug ara-C resulted in p53-induction and apoptosis in the human leukemia cell line BV173, only irradiation was capable of inducing p53-dependent CD95 expression *(41)*. Thus, the susceptibility of CD95 to p53-mediated upregulation is dependent on the genotoxic signal.

Regulation of CD95 by Biological Response Modifiers

TNF-α induces CD95 expression by activating NF-κB. This upregulation has been shown to be dependent on the RelA subunit of NF-κB *(47)*.

Binding of IFN-γ to its receptor leads to the activation of tyrosine kinases of the Janus family (JAK). Activated JAKs then phosphorylate subunit 1 of the IFN-γ receptor (IFNγR1), which subsequently serves as a docking site for signaling and transactivation (STAT) proteins, followed by their phosphorylation. The STAT proteins, mainly STAT1, form homo- or heterodimers, translocate to the nucleus, and regulate gene transcription by binding to gamma activating sequences (GAS elements) in the promoter of IFN-γ regulated genes *(48)*. IFN-γ has been shown to upregulate CD95 in cells from various tumors, including gliomas, Ewing's sarcoma, colon cancer, and in normal epithelial cells *(49–52)*. The dependency of IFN-γ- induced CD95 upregulation on STAT1 was demonstrated in the colon cancer cell line HT29. No increase in CD95 was observed in STAT1-deficient cells, but transfection of STAT1 restored CD95 responsiveness to IFN-γ in these cells *(53)*.

IL-12 has been shown to directly upregulate surface expression of CD95 in the human osteosarcoma cell line SAOS and the human breast cancer cell lines MDB-MB-231 *(54)*. There is preliminary evidence that this increase in CD95 expression involves the NF-κB pathway *(54)*. Stimulation of CD95 may add to the antitumor activity of IL12 in several preclinical animal tumor models *(55)*.

In lung cancer cells, the synthetic retinoid CD437 induces increased CD95 expression, which is dependent on wild-type p53 *(56)*.

EXPRESSION OF DEATH RECEPTOR DR3

Activation of death receptor (DR)3 is capable of inducing both NF-κB and apoptosis *(57)*. The DR3 gene locus is located on human chromosome band 1p36.2-p36.3 *(58)*. This gene locus is frequently deleted in neuroblastoma and other neuroectodermal tumors. In medulloblastoma/PNET, expression of DR3 is significantly associated with survival *(59)*. The DR3 promoter and its regulation have not yet been described.

THE TRAIL RECEPTORS DR4 AND DR5

TNF-related apoptosis-inducing ligand (TRAIL, also known as APO2L) interacts specifically with five different receptors. Death receptors DR4 (also known as TRAIL-R1) and DR5 (also known as TRAIL-R2, TRICK2, and KILLER) are type I transmembrane proteins, which contain an intracellular death domain *(60)*. Binding of TRAIL to receptors DR4 and DR5 leads to apoptosis via recruitment of adaptor proteins such as Fas-associated death domain (FADD), resulting in activation of the caspase system. Decoy receptor DcR1 (also known as TRAIL-R3 or TRID), a glycosylphosph-atidylinositol-linked protein, DcR2 (also known as TRAIL-R4 or TRUNDD), and osteoprotegerin contain either no cytoplasmic death domain or a truncated death domain. Therefore binding of TRAIL to these receptors does not result in apoptosis.

Regulation of DR4 and DR5

The DR4 Promoter

The 5' flanking region of the DR4 gene has been recently characterized *(61)*. Three putative binding sites for AP-1 were identified, with the site located at –350/–344 being tested and shown to be functionally active. TPA, a strong inducer of AP-1, enhanced the binding of this DR4 AP-1 site to nuclear extracts and increased transcription of DR4.

There is evidence that DR4 is a DNA-damage-inducible gene that is p53-regulated in some types of cancer cells *(62)*. When HPV E6 was transfected into wild-type p53 lung cancer cells, leading to decreased levels of p53 protein, DR4 induction by DNA-damaging agents was suppressed. Conversely, transfection of exogenous wild-type p53 led to the upregulation of endogenous DR4 in cells with mutant p53.

The DR5 Promoter

As in TNFR, CD95, and DR4 genes, DR5 contains a TATA-less promoter. There are two SP1 sites responsible for basal transcriptional activity. Transient transfection assays with serial 5' deletion mutants identified the minimal promoter region between –198 and –116 *(63)*.

DR5 and p53

Exposure of various human cancer cell lines to doxorubicin, etoposide, or irradiation led to induction of DR5 in cells with wild-type p53 status, but not in cells with mutant p53 *(64)*. Overexpression of wild-type p53 in p53-deficient cells caused induction of DR5. A p53 DNA-binding site was identified within intron 1, and mutation of this binding site led to loss of DR5 inducibility in reporter gene assays *(65)*. Interestingly, p53-dependent upregulation of DR5 seems to be restricted to wild-type p53 cells undergoing apoptosis but not cell-cycle arrest when exposed to DNA-damaging agents *(66)*.

Regulation of DR4 and DR5 Through NF-κB

Etoposide has been shown to upregulate DR4 and DR5 expression in epithelial cells such as breast cancer and human embryonic kidney cells *(67)*. The induction involves the nuclear factor κB (NF-κB) pathway and can be blocked by expression of kinase-inactive MEK kinase 1 (MEKK1) or dominant-negative inhibitor of NF-κB (IκB). Ravi et al. demonstrated that TNF-α increased expression of DR4 and DR5 by inducing degradation of IκB and subsequent activation of NF-κB *(68)*. This upregulation was dependent on the c-Rel subunit of NF-κB. Upregulation of DR5 but not DR4 through NF-κB has been described in various epithelial cell lines after exposure to TRAIL *(69)*. In fact, a NF-κB binding site has been described between +385 and +394 in intron 1 of the DR5 gene *(63)*.

Regulation of DR4 and DR5 by Chemotherapy

In prostate cancer cells, protein levels of DR4 and DR5 were upregulated up to eight-fold when cells were treated with paclitaxel *(70)*. Interestingly, protein induction was not associated with an increase in mRNA compatible with a posttranscriptional mechanism. Treatment of human leukemic cells with etoposide, Ara-C, or doxorubicin increased DR5 protein expression but not DR4 expression *(71)*. When cells were pretreated with these drugs at clinically achievable concentrations, apoptosis induced by TRAIL was significantly increased.

Regulation of DR4 and DR5 by Biological Response Modifiers

IFN-γ was shown to downregulate mRNA and surface expression of DR4 and DR5 in human fibroblasts *(72)*. This effect was associated with inhibition of NF-κB. In contrast, in various tumor cell lines, DR5 expression is stimulated by IFN-γ *(73)* independently from the p53 status, and is delayed in STAT1-null cells. Likewise, the glucocorticoid dexamethasone has been demonstrated to elevate DR5 mRNA expression by a mechanism unrelated to p53 in cancer cell lines *(73)*. Interestingly, the glucocorticoid prednisone, though also inducing apoptosis, did not induce DR5 transcription.

Influence of Viral Infection on TRAIL Receptor Expression

Human herpes virus 7 (HHV-7) is endemic in the adult population and represents a potential opportunistic agent in immunocompromised individuals. HHV preferentially infects CD4+ T-cells. Infection of T-cells is associated with marked downregulation of DR4, making cells resistant to TRAIL-mediated apoptosis *(74)*. In contrast, infection of human fibroblasts with cytomegalovirus (CMV) leads to increased DR4 and DR5 expression *(72)*. Interestingly, CMV infection activates NF-κB, which in turn has been shown to signal upregulation of DR4 and DR5 *(67,75)*.

Expression of TRAIL Receptors in Cancer and Nonmalignant Disease

In colon cancer, the inducible cyclooxygenase-2 (COX-2) gene, which regulates prostaglandin biosynthesis, is upregulated *(76)*. When HCT-15 colon cancer cells lacking endogenous COX-2 were transfected with COX-2 cDNA, TRAIL-induced apoptosis was attenuated, accompanied by transcriptional downregulation of DR5 and by increased Bcl-2 expression *(77)*. The nonsteroidal antiinflammatory drug sulindac sulfide inhibited COX-2 enzymatic activity and reversed COX-2-mediated downregulation of DR5 mRNA and protein.

Toxic bile salts promote liver injury and the development of liver cirrhosis *(78)*. The toxic bile salt glycochenodeoxycholate (GCDC) was shown to induce apoptosis in a hepatocellular carcinoma cell line, which was associated with increased expression and aggregation of DR5 but not DR4 *(79)*.

REGULATION OF DEATH RECEPTOR DR6

The death receptor DR6 has been characterized by Pan et al. *(80)*. DR6 is expressed in most human tissues. In LnCAP prostate cancer cells, TNF-α induced DR6 mRNA and protein levels *(81)*. This induction could be blocked by inhibiting NF-κB activation. Increased expression of DR6 has been described in late-stage prostate tumors compared to normal tissue and tumor cell lines derived from less advanced prostate cancers.

DECOY RECEPTORS (DCR)

The TRAIL-binding receptors DcR1 and DcR2, as well as the Fas ligand-binding receptor DcR3, are called decoys because they do not contain an intracellular death domain and protect cells from the cytotoxic effect of the respective death ligand *(82)*.

Promoter Structure of DcR1

The promoter structure of the human DcR1 gene has been investigated by Ruiz et al. *(83)*. The promoter contains a TATA-consensus box. Deletion analysis identified a minimal promoter region within the first 33 nucleotides upstream of the transcription initiation site. Transcriptional activity increases with extended size of 5' fragments, suggesting functional binding sites for additional, not yet identified transcription factors that cooperate with the basal transcription machinery in the regulation of the DcR1 gene.

Regulation of Expression of Decoy Receptors

Sheikh et al. demonstrated that DcR1 is upregulated in p53 wild-type but not p53-negative cell lines after exposure to X-ray *(84)*. When a human temperature-sensitive p53 was transfected into p53-null H1299 lung carcinoma cells, DcR1 was upregulated upon shift to the permissive temperature. Also, doxorubicin, a p53-inducing drug, was able to activate a DcR1 promoter construct in MCF7 cells *(83)*. However, abrogation of p53 activity by HPV E6 protein through proteasome-dependent degradation did not affect the transcriptional activity of this promoter fragment, indicating that the p53-responsive site must be located outside the promoter region of –502, +42.

Overexpression of cRel, a member of the Rel/NF-κB family of transcription factors leads to upregulation of DcR1 in HeLa cells and to resistance against TRAIL-induced apoptosis *(85)*. Upregulation of DcR1 was also achieved by TNF-α via activation of endogenous Rel/NF-κB factors.

Maeda et al. demonstrated upregulation of DcR2 and downregulation of DcR3 in human keratinocytes after exposure to ultraviolet B irradiation by a mechanism that remains to be identified *(86)*.

Fresh neuroblastoma cells and various tumor cell lines have been shown not to express DcR1 and DcR2. This lack of decoy receptor expression was demonstrated to be associated with dense hypermethylation of their promoter regions *(87)*. Treatment with 5-aza-2'deoxycytidine resulted in partial demethylation and restored mRNA expression of DcR1 and DcR2.

Abundant levels of DcR1 and DcR3 have been observed in tumors of the gastrointestinal tract *(84,88)*. It is hypothesized that this overexpression confers growth advantage by inhibiting TRAIL- and CD95-mediated destruction of tumor cells.

CONCLUSION

Although control and fine-tuning of death receptor transcription and activity is complex and cell-type specific, several regulatory proteins seem to play key roles. Among them p53 and NFκB are frequently involved in the regulation of several death receptors and may contribute to the cytotoxicity of chemo- and radiotherapeutic agents. Therefore, restoration of function of these regulatory proteins, which is frequently compromised in cancer cells, is a major goal in the development of biology-based new tumor-treatment strategies.

REFERENCES

1. Tartaglia LA, Goeddel DV. Two TNF receptors. Immunol Today 1992;13(5):151–153.
2. Grell M, Zimmermann G, Hulser D, Pfizenmaier K, Scheurich P. TNF receptors TR60 and TR80 can mediate apoptosis via induction of distinct signal pathways. J Immunol 1994;153(5):1963–1972.
3. Santee SM, Owen-Schaub LB. Human tumor necrosis factor receptor p75/80 (CD120b) gene structure and promoter characterization. J Biol Chem 1996;271(35):21,151–21,159.
4. Winzen R, Wallach D, Engelmann H, et al. Selective decrease in cell surface expression and mRNA level of the 55-kDa tumor necrosis factor receptor during differentiation of HL-60 cells into macrophage-like but not granulocyte-like cells. J Immunol 1992;148(11):3454–3460.
5. Kemper O, Wallach D. Cloning and partial characterization of the promoter for the human p55 tumor necrosis factor (TNF) receptor. Gene 1993;134(2):209–216.
6. Kuhnert P, Kemper O, Wallach D. Cloning, sequencing and partial functional characterization of the 5' region of the human p75 tumor necrosis factor receptor-encoding gene (TNF-R). Gene 1994;150(2): 381–386.
7. Kalthoff H, Roeder C, Brockhaus M, Thiele HG, Schmiegel W. Tumor necrosis factor (TNF) up-regulates the expression of p75 but not p55 TNF receptors, and both receptors mediate, independently of each other, up-regulation of transforming growth factor alpha and epidermal growth factor receptor mRNA. J Biol Chem 1993;268(4):2762–2766.

8. Dickensheets HL, Freeman SL, Smith MF, Donnelly RP. Interleukin-10 upregulates tumor necrosis factor receptor type-II (p75) gene expression in endotoxin-stimulated human monocytes. Blood 1997;90(10):4162–4171.
9. Ware CF, Crowe PD, VanArsdale TL, Andrews JL, et al. Tumor necrosis factor (TNF) receptor expression in T lymphocytes. Differential regulation of the type I TNF receptor during activation of resting and effector T cells. J Immunol 1991;147(12):4229–4238.
10. Kohno T, Brewer MT, Baker SL, et al. A second tumor necrosis factor receptor gene product can shed a naturally occurring tumor necrosis factor inhibitor. Proc Natl Acad Sci USA 1990;87(21):8331–8335.
11. Van Zee KJ, Kohno T, Fischer E, Rock CS, Moldawer LL, Lowry SF. Tumor necrosis factor soluble receptors circulate during experimental and clinical inflammation and can protect against excessive tumor necrosis factor alpha in vitro and in vivo. Proc Natl Acad Sci USA 1992;89(11):4845–4849.
12. Reddy P, Slack JL, Davis R, et al. Functional analysis of the domain structure of tumor necrosis factor-alpha converting enzyme. J Biol Chem 2000;275(19):14,608–14,614.
13. Hino T, Nakamura H, Abe S, et al. Hydrogen peroxide enhances shedding of type I soluble tumor necrosis factor receptor from pulmonary epithelial cells. Am J Respir Cell Mol Biol 1999;20(1):122–128.
14. Zhang Z, Kolls JK, Oliver P, et al. Activation of tumor necrosis factor-alpha-converting enzyme-mediated ectodomain shedding by nitric oxide. J Biol Chem 2000;275(21):15,839–15,844.
15. Madge LA, Sierra-Honigmann MR, Pober JS. Apoptosis-inducing agents cause rapid shedding of tumor necrosis factor receptor 1 (TNFR1). A nonpharmacological explanation for inhibition of TNF-mediated activation. J Biol Chem 1999;274(19):13,643–13,649.
16. Joyce DA, Gibbons DP, Green P, Steer JH, Feldmann M, Brennan FM. Two inhibitors of pro-inflammatory cytokine release, interleukin-10 and interleukin-4, have contrasting effects on release of soluble p75 tumor necrosis factor receptor by cultured monocytes. Eur J Immunol 1994;24(11):2699–2705.
17. Philippe C, Roux-Lombard P, Fouqueray B, Perez J, Dayer JM, Baud L. Membrane expression and shedding of tumour necrosis factor receptors during activation of human blood monocytes: regulation by desferrioxamine. Immunology 1993;80(2):300–305.
18. Joyce DA, Kloda A, Steer JH. Dexamethasone suppresses release of soluble TNF receptors by human monocytes concurrently with TNF-alpha suppression. Immunol Cell Biol 1997;75(4):345–350.
19. Ding AH, Sanchez E, Srimal S, Nathan CF. Macrophages rapidly internalize their tumor necrosis factor receptors in response to bacterial lipopolysaccharide. J Biol Chem 1989;264(7):3924–3929.
20. Alsalameh S, Mattka B, Al Ward R, et al. Preferential expression of tumor necrosis factor receptor 55 (TNF-R55) on human articular chondrocytes: selective transcriptional upregulation of TNF-R75 by proinflammatory cytokines interleukin 1beta, tumor necrosis factor-alpha, and basis fibroblast growth factor. J Rheumatol 1999;26(3):645–653.
21. Holtmann MH, Douni E, Schutz M, et al. Tumor necrosis factor-receptor 2 is up-regulated on lamina propria T cells in Crohn's disease and promotes experimental colitis in vivo. Eur J Immunol 2002;32(11):3142–3151.
22. Goetz M, Schiel X, Heussel H, Steinmetz T, Hiddemann W, Weiss M. Elevation of soluble tumor necrosis factor receptor II in non-febrile patients with acute myeloid leukemia. Eur J Med Res 2002;7(11):487–490.
23. Metkar SS, Naresh KN, Manna PP, Srinivas V, Advani SH, Nadkarni JJ. Circulating levels of TNF alpha and TNF receptor superfamily members in lymphoid neoplasia. Am J Hematol 2000;65(2):105–110.
24. Tesarova P, Kvasnicka J, Umlaufova A, Homolkova H, Jirsa M, Tesar V. Soluble TNF and IL-2 receptors in patients with breast cancer. Med Sci Monit 2000;6(4):661–667.
25. Leithauser F, Dhein J, Mechtersheimer G, et al. Constitutive and induced expression of APO-1, a new member of the nerve growth factor/tumor necrosis factor receptor superfamily, in normal and neoplastic cells. Lab Invest 1993;69(4):415–429.
26. Cheng J, Liu C , Koopman WJ, Mountz JD. Characterization of human Fas gene. Exon/intron organization and promoter region. J Immunol 1995;154(3):1239–1245.
27. Behrmann I, Walczak H, Krammer PH. Structure of the human APO-1 gene. Eur J Immunol 1994;24(12):3057–3062.
28. Xiang H, Fox JA, Totpal K, et al. Enhanced tumor killing by Apo2L/TRAIL and CPT-11 co-treatment is associated with p21 cleavage and differential regulation of Apo2L/TRAIL ligand and its receptors. Oncogene 2002;21(22):3611–3619.
29. Azizkhan JC, Jensen DE, Pierce AJ, Wade M. Transcription from TATA-less promoters: dihydrofolate reductase as a model. Crit Rev Eukaryot Gene Expr 1993;3(4):229–254.

30. Wada N, Matsumura M, Ohba Y, Kobayashi N, Takizawa T, Nakanishi Y. Transcription stimulation of the Fas-encoding gene by nuclear factor for interleukin-6 expression upon influenza virus infection. J Biol Chem 1995;270(30):18,007–18,012.
31. Rudert F, Visser E, Forbes L, Lindridge E, Wang Y, Watson J. Identification of a silencer, enhancer, and basal promoter region in the human CD95 (Fas/APO-1) gene. DNA Cell Biol 1995;14(11):931–937.
32. Lasham A, Lindridge E, Rudert F, Onrust R, Watson J. Regulation of the human fas promoter by YB-1, Puralpha and AP-1 transcription factors. Gene 2000;252(1–2):1–13.
33. Li XR, Chong AS, Wu J, et al. Transcriptional regulation of Fas gene expression by GA-binding protein and AP-1 in T cell antigen receptor.CD3 complex-stimulated T cells. J Biol Chem 1999;274(49):35,203–35,210.
34. Miyawaki T, Uehara T, Nibu R, et al. Differential expression of apoptosis-related Fas antigen on lymphocyte subpopulations in human peripheral blood. J Immunol 1992;149(11):3753–3758.
35. van Leeuwen JE, Samelson LE. T cell antigen-receptor signal transduction. Curr Opin Immunol 1999;11(3):242–248.
36. Chan H, Bartos DP, Owen-Schaub LB. Activation-dependent transcriptional regulation of the human Fas promoter requires NF-kappaB p50-p65 recruitment. Mol Cell Biol 1999;19(3):2098–2108.
37. Takizawa T, Fukuda R, Miyawaki T, Ohashi K, Nakanishi Y. Activation of the apoptotic Fas antigen-encoding gene upon influenza virus infection involving spontaneously produced beta-interferon. Virology 1995;209(2):288–296.
38. Kaufmann SH, Earnshaw WC. Induction of apoptosis by cancer chemotherapy. Exp Cell Res 2000;256(1):42–49.
39. Owen-Schaub LB, Zhang W, Cusack JC, et al. Wild-type human p53 and a temperature-sensitive mutant induce Fas/APO-1 expression. Mol Cell Biol 1995;15(6):3032–3040.
40. Muller M, Wilder S, Bannasch D, et al. p53 activates the CD95 (APO-1/Fas) gene in response to DNA damage by anticancer drugs. J Exp Med 1998;188 (11):2033–2045.
41. Kobayashi T, Ruan S, Jabbur JR, et al. Differential p53 phosphorylation and activation of apoptosis-promoting genes Bax and Fas/APO-1 by irradiation and ara-C treatment. Cell Death Differ 1998;5(7):584–591.
42. Lorenzo E, Ruiz-Ruiz C, Quesada AJ, et al. Doxorubicin induces apoptosis and CD95 gene expression in human primary endothelial cells through a p53-dependent mechanism. J Biol Chem 2002;277(13): 10,883–10,892.
43. Lowe SW. Cancer therapy and p53. Curr Opin Oncol 1995;7(6):547–553.
44. Kastan MB, Zhan Q, El Deiry WS, et al. A mammalian cell cycle checkpoint pathway utilizing p53 and GADD45 is defective in ataxia-telangiectasia. Cell 1992;71(4):587–597.
45. El Deiry WS, Tokino T, Velculescu VE, et al. WAF1, a potential mediator of p53 tumor suppression. Cell 1993;75(4):817–825.
46. Munsch D, Watanabe-Fukunaga R, Bourdon JC, et al. Human and mouse Fas (APO-1/CD95) death receptor genes each contain a p53-responsive element that is activated by p53 mutants unable to induce apoptosis. J Biol Chem 2000;275(6):3867–3872.
47. Ouaaz F, Li M, Beg AA. A critical role for the RelA subunit of nuclear factor kappaB in regulation of multiple immune-response genes and in Fas-induced cell death. J Exp Med 1999;189(6):999–1004.
48. Platanias LC, Fish EN. Signaling pathways activated by interferons. Exp Hematol 1999;27(11): 1583–1592.
49. Weller M, Frei K, Groscurth P, Krammer PH, Yonekawa Y, Fontana A. Anti-Fas/APO-1 antibody-mediated apoptosis of cultured human glioma cells. Induction and modulation of sensitivity by cytokines. J Clin Invest 1994;94(3):954–964.
50. Ossina NK, Cannas A, Powers VC, et al. Interferon-gamma modulates a p53-independent apoptotic pathway and apoptosis-related gene expression. J Biol Chem 1997;272(26):16,351–16,357.
51. Kontny HU, Lehrnbecher TM, Chanock SJ, Mackall CL. Simultaneous expression of Fas and nonfunctional Fas ligand in Ewing's sarcoma. Cancer Res 1998;58(24):5842–5849.
52. Ruemmele FM, Russo P, Beaulieu J, et al. Susceptibility to FAS-induced apoptosis in human nontumoral enterocytes: role of costimulatory factors. J Cell Physiol 1999;181(1):45–54.
53. Xu X, Fu XY, Plate J, Chong AS. IFN-gamma induces cell growth inhibition by Fas-mediated apoptosis: requirement of STAT1 protein for up-regulation of Fas and FasL expression. Cancer Res 1998;58(13):2832–2837.
54. Lafleur EA, Jia SF, Worth LL, Zhou Z, Owen-Schaub LB, Kleinerman ES. Interleukin (IL)-12 and IL-12 gene transfer up-regulate Fas expression in human osteosarcoma and breast cancer cells. Cancer Res 2001;61(10):4066–4071.

55. Siders WM, Wright PW, Hixon JA, et al. T cell- and NK cell-independent inhibition of hepatic metastases by systemic administration of an IL-12-expressing recombinant adenovirus. J Immunol 1998;160(11): 5465–5474.
56. Sun SY, Yue P, Hong WK, Lotan R. Induction of Fas expression and augmentation of Fas/Fas ligand-mediated apoptosis by the synthetic retinoid CD437 in human lung cancer cells. Cancer Res 2000;60(22):6537–6543.
57. Chinnaiyan AM, O'Rourke K, Yu GL, et al. Signal transduction by DR3, a death domain-containing receptor related to TNFR-1 and CD95. Science 1996;274(5289):990–992.
58. Grenet J, Valentine V, Kitson J, Li H, Farrow SN, Kidd VJ. Duplication of the DR3 gene on human chromosome 1p36 and its deletion in human neuroblastoma. Genomics 1998;49(3):385–393.
59. Eggert A, Grotzer MA, Zuzak TJ, Ikegaki N, Zhao H, Brodeur GM. Expression of Apo-3 and Apo-3L in primitive neuroectodermal tumours of the central and peripheral nervous system. Eur J Cancer 2002;38(1):92–98.
60. Smyth MJ, Takeda K, Hayakawa Y, Peschon JJ, van den Brink MR, Yagita H. Nature's TRAIL—on a path to cancer immunotherapy. Immunity 2003;18(1):1–6.
61. Guan B, Yue P, Lotan R, Sun SY. Evidence that the human death receptor 4 is regulated by activator protein 1. Oncogene 2002;21(20):3121–3129.
62. Guan B, Yue P, Clayman GL, Sun SY. Evidence that the death receptor DR4 is a DNA damage-inducible, p53-regulated gene. J Cell Physiol 2001;188(1):98–105.
63. Yoshida T, Maeda A, Tani N, Sakai T. Promoter structure and transcription initiation sites of the human death receptor 5/TRAIL-R2 gene. FEBS Lett 2001;507(3):381–385.
64. Wu GS, Burns TF, McDonald ER, III, et al. KILLER/DR5 is a DNA damage-inducible p53-regulated death receptor gene. Nat Genet 1997;17(2):141–143.
65. Takimoto R, El Deiry WS. Wild-type p53 transactivates the KILLER/DR5 gene through an intronic sequence-specific DNA-binding site. Oncogene 2000;19(14):1735–1743.
66. Wu GS, Burns TF, McDonald ER, III, et al. Induction of the TRAIL receptor KILLER/DR5 in p53-dependent apoptosis but not growth arrest. Oncogene 1999;18(47):6411–6418.
67. Gibson SB, Oyer R, Spalding AC, Anderson SM, Johnson GL. Increased expression of death receptors 4 and 5 synergizes the apoptosis response to combined treatment with etoposide and TRAIL. Mol Cell Biol 2000;20(1):205–212.
68. Ravi R, Bedi GC, Engstrom LW, et al. Regulation of death receptor expression and TRAIL/Apo2L-induced apoptosis by NF-kappaB. Nat Cell Biol 2001;3(4):409–416.
69. Shetty S, Gladden JB, Henson ES, et al. Tumor necrosis factor-related apoptosis inducing ligand (TRAIL) up-regulates death receptor 5 (DR5) mediated by NFkappaB activation in epithelial derived cell lines. Apoptosis 2002;7(5):413–420.
70. Nimmanapalli R, Perkins CL, Orlando M, O'Bryan E, Nguyen D, Bhalla KN. Pretreatment with paclitaxel enhances apo-2 ligand/tumor necrosis factor-related apoptosis-inducing ligand-induced apoptosis of prostate cancer cells by inducing death receptors 4 and 5 protein levels. Cancer Res 2001;61(2):759–763.
71. Wen J, Ramadevi N, Nguyen D, Perkins C, Worthington E, Bhalla K. Antileukemic drugs increase death receptor 5 levels and enhance Apo-2L-induced apoptosis of human acute leukemia cells. Blood 2000;96(12):3900–3906.
72. Sedger LM, Shows DM, Blanton RA, et al. IFN-gamma mediates a novel antiviral activity through dynamic modulation of TRAIL and TRAIL receptor expression. J Immunol 1999;163(2):920–926.
73. Meng RD, El Deiry WS. p53-independent upregulation of KILLER/DR5 TRAIL receptor expression by glucocorticoids and interferon-gamma. Exp Cell Res 2001;262(2):154–169.
74. Secchiero P, Mirandola P, Zella D, et al. Human herpesvirus 7 induces the functional up-regulation of tumor necrosis factor-related apoptosis-inducing ligand (TRAIL) coupled to TRAIL-R1 down-modulation in CD4(+) T cells. Blood 2001;98(8):2474–2481.
75. Yurochko AD, Kowalik TF, Huong SM, Huang ES. Human cytomegalovirus upregulates NF-kappa B activity by transactivating the NF-kappa B p105/p50 and p65 promoters. J Virol 1995;69(9):5391–5400.
76. Eberhart CE, Coffey RJ, Radhika A, Giardiello FM, Ferrenbach S, DuBois RN. Up-regulation of cyclooxygenase 2 gene expression in human colorectal adenomas and adenocarcinomas. Gastroenterology 1994;107(4):1183–1188.
77. Tang X, Sun YJ , Half E, Kuo MT, Sinicrope F. Cyclooxygenase-2 overexpression inhibits death receptor 5 expression and confers resistance to tumor necrosis factor-related apoptosis-inducing ligand-induced apoptosis in human colon cancer cells. Cancer Res 2002;62(17):4903–4908.

78. Greim H, Trulzsch D, Czygan P, et al. Mechanism of cholestasis. 6. Bile acids in human livers with or without biliary obstruction. Gastroenterology 1972;63(5):846–850.
79. Higuchi H, Bronk SF, Takikawa Y, et al. The bile acid glycochenodeoxycholate induces trail-receptor 2/DR5 expression and apoptosis. J Biol Chem 2001;276(42):38,610–38,618.
80. Pan G, Bauer JH, Haridas V, et al. Identification and functional characterization of DR6, a novel death domain-containing TNF receptor. FEBS Lett 1998;431(3):351–356.
81. Kasof GM, Lu JJ, Liu D, et al. Tumor necrosis factor-alpha induces the expression of DR6, a member of the TNF receptor family, through activation of NF-kappaB. Oncogene 2001;20(55):7965–7975.
82. Mantovani A, Locati M, Vecchi A, Sozzani S, Allavena P. Decoy receptors: a strategy to regulate inflammatory cytokines and chemokines. Trends Immunol 2001;22(6):328–336.
83. Ruiz dA, Lopez-Rivas A, Redondo JM, Rodriguez A. Transcription initiation sites and promoter structure of the human TRAIL-R3 gene. FEBS Lett 2002;531(2):304–308.
84. Sheikh MS, Huang Y, Fernandez-Salas EA, et al. The antiapoptotic decoy receptor TRID/TRAIL-R3 is a p53-regulated DNA damage-inducible gene that is overexpressed in primary tumors of the gastrointestinal tract. Oncogene 1999;18(28):4153–4159.
85. Bernard D, Quatannens B, Vandenbunder B, Abbadie C . Rel/NF-kappaB transcription factors protect against tumor necrosis factor (TNF)-related apoptosis-inducing ligand (TRAIL)-induced apoptosis by up-regulating the TRAIL decoy receptor DcR1. J Biol Chem 2001;276(29):27,322–27,328.
86. Maeda T, Hao C , Tron VA. Ultraviolet light (UV) regulation of the TNF family decoy receptors DcR2 and DcR3 in human keratinocytes. J Cutan Med Surg 2001;5(4):294–298.
87. van Noesel MM, van Bezouw S, Salomons GS, et al. Tumor-specific down-regulation of the tumor necrosis factor-related apoptosis-inducing ligand decoy receptors DcR1 and DcR2 is associated with dense promoter hypermethylation. Cancer Res 2002;62(7):2157–2161.
88. Bai C, Connolly B, Metzker ML, et al. Overexpression of M68/DcR3 in human gastrointestinal tract tumors independent of gene amplification and its location in a four-gene cluster. Proc Natl Acad Sci USA 2000;97(3):1230–1235.

10 Regulation of Trail Receptor Expression in Human Melanoma

Peter Hersey, FRACP, DPhil,
Si Yi Zhang, PhD,
and Xu Dong Zhang, MD, PhD

SUMMARY

In previous studies we have shown that the level of expression of tumor necrosis factor-related apoptosis-inducing ligand (TRAIL) death receptor R2 was a major determinant of the sensitivity of melanoma cell lines to TRAIL-induced apoptosis. Transcriptional events regulating TRAIL death receptor expression have been the focus of much study, but our investigations point to a more important role for posttranscriptional events in regulation of TRAIL death receptors. First, although there was a wide variation in TRAIL-R2 expression between melanoma cell lines, this did not correlate with mRNA expression assessed by real-time PCR. Similarly, early passage primary cultures from patients tended to have low TRAIL-R2 protein expression compared to cells in later passage cultures, even though TRAIL-R2 mRNA expression was similar in early and late passages. Second, generation of TRAIL-resistant melanoma lines by culture in TRAIL was also associated with decreased expression of TRAIL-R2 protein, but TRAIL-R2 mRNA levels were similar to those in parental high-TRAIL-R2 expressing cells. The latter model was used to explore post-transcriptional regulation of TRAIL-R2. Expression from a luciferase reporter gene construct with the 3' untranslated region (UTR) (but not the 5'UTR) of TRAIL-R2 was suppressed when transfected into the TRAIL-selected (resistant) melanoma lines and in early passage (resistant) primary melanoma cultures. RNA gel shift assays demonstrated protein(s) binding to the 3'UTR but not the 5'UTR of TRAIL-R2 mRNA. These results suggest that TRAIL-R2 expression in melanoma cell lines is determined in large part by posttranscriptional events and that protein(s) binding to the 3'UTR region of TRAIL-R2 mRNA may play a key role in this regulation. Decoy receptors appeared to play little or no role in regulation of TRAIL-mediated apoptosis of melanoma.

From: *Cancer Drug Discovery and Development: Death Receptors in Cancer Therapy*
Edited by: W. S. El-Deiry © Humana Press Inc., Totowa, NJ

INTRODUCTION

TRAIL is one of several members of the tumor necrosis factor (TNF) family that can induce apoptosis by interaction with receptors on the cell surface, which contain so-called death domains (DDs). TRAIL is of particular importance in that it appears to induce apoptosis in a wide variety of cancer cell lines but not in cultures from normal tissues *(1,2)*. One form of TRAIL (amino acids 114–281 fused to an amino-terminal polyhistidine tag) was found to induce apoptosis in normal human liver cells *(3)*, but other forms, such as the zinc-bound 114–281 form or 95–281 amino acid fused to the leucine zipper from yeast, have not been toxic to a range of normal cells in vitro, and the zinc-bound form has not been toxic in nonhuman primates *(4,5)*.

The physiological role of TRAIL is not well established. It is expressed on CD4 T-cells *(6)*, natural killer (NK) cells, monocytes *(7)*, and to a lesser extent CD8 T-cells. It is upregulated by type I interferons and interleukin (IL)-2 *(8,9)*, and may play a role in control of viral infections *(10)*. In animal models, TRAIL was shown to mediate natural killer-cell surveillance against development of liver metastases *(11,12)*. TRAIL knockout or TRAIL antibody-treated mice were more susceptible to development of chemically induced tumors and to development of metastases in liver or lungs *(13,14)*. TRAIL knockout mice were developmentally normal but had less resistance to lymphomas, particularly from metastases to liver *(15)*. From these studies and the expression of TRAIL on effector lymphocytes, the main role of TRAIL appears to be as a defense mechanism against viral infections and tumor-cell development or progression. It may therefore be a second cytotoxic mechanism that acts in addition to or in place of the perforin granzyme system used by CD8 cytotoxic T-lymphocytes (CTL) and NK cells. It is not clear why TRAIL is more effective than FasL against tumor cells, but one study suggested that the apoptotic pathway induced by TRAIL was able to bypass an inhibitor of tBid that blocked binding to mitochondria in FasL-stimulated cells *(16)*.

RECEPTORS FOR TRAIL

TRAIL differs from other members of the TNF family in having a relatively complex set of receptors. This includes two death receptors, TRAIL-R1 (death receptor [DR]4) and -R2 (DR5), and two decoy receptors (DcRs), TRAIL-R3 (DcR1) and -R4 (DcR2). A third decoy receptor, osteoprotegerin receptor (OPG), was initially described as a receptor for receptor activator of NF-κB (RANKL), and was subsequently shown to bind to TRAIL, albeit with low affinity.

TRAIL-R2 appears to be relatively more important than TRAIL-R1 in induction of apoptosis, and to have higher affinity for TRAIL *(17)*. TRAIL-R2 may also be more stringent in its activation requirements, in that TRAIL-R1 was reported to be activated by soluble forms of TRAIL whereas activation of TRAIL-R2 needed membrane-bound or crosslinked forms of TRAIL *(18)*. Both death receptors are believed to form trimers in the membrane and induce apoptosis by recruitment of the adaptor protein FADD, which binds to the death domains in the receptor. Death effector domains in FADD then interact with similar domains in procaspase 8, leading to downstream events that induce apoptosis *(19,20)*.

TRAIL-R1, -R2, and -R4 can activate the transcription factor NF-κB and c-Jun N-terminal kinase (JNK). This involves recruitment of receptor interacting protein (RIP) and TRAF-2

(TNFR-associated factor 2) *(21)*. However, activation of JNK by signals through TRAIL-R1 may involve the MEKK1-MKK4 pathway *(22)*. Activation of this pathway may have both pro- and antiapoptotic effects, in that activation of MEKK1 may amplify apoptosis by caspase activation in a feedback loop *(23)*. In contrast, TRAIL activation of Erk1/2 may override the TRAIL-induced apoptosis pathway *(24)*.

Regulation of TRAIL Receptor Expression

Information about the regulation of TRAIL-R expression is still incomplete. In some cell types, chemotherapy and irradiation were shown to upregulate TRAIL-R2/DR5 expression by activation of p53 *(25)*, whereas in other cell types p53-independent mechanisms were involved *(26)*. TRAIL-R2 expression in non-small-cell carcinoma of the lung was not related to its p53 status *(27)*. Upregulation of TRAIL-R2 by dexamethasone and interferon-γ (IFN-γ) was independent of p53 *(26)*. TRAIL-R1 (DR4) appeared to be regulated by p53 *(28)*. Similarly, the decoy receptor TRAIL-R3 (DcR1) appeared to be upregulated by p53 *(29)*.

IFN-γ downregulated activation of NF-κB and increased TRAIL-R1 and TRAIL-R2 expression in normal fibroblasts, whereas cytomegalovirus (CMV) infection of fibroblasts down-regulated TRAIL-R1 and -R2 expression *(10)*. Activation of NF-κB or overexpression of c-Rel was associated with upregulation of the decoy receptor TRAIL-R3 (DcR1) in HeLa cells *(30)*, and the c-Rel subunit of NF-κB was reported to upregulate TRAIL-R1 and -R2 *(31)*. Activation of NF-κB by TRAIL was also shown to upregulate TRAIL-R2 (DR5) in epithelial cell lines *(32)*. In contrast, overexpression of cyclooxygenase-2 inhibited TRAIL-R2 (DR5) in colon carcinoma cells *(33)*.

The DNA-binding sites for p53 were found to be located at three sites in the genomic locus of TRAIL-R (DR5), either upstream of the ATG site or within intron 1 or intron 2. The latter appeared to be the main site involved in p53 upregulation of DR5 *(34)*. The promoter region of the DR5 gene was found to have transcription start sites 122 and 137 base pairs upstream of the initiation codon. Two SP1 sites were responsible for the basal transcriptional activity *(35)* and it was speculated that agents binding to the SP1 sites (such as certain histone deacetylase inhibitors) may upregulate TRAIL-R2 expression. The promoter region for TRAIL-R1 (DR4) contained several AP-1 binding sites. The latter is a target for the JNK pathway that can be activated by several chemotherapeutic agents *(36)*.

TRAIL-INDUCED APOPTOSIS OF MELANOMA

Our interest in the potential therapeutic role of TRAIL was stimulated by the discovery that TRAIL, but not TNF-α or FasL, was a key molecule in killing of melanoma by CD4 T-cells, and was able to induce apoptosis in a wide range of melanoma cell lines. Importantly, it was found that melanoma cells resistant to TRAIL were also resistant to killing by CD4 T-cells *(6,37)*. One of the implications of these findings was that understanding the basis for resistance of melanoma cells to TRAIL may provide therapeutic approaches that would sensitize melanoma cells not only to killing by TRAIL, but also to killing by CD4 T-cells stimulated by vaccines or cytokines such as IL-2 or IFN-α and β.

Type 1 IFNs appear particularly important in upregulation of TRAIL expression on human blood lymphocytes *(8)*. TRAIL could also be upregulated on activated T–cells, and this appeared to be due to activation of NF-κB via the T-cell receptor *(38)*. The induced expression of TRAIL was linked to a c-Rel binding site in the proximal TRAIL promoter. Studies on blood lymphocytes from patients with melanoma demonstrated constitutive expression of TRAIL in such patients, and this was markedly increased by exposure to IFN-α2 and to a lesser extent by IFN-γ *(9)*. There was marked variation among patients, and supernatants from some melanoma could completely inhibit TRAIL expression. The factors in the supernatants involved in inhibition of expression are as yet unknown.

Is the Variable Response of Melanoma to TRAIL Due to Variation in TRAIL Receptor Expression?

We explored whether the variable response of melanoma to TRAIL was related to the level of expression of TRAIL death or decoy receptors. Studies on a large number of melanoma cell lines showed that the presence or absence of decoy receptors, including the OPG receptor *(39)*, had little or no relation to the killing of melanoma cells by TRAIL. Subsequent studies also showed that in cells expressing TRAIL-R2, activation of caspase 8 and Bid by TRAIL proceeded normally *(40)*. Studies on the expression of death receptors by polymerase chain reaction (PCR) and specific monoclonal antibodies showed heterogeneity in their expression, with some lines expressing only TRAIL-R1 or -R2. There was, however, an overall correlation of the level of TRAIL-induced apoptosis with death receptor expression, particularly that of TRAIL-R2. Not surprisingly, melanoma cells with no death receptors were not killed by TRAIL. There was a relatively high percentage of melanoma cell lines in the latter category, consistent with TRAIL-mediated selection of TRAIL-R-negative melanoma cells by the immune system. Many other lines had lost either TRAIL-R1 or -R2. In addition, a number of established cell lines had relatively low expression of TRAIL-R1 and -R2, and these lines had correspondingly low sensitivity to TRAIL-induced apoptosis *(39)*.

Of particular concern was the finding that freshly isolated melanoma cells from surgical biopsies and early passage cultures from the biopsies had low or no TRAIL receptor expression and low sensitivity to TRAIL. With increasing duration in culture, the expression of TRAIL-R1 and -R2 receptors increased in the melanoma cells, as did their sensitivity to TRAIL-induced apoptosis *(41)*.

To better understand the resistance of fresh isolates of melanoma cells to TRAIL, we developed a model based on growth of sensitive melanoma lines in the presence of TRAIL. The majority of the cells in such cultures were killed, but over several weeks, TRAIL-resistant cells grew out. These cells had low TRAIL receptor expression and were resistant to TRAIL-induced apoptosis. We considered that such cultures may provide a possible model for melanoma cells isolated from patients that may have had similar exposure to TRAIL in vivo. Growth of the cells in the absence of TRAIL resulted in recovery of TRAIL-R expression and partial recovery of sensitivity to TRAIL. This argued against low TRAIL-R expression owing to selection of melanoma cells with somatic mutations, and was more consistent with phenotypic changes due to activation of signal pathways or processing of TRAIL receptors. The latter was considered possible as interaction of TRAIL with death receptors was shown to result in rapid endocytosis of the receptor. Re-expression of the receptors depended on synthesis and export of new receptors from the Golgi apparatus *(42)*.

Regulation of TRAIL Death Receptor Expression in Melanoma is Largely Due to Posttranscriptional Events

The observation made from studies on the three models referred to above—i.e., varying sensitivity to TRAIL in cell lines with different levels of TRAIL-R expression, low death receptor expression in fresh isolates of melanoma, and low death receptor expression in TRAIL-selected resistant lines—would be consistent with either transcriptional or post-transcriptional control. To answer this question, mRNA levels for TRAIL-R2 were studied by real-time PCR. An example of such studies in TRAIL-selected lines and fresh melanoma isolates is shown in Fig. 1.

mRNA levels were similar irrespective of the level of TRAIL-R2 protein expression. Several trivial explanations did not apply—e.g., the protein receptors were not located in the cytosol, as the receptors could not be identified in permeabilized cells or in Western blots. The surface expression was not masked by other proteins, in that low pH acetate buffers (pH 3.8) or trypsin treatment did not expose the receptors. The results therefore pointed to posttranscriptional control of receptor expression as being a key determinant of TRAIL-R2 (DR5) expression.

There are now many precedents for the control of translation by proteins that bind to the 5' or 3'UTR of mRNA. These proteins may be specific for particular mRNAs or mRNAs in general *(43)*. Binding of the 5'UTR region of mRNA for CDK4 by p53 downregulates this particular protein *(44)*. TNF-α protein expression is regulated by proteins binding to AU-rich elements in the 3'UTR of its mRNA. T-cell intracellular antigen-1 (TIA-1) and TIA-1-related protein (TIAR) act as translational silencers. Tristetrapolin (TTP) binding is dependent on lipopolysaccharide (LPS) stimulation of macrophages, and binding is abrogated by treatment with phosphatases *(45)*. Table 1 summarizes a selection of some known RNA binding proteins (RBP).

We examined melanoma cells for the presence of RBP using riboprobes corresponding to the 3' or 5'UTR of TRAIL-R2 in RNA-gel shift assays. This identified a protein that was present in the TRAIL-selected resistant lines and in early passage TRAIL-resistant fresh isolates, but not in the parental sensitive lines or late passages of fresh isolates (Fig. 2). Proteins binding to the 5'UTR were not identified. Transfection of a firefly luciferase reporter construct containing the 3'UTR of TRAIL-R into parental and TRAIL-selected lines showed that expression relative to a control *Renilla* luciferase vector was suppressed in the TRAIL-selected resistant lines. The nature of the protein binding to the 3'UTR and the RNA sequence bound are under investigation. Actinomycin D chase experiments suggested that binding of the protein to TRAIL-R2 mRNA was associated with more rapid degradation of the mRNA *(45a)*. These results are consistent with inhibition of translation from TRAIL-R2 mRNA due to protein(s) binding to the 3'UTR of the mRNA.

Much more work is needed to study the factors involved in regulation of translation, but the results raise the prospects of therapeutic interventions based on use of immunomodulatory peptides to inhibit binding of proteins to the 3'UTR, as described for regulation of mRNA for TNF-α *(46)*. Another approach is the use of RNA mimics of the 3'UTR region. The signal pathways involved in regulation of RBPs have received relatively little attention. Proinflammatory stimuli, such as LPS and IL-1, induced stabilization of mRNA transcripts containing AU elements by activation of p38 MAP kinase and its substrate, MAP kinase activated protein kinase (MK2) *(47)*. Examples of such regulation are the production of TNF-α and IL-6 in response to LPS *(48)*.

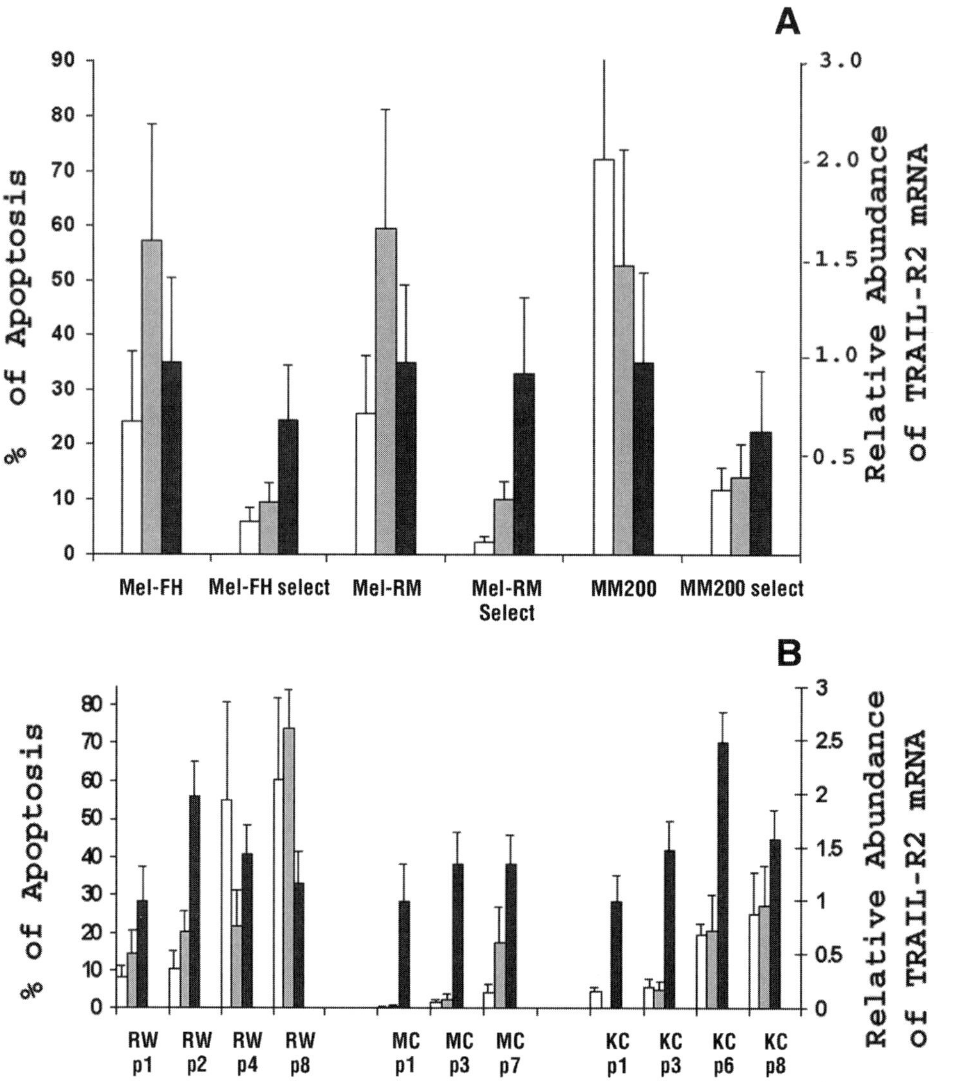

Fig. 1. (**A**) TRAIL-R2 mRNA in melanoma cell lines before and after selection by culture in TRAIL (Mel-FH select, Mel-RM select, M200 select. Assays carried out from 3 to 7 d after culture in the absence of TRAIL). TRAIL-R2 protein expression was at low levels in the selected lines but mRNA levels were little changed. (**B**) TRAIL-R2 mRNA and protein expression in successive passages of three primary isolates (RW, KC, and MC were from lymph node metastases). mRNA was present in early passages even though TRAIL-R2 protein was absent or at low levels of expression.

TRAIL Decoy Receptors

The discovery of two receptors for TRAIL that did not have death domains and the finding that transfection of the receptors into cells reduced sensitivity to TRAIL, gave rise to the concept that they were responsible for protection of normal cells against TRAIL-induced apoptosis *(49,50)*. TRAIL mRNA is also widely distributed in tissues except

Table 1
RNA Binding Proteins (RBP)

Name of RBP	*Tissue Specificity*	*Sequence of UTR*	*Function*	*Refere*
(ELAV family) HuR	Ubiquitous	ARE (AU-rich elements)	Stabilization of mRNA for c-fos, VEGF, p21, TNF-α, C-myc & IL-3	*57–*
Hel-N1, Huc, HuD	Neural tissue	AU-rich sequences	Autoimmunity	*60,6*
Poly A binding protein	Ubiquitous (70kD)	Poly A tail & AU-rich regions	mRNA stability	*59,6*
TTP	Macrophages	3'UTR UUAUUUAUU	LPS Induction of TNF-α	*63*
TIAR/TIA-1	Macrophages Neural tissue Gonads	3'UTR clustered AUUUA Pentamers	Inhibition of translation during stress Proapoptotic, regulator of splicing	*64*
CRD-BP	Breast & Colon Ca	C-Myc RNA	Stabilizes c-Myc	*65*
P53	Various	5'UTR -100 to -64 of CDK4	Inhibits CDK4 synthesis	*44*

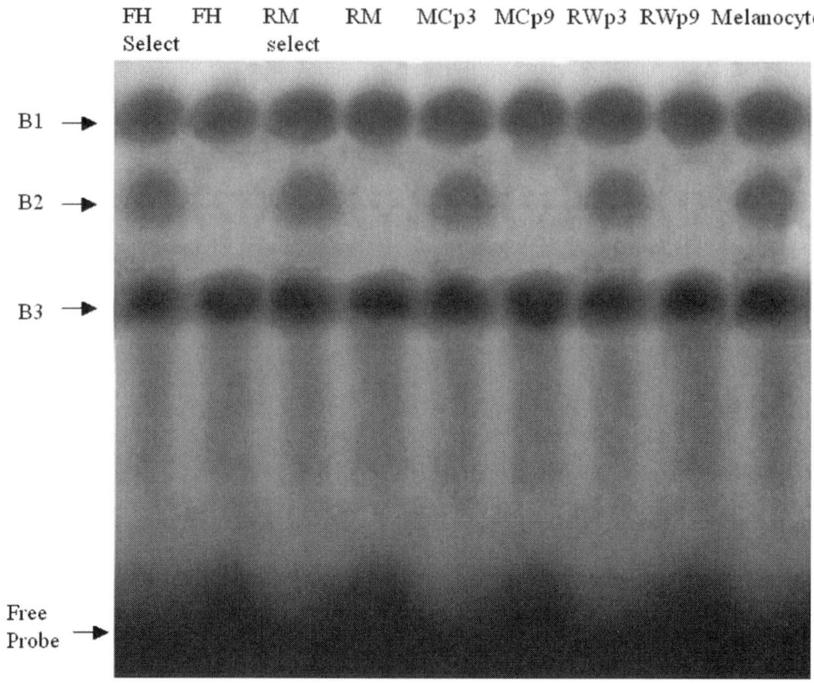

Fig. 2. Identification of proteins binding to the 3'UTR of mRNA for TRAIL-R2. RNA gel retardation assay using 32P labeled 3'UTR of R2 and cytosolic extracts from Mel-FH, Mel-FH select, Mel-RM, Mel-RM select, Mel-MC passage 3 and 9, Mel-RM passage 3 and 9, and cultured melanocytes. Two RNA-protein complexes were formed with one extra band (B2) found in the TRAIL insensitive cells having low TRAIL-R2 protein expression, including Mel-FH select, Mel-RM select, Mel-MC passage 3, Mel-RWp3, and melanoctyes. The upper band was not inhibitable by the unlabeled 3'UTR probe and represents nonspecific binding to cytosolic proteins. This is indicated as (B1) in the figure.

brain, liver, and testes *(1)*. This hypothesis conveniently explained why normal tissues were not damaged by TRAIL despite the widespread expression of mRNA for TRAIL-R1 (DR4) and TRAIL-R2 (DR5) in most tissues.

A corollary of this hypothesis was that tumor cells may be resistant to TRAIL because of their expression of decoy receptors. We tested this hypothesis in a wide panel of melanoma cell lines and found no correlation between decoy receptor expression and sensitivity to TRAIL-induced apoptosis—e.g., some lines with high sensitivity to TRAIL in apoptosis assays had expression of both decoy receptors, and conversely some lines with low sensitivity to TRAIL had no detectable TRAIL decoy receptor expression *(39)*. These studies demonstrated, however, that decoy receptors were located predominantly within the nuclei of the melanoma cells. In contrast, the death receptors were located in both the cell membranes and the cytosol. Results from confocal microscopy confirmed that the decoy receptors were located in the nucleus. After exposure of the cells to TRAIL, the decoy receptors underwent rapid relocation to the cytosol and cell membranes. This relocation was dependent on signals transmitted from the death receptors TRAIL-R1 and -R2, and appeared to involve activation of NF-κB *(42)*. This pattern of receptor distribution was different from that of the death receptors, which were located in the cell membrane and trans Golgi apparatus in resting cells. After exposure to TRAIL, the death receptors were internalized into endosomes, and cell-surface expression was markedly decreased. The latter pattern of distribution is similar to that described for TNF-R1 and Fas *(51)*.

The lack of protection of melanoma cells by decoy receptors against TRAIL-mediated apoptosis indicated that the original hypothesis regarding protection of cells by decoy receptors might be incorrect. When we transfected TRAIL-R4 into melanoma cells, there was good surface expression of the receptor and partial suppression of TRAIL-induced apoptosis. (Transfection of TRAIL-R3 resulted in cell-surface expression but very little suppression of apoptosis.) Moreover, when we examined TRAIL-induced apoptosis of normal cultured endothelial cells, we found, as reported by Sheridan et al. (1997), that expression of TRAIL-R3 was essential to protect endothelial cells from TRAIL-mediated apoptosis. TRAIL-R3 in these cells was located in the cytosol and cell membranes, which may indicate that this localization is needed to inhibit TRAIL-induced apoptosis.

Studies on other cell types indicated that decoy receptors appeared to play little or no role in protection against TRAIL. Melanocytes had very low expression of TRAIL-R2, and caspase-3 was not activated after exposure to TRAIL. This suggested that TRAIL-R2 expression was too low to initiate the apoptotic pathway. In contrast, fibroblasts had normal levels of TRAIL-R2 and caspase-3 was activated after exposure to TRAIL. TRAIL-R3 was located in the nucleus and played no role in protection against TRAIL. We presume the cells were protected by mechanisms downstream of caspase-3, such as XIAP, but this has not been confirmed. Clearly, protection of normal tissues by decoy receptors is not applicable to all tissues, and other mechanisms, such as low TRAIL death receptor expression or inhibitor of apoptosis proteins (IAPs), may be important in other tissues.

The mechanism of inhibition of TRAIL-induced apoptosis by decoy receptors is largely unknown. The idea that they act as decoys or "sinks" for TRAIL seems unlikely, as there would need to be an excess of the decoy compared to death receptors. Inhibition of apoptosis by activation of the transcription factor NF-κB by TRAIL-R4 has also been proposed *(52)*. NF-κB upregulates a number of antiapoptotic proteins, such as IAP-1 and -2, XIAP, and the antiapoptotic Bcl-2 family proteins, Bcl-XL and A1. However, the kinetics of activation of NF-κB and transcription of these proteins would be too slow to account for the relatively rapid induction of apoptosis by TRAIL. After exposure to TRAIL, caspase-8 and Bid were activated by 30 min, and changes in mitochondrial permeability fully evident by 1 h *(40)*. Further study is needed to determine how decoy receptors function.

DISCUSSION

The possibility of using TRAIL as a therapeutic agent has attracted much attention, mainly because of its relative lack of toxicity against most normal tissues. Much work has already been done on the optimal pharmacological form of the drug, and initial reports suggest that the 114–281 amino acid form that has been stabilized with zinc appears optimal *(4,53)*. The half-life in nonhuman primates was, however, only 23–31 min, and most was excreted via the kidneys *(5)*.

In view of this, the use of agonistic antibodies against the death receptors TRAIL-R1 or -R2, which have a much longer half-life, has attracted much attention and was shown to be effective against human colon carcinoma xenografts in NOD/SCID mice *(54)*. A theoretical limitation to the use of agonistic antibodies is the possible induction of apoptosis in normal cells that depend on activation of decoy receptors for their survival against TRAIL—e.g., cultured endothelial cells express both TRAIL-R1 and -R2 death receptors but are protected from TRAIL-induced apoptosis by the decoy receptor TRAIL-R3 *(42,50)*. Activation of the death receptor by antibodies without activation of TRAIL-R3 would be expected to induce death of endothelial cells and toxicity to the host. TRAIL expression may also be stimulated indirectly with cytokines such as IFN-α and β, and IL-2. We have shown that treatment of melanoma patients with long-acting pegylated interferon (PEG-intron) induces TRAIL expression on lymphocytes, but this varied considerably among patients (unreported data). Cytokine-mediated induction of TRAIL may therefore be unreliable due to immunomodulatory effects of the tumor.

The present studies show that the main limitations of treatment with TRAIL may be the level of expression of the death receptors. Some melanoma had lost expression of all TRAIL receptors, presumably due to genetic loss of the region on chromosome 8p 22-21 coding for the receptors *(55)*. In some cell lines, expression of the death receptors was at low levels. More importantly, most fresh isolates of human melanoma cells had low or undetectable TRAIL-R expression, and this was associated with low or no sensitivity to TRAIL-induced apoptosis. However, mRNA for the main death receptor TRAIL-R2 was present at similar levels to that in melanoma cells that had normal levels of TRAIL-R2 protein expression. Similarly, it was shown that mRNA levels were normal in melanoma lines selected for resistance to TRAIL by culture in TRAIL, even though TRAIL-R2 protein expression was at low levels. These studies clearly pointed to translational control as a key factor in regulation of TRAIL death receptor expression. This level of control is well recognized for the production of a number of cytokines, such as TNF-α, but has not previously received attention in respect to TRAIL receptor expression.

Very little is known about the signal pathways involved in regulation of translation. Inflammatory stimuli were reported to activate MAP kinase activated protein kinase (MK2), and the latter stabilized mRNA transcripts containing AU elements in the 3'UTR, as described for TNF-α *(56)*. Ultraviolet radiation had a stabilizing effect on mRNA in general, and this did not involve MK2 activation *(47)*. We have identified a protein binding to the 3'UTR of TRAIL-R2 that appears to be associated with more rapid turnover of mRNA for TRAIL-R2 and inhibition of TRAIL-R2 protein expression. Much work remains, however, to determine the mechanism involved in inhibition of TRAIL-R2 protein expression, the nature of the protein(s) involved, and signals involved in regulation of protein binding to the 3'UTR.

A major question will then be whether therapeutic initiatives designed to upregulate TRAIL-R expression will be specific for tumor cells or also act on normal tissues. Melanocytes have very low levels of TRAIL-R2 protein expression, but “normal” levels of TRAIL-R2 mRNA. Translational control might therefore be a general phenomenon that protects normal tissue from TRAIL-induced apoptosis. If this is the case, then therapeutic prospects based on upregulation of TRAIL death receptors may be limited.

REFERENCES

1. Wiley SR, Schooley K, Smolak PJ, et al. Identification and characterization of a new member of the TNF family that induces apoptosis. Immunity 1995;3:673–682.
2. Pitti RM, Marsters SA, Ruppert S, Donahue CJ, Moore A, Ashkenazi A. Induction of apoptosis by Apo-2 ligand, a new member of the tumor necrosis factor cytokine family. J Biol Chem 1996;271:12,687–12,690.
3. Jo M, Kim T-H, Seol D-W, et al. Apoptosis induced in normal human hepatocytes by tumor necrosis factor-related apoptosis-inducing ligand. Nature Medicine 2000;6:564–567.
4. Ashkenazi A. Targeting death and decoy receptors of the tumour-necrosis factor superfamily. Nat Rev Cancer 2002;2:420–430.
5. Kelley SK, Harris LA, Xie D, et al. Preclinical studies to predict the disposition of Apo2L/tumor necrosis factor-related apoptosis-inducing ligand in humans: characterization of in vivo efficacy, pharmacokinetics, and safety. J Pharmacol Exp Ther 2001;299:31–38.
6. Thomas WD, Hersey P. TNF-related apoptosis-inducing ligand (TRAIL) induces apoptosis in Fas ligand-resistant melanoma cells and mediates CD4 T cell killing of target cells. J Immunol 1998;161:2195–2200.
7. Griffith TS, Wiley SR, Kubin MZ, Sedger LM, Maliszewski CR, Fanger NA. Monocyte-mediated tumoricidal activity via the tumor necrosis factor–related cytokine, TRAIL. J Exp Med 1999;189:1343–1353.
8. Kayagaki N, Yamaguchi N, Nakayama M, Eto H, Okumura K, Yagita H. Type I interferons (IFNs) regulate tumor necrosis factor-related apoptosis-inducing ligand (TRAIL) expression on human T cells: A novel mechanism for the antitumor effects of type I IFNs. J Exp Med 1999;189:1451–1460.
9. Nguyen T, Thomas W, Zhang XD, Gray C, Hersey P. Immunologically-mediated tumour cell apoptosis: the role of TRAIL in T cell and cytokine-mediated responses to melanoma. Forum (Genova) 2000;10:243–252.
10. Sedger LM, Shows DM, Blanton RA, et al. IFN-gamma mediates a novel antiviral activity through dynamic modulation of TRAIL and TRAIL receptor expression. J Immunol 1999;163:920–926.
11. Takeda K, Hayakawa Y, Smyth MJ, et al. Involvement of tumor necrosis factor–related apoptosis-inducing ligand in surveillance of tumor metastasis by liver natural killer cells. Nature Medicine 2001;7:94–100.
12. Smyth MJ, Cretney E, Takeda K, et al. Tumor necrosis factor-related apoptosis-inducing ligand (TRAIL) contributes to interferon gamma-dependent natural killer cell protection from tumor metastasis. J Exp Med 2001;193:661–70.
13. Cretney E, Takeda K, Yagita H, Glaccum M , Peschon JJ, Smyth MJ. Increased susceptibility to tumor initiation and metastasis in TNF-related apoptosis-inducing ligand-deficient mice. J Immunol 2002;168:1356–1361.
14. Takeda K, Smyth MJ, Cretney E, et al. Critical role for tumor necrosis factor-related apoptosis-inducing ligand in immune surveillance against tumor development. J Exp Med 2002;195:161–169.
15. Sedger LM, Glaccum MB, Schuh JCL, et al. Characterization of the in vivo function of TNF-α-related apoptosis-inducing ligand, TRAIL/Apo2L, using TRAIL/Apo2L gene-deficient mice. Eur J Immunol 2002;32:2246–2254.
16. Werner AB, de Vries E, Tait SW, Bontjer I, Borst J. TRAIL receptor and CD95 signal to mitochondria via FADD, caspase-8/10, Bid, and Bax but differentially regulate events downstream from truncated Bid. J Biol Chem 2002;277:40,760–40,767.
17. Truneh A, Sharma S, Silverman C, et al. Temperature-sensitive differential affinity of TRAIL for its receptors. DR5 is the highest affinity receptor. J Biol Chem 2000;275:23,319–23,325.
18. Wajant H, Moosmayer D, Wuest T, et al. Differential activation of TRAIL-R1 and -R2 by soluble and membrane TRAIL allows selective surface antigen-directed activation of TRAIL-R2 by a soluble TRAIL derivative. Oncogene 2001;20:4101–4106.
19. Kischkel FC, Lawrence DA, Chuntharapai A, Schow P, Kim KJ, Ashkenazi A. Apo2L/TRAIL-dependent recruitment of endogenous FADD and caspase-8 to death receptors 4 and 5. Immunity 2000;12:611–620.
20. Sprick MR, Weigand MA, Rieser E, et al. FADD/MORT1 and caspase-8 are recruited to TRAIL receptors 1 and 2 and are essential for apoptosis mediated by TRAIL receptor 2. Immunity 2000;12:599–609.
21. Lin Y, Devin A, Cook A, et al. The death domain kinase RIP is essential for TRAIL (Apo2L)-induced activation of IkappaB kinase and c-Jun N-terminal kinase. Mol Cell Biology 2000;20:6638–6645.

22. Hu WH, Johnson H, Shu HB. Tumor necrosis factor–related apoptosis-inducing ligand receptors signal NF-kappa B and JNK activation and apoptosis through distinct pathways. J Biol Chem 1999;274:30,603–30,610.
23. Bild AH, Mendoza FJ, Gibson EM, et al. MEKK1-induced apoptosis requires TRAIL death receptor activation and is inhibited by AKT/PKB through inhibition of MEKK1 cleavage. Oncogene 2002;21:6649–6656.
24. Tran SEF, Holmstrom TH, Ahonen M, Kahari V-M, Eriksson JE. MAPK/ERK overrides the apoptotic signaling from Fas, TNF, and TRAIL receptors. J Biol Chem 2001;276:16,484–16,490.
25. Sheikh MS, Burns TF, Huang Y, et al. p53-dependent and -independent regulation of the death receptor KILLER/DR5 gene expression in response to genotoxic stress and tumor necrosis factor alpha. Cancer Res 1998;58:1593–1598.
26. Meng RD, el-Deiry WS. p53-independent upregulation of KILLER/DR5 TRAIL receptor expression by glucocorticoids and interferon-gamma. Experimental Cell Research 2001;262:154–169.
27. Wu WG, Soria JC, Wang L, Kemp BL, Mao L. TRAIL-R2 is not correlated with p53 status and is rarely mutated in non-small cell lung cancer. Anticancer Res 2000;20:4525–4529.
28. Guan B, Yue P, Lotan R, Sun SY. Evidence that the human death receptor 4 is regulated by activator protein 1. Oncogene 2002;21:3121–3129.
29. Sheikh MS, Fornace AJ Jr. Death and decoy receptors and p53-mediated apoptosis. Leukemia 2000;14:1509–1513.
30. Bernard D, Quatannens B, Vandenbunder B, Abbadie C. Rel/NF-kappaB transcription factors protect from TRAIL-induced apoptosis by up-regulating the TRAIL decoy receptor DcR1. J Biol Chem 2001;276:27,322–27,328.
31. Ravi R, Bedi GC, Engstrom LW, et al. Regulation of death receptor expression and TRAIL/Apo2L-induced apoptosis by NF-kappaB. Nat Cell Biol 2001;3:409–416.
32. Shetty S, Gladden JB, Henson ES, et al. Tumor necrosis factor–related apoptosis inducing ligand (TRAIL) up-regulates death receptor 5 (DR5) mediated by NFkappaB activation in epithelial derived cell lines. Apoptosis 2002;7:413–420.
33. Tang X, Sun YJ, Half E, Kuo MT, Sinicrope F. Cyclooxygenase-2 overexpression inhibits death receptor 5 expression and confers resistance to tumor necrosis factor-related apoptosis-inducing ligand-induced apoptosis in human colon cancer cells. Cancer Res 2002;62:4903–4908.
34. Takimoto R, El-Deiry WS. Wild-type p53 transactivates the KILLER/DR5 gene through an intronic sequence-specific DNA-binding site. Oncogene 2000;19:1735–1743.
35. Yoshida T, Maeda A, Tani N, Sakai T. Promoter structure and transcription initiation sites of the human death receptor 5/TRAIL-R2 gene. FEBS Lett 2001;507:381–385.
36. Guan B, Yue P, Clayman GL, Sun SY. Evidence that the death receptor DR4 is a DNA damage-inducible, p53-regulated gene. J Cell Physiol 2001;188:98–105.
37. Thomas WD, Hersey P. CD4 T cells kill melanoma cells by mechanisms that are independent of Fas (CD95). Int J Cancer 1998;75:1–7.
38. Baetu TM, Kwon H, Sharma S, Grandvaux N , Hiscott J. Disruption of NF-κB signaling reveals a novel role for NF-κB in the regulation of TNF-related apoptosis-inducing ligand expression. J Immunol 2001;167:3164–3173.
39. Zhang XD, Franco A, Myers K, Gray C, Nguyen T, Hersey P. Relation of TNF-related apoptosis-inducing ligand (TRAIL) receptor and FLICE-inhibitory protein expression to TRAIL-induced apoptosis of melanoma. Cancer Research 1999;59:2747–2753.
40. Zhang XD, Zhang XI, Gray CP, Nguyen T, Hersey P. Tumor necrosis factor-related apoptosis-inducing ligand-induced apoptosis of human melanoma is regulated by Smac/DIABLO release from mitochondria. Cancer Res 2001;61:7339–7348.
41. Nguyen T, Zhang XD, Hersey P. Relative resistance of fresh isolates of melanoma to tumor necrosis factor-related apoptosis-inducing ligand (TRAIL) induced apoptosis [abstr]. Clin Cancer Res 2001;7:966s–973s.
42. Zhang XD, Franco AV, Nguyen T, Gray CP, Hersey P. Differential localization and regulation of death and decoy receptors for TNF-related apoptosis-inducing ligand (TRAIL) in human melanoma cells. J Immunol 2000;164:3961–3970.
43. Cazzola M, Skoda RC. Translational pathophysiology: a novel molecular mechanism of human disease. Blood 2000;95:3280–3288.
44. Miller SJ, Suthiphongchai T, Zambetti GP, Ewen ME. p53 binds selectively to the 5' untranslated region of cdk4, an RNA element necessary and sufficient for transforming growth factor β- and p53-mediated translational inhibition of cdk4. Mol Cell Biol 2000;20:8420–8431.

45. Zhang T, Kruys V, Huez G, Gueydan C. AU-rich element-mediated translational control: complexity and multiple activities of trans-activating factors. Biochem Soc Trans 2001;30:952–958.
45a. Zhang XY, Zhang XD, Borrow JM, Nguyen T, Hersey P. Translational control of tumor necrosis factor-related apoptosis-inducing ligand (TRAIL) death receptor expression in melanoma cells. J Biol Chem 2004;279:10,606–10,614.
46. Iyer S, Kontoyiannis D, Chevrier D, et al. Inhibition of tumor necrosis factor mRNA translation by a rationally designed immunomodulatory peptide. J Biol Chem 2000;275:17,051–17,057.
47. Bollig F, Winzen R, Kracht M, et al. Evidence for general stabilization of mRNAs in response to UV light. Eur J Biochem 2002;269:5830–5839.
48. Neininger A, Kontoyiannis D, Kotlyarov A, et al. MK2 targets AU-rich elements and regulates biosynthesis of tumor necrosis factor and interleukin-6 independently at different post-transcriptional levels. J Biol Chem 2002;277:3065–3068.
49. Gura T. How TRAIL kills cancer cells, but not normal cells. Cancer Research 1997;277:768.
50. Sheridan JP, Marsters SA, Pitti RM, et al. Control of TRAIL-induced apoptosis by a family of signaling and decoy receptors. Science 1997;277:818–821.
51. Jones SJ, Ledgerwood EC, Prins JB, et al. TNF recruits TRADD to the plasma membrane but not the trans-Golgi network, the principal subcellular location of TNF-R1. J Imunol 1999;162:1042–1048.
52. Degli-Esposti MA, Dougall WC, Smolak PJ, Waugh JY, Smith CA, Goodwin RG. The novel receptor TRAIL-R4 induces NF-kappaB and protects against TRAIL-mediated apoptosis, yet retains an incomplete death domain. Immunity 1997;7:813–820.
53. Lawrence D, Shahrokh Z, Marsters S, et al. Differential hepatocyte toxicity of recombinant Apo2L/TRAIL versions. Nat Med 2001;7:383–385.
54. Odoux C, Albers A, Amoscato AA, Lotze MT , Wong MK. TRAIL, FasL and a blocking anti-DR5 antibody augment paclitaxel-induced apoptosis in human non-small-cell lung cancer. Int J Cancer 2002;97:458–465.
55. Walczak H, Degli-Esposti MA, Johnson RS, et al. TRAIL-R2: a novel apoptosis-mediating receptor for TRAIL. The EMBO Journal 1997;16:5386–5397.
56. Kotlyarov A, Gaestel M. Is MK2 (mitogen-activated protein kinase-activated protein kinase 2) the key for understanding post-transcriptional regulation of gene expression? Biochem Soc Trans 2001;30:959–963.
57. Di Marco S, Hel Z, Lachance C, Furneaux H, Radzioch D. Polymorphism in the 3'-untranslated region of TNFalpha mRNA impairs binding of the post-transcriptional regulatory protein HuR to TNFalpha mRNA. Nucleic Acid Res 2001;29:863–871.
58. Sakai K, Kitagawa Y, Hirose G. Binding of neuronal ELAV-like proteins to the uridine-rich sequence in the 3'-untranslated region of tumor necrosis factor-α messenger RNA. FEBS Lett 1999;446:157–162.
59. Fan XC, Steitz JA. Overexpression of HuR, a nuclear-cytoplasmic shuttling protein, increases the in vivo stability of ARE-containing mRNAs. EMBO J 1998;17:3448–3460.
60. Akamatsu W, Okana HJ, Osumi N, et al. Mammalian ELAV-like neuronal RNA-binding proteins HuB and HuC promote neuronal development in both the central and the peripheral nervous system. Proc Natl Acad Sci USA 1999;96:9885–9890.
61. Levine TD, Gao F, King PH, Andrews LG, Keene JD. Hel-N1: an autoimmune RNA-binding protein with specificity for 3' uridylate-rich untranslated regions of growth factor mRNAs. Mol Cell Biol 1993;13:3494–3504.
62. Khaleghpour K, Kahvejian A, De Crescenzo G, et al. Dual interactions of the translational repressor Paip2 with poly (A) binding protein. Mol Cell Biol 2001;21:5200–5213.
63. Gueydan C, Droogmans L, Chalon P, Huez G, Caput D, Kruys V. Identification of TIAR as a protein binding to the translational regulatory AU-rich element of tumor necrosis factor α MRN. J Biol Chem 1999;274:2322–2326.
64. Piecyk M, Wax S, Beck AR, et al. TIA-1 is a translational silencer that selectively regulates the expression of TNF-alpha. EMBO J 2000;19:4154–4163.
65. Ross J, Lemm I, Berberet B. Overexpression of an mRNA-binding protein in human colorectal cancer. Oncogene 2001;20:6544–6550.

11 Regulation of Death Receptors by Synthetic Retinoids

Shi-Yong Sun, PhD

THERAPEUTIC RETINOIDS AND THEIR ACTION MECHANISMS

The term *retinoids* refers to an entire group of natural and synthetic retinol (vitamin A) metabolites and analogs. They exert profound effects on growth, differentiation, and apoptosis of many cell types *(1)*. Thus, they play important roles in regulating, among other things, embryonic development, hematopoiesis, bone formation, glucose and lipid metabolism, and carcinogenesis *(1)*. Currently, retinoids are used clinically in the treatment of skin disorders such as acne and psoriasis, and in the prevention or treatment of certain types of cancer, such as the treatment of acute promyelocytic leukemia (APL) and cutaneous T-cell lymphoma, reversal of premalignant lesions, and inhibition of the development of second primary tumors *(2,3)*.

Nuclear Retinoid Receptors

For several decades, extensive research has been dedicated to elucidating the molecular and cellular mechanism of the retinoids' action. In particular, the discovery and cloning of the retinoid receptors has revolutionized our understanding of how retinoids exert their pleiotropic effects. It is generally thought that the effects of the retinoids are mainly mediated by nuclear retinoid receptors, which are members of the steroid hormone receptor superfamily *(4,5)*. There are two types of retinoid receptor: retinoic acid receptors (RARs), which bind to all-*trans*-retinoic acid (ATRA) and 9-*cis*-retinoic acid (9CRA) with similar affinity, and retinoid X receptors (RXRs), which bind 9CRA. Each type of nuclear retinoid receptor includes three subtypes: α, β, and γ, with distinct amino- and carboxy-terminal domains *(4,5)*. Each subtype is encoded by a specific gene, from which usually multiple isoforms can be generated involving differential splicing and multiple promoters. The receptor subtypes and isoforms are expressed in a developmental and tissue-specific manner, suggesting that each of them has specific tasks in the regulation of developmental and cell-type or tissue-specific biological processes *(4,5)*. Like other members of this family, the retinoid receptors are ligand-activated, DNA-

From: *Cancer Drug Discovery and Development: Death Receptors in Cancer Therapy*
Edited by: W. S. El-Deiry © Humana Press Inc., Totowa, NJ

binding, *trans*-acting, transcription-modulating proteins. RARs can form heterodimers with RXRs. The heterodimers can bind to specific DNA sequence retinoic acid response elements (RARE), characterized by direct repeats of (A/G)GGTCA separated by five nucleotides (DR5) (e.g., RARβ2 gene) or by one or two nucleotides (DR1 or DR2) (e.g., CRABP II and CRBP I genes), with RXR bound in the 5' and RAR in the 3' position *(4,5)*.

The recent discovery of nuclear receptor-associated proteins (coactivators and corepressors) provided details on how DNA-bound unliganded and liganded receptor dimers influence transcription of target genes. In the absence of an RAR ligand (e.g., ATRA), the RXR/RAR heterodimer recruits nuclear receptor corepressor proteins N-CoR or SMRT, Sin3, and histone deacetylase *(4,5)*. This may lead to histone deacetylation and formation of an inactive chromatin structure, preventing transcription. Ligand binding causes the dissociation of corepressor proteins and promotes the association of coactivators (e.g., CBP/p300 and ACTR) with the liganded receptors. This binding results in chromatin decondensation and activation of gene transcription *(4,5)*. It is remarkable that several coactivators and corepressors are shared by multiple signaling pathways. For example, CBP has been implicated in AP-1, p53, and STAT signaling, among others, and Sin3 and HDAC-1 are involved in Mad-Max signaling *(6,7)*. This model of transcriptional activation and repression by nuclear receptors and their cofactors provides a direct link not only among multiple signaling pathways critical in cellular proliferation, differentiation, and apoptosis, but also among these pathways and the chromatin structure of target genes.

In addition to forming heterodimers with RARs, RXRs can form heterodimers with several other nuclear receptors, including thyroid hormone receptors (TRs), vitamin D receptors (VDRs), peroxisomal proliferator-activator receptors (PPARs), farnesoid X receptors (FXRs), and liver X receptors (LXRs). Thus, RXR is a common partner in at least 11 distinct signaling pathways *(6)*. When RXRs form heterodimers with RARs, TRs, or VDRs (i.e., nonpermissive heterodimers), they function mostly as silent partners. However, RXRs can function as ligand-responsive receptors when they form heterodimers with PPARγ, LXR, or FXR (i.e., permissive heterodimers) *(8)*. In this regard, these heterodimers can be activated by either RXR-selective ligands or by the partner's ligand, such as thiazolidinediones (for PPARγ). Therefore, RXR-selective retinoids may have clinical applications for the prevention and treatment of diseases other than cancer, such as diabetes, obesity, and atherosclerosis.

Development of Novel Synthetic Retinoids With Therapeutic Potentials

The pleiotropic biological activities of retinoids also mean that they have a correspondingly large potential for inducing unwanted effects. Indeed, animal studies and clinical practice have revealed receptor-mediated acute and chronic toxicity and adverse effects, including skeletal abnormalities, mucocutaneous toxicity, hypertriglyceridemia, hypothyroidism, and teratogenesis *(3)*. Although retinoids have shown considerable promise in dermatological and oncological indications, these adverse effects have hampered or restricted their use, particularly as preventive agents for chronic administration. Therefore, great efforts have been made for the past decades to design and synthesize novel retinoids with a more favorable therapeutic index and with reduced risk of adverse effects and teratogenesis. In fact, the discovery of six nuclear retinoid receptors that mediate the major biological effects of retinoids may allow us to synthesize receptor-selective retinoids, which will have a narrower range of adverse effects while maintaining specific therapeutic activities. By far, the efforts in this respect have successfully resulted in two receptor-selective retinoids, tazorac/zorac (tazarotene, AGN190168) and Differin (adapalene, CD271), which are topical drugs for the treatment of psoriasis and acne *(3,9)*.

Generally speaking, retinoids inhibit the proliferation of premalignant and malignant cells. Some of them in fact are inducers of apoptosis in a variety of cancer cells. However, most solid tumor cells are resistant to natural retinoids such as ATRA *(10–12)*. Among synthetic retinoids, some are effective in inhibiting the growth or inducing the death of cancer cells, including those resistant to natural retinoids. One such compound is *N*-(4-hydroxyphenyl)retinamide (4HPR), which induces apoptosis in various types of cancer cells and has been tested as a chemopreventive and therapeutic agent in many clinical trials *(13)*. Recently, a novel group of synthetic retinoids with an adamantyl group, such as CD437, CD271, CD2325, and MX335 (Fig. 1), have been identified as more effective than others in inhibiting the growth and inducing apoptosis of most cancer cells *(12,14)*. Among these retinoids, CD271 (adapalene) is the first of this class of synthetic retinoids that is currently being used clinically for the treatment of certain skin disorders *(15)*. Importantly, this compound has recently been demonstrated to be effective in treating cervical intraepithelial neoplasia in clinical trial *(16)*, suggesting a potential for chemoprevention of cervical cancer. These retinoids not only exert an anticancer effect in vitro but also inhibit the growth of several human tumor xenografts in nude mice *(17–19)*.

The Synthetic Retinoids CD437 and Its Analogs As Inducers of Apoptosis in Human Cancer Cells

Currently, CD437 represents the most potent synthetic retinoid that induces apoptosis of human cancer cells. It induces apoptosis in a variety of cancer cells, including lung, head and neck, prostate, breast, ovarian, and cervical cancer cells, leukemia cells, and melanoma cells *(14,18–31)*. More importantly, we recently found that CD437 selectively induced apoptosis in malignant but not in normal human lung epithelial cells *(32)*. Similar results were also observed in malignant and normal human epidermal keratinocytes *(33)*. These results warrant further study on its clinical potential as a cancer therapeutic agent. CD437 and its analogs were originally characterized as RAR-γ or -β/γ selective retinoids *(12)*. However, their effects on induction of apoptosis are independent of RARs, largely because they effectively induce apoptosis in retinoic acid-resistant cells *(24,27)* independently of nucleus *(34)*, and RAR-specific antagonists failed to block their effects on modulation of apoptosis-related genes and induction of apoptosis *(20)*. Thus, CD437 and its analogs represent a novel type of retinoid that induces apoptosis via unique but receptor-independent mechanisms.

CD437 and its analog MX335 induce apoptosis in human cancer cells regardless of p53 status *(14,17,21–25)*. However, in some types of cancer cell, such as lung cancer cells, we found that cell lines with wild-type p53 were more sensitive to CD437-induced apoptosis than those with mutant p53 *(35,36)*. Several p53-regulated genes, such as p21, Bax, Fas, and death receptor 5 (DR5), were induced only in lung cancer cell lines having wild-type p53 *(36,37)*. Moreover, targeting degradation of p53 protein by overexpression of HPV-16 E6 inhibited CD437-induced expression of several p53-regulated genes and apoptosis *(36,37)*. Similar results were obtained when lung cancer cells were treated with other CD437' analogs, including CD2325 and MX335 (our unpublished data). There-

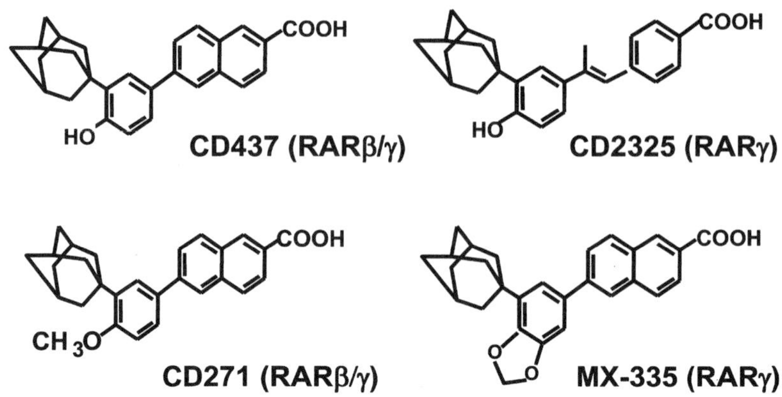

Fig. 1. Chemical structures and receptor selectivity of the synthetic retinoids CD437 and its analogs.

fore, our results indicate that a p53-mediated pathway is involved in apoptosis induced by CD437 and its analogs in certain types of cancer cells containing wild-type p53. Interestingly, some human prostate carcinoma cell lines with mutant p53 were even more sensitive than cells having wild-type p53 to CD437-induced apoptosis, implying that other mechanisms are involved in CD437-induced apoptosis in human prostate carcinoma cells *(21)*. Thus, CD437 can induce p53-dependent and/or -independent apoptosis depending on cell types. Other than p53, CD437 regulates the expression of several other important apoptosis-related genes, including AP-1 (Fos and Jun), Nur77, and c-Myc, which have been demonstrated to be essential for CD437-induced apoptosis *(21,22,24,38)*. Thus, it appears that CD437 induces apoptosis via multiple mechanisms depending on cell types.

P53-DEPENDENT AND -INDEPENDENT REGULATION OF DEATH RECEPTORS

p53-Dependent Regulation of Death Receptors

The p53 tumor suppressor gene plays a crucial role in protecting organisms from developing cancer *(39)*. p53 levels rise in response to different forms of stress, such as DNA damage and hypoxia, causing the cells to undergo either G1 arrest or apoptosis. p53 acts as a transcription factor and induces apoptosis by modulating the expression of downstream target genes *(40,41)*. Among these target genes, Fas was the first death receptor found to be regulated by p53 *(42–44)* and may be an important mediator of p53-mediated apoptosis *(45)*. Fas expression can be directly induced by wild-type p53 through p53-binding sites in the promoter and first intron of the Fas gene *(46)*. Recently, DR5 was demonstrated to be induced by DNA-damaging agents in a p53-dependent fashion *(47)*, and its transcription is directly transactivated by p53 through an intronic sequence-specific p53 DNA-binding site *(48)*. Interestingly, we recently have demonstrated that DR4 is also a DNA damage-inducible, p53-regulated gene, although we have not identified p53-binding sites in its promoter or intron region *(49)*. Our results show that DNA-damaging agents, such as the chemotherapeutic agents doxorubicin and etoposide and irradiation, induced a p53-dependent DR4 expression, which could be suppressed by enhancing the degradation of p53 protein using a HPV-16 E6 transfection strategy. Moreover, introduction of exogenous p53 by adenoviral infection resulted in upregulation of DR4 expression, which paralleled the induction of Fas and DR5 expression *(49)*.

p53-Independent Regulation of Death Receptors

Studies on characterization of the Fas gene revealed consensus sequences for several transcription factors, including AP-1, Sp-1, NF-κB, and NFAT, in its promoter region *(50,51)*. Thus, it is plausible that Fas expression may be regulated by p53-independent mechanisms. Indeed, interferon (IFN)-γ was reported to induce Fas expression independently of p53 in colon cancer cells *(52)*. Several studies have demonstrated that NF-κB transcriptionally regulates Fas expression *(53–55)*, which is involved in IFN-γ or tumor necrosis factor (TNF)-α-mediated upregulation of Fas expression in glial cells *(56)*. Moreover, transcriptional regulation of Fas expression by AP-1 was also reported recently *(57,58)*. There have been only a few studies dealing with p53-independent regulation of DR4 or DR5. Sheikh et al. *(59)* reported that TNF-α, a potent NF-κB activator, induced DR5 expression in a number of cancer cell lines independently of p53. Ravi et al. *(60)* reported that NF-κB induced expression of DR4 and DR5. We cloned and characterized the promoter region of DR4 and found some consensus sequences for Sp-1, AP-1 c-Myc, NF-κB and NFAT *(61)*. Moreover, phorbol 12-myristate 13-acetate (TPA), a potent AP-1 activator, increased AP-1 binding of DR4 promoter and induced DR4 expression in cancer cell lines with mutant p53 *(61)*, indicating a p53-independent regulation of DR4. We have demonstrated that this effect is mediated by an AP-1 site in the 5'-flanking region of DR4 gene *(61)*. Similarly, TPA also upregulated DR5 expression in these cell lines (our unpublished data). In addition, we recently found that overexpression of exogenous c-Myc upregulated expression of endogenous DR4 gene and DR5 in human cancer cells (our unpublished data). Therefore, it appears that the expression of death receptors can be regulated independent of the p53-mediated mechanism, possibly through mechanisms such as activation of AP-1, NF-κB, and/or c-Myc.

REGULATION OF DEATH RECEPTORS BY SYNTHETIC RETINOIDS

p53-Dependent and -Independent Induction of Death Receptors by CD437 and Its Analogs

While we found that CD437 increased p53 protein and upregulated the expression of several p53-regulated genes such as p21 and Bax in human lung cancer cells, the DR5 was cloned *(47,62)* and subsequently identified to be a p53-regulated gene *(47)*. Considering that Fas and DR5 are death-related and p53-regulated genes, we hypothesized that CD437 should be able to induce Fas and DR5 expression, possibly through a p53-mediated mechanism, in human lung cancer cells. Indeed, we found that CD437 strongly induced Fas and DR5 expression, mainly in lung cancer cell lines with wild-type p53, which correlated to its potencies in induction of apoptosis in these cell lines *(35–37)*. Moreover, degradation of p53 protein by transfection of HPV-16 E6 almost completely abolished CD437-induced upregulation of Fas and DR5 expression *(36,37)* as well as CD437-induced apoptosis *(36)*. Therefore, it appears that CD437 induces Fas and DR5 expression via a p53-mediated mechanism, at least in human lung cancer cells.

DR4, like DR5, also binds to TNF-related apoptosis-inducing ligand (TRAIL), leading to induction of apoptosis *(63)*. Therefore, we examined whether CD437 exerted any regulatory effect on DR4 expression in these cell lines. What we expected was that CD437 selectively induces DR5 but not DR4 expression, because DR4 was not reported to be a p53-regulated gene at the time when we started our work. However, we found that CD437 also induced DR4 expression in human lung cancer cells in a p53-dependent fashion, because CD437 significantly induced DR4 expression only in cell lines with wild-type p53, and targeting degradation of p53 protein by overexpression of HPV-16 E6 abolished CD437-induced DR4 expression (Fig. 2). This work led to our finding that DR4 is a DNA damage-inducible, p53-regulated gene *(49)*.

As in the induction of apoptosis, we found that p53 was not important for upregulation of death receptors by CD437 in human prostate and head and neck cancer cells, because CD437 induced the expression of death receptors regardless of p53 status in these cell lines *(14,21)*. Thus, it appears that CD437 induces a p53-dependent and/or -independent death receptor expression, depending on cell types or even different cell lines. Currently, it remains unclear how CD437 upregulates the expression of death receptors through p53-independent mechanism(s).

Because p53 plays a critical role in mediating upregulation of death receptors and induction of apoptosis by CD437 in lung cancer cells *(35,36)*, we wondered whether CD437 also induced the expression of death receptors and apoptosis in normal human lung epithelial cells, which possess wild-type p53. Importantly, we found that CD437 failed to induce the expression of death receptors, including Fas, DR4, and DR5, as well as apoptosis, in both normal human bronchial epithelial (NHBE) cells and small airway epithelial cells (SAEC) *(32)*. The failure of CD437 to induce death receptor expression and apoptosis in normal lung epithelial cells may be related to its inability to increase or stabilize p53 protein in these cells *(32)*.

Transcription-Dependent But Nuclear Retinoid Receptor-Independent Induction of Death Receptors by CD437

It is generally thought that nuclear retinoid receptors mediate the major biological effects of retinoids. To determine whether nuclear retinoid receptors play any role in mediating upregulation of death receptors by CD437, we examined the effect of CD437 on the expression of death receptors in the presence of the pan RAR-specific antagonist AGN193109. We found that AGN193109 failed to block or suppress Fas, DR4, or DR5 induction by CD437, indicating that CD437 induces death receptor expression independent of nuclear retinoid receptors (*47* and our unpublished data). This conclusion is further supported by the result that other receptor-selective retinoids, except for those having similar parent structures to CD437, failed to induce the expression of death receptors (*47* and our unpublished data).

Although transcription-independent induction of apoptosis has been reported *(64)*, we have demonstrated that transcription is required for CD437-induced apoptosis in our system, because the transcription inhibitor actinomycin D (Act D) sufficiently blocked CD437-induced apoptosis *(47)*. To determine whether transcription is required for the upregulation of death receptors by CD437, we examined mRNA stabilities of death receptors in the presence of CD437 and the effects of Act D on CD437-induced death receptor expression. We found that CD437 did not alter the mRNA stabilities of death receptors and

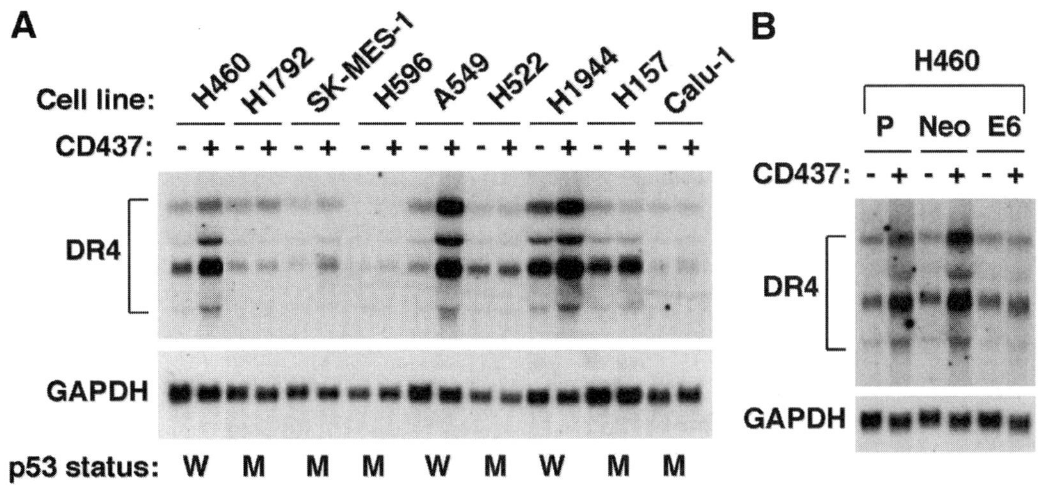

Fig. 2. p53-dependent induction of DR4 expression by CD437 in human lung cancer cells. (**A**) CD437 strongly induced DR4 expression in lung cancer cell lines with wild-type p53. (**B**) Targeting degradation of p53 protein by overexpression of HPV-16 E6 abolished CD437's ability to induce DR4 expression. After a 15-h treatment with 1-μM CD437, cells were harvested for preparation of total RNA for Northern blot analysis. W, wild-type; M, mutant; P, parental; GAPDH, glyceraldehydes-3-phosphate dehydrogenase.

Act D completely abrogated CD437-induced expression of death receptors (*47* and our unpublished data), demonstrating that CD437 upregulates death receptor expression at the transcriptional level.

p53-Independent Induction of Death Receptor Expression by CD437 and Its Analogs

It appears that CD437, as well as its analogs, induces a p53-independent upregulation of death receptor expression in certain types of cancer cells. However, the mechanism underlying p53-independent induction of death receptors by CD437 and its analogs remains unclear. It has been demonstrated that CD437 induces c-Myc expression and activates AP-1 by upregulation of c-Jun and c-Fos, which are essential for CD437-induced apoptosis *(24,38)*. Because of the roles of AP-1 and c-Myc in regulation of death receptor expression (*61* and our unpublished data), it is plausible to speculate that CD437 and its analogs induce p53-independent expression of death receptors through upregulation of c-Myc and activation of AP-1 in some cancer cell lines. More recently, Ponzanelli et al. *(65)* showed that CD437 increased the binding of nuclear extracts from CD437-sensitive NB4 leukemia cells, but not from CD437-resistant NB4 cells, to the NF-κB consensus sequence, indicating that CD437 activates NF-κB. A similar result was also obtained when we used nuclear extracts from CD437-treated prostate cancer cells (our unpublished data). Considering that NF-κB is also a regulator of death receptor expression, we hypothesize that CD437 and its analogs may also induce the expression of death receptors via activation of NF-κB. These possible mechanisms that mediate p53-independent upregulation of death receptors are summarized in Fig. 3.

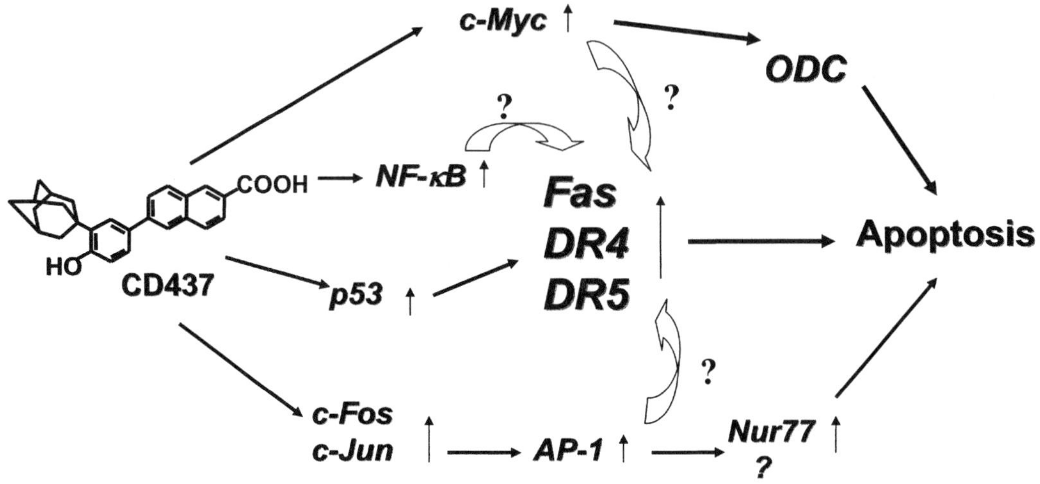

Fig. 3. A schema for proposed mechanisms by which CD437 and its analogs exert p53-dependent and/or -independent effects on induction of death receptors and apoptosis in human cancer cells. The pathways where there are question marks are speculated and need to be investigated. ODC, ornithine decarboxylase.

IMPLICATION OF THE INDUCTION OF DEATH RECEPTORS BY RETINOIDS IN CANCER CHEMOPREVENTION AND THERAPY

Death receptor and death ligand interaction activates a major apoptotic pathway *(66)*. In death ligand-expressing premalignant or malignant cells, binding of death ligands such as Fas ligand (FasL) and TRAIL to the increased number of death receptors due to retinoid treatment triggers the apoptotic signal leading to the killing of these abnormal cells. Furthermore, selective upregulation of death receptors in premalignant or malignant cells may make these cells become susceptible targets for immune cells (e.g., NK and T-cells), which express and secrete death ligands such as TRAIL *(67)*. Therefore, in addition to their direct cytotoxic effects, death receptor-inducing retinoids can sensitize premalignant and malignant cells to death receptor-mediated immune clearance, as well as enhance death receptor/death ligand-based immunotherapy *(67)*.

TRAIL has been considered to be a tumor-selective apoptosis-inducing cytokine and a promising new candidate for cancer therapy *(67–69)*. Many studies have demonstrated that TRAIL-induced apoptosis can be augmented by certain types of anticancer agents in a variety of cancer types both in vitro *(70,80)* and in vivo *(71,72,81)*. The mechanism underlying the augmentation of TRAIL-induced apoptosis by many agents is related to their ability to upregulate the expression of TRAIL receptors (i.e., DR4 and DR5) *(70,72,74)*. Our study has shown that CD437 selectively induced DR4 and DR5 in lung cancer cells but not in normal lung epithelial cells. In contrast, it upregulates DcR1 and DcR2 in normal lung epithelial cells but not in human lung cancer cells *(32)*. Therefore, CD437 and its analogs should be ideal agents for enhancing TRAIL-induced apoptosis in cancer cells while sparing normal cells. Indeed, we found that CD437 augmented TRAIL-induced apoptosis in cancer cells but not in normal cells *(21,82)*.

It has been demonstrated that TRAIL expression can be induced by several types of cancer therapeutic agents, such as retinoid acid *(83)*, IFNs *(84,85)*, and PI3 kinase inhibitors *(86)*. Therefore, it is plausible to propose that a combination of a TRAIL receptor-inducing retinoid such as CD437 with a TRAIL-inducing agent may exert augmented cell-killing via TRAIL/TRAIL receptor-mediated apoptosis. The study in this aspect may develop an effective and mechanism-based combination regimen for chemoprevention and/or chemotherapy.

REFERENCES

1. Gudas LJ, Sporn MB, Roberts AB. Cellular biology and biochemistry of the retinoids. In: Sporn MB, Roberts AB, Goodman DS (eds), The Retinoids, 2nd ed. Raven Press, New York: 1994:443–520.
2. Sun SY, Lotan R. Retinoids and their receptors in cancer development and chemoprevention. Crit Rev Oncol Hematol 2002;41:41–55.
3. Thacher SM, Vasaudevan J, Chandrartna RA. Therapeutic applications for ligands of retinoid receptors. Curr Pharm Des 2000;6:25–58.
4. Chambon P. A decade of molecular biology of retinoic acid receptors. FASEB J 1996;10:940–945.
5. Piedrafita FJ, Pfahl M. Nuclear retinoid receptors and mechanism of action. In: Nau H, Blaner WS (eds), Retinoids: The Biochemical and Molecular Basis of Vitamin A and Retinoid Action. Springer-Verlag, Berlin: 1999:153–184.
6. Blumberg B, Evans RM. Orphan nuclear receptors—new ligands and new possibilities. Genes Dev 1998;12:3149–3155.
7. Freedman LP. Increasing the complexity of coactivation in nuclear receptor signaling. Cell 1999;97:5–8.
8. Schulman IG, Crombie D, Bissonnette RP, et al. RXR-specific agonists and modulators: a new retinoid pharmacology. In: Nau H, Blaner WS (eds), Retinoids: The Biochemical and Molecular Basis of Vitamin A and Retinoid Action. Springer-Verlag, Berlin: 1999:215–235.
9. Shroot, Gibson DFC, Lu XP: Retinoid receptor–selective agonists and their action in skin. In: Nau H, Blaner WS (eds), Retinoids: The Biochemical and Molecular Basis of Vitamin A and Retinoid Action. Springer-Verlag, Berlin: 1999:539–559.
10. Geradts J., Chen JY, Russell EK, Yankaskas JR, Nieves L, Minna JD. Human lung cancer cells exhibit resistance to retinoic acid treatment. Cell Growth Differ 1993;4:799–809.
11. Sun SY, Yue P, Lotan R. Induction of apoptosis by N-(4-hydroxyphenyl)retinamide and its association with reactive oxygen species, nuclear retinoic acid receptors, and apoptosis-related genes in human prostate carcinoma cells. Mol Pharmacol 1999;55:403–410.
12. Sun SY, Yue P, Shroot B., et al. Differential effects of synthetic nuclear retinoid receptor-selective retinoids on the growth of human non-small cell lung carcinoma cells. Cancer Res 1997;57:4931–4939.
13. Ulukaya E, Wood EJ. Fenretinide and its relation to cancer. Cancer Treat Rev 1999;25:229–235.
14. Sun SY, Yue P, Mao L, et al. Identification of receptor-selective retinoids that are potent inhibitors of the growth of human head and neck squamous cell carcinoma cells. Clin Cancer Res 2000;6:1563–1573.
15. Brogden RN, Goa KE. Adapalene. A review of its pharmacological properties and clinical potential in the management of mild to moderate acne. Drugs 1997;53:511–519.
16. DiSilvestro PA, DiSilvestro JM, Lernhardt W, Pfahl M, Mannel RS. Treatment of cervical intraepithelial neoplasia levels 2 and 3 with adapalene, a retinoid-related molecule. J Lower Genital Tract Dis 2001;5:33–37.
17. Lu XP, Fanjul A, Picard N, et al. Novel retinoid-related molecules as apoptosis inducers and effective inhibitors of human lung cancer cells in vivo. Nat Med 1997;3:686–690.
18. Schadendorf D, Kern MA, Artuc M, et al. Treatment of melanoma cells with the synthetic retinoid CD437 induces apoptosis via activation of AP-1 in vitro, and causes growth inhibition in xenografts in vivo. J Cell Biol 1996;135:1889–1898.
19. Langdon SP, Rabiasz GJ, Ritchie AA, et al. Growth-inhibitory effects of the synthetic retinoid CD437 against ovarian carcinoma models in vitro and in vivo. Cancer Chemother Pharmacol 1998;42:429–432.
20. Sun S-Y, Yue P, Shroot B, Hong WK, Lotan R. Induction of apoptosis in human non-small cell lung carcinoma cells by a novel synthetic retinoid CD437. J Cell Physiol 1997;173:279–284.
21. Sun SY, Yue P, Lotan R. Implication of multiple mechanisms in apoptosis induced by the synthetic retinoid CD437 in human prostate carcinoma cells. Oncogene 2000;19:4513–4522.

22. Sun S-Y, Yue P, Chandraratna RAS, Tesfaigzi Y, Hong WK, Lotan R. Dual mechanisms of action of the retinoid CD437: nuclear retinoic acid receptor-mediated suppression of squamous differentiation and receptor-independent induction of apoptosis in UMSCC22B human head and neck squamous cell carcinoma cells. Mol Pharmacol 2000;58:508–514.
23. Adachi H, Preston G, Harvat B, Dawson MI, Jetten A. Inhibition of cell proliferation and induction of apoptosis by the retinoid AHPN in human lung carcinoma cells. Am J Respir Cell Mol 1998;18:823–333.
24. Li Y, Lin B, Agadir A, et al. Molecular determination of AHPN (CD437)-induced growth arrest and apoptosis in human lung cancer cell lines. Mol Cell Biol 1998;18:4719–4731.
25. Shao Z-M, Dawson MI, Li XS, et al. p53 independent G0/G1 arrest and apoptosis induced by a novel retinoid in human breast cancer cells. Oncogene; 1995;11:493–504.
26. Oridate N, Higuchi M, Suzuki S, Shroot B, Hong WK, Lotan R. Rapid induction of apoptosis in human C33A cervical carcinoma cells by the synthetic retinoid 6[3-(1-adamantyl)-4-hydroxyphenyl]-2-naphthalene carboxylic acid (CD437). Int J Cancer 1997;70:484–487.
27. Hsu, CA, Rishi AK, Li X-S, et al. Retinoid induced apoptosis in leukemia cells through a retinoic acid nuclear receptor-independent pathway. Blood 1997;89:4470–4479.
28. Gianni M, de The H. In acute promyelocytic leukemia NB4 cells, the synthetic retinoid CD437 induces contemporaneously apoptosis, a caspase-3-mediated degradation of PML/RARalpha protein and the PML retargeting on PML-nuclear bodies. Leukemia 1999;13:739–749.
29. Mologni L, Ponzanelli I, Bresciani F, et al. The novel synthetic retinoid 6-[3-adamantyl-4-hydroxyphenyl]-2-naphthalene carboxylic acid (CD437) causes apoptosis in acute promyelocytic leukemia cells through rapid activation of caspases. Blood 1999;93:1045–1061.
30. Liang JY, Fontana JA, Rao JN, et al. Synthetic retinoid CD437 induces S-phase arrest and apoptosis in human prostate cancer cells LNCaP and PC-3. Prostate 1999;38:228–236.
31. Zhang Y, Dawson MI, Mohammad R, et al. Induction of apoptosis of human B-CLL and ALL cells by a novel retinoid and its nonretinoidal analog. Blood 2002;100:2917–2925.
32. Sun SY, Yue P, Chen X, Hong WK, Lotan R. The synthetic retinoid CD437 selectively induces apoptosis in human lung cancer cells while sparing normal human lung epithelial cells. Cancer Res 2002;62:2430–2436.
33. Hail N Jr, Lotan R. Synthetic retinoid CD437 promotes rapid apoptosis in malignant human epidermal keratinocytes and G1 arrest in their normal counterparts. J Cell Physiol 2001;186:24–34.
34. Marchetti P, Zamzami N, Joseph B, et al. The novel retinoid 6-[3-(1-adamantyl)-4-hydroxyphenyl]-2-naphtalene carboxylic acid can trigger apoptosis through a mitochondrial pathway independent of the nucleus. Cancer Res 1999;59:6257–6266.
35. Sun S-Y, Yue P, Wu GS, et al. Mechanisms of apoptosis induced by the synthetic retinoid CD437 in human non-small cell lung carcinoma cells. Oncogene 1999;18:2357–2365.
36. Sun S-Y, Yue P, Wu GS, et al. Implication of p53 in growth arrest and apoptosis induced by the synthetic retinoid CD437 in human lung cancer cells. Cancer Res 1999;59:2829–2833.
37. Sun S-Y, Yue P, Hong WK, Lotan R. Induction of Fas expression and augmentation of Fas/FasL-mediated apoptosis by the synthetic retinoid CD437 in human lung cancer cells. Cancer Res 2000;60:6537–6543.
38. Sun S-Y, Yue P, Shroot B, Hong WK, Lotan R. Implication of c-Myc in apoptosis induced by the synthetic retinoid CD437 in human non-small cell lung carcinoma cells. Oncogene 1999;18:3894–3901.
39. Levine AJ. p53, the cellular gatekeeper for growth and division. Cell 1997;88:323–331.
40. Gottlieb TM, Oren M. p53 and apoptosis. Semi Cancer Biol 1998;8:359–368.
41. El-Deiry WS. Regulation of p53 downstream genes. Semi Cancer Biol 1998;8:345–357.
42. Owen-Schaub LB, Zhang W, Cusack JC, et al. Wild-type human p53 and a temperature-sensitive mutant induce Fas/APO-1 expression. Mol Cell Biol 1995;15:3032–3040.
43. Sheard MA, Vojtesek B, Janakova L, Kovarik J, Zaloudik J. Up-regulation of Fas (CD95) in human p53 wild-type cancer cells treated with ionizing radiation. Int J Cancer 1997;73:757–762.
44. Muller M, Strand S, Hug H, et al. Drug-induced apoptosis in hepatoma cells is mediated by the CD95 (APO-1/Fas) receptor/ligand system and involves activation of wild-type p53. J Clin Invest 1997;99:403–413.
45. Bennett M, Macdonald K, Chan SW, Luzio JP, Simari R, Weissberg P. Cell surface trafficking of Fas: a rapid mechanism of p53-mediated apoptosis. Science 1998;282:290–293.
46. Muller M, Wilder S, Bannasch D, et al. p53 activates the CD95 (APO-1/Fas) gene in response to DNA damage by anticancer drugs. J Exp Med 1998;188:2033–4205.
47. Wu GS, Burns TF, McDonald ER 3rd, et al. KILLER/DR5 is a DNA damage-inducible p53-regulated death receptor gene. Nat Genet 1997;17:141–143.

48. Takimoto R, El-Deiry WS. Wild-type p53 transactivates the KILLER/DR5 gene through an intronic sequence-specific DNA-binding site. Oncogene 2000;19(14):1735–1743.
49. Guan B, Yue P, Clayman GL, Sun S-Y. Evidence that death receptor DR4 is a DNA damage-inducible, p53-regulated gene. J Cell Physiol 2001;188:98–105.
50. Cheng J, Liu C, Koopman WJ, Mountz JD. Characterization of human Fas gene. Exon/intron organization and promoter region. J Immunol 1995;154:1239–1245.
51. Behrmann I, Walczak H, Krammer PH. Structure of the human APO-1 gene. Eur J Immunol 1994;24:3057–3062.
52. Ossina NK, Cannas A, Powers VC, et al. Interferon-gamma modulates a p53-independent apoptotic pathway and apoptosis-related gene expression. J Biol Chem 1997;272:16,351–16,357.
53. Chan H, Bartos DP, Owen-Schaub LB. Activation-dependent transcriptional regulation of the human Fas promoter requires NF-kappaB p50-p65 recruitment. Mol Cell Biol 1999;19:2098–2108.
54. Dudley E, Hornung F, Zheng L, Scherer D, Ballard D, Lenardo M. NF-kappaB regulates Fas/APO-1/CD95- and TCR-mediated apoptosis of T lymphocytes. Eur J Immunol 1999;29:878–886.
55. Kuhnel F, Zender L, Paul Y, et al. NFkappaB mediates apoptosis through transcriptional activation of Fas (CD95) in adenoviral hepatitis. J Biol Chem, 2000;275:6421–6427.
56. Lee SJ, Zhou T, Choi C, Wang Z, Benveniste EN. Differential regulation and function of Fas expression on glial cells. J Immunol 2000;164:1277–1285.
57. Li XR, Chong AS, Wu J, et al. Transcriptional regulation of Fas gene expression by GA-binding protein and AP-1 in T cell antigen receptor.CD3 complex-stimulated T cells. J Biol Chem, 1999;274:35,203–35,210.
58. Lasham A, Lindridge E, Rudert1 F, Onrust R, Watson J. Regulation of the human fas promoter by YB-1, Puralpha and AP-1 transcription factors. Gene 2000;252:1–13.
59. Sheikh MS, Burns TF, Huang Y, et al. p53-dependent and -independent regulation of the death receptor KILLER/DR5 gene expression in response to genotoxic stress and tumor necrosis factor alpha. Cancer Res 1998;58:1593–1598.
60. Ravi R, Bedi GC, Engstrom LW, et al. Regulation of death receptor expression and TRAIL/Apo2L-induced apoptosis by NF-κB. Nat Cell Biol 2001;3:409–416.
61. Guan B, Yue P, Lotan R, Sun S-Y. Evidence that the death receptor 4 is regulated by activator protein 1. Oncogene 2002;21:3121–3129.
62. Pan G, Ni J, Wei YF, Yu G, Gentz R, Dixit VM. An antagonist decoy receptor and a death domain-containing receptor for TRAIL. Science 1997;277:815–818.
63. Pan G, O'Rourke K, Chinnaiyan AM, et al. The receptor for the cytotoxic ligand TRAIL. Science 1997;276:111–113.
64. Piedrafita FJ, Pfahl M. Retinoid-induced apoptosis and Sp1 cleavage occur independently of transcription and require caspase activation. Mol Cell Biol 1997;17:6348–6358.
65. Ponzanelli I, Gianni M, Giavazzi R, et al. Isolation and characterization of an acute promyelocytic leukemia cell line selectively resistant to the novel antileukemic and apoptogenic retinoid 6-[3-adamantyl-4-hydroxyphenyl]-2-naphthalene carboxylic acid. Blood 2000;95:2672–2682.
66. Hengartner MO. The biochemistry of apoptosis. Nature 2000;407:770–776.
67. Smyth MJ, Takeda K, Hayakawa Y, Peschon JJ, van den Brink MR, Yagita H. Nature's TRAIL—on a path to cancer immunotherapy. Immunity. 2003;18:1–6.
68. Ashkenazi A, Dixit VM. Apoptosis control by death and decoy receptors. Curr Opin Cell Biol 1999;11: 255–260.
69. Ashkenazi A. Targeting death and decoy receptors of the tumour-necrosis factor superfamily. Nat Rev Cancer 2002;2:420–430.
70. Gibson SB, Oyer R, Spalding AC, Anderson SM, Johnson GL. Increased expression of death receptors 4 and 5 synergizes the apoptosis response to combined treatment with etoposide and TRAIL. Mol Cell Biol 2000;20:205–212.
71. Gliniak B, Le T. Tumor necrosis factor-related apoptosis-inducing ligand's antitumor activity in vivo is enhanced by the chemotherapeutic agent CPT-11. Cancer Res 1999;59:6153–6158.
72. Nagane M, Pan G, Weddle JJ, Dixit VM, Cavenee WK, Huang HJ. Increased death receptor 5 expression by chemotherapeutic agents in human gliomas causes synergistic cytotoxicity with tumor necrosis factor-related apoptosis-inducing ligand in vitro and in vivo. Cancer Res 2000;60:847–853.
73. Mizutani Y, Nakao M, Ogawa O, Yoshida O, Bonavida B, Miki T. Enhanced sensitivity of bladder cancer cells to tumor necrosis factor related apoptosis inducing ligand mediated apoptosis by cisplatin and carboplatin. J Urol 2001;165:263–270.

74. Nimmanapalli, R, Perkins CL, Orlando M, O'Bryan E, Nguyen D, Bhalla KN. Pretreatment with paclitaxel enhances apo-2 ligand/tumor necrosis factor-related apoptosis-inducing ligand-induced apoptosis of prostate cancer cells by inducing death receptors 4 and 5 protein levels. Cancer Res 2001;61:759–763.
75. Nimmanapalli R, Porosnicu M, Nguyen D, 'et al. Cotreatment with STI-571 enhances tumor necrosis factor alpha-related apoptosis-inducing ligand (TRAIL or apo-2L)-induced apoptosis of Bcr-Abl-positive human acute leukemia cells. Clin Cancer Res 2001;7:350–357.
76. Lacour S, Hammann A, Wotawa A, Corcos L, Solary E, Dimanche-Boitrel MT. Anticancer agents sensitize tumor cells to tumor necrosis factor-related apoptosis-inducing ligand-mediated caspase-8 activation and apoptosis. Cancer Res 2001;61:1645–1651.
77. Lee YJ, Lee KH, Kim HR, et al. Sodium nitroprusside enhances TRAIL-induced apoptosis via a mitochondria-dependent pathway in human colorectal carcinoma CX-1 cells. Oncogene 2001;20:1476–1485.
78. Cuello M, Ettenberg SA, Nau MM, Lipkowitz S. Synergistic induction of apoptosis by the combination of trail and chemotherapy in chemoresistant ovarian cancer cells. Gynecol Oncol 2001;81:380–390.
79. Cuello M, Ettenberg SA, Clark AS, et al. Down-regulation of the erbB-2 receptor by trastuzumab (herceptin) enhances tumor necrosis factor-related apoptosis-inducing ligand–mediated apoptosis in breast and ovarian cancer cell lines that overexpress erbB-2. Cancer Res 2001;61:4892–4900.
80. Rohn TA, Wagenknecht B, Roth W, et al. CCNU-dependent potentiation of TRAIL/Apo2L-induced apoptosis in human glioma cells is p53-independent but may involve enhanced cytochrome c release. Oncogene 2001;20:4128–4137.
81. Ashkenazi A, Pai RC, Fong S, et al. Safety and antitumor activity of recombinant soluble Apo2 ligand. J Clin Invest 1999;104:155–162.
82. Sun SY, Yue P, Hong WK, Lotan R. Augmentation of tumor necrosis factor–related apoptosis-inducing ligand (TRAIL)-induced apoptosis by the synthetic retinoid 6-[3-(1-adamantyl)-4-hydroxyphenyl]-2-naphthalene carboxylic acid (CD437) through up-regulation of TRAIL receptors in human lung cancer cells. Cancer Res 2000;60:7149–7155.
83. Altucci L, Rossin A, Raffelsberger W, Reitmair A, Chomienne C, Gronemeyer H. Retinoic acid-induced apoptosis in leukemia cells is mediated by paracrine action of tumor-selective death ligand TRAIL. Nat Med 2001;7:680–686.
84. Wang Q, Ji Y, Wang X, Evers BM. Isolation and molecular characterization of the 5'-upstream region of the human TRAIL gene. Biochem Biophys Res Commun 2000;276:466–471.
85. Gong B, Almasan A. Genomic organization and transcriptional regulation of human Apo2/TRAIL gene. Biochem Biophys Res Commun 2000;278:747–752.
86. Wang Q, Wang X, Hernandez A, Hellmich MR, Gatalica Z, Evers BM. Regulation of TRAIL expression by the phosphatidylinositol 3-kinase/Akt/GSK-3 pathway in human colon cancer cells. J Biol Chem 2002;277:36,602–36,610.

12 Role of p53 in Regulation of Death Receptors

Rishu Takimoto, MD, PhD

INTRODUCTION

p53 functions in the cellular response to DNA damage, thereby preventing accumulation of potentially oncogenic mutations and genomic instability *(1)*. Activation of p53 leads to suppression of cell growth or apoptosis to prevent the propagation of mutated genes *(1,2)*. p53 has also been implicated in differentiation *(3)*, senescence *(4)*, and inhibition of angiogenesis *(5)*. Although we do not yet fully understand how p53 elicits its effects upon cells, it is clear that the transcriptional activation function of p53 is a major component of its biological effects. Activated p53 binds to a specific DNA sequence and activates transcription. The importance of the DNA-binding is underscored by the fact that the vast majority of p53 mutations derived from tumors map within the domain required for sequence-specific DNA binding. p53 normally recognizes a 20-base-pair response element that has an internal symmetry. The consensus DNA sequence for p53 binding is 5'-PuPuPuC(A/T-A/T)GPyPyPy- N(0-13)-PuPuPuC(A/T-A/T)GPyPyPy-3', with the third C and seventh G being highly conserved in the 10-base-pair half-sites *(6)*. Identification of transcriptional targets of p53 has been critical in dissecting pathways by which p53 functions *(1,7)*. A growing number of genes have been found to contain p53-binding sites and/or response elements, and thus to have the potential to mediate the effects of p53 on cells, through upregulation of their expression and function. In this chapter, we review how p53 is activated, and how it emits a signal in response to DNA damage and death receptors induced by p53.

ACTIVATION OF P53

In order to emit the signal of p53, p53 has to be activated, and several activation mechanisms of p53 have been reported. Most of them are posttranslational modification of p53. It has been shown that ubiquitin-mediated proteolysis plays a role in the rapid turnover of p53 protein. But once several stressful conditions have appeared, p53 is stabilized and activated (Fig. 1). DNA damage, e.g., double-strand DNA breaks following ionizing irradiation (IR), thymine dimers produced by ultraviolet irradiation, or chemi-

From: *Cancer Drug Discovery and Development: Death Receptors in Cancer Therapy*
Edited by: W. S. El-Deiry © Humana Press Inc., Totowa, NJ

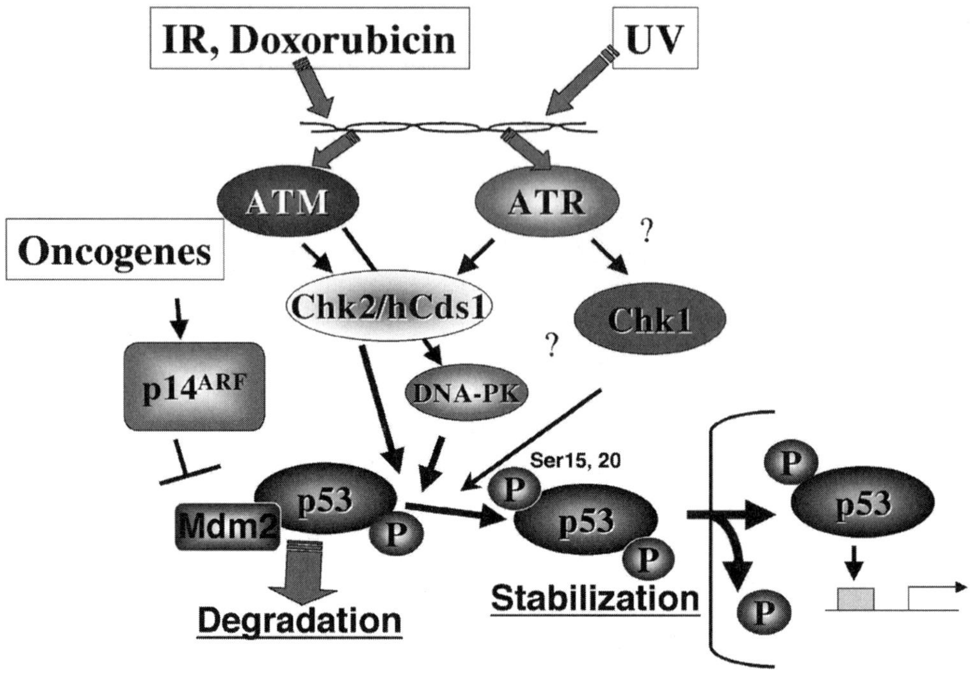

Fig. 1. Model for activation of p53 in response to DNA damage.

cal damage to DNA bases can lead to p53 activation. Hypoxia, heat-shock, radioactive chemicals, DNA transfection, and expression of viral and cellular oncogenes have also been shown to activate p53. Posttranslational modifications of the C-terminus of p53, including phosphorylation, dephosphorylation, acetylation, antibody binding, deletion of the C-terminus, or addition of a C-terminus peptide can induce sequence-specific DNA binding of p53.

Now two protein kinases, ATM (for ataxia telangiectasia mutated) and Chk2, are found to play an important role in p53 activation upon DNA damage such as double-strand breaks induced by IR. Specific phosphorylation, dephosphorylation, and acetylation events have been reported to activate p53 *(1,2,7)*. MDM2 protein, which was originally found to interact with and inhibit p53-dependent transcriptional activity, has recently been found to promote rapid degradation of p53. It has become clear that this MDM2-dependent degradative pathway contributes to the maintenance of low levels of p53 in normal cells *(8,9)*. DNA damage causes phosphorylation of serine residues in the amino terminus of p53. ATM, Chk1, and Chk2 phosphorylate p53 at amino termini that are close to the MDM2 binding site. Upon DNA damage, these kinases phosphorylate the p53 and thereby inhibit its interaction with MDM2, resulting in stabilization of p53. In particular, serine-15 has been found to be phosphorylated in response to DNA damage by IR or ultraviolet (UV) irradiation. *Ataxia telangiectasia* (AT)cells show delayed phosphorylation of serine-15 in response to IR, but show normal phosphorylation after UV irradiation, suggesting that ATM kinase is involved in the serine-15 phosphorylation after IR, although it is not absolutely required *(10)*. However, recent data suggest that serine-20 may be the critical residue regulating p53 stability, whereas serine-15 phosphorylation may be activating transcription by p53 without directly affecting protein stability *(11)*.

ATM also appears to be required for IR-induced dephosphorylation of p53. Serine-376, which allows specific binding of 14-3-3σ proteins to p53 and leads to an increase in the sequence-specific DNA-binding activity of p53 *(12)*. Acetylation of the C-terminus of p53 by CREB-binding protein (p300/CBP) was shown to enhance sequence-specific DNA binding by p53 *(13)*. p300/CBP are closely related histone acetyl transferases (HATs) *(14)* that interact with p53 and function as coactivators for p53-mediated transcription *(13–17)*. The activation of sequence-specific DNA-binding by p53 following DNA damage may involve sequential amino-terminal phosphorylation followed by carboxy-terminal acetylation by the coactivator p300 following DNA damage *(18)*. With the use of phosphorylated or acetylated peptide-specific antibodies, p300 has been shown to acetylate Lys-382 while the p300/CBP-associated factor (PCAF) acetylates Lys-320 of p53, and that either acetylation leads to enhance sequence-specific DNA-binding in vitro. p53 was found to be acetylated at Lys-382 and phosphorylated at Ser-33 and Ser-37 in vivo after exposure of cells to UV light or ionizing radiation. Interestingly, acetylation of p53 by p300 and PCAF was strongly inhibited by phosphopeptides corresponding to the amino terminus of p53 phosphorylated at Ser-37 and/or Ser-33, suggesting that phosphorylation in response to DNA damage may enhance the interaction of p300 and PCAF, thereby driving p53 acetylation. Recent studies also suggest that HDAC1-dependent deacetylation of p53 can reduce its transcriptional activity as well as its growth-suppressive and death-promoting actions *(19)*.

Several viral and cellular oncogenes have been shown to stabilize p53. Viral oncogenes including SV40 T antigen, adenovirus E1A, and human papilloma virus 16 E7 stabilize p53 *(20,21)*. This stabilization does not translate into the activation of p53, but rather a physiologically inactive p53 that is functionally inhibited. On the other hand, adenovirus has other cooperating oncogenes, like E1B and E4, which bind to p53 and inhibit apoptosis and/or growth arrest, thereby leading to successful viral DNA replication and cellular transformation. E1A can also inhibit transcriptional activation by p53 through interaction with CBP/p300, which may inhibit p53-mediated growth arrest and/or apoptosis *(22,23)*. The E6 gene product encoded by HPV16 binds to p53, which results in degradation of p53 and suppression of negative growth signals from p53.

The mechanism of p53 stabilization in response to viral oncogene expression has not been clearly understood until recently, when p19ARF (p14ARF in human), a product of INK4a/ARF locus translated in an alternate reading frame *(24)*, was identified. It was found that the ability of E1A to stabilize p53 is severely compromised in p19ARF-null cells *(25)*. p19ARF is a tumor suppressor, which can induce cell-cycle arrest in a p53-dependent as well as p53-independent manner *(26)*. It has been shown that p14ARF appears to sequester MDM2 into the nucleolus, keeping MDM2 away from p53.

These mechanisms contribute to p53 stabilization and transactivation of its target genes.

DEATH RECEPTORS OF P53 TARGET MOLECULES

Many target molecules of p53 has been identified. Most of them are related to apoptosis, cell-cycle arrest, anti-angiogenesis, and DNA repair (Fig. 2). In this issue, three major death receptors that have been described as p53 target molecules are reviewed.

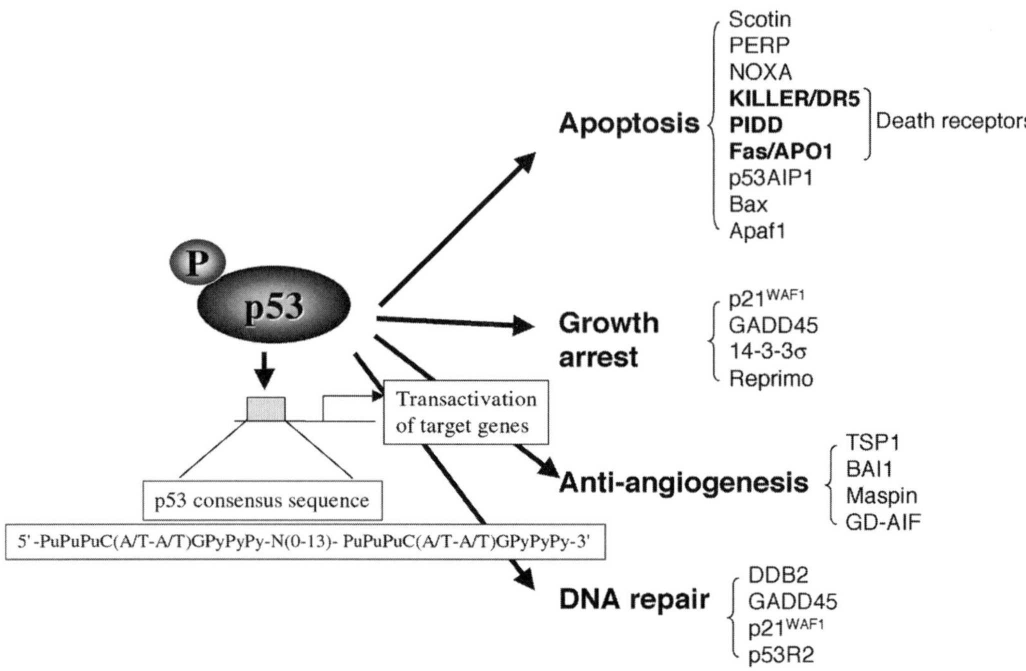

Fig. 2. p53 targets genes

Fas/APO-1

Fas/APO1 is a potent inducer of apoptosis in hematopoietic or liver cells exposed to Fas ligand *(27)*. Upon Fas ligand binding to the Fas receptor, the Fas receptor trimerizes. The death domain of Fas/APO1 recruits the Fas-associated death domain (FADD) adaptor, which recruits initiator caspase-8 to the death-inducing signaling complex (DISC), resulting in the activation of the caspase cascade. Fas/APO1 is not absolutely required for p53 to induce apoptosis, because cells that are deficient for Fas/APO1 are proficient in inducing apoptosis upon p53 activation (*see* Chapter 1). Muller et al. *(28)* have reported that Fas/APO1 was induced by chemotherapeutic agents in a p53-dependent manner. They could sensitize the cancer cells to Fas/APO1-mediated apoptosis after DNA damage. Furthermore, they identified a p53-responsive element within the first intron of the *Fas/APO1* gene, as well as three putative elements within the promoter. The intronic element conferred transcriptional activation by p53 and cooperated with p53-responsive elements in the promoter of the *Fas/APO1* gene. They demonstrated that only wt-p53 protein could bind and transactivate the *Fas/APO1*, but mt-p53 failed to induce apoptosis through Fas/APO1 activation. They concluded that loss of function of p53 contributes to tumor progression and to resistance of cancer cells to the Fas/APO1-mediated cell-killing signal.

p53-Induced Protein With a Death Domain (PIDD)

p53-induced protein with a death domain (*PIDD*) was discovered by differential display methods using Friend-virus-transformed mouse erythroleukemia cells that lack endogenous p53 expression and express a transfected temperature-sensitive (ts) p53 *(29)*.

PIDD was found to be upregulated upon DNA damage in a p53-dependent manner. The size of cDNA of the *PIDD* was estimated to be 4.2 Kb, and its predicted amino acid content appeared to be 915. An N-terminal seven tandem leucin-rich repeats and a death domain in the C-terminal region were found in the PIDD protein. The p53-consensus binding site was found in a *PIDD* promoter lesion. Overexpression of PIDD can suppress cell growth and promote apoptosis in p53-null cell lines K562 and Saos2, indicating that PIDD mediates p53-dependent apoptosis. However, its ligand and how PIDD induces apoptosis in the cell remains unclear.

KILLER/DR5

KILLER/DR5 is a death-domain-containing proapoptotic member of a recently discovered family of tumor necrosis factor-related apoptosis inducing ligand (TRAIL) receptors *(30)* (*see also* Chapter 1). Expression of KILLER/DR5 appears to be increased following exposure of wild-type p53-expressing cells to cytotoxic DNA-damaging agents such as γ-radiation, doxorubicin, or etoposide *(31)*. Indeed, a p53-responsive element was found within intron 1 in the *KILLER/DR5* genomic locus *(32)*. Like the Fas/APO1 receptor, signaling through proapoptotic TRAIL receptors involves downstream caspase activation *(33,34)*.

Enhancement of TRAIL sensitivity by p53 overexpression may increase the cancer cell killing. Kim et al. *(35)* reported that overexpression of p53 by adenovirus could sensitize the cancer cells to TRAIL through induction of KILLER/DR5. This combination cancer therapy may provide a new strategy for cancer cell killing without affecting normal human cells.

REFERENCES

1. Vogelstein B, Lane D, Levine AJ. Surfing the p53 network. Nature 2000;408:307–310.
2. Carr AM. Cell cycle. Piecing together the p53 puzzle. Science 2000;287:1765–1766.
3. Aloni-Grinstein R, Schwartz D, Rotter V. Accumulation of wild-type p53 protein upon gamma-irradiation induces a G2 arrest-dependent immunoglobulin kappa light chain gene expression. EMBO J 1995;14:1392–1401.
4. Atadja P, Wong H, Garkavtsev I, Veillette C, Riabowol K. Increased activity of p53 in senescing fibroblasts. Proc Natl Acad Sci USA 1995;92:8348–8352.
5. Dameron KM, Volpert OV, Tainsky MA, Bouck N. Control of angiogenesis in fibroblasts by p53 regulation of thrombospondin-1. Science 1994;265:1582–1584.
6. El-Deiry WS, Kern SE, Pietenpol JA, Kinzler KW, Vogelstein B. Definition of a consensus binding site for p53. Nat Genet 1992;1:45–49.
7. El-Deiry WS. Regulation of p53 downstream genes. Semin Cancer Biol. 1998;8:3916–3928.
8. Kubbutat MH, Jones SN, Vousden KH. Regulation of p53 stability by Mdm2. Nature 1997;387:299–303.
9. Haupt Y, Maya R, Kazaz A, Oren M. Mdm2 promotes the rapid degradation of p53. Nature 1997;387:296–299.
10. Canman CE, Lim DS, Cimprich KA, et al. Activation of the ATM kinase by ionizing radiation and phosphorylation of p53. Science 1998;281:1677–1679.
11. Hirao A, Kong YY, Matsuoka S, et al. DNA damage–induced activation of p53 by the checkpoint kinase Chk2. Science 2000;287:1824–1827.
12. Waterman MJ, Stavridi ES, Waterman JL, Halazonetis TD. ATM-dependent activation of p53 involves dephosphorylation and association with 14-3-3 proteins. Nat Genet 1998;19:175–178.
13. Gu W, Roeder RG. Activation of p53 sequence-specific DNA binding by acetylation of the p53 C-terminal domain. Cell 1997;90:595–606.
14. Bannister AJ, Kouzarides T. The CBP co-activator is a histone acetyltransferase. Nature 1996;384:641–643.

15. Avantaggiati ML, Ogryzko V, Gardner K, Giordano A, Levine AS, Kelly K. Recruitment of p300/CBP in p53-dependent signal pathways. Cell 1997;89:1175–1184.
16. Lill NL, Grossman SR, Ginsberg D, DeCaprio J, Livingston DM. Binding and modulation of p53 by p300/CBP coactivators. Nature 1997;387:823–827.
17. Wang T, Kobayashi T, Takimoto R, et al. hADA3 is required for p53 activity. EMBO J 2001;20:6404–6413.
18. Sakaguchi K, Herrera JE, Saito S, et al. DNA damage activates p53 through a phosphorylation-acetylation cascade. Genes Dev 1998;12:2831–2841.
19. Luo J, Su F, Chen D, Shiloh A, Gu W. Deacetylation of p53 modulates its effect on cell growth and apoptosis. Nature 2000;408:377–381.
20. Lowe SW, Ruley HE. Stabilization of the p53 tumor suppressor is induced by adenovirus 5 E1A and accompanies apoptosis. Genes Dev 1993;7:535–545.
21. Demers GW, Halbert CL, Galloway DA. Elevated wild-type p53 protein levels in human epithelial cell lines immortalized by the human papillomavirus type 16 E7 gene. Virology 1994;198:169–174.
22. Steegenga WT, van Laar T, Riteco N, et al. Adenovirus E1A proteins inhibit activation of transcription by p53. Mol Cell Biol 1996;16:2101–2109.
23. Somasundaram K, El-Deiry WS. Inhibition of p53-mediated transactivation and cell cycle arrest by E1A through its p300/CBP-interacting region. Oncogene 1997;14:1047–1057.
24. Kamijo T, Zindy F, Roussel MF, et al. Tumor suppression at the mouse INK4a locus mediated by the alternative reading frame product p19ARF. Cell 1997;91:649–659.
25. de Stanchina E, McCurrach ME, Zindy F, et al. E1A signaling to p53 involves the p19(ARF) tumor suppressor. Genes Dev 1998;12:2434–2442.
26. Weber JD, Jeffers JR, Rehg JE, et al. p53-independent functions of the p19(ARF) tumor suppressor. Genes Dev 2000;14:2358–2365.
27. Nagata S. Fas ligand and immune evasion. Nat Med 1996;2:1306–1307.
28. Muller M, Wilder S, Bannasch D, et al. p53 activates the CD95 (APO-1/Fas) gene in response to DNA damage by anticancer drugs. J Exp Med 1998;188:2033–2045.
29. Lin Y, Ma W, Benchimol S. Pidd, a new death-domain-containing protein, is induced by p53 and promotes apoptosis. Nat Genet 2000;26:122–127.
30. Ashkenazi A, Dixit VM. Apoptosis control by death and decoy receptors. Curr Opin Cell Biol 1999;11:255–260.
31. Wu GS, Burns TF, McDonald ER, 3rd, et al. KILLER/DR5 is a DNA damage–inducible p53-regulated death receptor gene. Nat Genet 1997;17:141–143.
32. Takimoto R, El-Deiry WS. Wild-type p53 transactivates the KILLER/DR5 gene through an intronic sequence-specific DNA-binding site. Oncogene 2000;19:1735–1743.
33. Pan G, O'Rourke K, Chinnaiyan AM, et al. The receptor for the cytotoxic ligand TRAIL. Science 1997;276:111–113.
34. Sheridan JP, Marsters SA, Pitti RM, et al. Control of TRAIL-induced apoptosis by a family of signaling and decoy receptors. Science 1997;277:818–821.
35. Kim K, Takimoto R, Dicker DT, Chen Y, Gazitt Y, El-Deiry WS. Enhanced TRAIL sensitivity by p53 overexpression in human cancer but not normal cell lines. Int J Oncol 2001;18:241–247.

13 Proapoptotic Gene Silencing Via Methylation in Human Tumors

Tanya Tekautz, MD, *Tal Teitz,* PhD,
Jill M. Lahti, PhD,
and Vincent J. Kidd, PhD

This review is dedicated with love to the memory and scientific life achievements of Dr. Vincent J. Kidd, a major contributing author to this manuscript, who passed away unexpectedly May 7, 2004. Dr. Kidd was devoted to the field of molecular oncology and a leader in the studies of epigenetic-mediated regulation of death pathways in cancer and the role of CDK1-related kinases. His research contributions include the studies of normal and aberrant apoptotic signaling in human tumors and novel cell division control-related protein kinases in transcriptional and splicing regulation. Vince was an exceptional colleague, mentor, and friend whose infectious enthusiasm for life and belief in science continues to inspire all of us who were privileged to know him.

INTRODUCTION

Apoptosis, or programmed cell death (PCD), is an active process whereby individual cells, responding to internal and/or external stimuli, commit suicide. This process plays a crucial role in the normal life cycle of organisms, facilitating embryonic development, metamorphosis, cellular specialization; maintaining homeostasis *(1,2)*. Apoptosis is characterized by a complex set of tightly controlled biochemical and molecular events leading to cell death, disassembly of various cellular components, and eventual engulfment of the resulting cellular debris *(3,4)*. Inappropriate apoptosis has been associated with a variety of pathological conditions, such as neurodegenerative disorders, autoimmune phenomena, mitochondrial disorders, ischemic damage and cancer *(5,6)*.

A wealth of evidence has accumulated during the last 10 years establishing the concept that tumorigenesis often arises from alterations in the balance between the rate of cellular proliferation and cell death. Increases in cellular proliferation due to dysregulation of the cell cycle as a result of overexpression of oncoproteins (e.g., c-Myc, N-Myc) involved in proliferation and/or the expression of oncogenes involved in cellular transformation

From: *Cancer Drug Discovery and Development: Death Receptors in Cancer Therapy*
Edited by: W. S. El-Deiry © Humana Press Inc., Totowa, NJ

(e.g., Ras) are clearly essential for the growth of tumors *(7)*. More recently, it has become evident that decreasing the rate of cell death by inactivating apoptotic signaling is also an important component of tumor cell growth. The ability to silence specific proapoptotic genes, such as those encoding procaspase-8 (i.e., *CASP8*) and the procaspase-9 modifying protein Apaf-1 (i.e., *Apaf-1*) *(8–10)*, may be of critical importance to this process for several reasons. First, because many, if not all, chemotherapeutic agents function through apoptotic signaling pathways, alterations in the ability to signal cell death will likely affect the outcome of treatment. Second, the classical view of why apoptotic pathways normally exist within a cell is to help facilitate tissue remodeling and the events associated with this process, including wound healing, inflammation, reproductive cycling, and normal organ development *(11)*. For example, there is strong evidence demonstrating that unligated integrins (e.g., β integrin tails) recruit and activate procaspase-8 in a death receptor-independent manner *(12)*, revealing an unexpected role for integrins and caspase-8 in the regulation of tumor cell apoptosis and tissue remodeling. Here we will provide an overview of recent literature detailing the epigenetic alterations in selected proapoptotic pathways within certain tumor cells, as well as the role of apoptosis in the chemotherapeutic and growth responses of those cancer cells.

For the purpose of this review, the second section will cover specific alterations in the expression or function of certain proapoptotic molecules (e.g., caspases 8 and 9, Apaf-1) that occur due to gene silencing in neural crest cell tumors (e.g., neuroblastoma and melanoma). Emphasis will be placed upon studies from our own, and other, laboratories demonstrating that *CASP8* gene expression can be extinguished in neuroblastoma tumor cells due to methylation of important 5' regulatory sequences. In addition, we will detail the spectrum of different tumor types in which the silencing of *CASP8* via methylation has now been observed. Furthermore, the results demonstrating similar types of silencing by methylation of the *Apaf-1* gene in melanoma tumors *(9)*, as well as other proapoptotic and signaling genes in various pediatric tumors *(13)*, will be discussed. The third section will provide an overview regarding current information on the chemotherapeutic response of cancer cells, particularly those in which caspase-8 is no longer expressed, and how caspase-8 is linked to the intrinsic mitochondrial cell-death pathway as part of an "apoptotic amplification loop," as well as how caspase-8 may be linked to integrin-mediated survival of tumor cells. The third section will summarize how the normal function of the cellular apoptotic machinery may be crucial to the mechanism(s) of action of chemotherapeutic drugs to selectively eliminate transformed cells via cell death, as well as explain how unligated integrins might function as proapoptotic biosensors to provide positive feedback to the cell during "productive" interactions (i.e., in a permissive ECM) while inducing apoptosis by triggering caspase recruitment/activation in cells entering an inappropriate microenvironment.

Elucidation of apoptotic pathways and their associated regulatory mechanisms has contributed greatly to our understanding of pharmacologically mediated cell death. Until recently, it was believed that all chemotherapeutic agents functioned in a similar manner to induce apoptosis; that is, they exert their effects by inducing cell death through the intrinsic or mitochondrial pathway. With the identification of specific alterations in proapoptotic molecules within individual tumors and the apparent function of these molecules as tumor suppressors commonly modified by epigenetic events, it is clear that the intrinsic pathway likely constitutes only one avenue within the repertoire of death pathways that may be induced via chemotherapeutic agents.

CASPASES-8 AND APAF-1 ARE FREQUENTLY SILENCED IN TUMORS VIA METHYLATION

Both internal and external stimuli can trigger the apoptotic process. The key mediators of most apoptotic signaling pathways in mammalian cells are enzymes known as caspases. Caspases are cysteine proteases with precise amino acid cleavage specificities that were formerly referred to as the interleukin-1-β-converting (ICE) family of enzymes *(14)*. The caspases are synthesized as zymogens, and referred to as procaspases. Each procaspase consists of a single polypeptide with an amino-terminal prodomain and two subunits, referred to as large and small domains, frequently separated by a linker sequence. The large subunit contains the active site of the cysteine protease. Activation of the procaspase requires proteolytic cleavage to remove the prodomain as well as the linker region (if present) by cleavage at specific aspartic acid residues, as well a similar cleavage between the large and small subunits to form the processed enzyme. The two large and small subunits then assemble as heterotetramers, with two large and two small subunits, resulting in a functionally active caspase.

Presently there are 14 known members of the caspase family in mammals, of which 10 have been demonstrated to participate in apoptosis—caspases 1, 2, 3, 5, 6, 7, 8, 9, 10, 11, 12, 13, and 14 *(14–16)*. These caspases can be further divided into two groups, the initiator and effector caspases, based upon their function(s) in the apoptotic signaling process (Fig. 1). The initiator caspases (i.e., caspases 2, 8, 9, 10, and 12) function at the apical portion of an apoptotic cascade, transmitting an external cell-death stimulus, ultimately activating the effector caspases *(14,16)*. Once activated by the initiator caspase, the effector caspases (i.e., caspases 3, 5, 6, 7, 13, 14, and occasionally 8) exert their effects through the proteolysis of various intracellular substrates. In contrast to the initiator procaspases, the effector procaspases appear to have a much more restricted capacity for auto-activation, and as a result are triggered by either the activated initiator caspases or by a select group of other proteases to exert their effects during apoptosis. Caspase-8 appears to be unique in its ability to act as both an initiator and an effector caspase *(17,18)*.

Two distinct pathways are involved in the initiation and propagation of apoptotic signals in eukaryotic cells. The nature of the inciting stimulus and intrinsic cellular characteristics appear to determine which pathway is activated (Fig. 2). An appreciation of the two pathways involved in apoptosis has important implications for the understanding of the associated pathological conditions and consequent strategies for therapeutic interventions. Presently, caspases 2, 8, 9, and 10 are thought to exist as the most apical caspases in these signaling pathways. Caspase-8 and to a lesser extent caspase-10 are the primary initiator caspases involved in death receptor-mediated, or extrinsic, pathways, and both of these procaspases are activated through the binding of either receptor-specific ligands or immunoglobulins that interact with the extracellular domain of the death receptors (i.e. Fas/CD95, tumor necrosis factor receptor [TNFR]1, death receptor [DR]3, DR4, DR5, and DR6; Fig. 2A) *(14,16,19)*. A conformational change in the cytoplasmic domain of the death receptor occurs through ligand binding to the external domain of the receptor, or by antibody crosslinking of the protein (Fig. 2A) *(16)*. Engagement of the death receptor in this manner allows an adapter molecule, e.g., the Fas-associated death domain (FADD) for Fas/CD95 or the TNFR-associated death domain (TRADD), to this conformationally altered cytoplasmic domain. Procaspase-8 binds to FADD and then undergoes autoproteolysis to remove the prodomain and generate the large and small

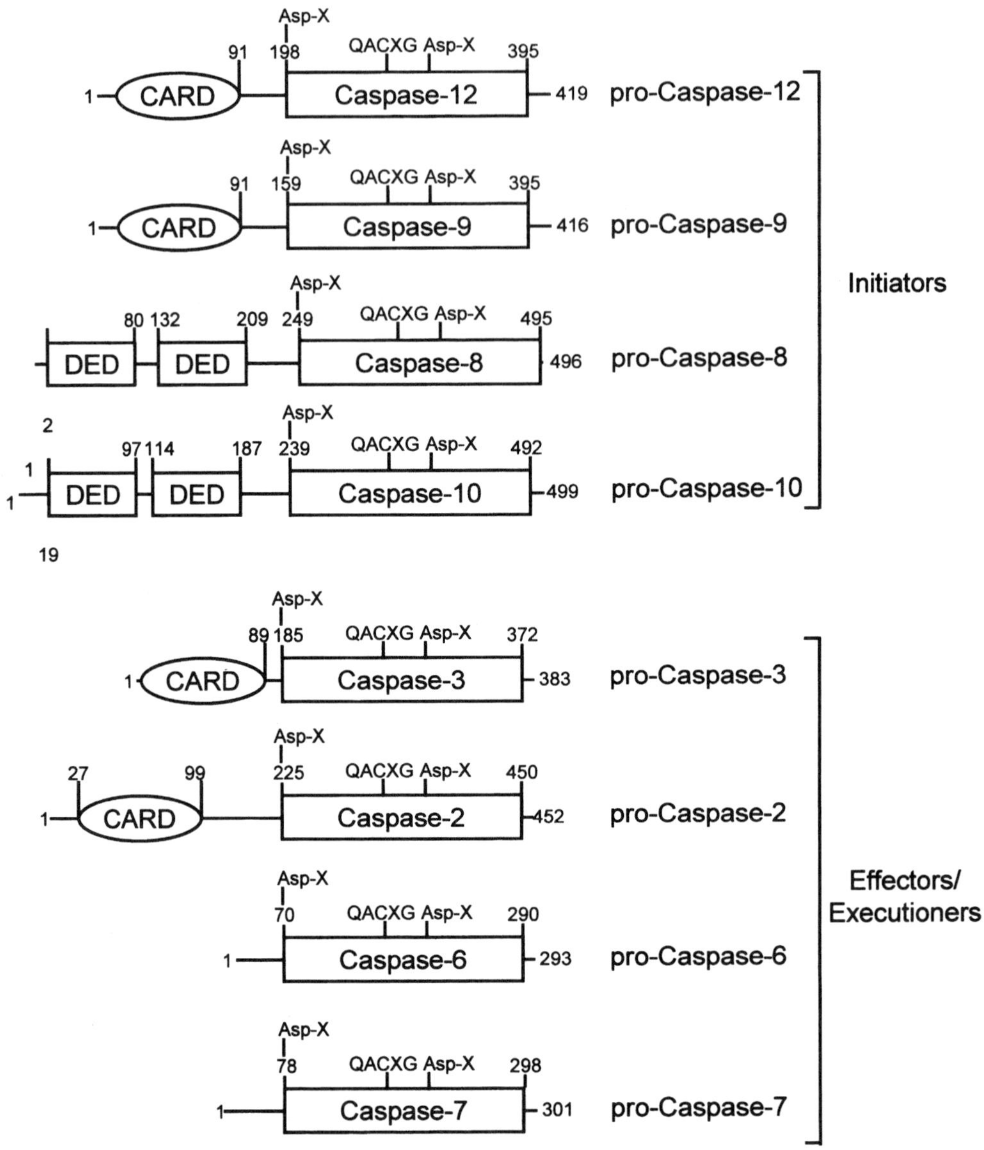

Fig. 1. Schematic representation of the various caspase structures. Both the initiator and executioner caspase structures are shown, with the various prodomains specific for each class (e.g., death effector domain, DED) and the sites of cleavage for processing of procaspases to remove the prodomains, as well as the Asp sites involved in generating the heteromeric large and small catalytic subunits of the active caspases. The active site of the enzyme is shown as the QACXG sequence above the protein, which is located in the larger subunit.

subunits that associate with another similarly modified procaspase-8 molecule to form the heterotetrameric active caspase-8 (Fig. 2A) *(14,16)*. Caspase-8 can then rapidly activate procaspases 6, 7, 13, and 14, in a so-called "caspase cascade," with the subsequent activation of procaspase-3 occurring via the action of caspase-6. It should be noted that there are different ligands and adapter molecules for the various death receptors; however, the ultimate sequence of events is similar irrespective of the death receptor that is stimulated. Cells that primarily employ this pathway in a rapid fashion (i.e., less than several seconds to recruit and activate the procaspase) during apoptosis are typically referred to as type I cells *(20)*.

A second, intrinsic, pathway that is involved in the initiation and propagation of apoptosis involves the mitochondria, cytochrome c release, and recruitment of cytochrome c and the procaspase-9 modifier Apaf-1, to the procaspase-9 molecule (Fig. 2B). These actions then result in the formation of a functional "apoptosome," which can then activate downstream effector caspases, such as caspase-3 *(21–23)*. Alternative stimuli also act upon the mitochondria, effecting a change in the mitochondrial transmembrane potential *(18)*. This results in an efflux of cytochrome c from the mitochondrial intermembrane space into the cytosol. The cytoplasmic cytochrome c binds to the apoptotic protease-activating factor-1 (Apaf-1), resulting in conformational changes in Apaf-1 that facilitate its binding to procaspase-9 and the subsequent autoproteolysis that generates active caspase-9 *(14)*. In addition, caspase-8 has been shown to activate this mitochondrial apoptotic signaling pathway through the cleavage of pro-Bid (Fig. 2B) *(14)*. Active Bid then translocates to the mitochondrial outer membrane and recruits Bax, resulting in a similar release of cytochrome c and activation of procaspase-9. Furthermore, active caspase-3 can trigger procaspase-8, leading to further enhancement of the mitochondrial apoptotic signaling pathway (Fig. 2B). The utilization of multiple apoptotic signaling pathways creates a so-called "apoptotic activation loop," effectively amplifying weaker apoptotic signals. Those cells that utilize intrinsic apoptotic signaling pathways in conjunction with the resulting, much slower, activation of death receptors are commonly referred to as type II cells *(18,20,24)*.

Irrespective of the inciting event involved in triggering apoptosis or the pathway invoked in the propagation of the apoptotic signal, the final events of cellular destruction and disassembly are the same, with the caveat that each pathway has unique proximal positive and negative regulators influencing the apoptotic process. More detailed information regarding the activation of the specific procaspases involved in the initiation of apoptosis (i.e., caspases 2, 8, and 9), as well as the possible alteration of their function during tumorigenesis, is presented in the next three sections.

Caspase-8 Involvement in Tumorigenesis Through Methylation of the CASP8 Gene

Caspase-8 has also been referred to as MACH1, FLICE, and Mch 5, depending upon the group that reported its discovery *(14)*. A simplified convention was adopted by researchers in the cell-death field that referred to these enzymes as caspases, where "c" indicates that the enzyme uses a cysteine protease mechanism, and "aspase" refers to the ability of these enzymes to cleave after aspartic amino acid residues *(25)*. Caspase-8 plays a central role in Fas/CD95-mediated apoptosis, acting as the primary initiator caspase in this signaling pathway. Caspase-8 has been shown to also function as an effector caspase once apoptosis is initiated *(17,18)*. Procaspase-8a is a 55.3-kDa protein of 496 amino acids, consisting of a 210-amino-acid prodomain followed by two homologous death-effector domains (DED) and a linker region, and then the two subunits p18 and p11, which form the functional enzyme (Fig. 1). In a manner somewhat similar to caspase-3, procaspase-8 appears to have a two-step processing scheme in type I cells, initially

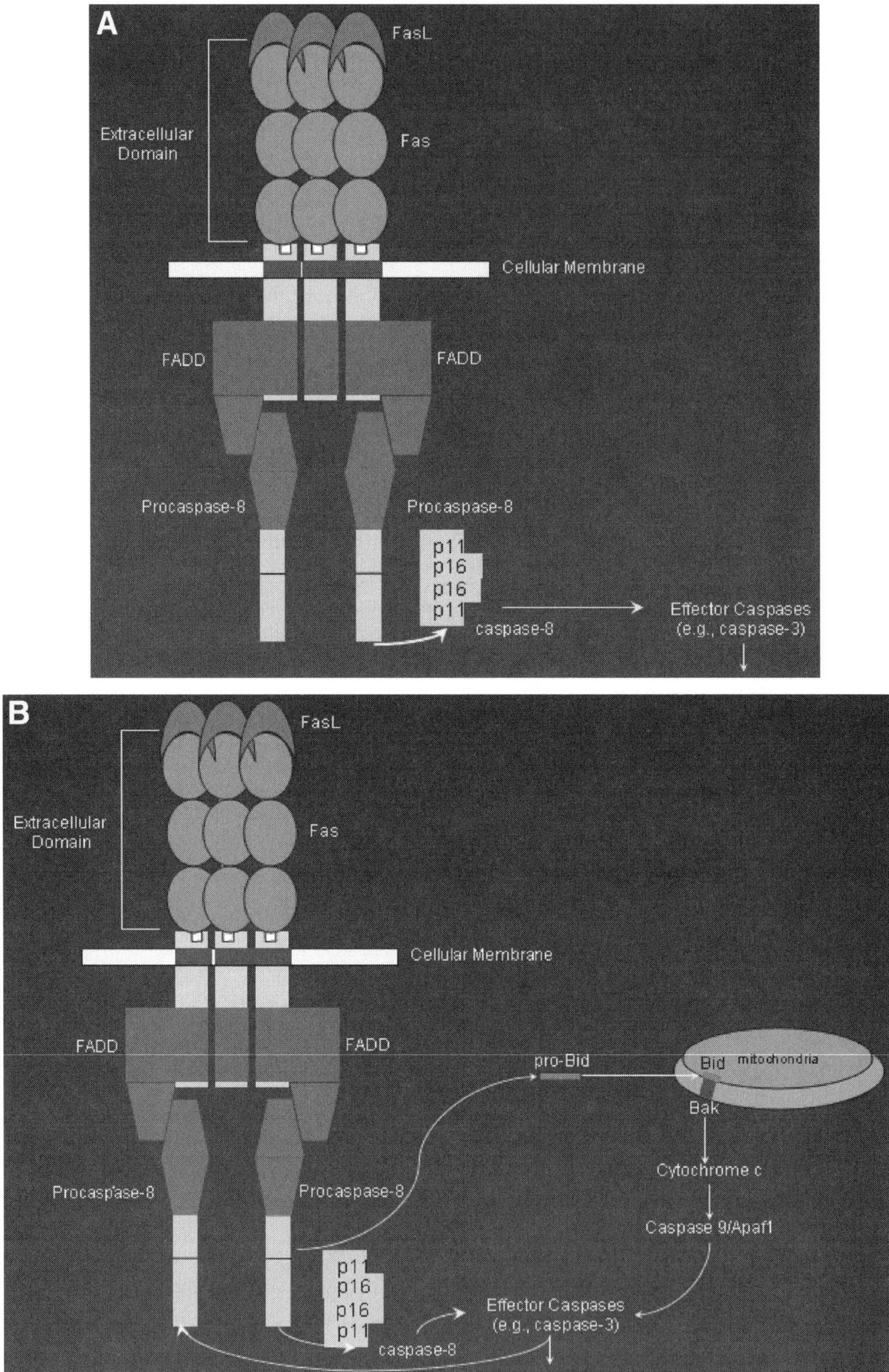
A
FasL
Extracellular
Domain
Fas
Cellular Membrane
FADD
FADD
Procaspase-8
Procaspase-8
p11
p16
p16
p11
caspase-8
Effector Caspases
(e.g., caspase-3)
B
FasL
Extracellular
Domain
Fas
Cellular Membrane
FADD
FADD
pro-Bid
Bid
mitochondria
Bak
Cytochrome c
Caspase 9/Apaf1
Procaspase-8
Procaspase-8
p11
p16
p16
p11
Effector Caspases
(e.g., caspase-3)
caspase-8

resulting in a larger p18 subunit, which is then further modified to create a smaller p16 large subunit (Fig. 2A). In contrast, type II cells appear to process the large subunit of procaspase-8 directly to a p16 large subunit without generating the p18 intermediate (Fig. 2B).

Procaspase-8 is normally activated through the binding of a ligand that is generated in response to stimulatory molecules or events, including cytokines, genotoxic drugs, and γ-irradiation, or a specific immunoglobulin generated to the same external domain of a cell-surface death receptor (i.e., CD95, TNFR1, NGFr, TNF-related apoptosis-inducing ligand [TRAIL], DR3, DR4, DR5, and DR6). In type I cells, using Fas/CD95 as an example, apoptosis is initiated by the trimerization of the Fas/CD95 receptor that is induced by the Fas/CD95 ligand or antagonist antibody by the rapid assembly of the death-inducing signaling complex (DISC) (Fig. 2A). Binding of the Fas/CD95 ligand to Fas/CD95 results in the recruitment of FADD to the intracellular portion of the receptor, the death domain (DD). Association of the death domain and FADD then recruits procaspase-8, which associates with the receptor complex and FADD via similar homologous regions (DDs) of its prodomain; the completely assembled DD/FADD/procaspase-8 complex is referred to as the DISC. Once the DISC is formed, procaspase-8 is autoproteolytically activated, and it is then capable of triggering the activation of other caspases in the apoptotic cascade (Fig. 2A).

In type II cells, the events triggering apoptosis occur at a much slower rate and involve the mitochondrial signaling pathway. The inciting stimulus precipitates the loss of the mitochondrial transmembrane potential, resulting in the release of cytochrome c from the mitochondrial intermembrane space *(20–23)*. In the cytosol, the cytochrome c and dATP binds with Apaf-1, exposing the caspase recruitment domain (CARD) of Apaf-1 so that it can then associate with a similar CARD region present in the sequence of procaspase-9 and result in its activation (Fig. 2B). Caspase-9 then activates procaspases 3 and 7, with caspase-3 triggering the activation of procaspases 2, 6, 7, and 9, and caspase-6 further activating any residual procaspase-8 (Fig. 2B) *(23,24,26–28)*. Caspase-8 is also capable of cleaving the proapoptotic Bcl-2 family member proBid, allowing it to recruit additional proapoptotic members of the Bcl2 family for the purpose

---

Fig. 2. (*opposite page*) Schematics representing the differences between the cellular activities of caspase-8 in the so-called type I and II cells. (A) Caspase-8 activation through the death-inducing signaling complex (DISC) in type I cells, where DISC formation occurs extremely rapidly. The various components of the DISC, including the Fas/CD95 receptor, the internal cellular death domain of the receptor crucial for the recruitment of the death adapter known as Fas-associated death domain (FADD), which was then responsible for the recruitment, and subsequent activation of procaspase-8 via the DED present in both FADD and procaspase-8. The heteromeric structure of the active caspase-8 enzyme, involving two large and two small subunits, each generated from a single procaspase-8 molecule. The subsequent activation of downstream executioner caspases (e.g., caspase-3) and the cleavage of important cellular components by these caspases are also shown. (B) Caspase-8 activation through the DISC in type II cells, where DISC formation occurs more slowly, requiring the recruitment of the mitochondrially-activated procaspase-9 through the cleavage of proBid by active caspase-8, and the subsequent ability of the Bid molecule to recruit and dimerize the proapoptotic Bcl-2 family member Bak. Activation of Bak results in the release of cytochrome c from mitochondria through the resulting pore, and activation of procaspase-9 via Apaf-a and cytochrome c association with the enzyme. The active caspase-9 then activates downstream effector caspases (e.g., caspase-3), as does active caspase-8, resulting in a caspase "amplification loop," which can amplify weaker cell death signals.

of activating the intrinsic pathway (*see* Fig. 2B and the discussion under the subheading "Caspase-8 Involvement in Death Receptor-Independent Apoptosis" below). Finally, an apparently novel mechanism of procaspase-8 activation that is death receptor-independent exists in certain cells and in response to specific types of death signals *(18,20,24)*.

Caspase-8$^{-/-}$ mice demonstrate apparently normal development until embryonic d 11.5, when they begin to die *(29)*. Examination of the embryos reveals poorly developed heart muscle and extensive erythrocyte accumulation in liver, lung, lens of the eye, and mesenchymal spaces; in addition, the embryos appear to have decreased numbers of myeloid progenitor cells. Cultured embryonic fibroblasts from caspase-8$^{-/-}$ mice appear to be resistant to Fas/CD95, TNFR1, and DR3 receptor-mediated cytotoxic events, but they retain their sensitivity to serum withdrawal, ultraviolet (UV) irradiation, ceramide, staurosporine, and the chemotherapeutic drug etoposide *(29)*. Recently, others have reported that when they have generated caspase-8$^{-/-}$ mice of their own, not only did they observe similar embryonic lethality at d 11.5 from cardiac rupture due to apoptosis of cardiomyocytes in the embryos, but they also observed a reproducible defect in the neural tube *(30)*. These investigators reported that narrowing of the ventricular zone as well as expression of neurogenic cell markers in that region (e.g., Pax6, Mash1, and neurogenin-2) were diminished in the mutant embryos. Of possible importance as well, they were also unable to detect massive numbers of apoptotic cells in the neural tube of the mutant embryos. All of these findings regarding the abnormal development of the neural tube in the *caspase-8*$^{-/-}$ mutant embryos at d 11.5 of development may be significant with regard to the somewhat specific involvement of *CASP8* gene silencing in neuroblastoma tumors, as well as other tumors that are of neural crest cell origin. This will be a topic of obvious importance in future studies.

Caspase-8 plays a pivotal role in apoptotic regulation, with defects in caspase-8 function being implicated in the development of tumors and/or the resistance of tumors to chemotherapeutic agents *(8,31–39)*. The tumor types in which the *CASP8* gene has been found to be silenced, and the percentage of these tumors affected, include primarily pediatric tumors that are derived from the neural crest, including neuroblastomas (52%), retinoblastomas (59%), medulloblastomas (81%), and alveolar rhabdmyosarcomas (83%) *(8,10)*. Methylation as an important epigenetic modification in pediatric tumors was first revealed in studies of neuroblastoma tumors that were resistant to chemotherapy *(8)*. Stage 4 neuroblastoma (NB) tumors with amplified *MYCN* frequently contain two or more *CASP8* alleles that are methylated, resulting in the complete loss of normal caspase-8 function (Fig. 3) *(8)*. An apparently important regulatory sequence corresponding to a portion of the 5'' untranslated region of the human *CASP8* gene contained in exon 3 and extending into intron 3 was the target of methylation examined in the gene. The procedure for methylation-specific PCR that was used to examine the *CASP8* gene in neuroblastoma, as well as the results of the analysis of several NB cell lines, is shown in Fig. 3.

Methylation-mediated silencing of caspase-8 was first noted when neuroblastoma cells lines were examined for expression of caspase-8; we found that they frequently did not express any caspase-8 mRNA or protein (i.e., >90% of the examined cell lines), often contained amplified *MYCN* sequences (i.e., >70%), and overexpress N-Myc mRNA and protein *(8)*. The loss of caspase-8 expression in NB cell lines was due to either the deletion of one or both of the *CASP8* gene alleles, or more commonly the methylation of one or both alleles (Fig. 4A). Similar data were also obtained in two different studies of neuro-

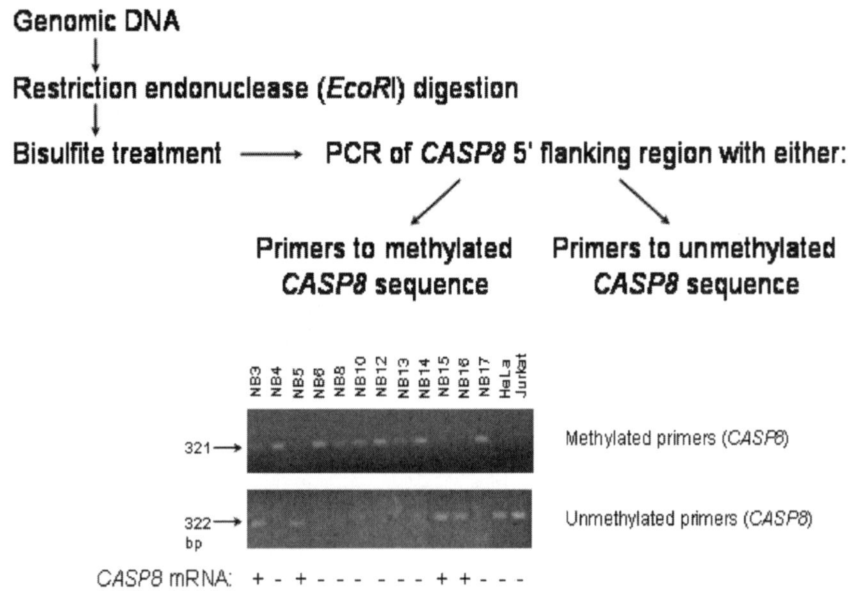

Fig. 3. Schematic representation of methylation-specific PCR analysis used to analyze the expression of *CASP8* in tumors of neural crest origin. The basic procedures involved in isolating and treating the genomic DNA from tumors, according to the procedure developed by Herman et al. *(101)*, so that both methylated and unmethylated regions corresponding to the exon 3-intron 3 region of the *CASP8* gene is shown as performed according to the procedure reported in the manuscript by Teitz et al. *(8)*. Examples of methylation-specific PCR analysis of completely methylated (i.e., the neuroblastoma cell lines NB4, NB6, NB8, NB10, NB12, NB13, NB14, and NB17), completely unmethylated (i.e., the neuroblastoma cell lines NB5, NB15, NB16, and HeLa and Jurkat cell lines), and finally partially methylated (i.e., the neuroblastoma cell line NB3) are also shown, and the production of caspase-8 mRNA as detected by RT-PCR is shown below the ethidium bromide-stained agarose gels (i.e., with a '+' indicating the presence of caspase-8 mRNA and a '–' indicating its absence).

blastoma patient tumors from North America and Japan, where 40–50% of the stage 4 patient tumor samples did not express caspase-8 due to the methylation of the corresponding *CASP8* genes and approx 66% of these methylated samples also contained amplified *MYCN (40)*. In contrast, very few (i.e., <4%) of the NB patient samples that expressed caspase-8 contained amplified *MYCN* genes. In addition, early-stage NB disease (i.e., stages 1–3) contained only partially methylated *CASP8* alleles, with the only example of complete *CASP8* methylation corresponding to a stage 3 NB tumor with amplified *MYCN* (Fig. 4B). In the Japanese study, possible genetic linkage to a region of human chromosome 2 band q33 was examined, since previous studies from this group had shown a high degree of complete loss of heterozygosity (LOH) in this area *(41)*, and the human *CASP8* gene had also been mapped to 2q33 *(42)*. Although no genetic linkage was obtained with regard to the 2q33 LOH that had been previously reported, this study did corroborate our previously published results *(8,40)*, with a large amount of epigenetic modification of the *CASP8* gene via methylation in the stage 4, and stage 4 with amplified *MYCN*, NB patient tumors.

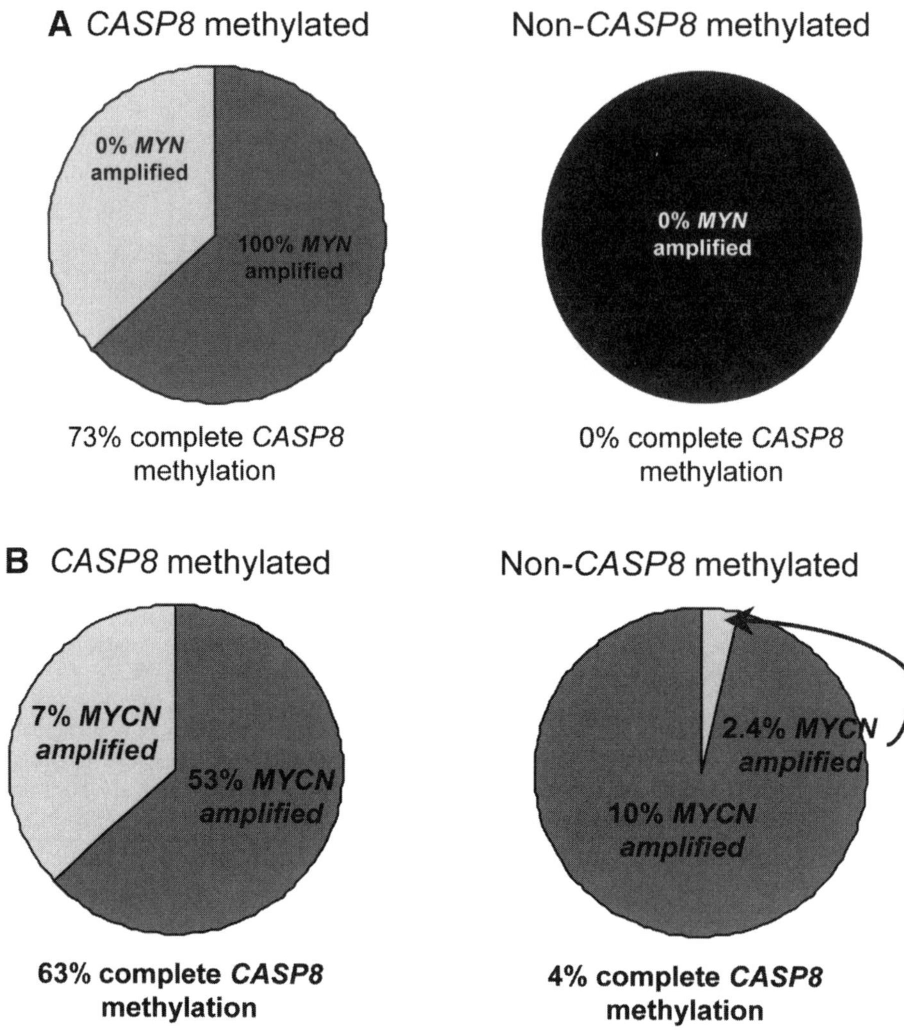

Fig. 4. Pie charts indicating the relative distribution of completely methylated *CASP8* alleles associated with amplified *MYCN* in both (A) neuroblastoma cell lines and (B) neuroblastoma patient samples. Data for these pie charts were derived from the original studies of neuroblastoma cell lines and patient samples reported in Teitz et al. *(8)*.

Myc dysregulation and associated silencing of *CASP8* expression has also been observed in small-cell lung carcinoma (SCLC), an adult tumor of neural crest cell origin (*[10,13]*; [Tekautz, Grenet, Teitz, Lahti, and Kidd, unpublished observation]). In these studies, caspase-8 expression was undetectable in approx 80% of the SCLC cell lines examined *(10)*. The loss of enzyme expression was found to be due to specific methylation of both alleles of the *CASP8* gene. Furthermore, much like what was observed in the NB tumor cell lines and patient samples, amplification of the *MYC* gene was observed in 100% of the SCLC cell lines that had silenced *CASP8* via methylation, and in 33% of the SCLC tumor cell lines that had not silenced *CASP8* (*[10]*; and unpublished observa-

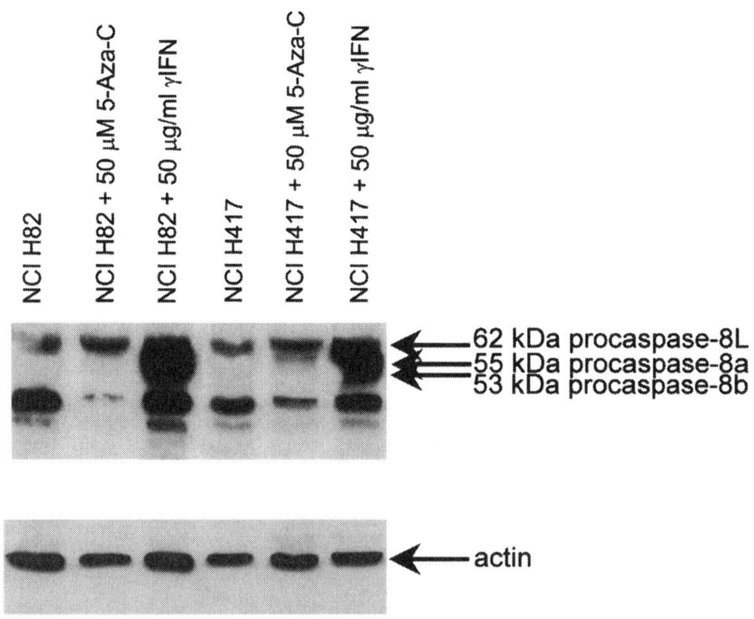

Fig. 5. Levels of the various procaspase-8 isoforms in small-cell lung carcinoma (SCLC) cell lines treated with either 5-Aza-deoxycytidine (5-Aza-C) or interferon (IFN)-γ. The SCLC cell lines NCI H82 and NCI H417 were treated as indicated above each lane. The top panel shows proteins from the cells immunoblotted with the human caspase-8 monoclonal antibody C15 and detection of increasing amounts of the largest caspase-8 isoform after treatment with IFN-γ. The lower panel represents the same proteins immunoblotted by a γ-actin antibody control.

tions). When caspase-8 enzyme function was restored in NB cell lines, either by treatment with either 5-azacytidine (i.e., a demethylating agent) or γ-interferon (Fig. 5), transduction of the NB tumor cells with caspase-8 retroviral expression vectors *(8,43)*, or microinjection of caspase-8 expression constructs in NB cells *(8)*, the resulting cells were re-sensitized to chemotherapeutic agents and underwent significantly greater cell death when exposed to these drugs. Taken together, these data strongly suggest that caspase-8 functions as a tumor suppressor in neuroblastoma. Thus, the data from the analyses of both human neuroblastoma and SCLC tumors suggest a potential correlation between the methylation of the *CASP8* gene and the ability of these tumor cells to tolerate the amplification of Myc mRNA and protein levels. Studies by others have shown that the overexpression of Myc creates cells that are extremely sensitized to apoptotic signals *(44–48)*. Thus, the inactivation of caspase-8 may prevent apoptosis in these tumor cells due to the administration of chemotherapeutic agents, and/or it may also play an important role in tumorigenesis by providing the tumor cells with a growth advantage in a particular microenvironment, possibly by allowing these cells to escape immune surveillance. The observation that *CASP8* gene expression can be reactivated by treatment of NB cell lines with de-methylating agents or γ-interferon suggests that these drugs may be clinically relevant to the treatment of neuroblastoma, particularly if used in conjunction with other conventional chemotherapeutic agents (see the subheading "Cancer Therapy").

Caspase-8 has also been suggested as a possible target for gene therapy *(8,43,48a)*. Initial trials in mice using the tert promoter (i.e., the human telomerase catalytic subunit promoter expressed in 90% of all tumor cells) are somewhat promising, with this promoter enhancing caspase-8 expression in tumor cells. Further, when these tumor cells are reintroduced into nude mice, they demonstrate a marked reduction in proliferative capacity.

The Involvement of Caspase-9 in Tumorigenesis

Caspase-9 is synonymous with ICE-LAP6 and Mch 6. Caspase-9 functions as an initiator caspase in the mitochondrial apoptotic signaling pathway (Fig. 2B). Procaspase-9 is a 416-amino-acid, 46-kDa protein with a 130-amino-acid N-terminal domain, a p17 large and a p10 small subunit (Fig. 1). Caspase-9 is the apical caspase in the intrinsic mitochondrial apoptotic pathway. Procaspase-9 is converted to caspase-9 through the actions of the Apaf-1/cytochrome c complex *(49–53)*, although it has been reported that procaspase-9 activation can take place in the absence of both cytochrome c and Apaf-1 *(54)*. Just how these data reflect possible cell-type specificity is unknown at this time. Once in its active form, caspase-9 is capable of activating the downstream caspases 3, 6, and 7, thereby propagating the apoptotic signal cascade, as described previously. More recent data indicate that caspase-9 may not be the initiator caspase in response to stress signals in some cells *(55)*. Instead, procaspase-2 appears to fulfill this role upstream of mitochondria as part of a much larger multi-protein complex that does not contain either Apaf-1 or cytochrome c. The data suggest that recruitment of procaspase-2 to this larger protein complex is sufficient to mediate its activation, perhaps via oligomerization of procaspase-2 independently of the Apaf-1 apoptosome, which is required for the activation of procaspase-9, rather than through the sequential cleavage and activation of the procaspase molecule *(56)*. This model of initiator procaspase activation is rather novel, and could also be relevant to the death receptor-independent activation of procaspase-8 that has been observed in a number of different circumstances.

Caspase-$9^{-/-}$ mice also die during early embryogenesis. These mutant embryos demonstrate abnormalities in brain development similar to those of caspase-$3^{-/-}$ null mice; however, the abnormalities in the *casp9*$^{-/-}$ mice are more severe *(57)*. Cells with the caspase-$9^{-/-}$ deficiency demonstrate normal mitochondrial cytochrome c release after UV irradiation, but caspase-3 is not processed normally in embryonic stem cells, embryonic fibroblasts, or cell lysates that have been isolated from neuronal or thymocyte cells of caspase-$9^{-/-}$ conditionally deficient mice. This lack of caspase-3 activation occurs even after the addition of exogenous cytochrome c and dATP, which suggests that caspase-9 is prerequisite for the activation of caspase-3 in this situation. Even though the human *CASP9* gene has been localized to chromosome 1 band p36.3 *(9)*, a chromosomal region believed to harbor one or more tumor suppressor genes *(58–60)*, thus far there has been no evidence that caspase-9 functions as a tumor suppressor itself. In fact, caspase-9 has been ruled out as a potential tumor suppressor in neuroblastoma *(61)* as well as other cancers *(62)*, suggesting that its role may be more that of a bystander rather than that of a direct participant in tumorigenesis. The role of caspase-9 as a bystander during tumorigenesis is based upon its association with, and functional dependence upon, the *Apaf-1* gene (another bona fide tumor suppressor that functions within the caspase machinery as a regulator of caspase-9) *(9)*.

Apaf-1 and Its Loss of Expression in Melanoma Tumors Due to the Methylation of Its Corresponding Gene

Apaf-1 is a mitochondria-associated protein that binds procaspase 9 and activates the enzyme (Fig. 2B). In order to bind caspase-9, Apaf-1 undergoes a significant conformational change. In most cell types, this conformational change requires the binding of cytochrome c, although in a few cell types the conformational change may be cytochrome c independent. Apaf-1 contains a CARD domain that shares homology with similar domains in caspase-2, and caspase-9 serves as the caspase recruitment domain. In addition to the CARD domain, Apaf-1 also contains a nucleotide binding domain, an oligomerization domain, and 12 WD repeats in the carboxyl-terminal domain that appear to function as a negative regulatory domain that keeps the protein inactive and prevents the binding of procaspase-9 to the apoptosome until Apaf-1 binds cytochrome c (Figs. 1 and 2B) *(63)*. Apaf-1 functions as an oligomer. Oligomerization of Apaf-1 is dependent on the presence of ATP or dATP *(51)*. The oligomerization site has been suggested as a possible site for the design of therapeutic drugs that would prevent activation of procaspase-9.

While *CASP9*$^{-/-}$ mice are embryonic lethal, *Apaf-1*$^{-/-}$ knockout mice are viable, and they exhibit a wide resistance to chemotherapeutic drugs and irradiation *(57)*. Despite their general resistance to chemotherapeutic drugs, *Apaf-1*$^{-/-}$ knockout mice are sensitive to Fas/CD95-mediated cell death, suggesting that Apaf-1 is essential only for the activation of the procaspase-9 intrinsic caspase pathway. Recently, an absence of Apaf-1 expression was detected in a subset of human melanoma patients *(9)*. Much like the absence of caspase-8 expression in neuroblastoma, *Apaf-1* gene expression was extinguished through epigenetic means, via the methylation of promoter sequences in the gene. Therefore, *Apaf-1* can now be considered as a second bona fide example of a proapoptotic gene product functioning as a tumor suppressor in human tumor cells, and whose gene is preferentially silenced in a subset of human tumors via methylation of a portion of the gene.

Caspase-8 Involvement in Death Receptor-Independent Apoptosis

In the mitochondrial pathway, caspase-8 can also act as an effector caspase, acting independently to cleave certain cellular substrates (e.g., the cytolinker plectin) *(17)*. The mechanism(s) involved in the reported death receptor-independent activation of procaspase-8 is unknown. A number or reports have appeared indicating that procaspase-8 can be activated in various ways (e.g., unligated integrin recruitment of procaspase-8 to the cell membrane results in its activation) *(12)*, and caspase-3 has been suggested as an activator of procaspase-8 in MCF-7 cells *(18)* (Fig. 2B). Even though activated caspase-8 is not required for caspase-9-mediated apoptosis, it can significantly accelerate this apoptotic process, much like what has recently been proposed for procaspase-2 *(56)*, through the amplification of weaker death signals, ensuring that cell death occurs within an appropriate time frame (Fig. 2B). We and others now have additional data that support the concept that an "initiator" caspase can also function as an effector/executioner caspase. Several groups have shown that caspase-8-mediated cell death occurs in response to a variety of apoptotic stimuli, including chemotherapeutic drugs, independent of death receptor function as well *(31,32,34)*.

The intrinsic caspase-9-mediated mitochondrial apoptotic signaling pathway is also influenced by expression of the tumor suppressor p53, whereas the possible involvement of p53 in the caspase-8-mediated apoptotic pathway has not been well characterized *(64,65)*. Originally it was believed that cross-talk between the extrinsic (death receptor) and intrinsic (mitochondrial) cell-death pathways did not occur, and that these two pathways represented separate apoptotic signaling arms. In part, this independent pathway hypothesis contributed to some confusion regarding the experimental results of some investigators, including Debatin and colleagues, indicating that the Fas/CD95 pathway was involved in mediating drug-induced apoptosis of neuroblastoma, as well as other solid tumor cells *(35,43,66)*. These results were controversial because other investigators, primarily working with hematopoietic tumor cells, and not solid tumors, could not replicate their data, leading to the suggestion that the intrinsic pathway was exclusively responsible for the cell death observed in response to chemotherapeutic drug treatment *(67)*. However, new data from a number of laboratories indicates that the full activation of caspase-9 may also involve caspases 3 and 8 in certain cell types and for specific, perhaps weaker, apoptotic signals. Others have now reported that caspase-3 is essential for the activation of procaspase-8 and the generation of truncated proBid (tBid) upstream of caspase-9 activation*(18)*. These observations suggest the presence of a caspase signal amplification loop. Thus, the Fas/CD95 death receptor is not necessarily the important player in the results cited above, but rather the ability of caspase-8 to function in death receptor-independent manner. Consistent with these observations, Dr. S. Korsmeyer's laboratory has recently demonstrated that tBid is a ligand that inserts into the mitochondrial membrane, and then facilitates Bak oligomerization in the membrane as well as the subsequent release of cytochrome c from the resulting mitochondrial membrane pore *(68)*. Their results suggest that the ligand function of tBid, and subsequent Bak-mediated release of cytochrome c, may account for the dramatic differences between caspase-8 function in lymphoid and hepatic cells. Further discussion of caspase-8 and death receptor-independent apoptosis can be found in the next section, which deals with the possible role of integrins in caspase-8-mediated signaling of cell death.

How Unligated Integrins Function as Proapoptotic Biosensors With Activated Caspase-8

It has been demonstrated that death receptor-independent recruitment and activation of procaspase-8 are linked to the growth of certain nonadhesive tumor cells that express unligated integrins, a specific type of cell-adhesion receptor *(12)*. Figure 6 compares a normal (A) and a transformed cell (B) that no longer undergoes apoptosis. These unligated integrins, or γ- integrin tails, appear to recruit procaspase-8, when it is expressed, to the cellular membrane, where it is activated by an unknown mechanism (Fig. 6), resulting in apoptosis. However, in a number of tumor cells this is not the case. In these particular cells, the absence of procaspase-8 expression prevents transmission of the unligated integrin signals, resulting in enhanced cell survival *(8)*. This observation may be extremely important, particularly since the integrins are cell-surface receptors that are involved in numerous cellular functions, including cell survival, maintenance of cellular integrity, proliferation, and chemotaxis in response to signals coming from the surrounding extracellular matrix (ECM) *(69)*. With regard to the loss of caspase-8 expression and its recruitment to unligated integrins in the cell membrane, it is possible that this is not only

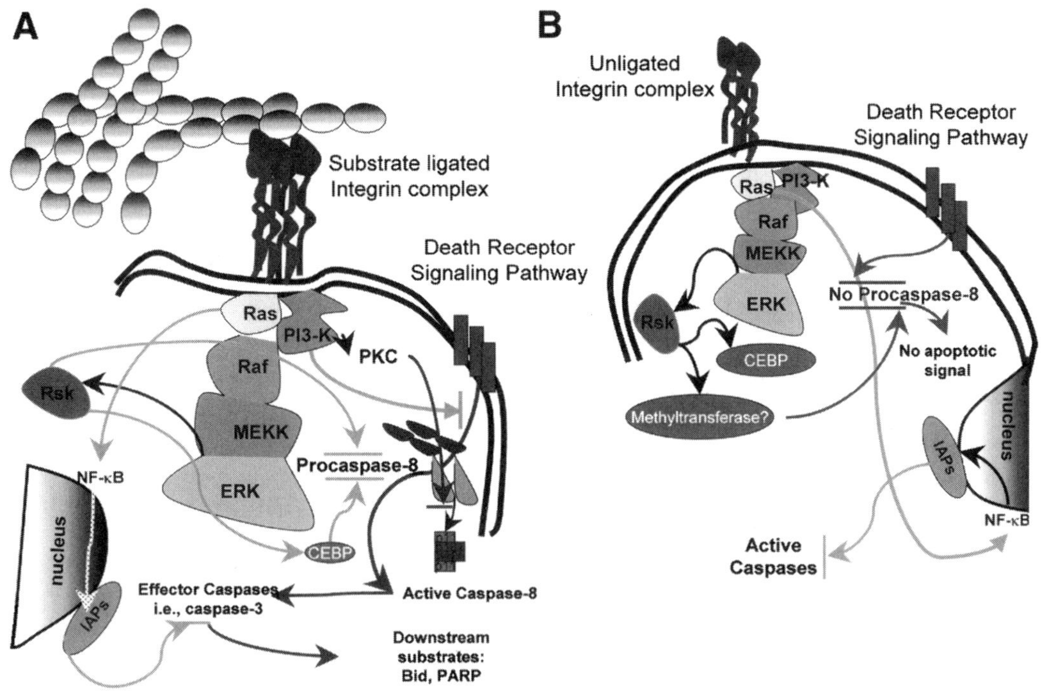

Fig. 6. Schematic representations of protein kinase activating pathways and death receptor signaling pathways in either (**A**) normal control cells with substrate ligated integrin complexes or (**B**) tumorigenic cells with unligated integrin complexes. The potential relationship between a putative methylatransferase and the extinguishing of procaspase-8 expression is shown in the putative tumor cell shown in panel B. Conversely, the ability of ligated integrins to activate procaspase-8 in a death receptor-independent manner is shown in the normal cells in panel A.

relevant to the persistence of that particular tumor cell (Fig. 6B), but to its ability to mobilize more easily to remote sites, and to survive hostile microenvironments within the body as well (Fig. 6). One of the earliest recognized functions for apoptosis was the elimination of cells from inappropriate cellular microenvironments. If this particular response were eliminated, the resulting tumor cell would not only have enhanced ability to survive stress and insults ranging from chemotherapeutic drugs to irradiation; this cell would also possess the unique ability to survive in cellular environments that would normally induce apoptosis (Fig. 6). In addition, since integrins help to induce wound healing through angiogenesis, and any tumor cell capable of inducing crucial angiogenic responses could create a vascular support network, ensuring that it would not only survive, but thrive, and would be well on its way to metastasis. Thus, it is clear that the ability of tumor cells to survive genotoxic insults and consequently adapt to hostile environments provides a significant survival advantage over the host's native, unaltered cells.

CANCER THERAPY

Cancer is, quite simply, the failure of normal cell growth and differentiation, resulting in an abnormal accumulation of cells with altered growth characteristics. This is due, at least in part, to a blunted (or absent) response to proapoptotic stimuli. Normal cell growth is a tightly regulated process with numerous regulatory checkpoints throughout the cell cycle. One function of these checkpoints is to ensure the genomic integrity of the cell. In the presence of DNA damage, cell division is halted until the acquired lesion is repaired; alternatively, if the genomic insult is irreparable, the cell undergoes apoptosis. Cancer cells are derived from a population of previously normal cells that have incurred numerous (i.e., at least two to three) genotoxic events. These events may be the result of constitutional gene defects resulting in genetic instability such as that seen with Rb gene mutations and retinoblastoma *(65)*. Viral infections have also been related with certain cancers, such as those associated with the human papilloma virus and cervical cancer, the Epstein–Barr virus and the resulting lymphomas related to immune suppression, and Burkitt's lymphoma *(70)*. Additionally, genetic mutations acquired due to environmental insults, such as exposure to vinyl chloride and the resulting hepatocellular carcinoma, cigarette smoking and lung cancer, ultraviolet irradiation and melanoma, or ionizing radiation and leukemia or brain tumors, are just a few of the tumors that may be the subsequent result. One of three potential fates may befall the cell during its lifetime: normal development, cell death, or, given the appropriate circumstances, progression to a tumor cell. Influences that promote tumor cell formation, whether environmental or chemical, are not typically carcinogenic, but may act as such when applied to mutated cells. These mutated cells have frequently altered their expression of those genes that stimulate (oncogenes) or inhibit (tumor suppressor genes) cell proliferation/apoptosis, thus allowing the mutant cell to persist and propagate despite normal cellular and environmental restraints. Failure of the normal intrinsic cellular mechanisms to abrogate propagation of these cells further contributes to neoplastic transformation by allowing genetically unstable cells to persist in the environment and acquire further gene mutations and/or epigenetic modifications. The net result is a population of genetically abnormal cells with altered growth characteristics that provide them a distinct growth advantage (i.e., decreased oxygen requirement, loss of contact inhibition, growth factor and hormone independence, and resistance to immune-based destruction).

Conventional cancer therapies have targeted neoplastic cells in a relatively nonspecific manner, predominantly by interfering with metabolic, synthetic, and/or mitotic processes in active cells and thus inducing apoptosis. This approach inevitably results in corruption of cell functions in very active, nonneoplastic cells such as gastrointestinal mucosal, epithelial, and hematopoetic cells with the concomitant sacrifice of these normal cells. Recent advances in our understanding of apoptosis and how it is altered in certain tumors have yielded an appreciation for the role of chemotherapy and irradiation in inducing apoptosis in these tumors. A number of studies have speculated that anticancer drugs initiate apoptosis via synthesis of Fas ligand (FasL) and upregulation of Fas/CD95, or through the intrinsic mitochondrial pathway mediated via p53. FasL binds to Fas/CD95 and activates the death receptor pathway in an autocrine or paracrine manner. Chemotherapeutic agents implicated in such apoptotic activation include doxorubicin, etoposide, teniposide, methotrexate, cyclophosphamide, cisplatin, carboplatin, and bleomycin *(8,9,71–75)*. This proposed mechanism of action is based upon the observed increase in FasL mRNA and Fas/CD95 expression in cancer cell lines after treatment with these agents *(76–78)*. Though this clearly demonstrates a temporal relationship between treatment with anti-cancer drugs and the upregulation of proapoptotic mediators, it does not convincingly identify the mechanism(s) of chemotherapy-induced apoptosis. Illustrative of this point, experiments using cells from a variety of tumors known to upregulate Fas/CD95 and FasL with chemotherapeutic agents, pretreatment of these tumors with anti-Fas or anti-FasL immunoglobulin has shown variable to no effect on subsequent chemotherapy-induced apoptosis *(79,80)*. A second example involves the use of dominant negative FADD$^{-/-}$ mutant cells or cells overexpressing FADD-like ICE (FLICE)- inhibitory protein (FLIP), which would normally prevent the receptor-initiated activation of procaspase-8 to caspase-8, which once again demonstrates minimal to absent ability to attenuate apoptosis following treatment of these pretreated cells with chemotherapeutic drugs *(81)*. Finally, tumor cells that lack Fas/CD95 and thus cannot respond to FasL, demonstrate normal apoptosis in response to chemotherapeutic drug therapy *(8)*. Further investigation has demonstrated mitochondrial perturbation (i.e., loss of transmembrane potential and elevated levels of cytosolic cytochrome c) occurring concomitantly with the upregulation of Fas/CD95 and/or FasL expression, suggesting potentially at least two sites where such drugs might influence the initiation of apoptosis.

Tumor Cell Resistance Involving Caspases-8 and -9

Tumor cell death induced by chemotherapy and irradiation is the result of the disruption in processes vital for the normal function, and life, of the cell. Drugs successfully used in cancer therapy include antimetabolites (methotrexate and 5-fluorouracil), DNA-damaging agents (doxorubicin, cyclophosphamide, and platinating agents), mitotic inhibitors (vincristine and vinblastine), nucleotide analogs (6-mercaptopurine and 6-thioguanine), and topoisomerase inhibitors (teniposide, etoposide, and topotecan). The net effect of this diverse group of compounds is the same: disruption of the processes requisite for cell survival, resulting in either cell-cycle arrest and DNA-damage repair or the death of the cell through the initiation of apoptosis *(82,83)*. Cancer cells should always be considered as damaged cells capable of prolonged survival, frequently due to their ability to evade these checkpoints.

Most DNA-damaging reagents, including danorubicin, doxorubicin, etoposide, and mitomycin C, as well as fludorabine and flavopiridol, kill cells through the activation of caspases *(82,83)*. Ionizing radiation causes tumor cell death via activation of caspase-8 *(84)*. Experiments with synthetic caspase inhibitors have shown that caspase-1, or a closely related caspase, is important for drug-induced apoptosis in glioma cells *(77,78,85)*. Other studies implicate different caspases (e.g., caspase-3 and -8) or all caspases sensitive to the universal caspase inhibitor ZVAD-Fmk, in the drug responses of other tumors *(71)*. Another universal caspase inhibitor, CrmA, which inhibits both caspase-1 and caspase-8 *(8,71,86)*, inhibits apoptosis mediated by both the Fas/CD95- and TNFR1 receptor-mediated pathways in response to drugs or γ-irradiation. Other studies on cells from knockout mice show that caspase-8$^{-/-}$ mice remain sensitive to certain chemotherapeutic drugs while cells from caspase-9$^{-/-}$ mice are highly resistant to the same drugs *(29,56)*. Based upon our own studies performed using caspase-8 null neuroblastoma tumor cells that overexpress N-myc (i.e., due to amplification of the *MYCN* gene), it appears that the effectiveness of certain chemotherapeutic drugs may be influenced directly by the presence/absence of pro- and antiapoptotic gene products, with the tumor cells appearing to be more sensitive to these agents once a normal apoptotic signaling pathway is restored (*[8]*; Houghton, Teitz and Kidd, unpublished results). The most encouraging news, however, is that the replacement of a particular procaspase, procaspase-8, absent in this particularly virulent form of neuroblastoma, seems to enhance their sensitivity to certain chemotherapeutic drugs *(8,38,42)*. Furthermore, it has been demonstrated that both 2-deoxy-azacytidine *(8,42)* and γ-interferon *(38)* dramatically enhance the endogenous levels of procaspase-8 within these neuroblastoma cells (Fig. 5), the former most likely due to demethylation of the *CASP8* gene in these tumors, and the latter for unknown mechanistic reasons probably related to the binding of unknown transcription factor(s) at important regulatory regions within the gene that may not be necessary for normal gene transcription. In fact, one study has linked the ability of γ-interferon to upregulate procaspase-8 levels in tumor cells to the Stat1 pathway *(87)*. A therapeutic trial combining one or both of these agents to chemotherapeutic drug treatment of this particular form of cancer may provide the appropriate combination to allow apoptosis to ensue. Similar combinations of de-methylating agents and/or γ-interferon with chemotherapeutic drugs may dramatically enhance the survival rate of those with tumors that have previously been thought to be of poor prognosis.

The levels of Bcl2 family members can also influence the tumor cell response to chemotherapeutic drugs. High levels of the anti-apoptotic protein Bcl2 can prolong tumor cell survival, whereas high levels of the proapoptotic molecule Bax can increase the effectiveness of chemotherapeutic agents. One approach to combating the protective effects of Bcl-2 has been to use Bcl-2 antisense therapies in both cell lines and primary tumor samples *(88,89)*. These studies showed that by using anti-sense Bcl-2 it was possible to increase apoptosis in certain circumstances. Based upon these results, Bcl-2 antisense therapy is currently being used in a phase 1 clinical trial with human subjects. Other approaches to modulating Bcl-2 levels are also being employed to treat human tumors. For example, all-trans retinoic acid downregulates both proapoptotic proteins Bcl-2 and Bcl-X_L as well as inducing phosphorylation of Bcl-2 that results in the loss of its protective capacity. Treatment with all-trans retinoic acid prior to the administration of drugs such as Ara-C enhances Ara-C-induced apoptosis *(90)*. The effectiveness of ribozymes directed against Bcl-2 and Bcl-X_L, which inactivate the protective effects of these Bcl-2 family members, as therapeutic tools is also being examined. Drugs such as bryostatin, UNC-01, taxol, and the retinoid analog 4-HPR also alter Bcl-2 function by inducing its phosphorylation, and thereby its inactivation *(91)*. Several drugs that inhibit mitochondrial permeability changes are also now being tested in clinical trials. Arsenic trioxide has significant therapeutic effect against promyelocytic leukemia and activates cytochrome c release and caspase activation in vitro as well as inducing a permeability transition pore complex using a cell-free system in a Bcl-2-inhibitable manner *(88,91)*. Other drugs in this category, including lonidamine, betulinic acid, and CD437 (a new retinoid acid receptor agonist) also cause permeabilization of isolated membranes, and rhodacyanine lipophilic cations including MKT-077 *(92,93)*. MKT-077 is a rhodacyanine dye that is selectively toxic to carcinoma cells, and may cause mitochondrial membrane potential changes as well. Currently in phase I trials, the use of londiamine enhances the apoptotic responses of tumor cells to cisplatin, cyclophosphamide, doxorubicin, paclitaxel, melphalan, and γ-irradiation both in vitro and in vivo. When londiamine is used in combination therapy in phase II and phase III trials in patients with metastatic breast cancer and inoperable non-small-cell lung cancer, patients show improvement in overall response, in tumor size, the increase in median time involved in tumor progression, and the median survival rate of patients *(93)*. Addition of londiamine to isolated mitochondria in vitro can cause dissipation of the mitochondrial membrane potential and the subsequent release of cyctochrome c, the effects of which are inhibited by recombinant Bcl2. Finally, the induction of Bax in vivo within targeted tumor cells may prove to be more useful than adenoviral p53 as an anticancer agent *(94)*.

Some of the cytostatic drugs used in chemotherapy to kill target tumor cells do so by upregulating Fas/CD95 as well as inducing FasL expression within the same cell. Tumor cells insensitive to Fas/CD95-mediated apoptosis are frequently resistant to these drugs. Cytotoxic drugs such as bleomycin, cis-platinin, and etoposide induce only Fas/CD95 expression in tumor cells *(30,33,95)*. In leukemic cells, doxorubicin and methotrexate (MTX) have both been demonstrated to work via the stimulation of FasL expression *(30,34)*. Thus, by blocking Fas/CD95 through methylation of a DISC component, including caspase-8, or a component of the intrinsic mitochondrial apoptotic signaling pathway, one can abolish the effects of these drugs.

Finally, the TRAIL receptor is an attractive target because 80% of human cancer cell lines are sensitive to TRAIL-induced apoptosis, at least to some extent, while normal cells do not express the TRAIL receptor *(95–97)*. In addition, TRAIL is capable of directly activating the caspases, without nearly as many intermediates involved along the way *(97)*. There are some data suggesting that tumor cells resistant to TRAIL-mediated cell death can be sensitized by subtoxic concentrations of drugs/cytokines, and the subsequently sensitized cells then undergo significant TRAIL-mediated apoptosis *(75)*. TRAIL has also been shown to have a synergistic effect when combined with TNF-α, etoposide, 5-flurouracil, and camptothecin in pilot studies *(98)*. The use of recombinant TRAIL to target death receptor signaling pathways may be especially important in p53-negative tumor cells, since the apoptotic response induced by TRAIL is not influenced by p53 *(99)*. TRAIL-induced apoptosis is also largely free from the influence of the anti-apoptotic Bcl2 family members. Preclinical work with xenographs using mammary and colon carcinomas as well as intracranial gliomas demonstrate that treatment of these mice with recombinant TRAIL significantly decreased the size of tumors. In fact, gliomas injected with recombinant TRAIL underwent complete disease regression that entirely ablated the tumor. Treatment of colon carcinoma xenographs with TRAIL in combination with existing chemotherapy has resulted in a substantial regression in tumor size, and in some cases remission *(100)*. Despite the positive results achieved using the human tumor cell lines and mouse xenograft models, the potential toxicity of TRAIL in humans is not known; however, TRAIL is not toxic in other primates *(97)*.

It is clear from the early work performed on the expression of procaspase-8 and Apaf-1 in tumors that by understanding how apoptotic signaling pathways work in transformed cells, as well as in response to various chemotherapeutic agents and irradiation, it should be possible to achieve significant advancements in cancer therapy. Thus, much like the progress in the treatment of particular metabolic disorders due to their molecular analysis, cancer treatment may also be specifically tailored to individual tumor types by using information concerning both the genetic makeup of these tumor cells and the mode of drug action, thereby allowing chemotherapy to function more effectively.

REFERENCES

1. Kerr JFR, Wyllie AH, Currie AR. Apoptosis: a basic biological phenomenon with wide-ranging implications in tissue kinetics. Br J Cancer 1972;26:239–257.
2. Wylie AH, Kerr JFR, Currie AR. Cell death: the significance of apoptosis. Int Rev Cytol 1981;68:251–305.
3. Raff MC. Social controls on cell survival and cell death. Nature 1992;356:397–400.
4. Ellis RE, Yuan JY, Horvitz HR. Mechanisms and functions of cell death. Ann Rev Cell Biol 1991: 663–698.
5. Ashkenazi A, Dixit VM. Death receptors: signaling and modulation. Science 1998;281:1305–1308.
6. Pothana S, Dong Z, Mikhailov V, Denton M, Venkatachalam M. Apoptosis: definition, mechanisms, and relevance to disease. Am J Med 1999;107:498–506.
7. Reed JC, Cuddy M, Haldar S, et al. BCL2-mediated tumorigenicity of a human T-lymphoid cell line: synergy with MYC and inhibition by BCL2-antisense. Proc Natl Acad Sci USA 1990;87:3660–3664.
8. Teitz T, Wei T, Valentine MB, et al. Caspase 8 is deleted or silenced preferentially in childhood neuroblastomas with amplification of *MYCN*. Nature Med 2000;6:529–535.
9. Soengas MS, Capodieci P, Polsky D, et al. Inactivation of the apoptosis effector Apaf-1 in malignant melanoma. Nature 2001;409:207–211.
10. Shivapurkar N, Reddy J, Matta H, et al. Loss of expression of death-inducing signaling complex (DISC) components in lung cancer cell lines and the influence of MYC amplification. Oncogene 2002;21:8510–8514.
11. Cohen GM. Caspases—the executioners of apoptosis. Biochem J 1997;326:1–16.
12. Stupack DG, Puente XS, Boutsaboualoy S, Storgard CM, Cheresh DA. .Apoptosis of adherent cells by recruitment of caspase-8 to unligated integrins. J Cell Biol 2001;155:459–470.
13. Harada K, Toyooka S, Shivapurkar N, et al. Deregulation of caspase 8 and 10 expression in pediatric tumors and cell lines. Cancer Res 2002;62:5897–5901.
14. Cryns VL, Yuan JY. Proteases to die for. Genes & Devel 1998;12:1551–1570.
15. Craen MV, Loo GV, Pype S, et al. Identification of a new caspase homologue: caspase-14. Cell Death & Diff 1998;5:838–846.
16. Salvesen GS, Dixit VM. Caspases: intracellular signaling by proteolysis. Cell 1997;91:443–446.
17. Stegh AH, Herrmann H, Lampel S, et al. Identification of the cytolinker plectin as a major early in vivo substrate for caspase 8 during CD95- and tumor necrosis factor receptor-mediated apoptosis. Mol Cell Biol 2000;20:5665–5679.
18. Tang D, Lahti JM, Kidd VJ. Caspase-8 activation and Bid cleavage contribute to MCF7 cellular execution in a caspase-3-dependent manner during staurosporine-mediated apoptosis. J Biol Chem 2000;275:9303–9307.
19. Kidd VJ. Proteolytic activities that mediate apoptosis. Ann Rev Physiol 1998;60:533–573.
20. Scaffidi C, Schmitz I, Zha J, Korsmeyer SJ, Krammer PH, Peter ME. Differential modulation of apoptosis sensitivity in CD95 type I and type II cells. J Biol Chem 1999;274:22,532–22,538.
21. Srinivasula SM, Ahmad MF, Fernandes-Alnemri T, Litwack G, Alnemri ES. Molecular ordering of the Fas-apoptotic pathways: the Fas/APO-1 protease Mch5 is a CrmA-inhibitable protease that activates multiple Ced3/ICE-like cysteine proteases. Proc Natl Acad Sci USA 1996;93:14,486–14,491.
22. Li P, Nijhawan D, Budihardjo I, Srinivasula SM, et al. Cytochrome c and dATP-dependent formation of Apaf-1/caspase-9 complex initiates an apoptotic protease cascade. Cell 1997;91:479–489.
23. Liu X, Kim CN, Yang J, Jemmerson R, Wang X. Induction of apoptotic program in cell-free extracts: requirement for dATP and cytochrome c. Cell 1996;86:147–157.
24. Kuwana T, Smith JJ, Muzio M, Dixit VM, Newmeyer DD, Kornbluth S. Apoptosis induction by caspase-8 is amplified through the mitochondrial release of cytochrome c. J Biol Chem 1998;273:16589–16594.
25. Alnemri ES, Livingston DJ, Nicholson DW, et al. Human ICE/CED-3 protease nomenclature. Cell 1996;87:171.
26. Zou H, Henzel WJ, Liu XS, Lutschg A, Wang XD. Apaf-1, a human protein homologous to *C. elegans* ced-4, participates in cytochrome c-dependent activation of caspase-3. Cell 1997;90(3):405–413.
27. Li F, Srinivasan A, Wang Y, Armstrong RC, Tomaselli KJ, Fritz LC. Cell-specific induction of apoptosis by microinjection of cyctochrome c. J Biol Chem 1997;272:30,299–30,305.
28. Green DR, Reed JC. Mitochondria and apoptosis. Science 1998;281:1309–1311.
29. Varfolomeev E, Schuchmann M, Luria V, et al. Targeted disruption of the mouse *caspase 8* gene ablates cell death induction by the TNF receptors, Fas/Apo1, and DR3 and is lethal prenatally. Immunity 1998;9:267–276.
30. Sakamaki K, Inoue T, Asano M, et al. *Ex vivo* whole-embryo culture of caspase-8 deficient embryos normalize their aberrant phenotypes in the developing neural tube and heart. Cell Death & Diff 2002;9:1196–1206.

31. Villunger A, Egle A, Kos M, et al. Drug-induced apoptosis is associated with enhanced Fas (Apo-1/CD95) ligand expression but occurs independently of Fas (Apo-1/CD95) signaling in human T-acute lymphatic leukemia cells. Cancer Res 1997;57:3331–3334.
32. Sun XM, MacFarlane M, Zhuang J, Wolf BB, Green DR, Cohen GM. Distinct caspase cascades are initiated in receptor-mediated and chemical-induced apoptosis. J Biol Chem 1999;274:5053–5060.
33. Fulda S, Lutz W, Schwab M, Debatin K-M. Myc-N sensitizes neuroblastoma cells for drug-induced apoptosis. Oncogene 1999;18:1479–1486.
34. Wesselborg S, Engels IH, Rossmann E, Los M, Schulze-Osthoff K. Anticancer drugs induce caspase-8/FLICE activation and apoptosis in the absence of CD95 receptor/ligand interaction. Blood 1999;93:3053–3063.
35. Fulda S, Strauss G, Meyer E, Debatin KM. Functional CD95 ligand and CD95 death-inducing signaling complex in activation-induced cell death and doxorubicin-induced apoptosis in leukemic T cells. Blood 2000;95:301–308.
36. Kluza J, Lansiaux A, Wattez N, Mahieu C, Osheroff N, Bailly C. Apoptotic response of HL-60 human leukemia cells to the antitumor drug TAS-103. Cancer Res 2000;60:4077–4084.
37. Hopkins-Donaldson S, Bodmer JL, Bourloud KB, Brognara CB, Tschopp J, Gross N. Loss of caspase-8 expression in highly malignant human neuroblastoma cells correlates with resistance to tumor necrosis factor–related apoptosis-inducing ligand-induced apoptosis. Cancer Res 2000;60:4315–4319.
38. Zuzak TJ, Steinhoff DF, Sutton LN, Phillips PC, Eggert A, Grotzer MA. Loss of *caspase-8* mRNA expression is common in childhood primitive neuroectodermal brain tumour/medulloblastoma. Eur J Cancer 2002;38:83–91.
39. Fulda S, Debatin KM. IFNg sensitizes for apoptosis by upregulating caspase-8 expression through the Stat1 pathway. Oncogene 2002;21:2295–2308.
40. Takita J, Yang HW, Chen YY, et al. Allelic imbalance on chromosome 2q and alterations of the caspase 8 gene in neuroblastoma. Oncogene 2001;20:4424–4432.
41. Takita J, Hayashi Y, Kohno Y, et al. Allelotype of neuroblastoma. Oncogene 1995;11:1829–1834.
42. Grenet J, Teitz T, Wei T, Valentine V, Kidd VJ. Structure and chromosome localization of the human *CASP8* gene. Gene 1999;226:225–232.
43. Fulda S, Kufer MU, Meyer E, van Valen F, Dockhorn-Dworniczak B, Debatin KM. Sensitization for death receptor- or drug-induced apoptosis by re-expression of caspase-8 through demethylation or gene transfer. Oncogene 2001;20:5865–5877.
44. Evan GI, Wyllie AH, Gilbert CS, et al. Induction of apoptosis in fibroblasts by c-myc protein. Cell 1992;69:119–128.
45. Hueber AO, Zornig M, Lyon D, Suda T, Nagata S, Evan GI. Requirement for the CD95 receptor-ligand pathway in c-myc-induced apoptosis. Science 1997;278:1305–1309.
46. Juin P, Evan G. Caspase 8: the killer you can't live without. Nature Med 2000;6:498–500.
47. Klefstrom J, Verschuren EW, Evan G. c-Myc augments the apoptotic activity of cytosolic death receptor signaling proteins by engaging the mitochondrial apoptotic pathway. J Biol Chem 2002;277:43,224–43,232.
48. Juin P, Hueber AO, Littlewood T, Evan GI. c-Myc-induced sensitization to apoptosis is mediated through cytochrome c release. Genes & Devel 1999;13:1367–1381.
48a. Koga S, Hirohata S, Kondo Y, et al. A novel telomerase-specific gene therapy: gene transfer of caspase-8 utilizing the human telomerase catalytic subunit gene promoter. Hum Gene Ther 2000;11:1397–1406.
49. Rodriguez J, Lazebnik Y. Caspase-9 and APAF-1 form an active holoenzyme. Genes & Devel 1999;13:3179–3184.
50. Budihardjo I, Oliver H, Lutter M, Luo X, Wang XD. Biochemical pathways of caspase activation during apoptosis. Annu Rev Cell Dev Biol 1999;15:269–290.
51. Saleh A, Srinivasula SM, Acharya S, Fishel R, Alnemri ES. Cytochrome c and dATP-mediated oligomerization of Apaf-1 is a prerequisite for procaspase-9 activation. J Biol Chem 1999;274:17,941–17,945.
52. Hu Y, Benedict MA, Ding L, Ez G. Role of cytochrome c and dATP/ATP hydrolysis in Apaf-1-mediated caspase- 9 activation and apoptosis. EMBO J 1999;18:3586–3595.
53. Shiozaki EN, Chai J, Shi Y. Oligomerization and activation of caspase-9, induced by Apaf-1 CARD. Proc Natl Acad Sci USA 2002;99:4197–4202.
54. Stennicke HR, Deveraux QL, Humke EW, Reed JC, Dixit VM, Salvesen GS. Caspase-9 can be activated without proteolytic processing. J Biol Chem 1999;274:8359–8362.

55. Rao RV, Castro-Obregon S, Frankowski H, et al. Coupling endoplasmic reticulum stress to the cell death program. An Apaf-1-independent intrinsic pathway. J Biol Chem 2002;277:21,836–21,842.
56. Read SH, Baliga BC, Ekert PG, Vaux DL, Kumar S. A novel Apaf-1-independent putative caspase-2 activation complex. J Cell Biol 2002;159:739–745.
57. Hakem R, Hakem A, Duncan GS, et al. Differential requirement for caspase 9 in apoptotic pathways in vivo. Cell 1998;94:339–352.
58. Caron HN, van Sluis P, van Hoeve M, et al. Allelic loss of chromosome 1p36 in neuroblastoma is of preferential maternal origin and correlates with N-myc amplication. Nature Gen 1993;4:187–190.
59. Bello MJ, deCampos JM, Kusak ME, et al. Allelic loss at 1p is associated with tumor progression of meningiomas. Genes, Chromosomes & Cancer 1994;9:296–298.
60. Caron HN, Peter M, van Sluis P, et al. Evidence for two tumor suppressor loci on chromosomal bands 1p35-36 involved in neuroblastoma: one probably imprinted, another associated with N-myc amplification. Hum Mol Genet 1995;4:535–539.
61. Teitz T, Wei T, Liu D, et al. Caspase-9 and Apaf-1 are expressed and functionally active in human neuroblastoma tumor cell lines with 1p36 LOH and amplified *MYCN*. Oncogene 2002;21:1848–1858.
62. Wolf BB, Schuler M, Li W, et al. Defective cytochrome c-dependent caspase activation in ovarian cancer cell lines due to diminished or absent apoptotic protease activating factor-1 activity. J Biol Chem 2001;276:34,244–34,251.
63. Adrain C, Slee EA, Harte MT, Martin SJ. Regulation of apoptotic protease activating factor-1 oligomerization and apoptosis by the WD-40 repeat region. J Biol Chem 1999;274:20,855–20,860.
64. Sitailo LA, Tibudan SS, Denning MF. Activation of caspase-9 is required for UV-induced apoptosis of human keratinocytes. J Biol Chem 2002;277:19,346–19,352.
65. Ding H, Lin I, McGill P, et al. Essential role for caspase-8 in transcription-independent apoptosis triggered by p53. J Biol Chem 2000;275:38,905–38,911.
66. Ferrari D, Stepczynska A, Los M, Wesselborg S, Schulze-Osthoff K. Differential regulation and ATP requirement for caspase-8 and caspase-3 activation during CD95- and anticancer drug–induced apoptosis. J Exp Med 1998;188:979–984.
67. Eischen CM, Kottke T, Martins LM, et al. Comparison of apoptosis in wild-type and Fas-resistant cells: chemotherapy-induced apoptosis is not dependent on Fas/Fas ligand interactions. Blood 1997;90:935–943.
68. Yin X-M, Wang K, Gross A, et al. Bid-deficient mice are resistant to Fas-induced hepatocellular apoptosis. Nature 1999;400:886–891.
69. Stupack DG, Cheresh DA. Get a ligand, get a life: integrins, signaling and cell survival. J Cell Science 2002;115:3729–3738.
70. Ben-Yosef T, Yanuka O, Halle D, Benvenisty N. Involvement of Myc targets in c-myc and N-myc induced human tumors. Oncogene 1998;17:165–171.
71. Barge RY, Willemze R, Vandenabeele P, Fiers W, Beyaert R. Differential involvement of caspases in apoptosis of myeloid leukemic cells induced by chemotherapy versus growth factor withdrawal. FEBS Lett 1997;409:207–210.
72. Herr I, Wilhelm D, Bohler T, Angel P, Debatin K-M. Activation of CD95 (APO-1/Fas) signaling by ceramide mediates cancer therapy-induced apoptosis. EMBO J 1997;16:6200–6208.
73. Liu JR, Opipari AW, Tan L, et al. Dysfunctional apoptosome activation in ovarian cancer: implications for chemoresistance. Cancer Res 2002;62:924–931.
74. Milner AE, Palmer DH, Hodgkin EA, et al. Induction of apoptosis by chemotherapeutic drugs: the role of FADD in activation of caspase-8 and synergy with death receptor ligands in ovarian carcinoma cells. Cell Death & Diff 2002;9:287–300.
75. Leverkus M, Yaar M, Gilchrest BA. Fas/Fas ligand interaction contributes to UV-induced apoptosis in human keratinocytes. Exp Cell Res 1997;232:255–262.
76. Brunner T, Mogil RJ, LaFace D, et al. Cell-autonomous Fas (CD95)/Fas-ligand interaction mediates activation-induced apoptosis in T-cell hybridomas. Nature 1995;373:441–444.
77. Ju S-T, Panks DJ, Cui HL, et al. Fas(CD95)/FasL interactions required for programmed cell death after T-cell activation. Nature 1995;373:444–448.
78. Griffith TS, Brunner T, Fletcher SM, Green DR, Ferguson TA. Fas ligand-induced apoptosis as a mechanism of immune privilege. Science 1995;270:1189–1192.
79. Peli J, Schröter M, Rudaz C, et al. Oncogenic Ras inhibits Fas ligand-mediated apoptosis by downregulating the expression of Fas. EMBO J 1999;18:1824–1831.

80. Petak I, Tillman DM, Harwood FG, Mihalik R, Houghton JA. Fas-dependent and -independent mechanisms of cell death following DNA damage in human colon carcinoma cells. Cancer Res 2000;60: 2643–2650.
81. Djerbi M, Screpanti V, Catrina AI, Bogen B, Biberfeld P, Grandien A. The inhibitor of death receptor signaling, FLICE-inhibitory protein defines a new class of tumor progression factors. J Exp Med 1999;190:1025–1032.
82. Gottesman MM. Mechanisms of cancer drug resistance. Annual Rev Medicine 2002;53:615–627.
83. Friesen C, Fulda S, Debatin K-M. Cytotoxic drugs and the CD95 pathway. Leukemia 1999;13:1854–1858.
84. Rehemtulla A, Hamilton CA, Chinnaiyan AM, Dixit VM. Ultraviolet radiation–induced apoptosis is mediated by activation of CD95 (Fas/APO-1). J Biol Chem 1997;272:25,783–25,786.
85. Selzer PM, Pingel S, Hsieh I, et al. Cysteine protease inhibitors as chemotherapy: Lessons from a parasite target. Proc Natl Acad Sci USA 1999;96:11,015–11,022.
86. Fulda S, Meyer E, Debatin KM. Metabolic inhibitors sensitize for CD95 (APO-1/Fas)-induced apoptosis by down-regulating Fas-associated death domain-like interleukin 1-converting enzyme inhibitory protein expression. Cancer Res 2000;60:3947–3956.
87. Fulda S, Debatin KM. IFNgamma sensitizes for apoptosis by upregulating caspase-8 expression through the Stat1 pathway. Oncogene 2002;21:2295–2308.
88. Reed JC, Tomaselli KJ. Drug discovery opportunities from apoptosis research. Current Opinion in Biotechnology 2001;11:586–592.
89. Konopleva M, Zhou S, Xie Z, et al. Apoptosis: molecules and mechanisms. In: Kaspers GJL, Pieters R, Veerman AJP (eds), Drug Resistance in Leukemia and Lymphoma III. Kluwer Academic/Plenum Publishers, Norwell, MA: 1999;217–236.
90. Kim CN, Wang XD, Huang Y, et al. Overexpression of bcl-x_L, inhibits ara-c-induced mitochondrial loss of cytochrome c and other perturbations that activate the molecular cascade of apoptosis. Cancer Res 1997;57(15):3115–3120.
91. Reed JC. Dysregulation of apoptosis in cancer. J Clin Onc 1999;17:2941–2953.
92. Fulda S, Friesen C, Los M, et al. Betulinic acid triggers CD95 (Apo-1/Fas)- and p53-independent apoptosis via activation of caspases in neuroectodermal tumors. Cancer Res 1997;57(21):4956–4964.
93. Houghton JA. Apoptosis and drug response. Curr Opinion Oncology 1999;11:475–481.
94. McPake CR, Tillman DM, Poquette C, George EO, Houghton JA, Harris LC. Bax is an important determinant of chemosensitivity in pediatric tumor cell lines independent of Bcl-2 expression and p53 status. Oncology Res 1998;10:235–244.
95. Gibson SB, Oyer R, Spalding AC, Anderson SM, Johnson GL. Increased expression of death receptors 4 and 5 synergizes the apoptosis response to combined treatment with etoposide and TRAIL. Mol Cell Biol 2000;20:205–212.
96. Walczak H, Krammer PH. The CD95 (APO-1/Fas) and the TRAIL (APO-2L) apoptosis systems. Exp Cell Res 2000;256:58–66.
97. Kim K, Fisher MJ, Xu S-Q, El-Diery WS. Molecular determinants of responses to TRAIL in killing normal and cancer cells. Clin Cancer Res 2000;6:335–346.
98. Walczak H, Miller RE, Ariail K, et al. Tumoricidal activity of tumor necrosis factor-related apoptosis-inducing ligand in vivo. Nature Med 1999;5:157–163.
99. Sheikh MS, Huang Y, Fernandes-Salas EA, et al. The antiapoptotic decoy receptor TRID/TRAIL-R3 is a p53-regulated DNA damage–inducible gene that is overexpressed in primary tumors of the gastrointestinal tract. Oncogene 1999;18:4153–4159.
100. Strater J, Hinz U, Walczak H, et al. Expression of TRAIL and TRAIL receptors in colon carcinoma: TRAIL-R1 is an independent prognostic parameter. Clin Cancer Res 2002;8:3734–3740.
101. Herman JG, Graff JR, Myohanen S, Nelkin BD, Baylin SB. Methylation-specific PCR: a novel PCR assay for methylation status of CpG islands. Proc Natl Acad Sci USA 1996;93:9821–9826.

14 Regulation of Death Receptor-Induced Apoptosis by NF-κB and Interferon Signaling Pathways

Implications for Cancer Therapy

Rajani Ravi, PhD and Atul Bedi, MD

INTRODUCTION

Programmed cell death, or apoptosis, enables the physiologic culling of excess cells during embryonic development as well as the selective attrition of cells for tissue remodeling, regeneration, and homeostasis. The vertebrate immune system uses apoptosis to delete lymphocytes with inoperative or auto-reactive receptors from its repertoire, and to reverse clonal expansion at the end of an immune response. Cytotoxic T-lymphocytes and natural killer (NK) cells induce apoptosis of target cells during innate and adaptive immune responses against intracellular pathogens, cancer cells, or transplanted tissues. The altruistic demise of cells in response to cellular stress or injury or genetic errors, serves to preserve genomic integrity and constitutes an important mechanism of tumor surveillance. Given the crucial role of apoptosis in such a diverse array of physiological functions, it is no surprise that aberrations of this process underlie a host of developmental, immune, degenerative, and neoplastic disorders. This appreciation has fuelled frenetic investigation of the molecular determinants and regulatory mechanisms of apoptosis *(1)*. The molecular execution of cell death involves activation of members of a family of cysteine-dependent aspartate-specific proteases (caspases). One mechanism of activating caspases, termed the *extrinsic* pathway, is triggered by engagement of cell surface *death receptors* by their specific ligands *(2)*. In this chapter, we review our current understanding of the molecular determinants of death receptor-induced apoptosis, and identify the key regulators of these death-signaling pathways. We also highlight the enormous promise of targeting death receptors or their regulatory circuits for treatment of human cancers.

From: *Cancer Drug Discovery and Development: Death Receptors in Cancer Therapy*
Edited by: W. S. El-Deiry © Humana Press Inc., Totowa, NJ

DEATH RECEPTORS AND LIGANDS

Death receptors are cell-surface receptors that trigger death signals following engagement with their cognate "death ligands"*(2)*. Death receptor-transduced signals play an instrumental role in "instructive apoptosis," a mechanism that has evolved to enable the deletion of cells in higher metazoans. Death receptors belong to the tumor necrosis factor receptor (TNFR) gene superfamily, whose members have cysteine-rich extracellular domains (CRDs) in their amino-terminal regions *(3)*. The death receptors constitute a subgroup of this family that also possess a homologous cytoplasmic sequence termed the *death domain (4,5)*. The best characterized death receptors are TNFR1 (also called p55 or CD120a) *(3)*, CD95 (also called Fas or Apo1) *(6)*, avian CAR1, death receptor 3 (DR3; also called Apo3, WSL-1, TRAMP, or LARD) *(7–11)*, TRAIL-R1 (also called DR4) *(12)*, TRAIL-R2 (also called DR5, Apo2, TRICK2, or KILLER) *(13–17)*, and DR6 *(18)*. These receptors are activated by ligands of the TNF gene superfamily; TNFR1 is ligated by TNF and lymphotoxin α, CD95 is bound by CD95L (FasL) *(6)*, DR3 interacts with Apo3 ligand (Apo3L, also called TWEAK) *(19,20)*, and TRAIL-R1 and TRAIL-R2 are engaged by Apo2 ligand (Apo2L, also called TNF-related apoptosis inducing ligand [TRAIL]) *(21,22)*.

INDUCTION OF APOPTOSIS BY DEATH RECEPTORS

The Molecular Machinery of Cell Death—Caspases

The molecular machinery of cell death comprises an evolutionarily conserved family of cysteine aspartate proteases (caspases) that execute cell disassembly via cleavage of critical substrates that maintain cytoskeletal and DNA integrity *(23)*. Caspases recognize specific tetrapeptide motifs in their target proteins and cleave their substrates at Asp-Xxx bonds (after aspartic acid residues) *(24)*. At least 14 caspases and more than 100 substrates have been identified *(23)*. Caspases are divided into distinct subfamilies based on their structural and sequence identities and their substrate specificity, determined by the specific pattern of four residues amino-terminal to the cleavage site (the P2–P4 positions). While caspases typically function by inactivating proteins by proteolytic cleavage, they can also, in some cases, activate the target by cleaving off a negative regulatory domain. Caspase-mediated cleavage of key substrates underlies many of the characteristic features of apoptosis, such as nuclear shrinkage *(25,26)*, plasma membrane blebbing *(27–29)*, and internucleosomal DNA fragmentation *(30–32)*. Deficiency of specific caspases or their inhibition can prevent apoptosis in response to diverse death stimuli *(23)*. As such, caspases represent the fundamental executioners of cell death.

Activation of Caspases by Death Receptors

Caspases are synthesized as inactive zymogens that comprise an N-terminal prodomain and two other domains, p20 and p10, which form the active mature enzyme upon cleavage between the p20 and p10 domains as well as between the p20 domain and the prodomain *(23)*. Since these Asp-X cleavage sites correspond to caspase substrate motifs, procaspases can be activated by either previously activated upstream caspases and/or by autocatalytic processing *(24)*. Members of the death receptor family share the same fundamental mechanism(s) of activating caspases and amplifying this enzymatic cascade (Fig. 1). These sequential steps and signaling pathways are dissected below.

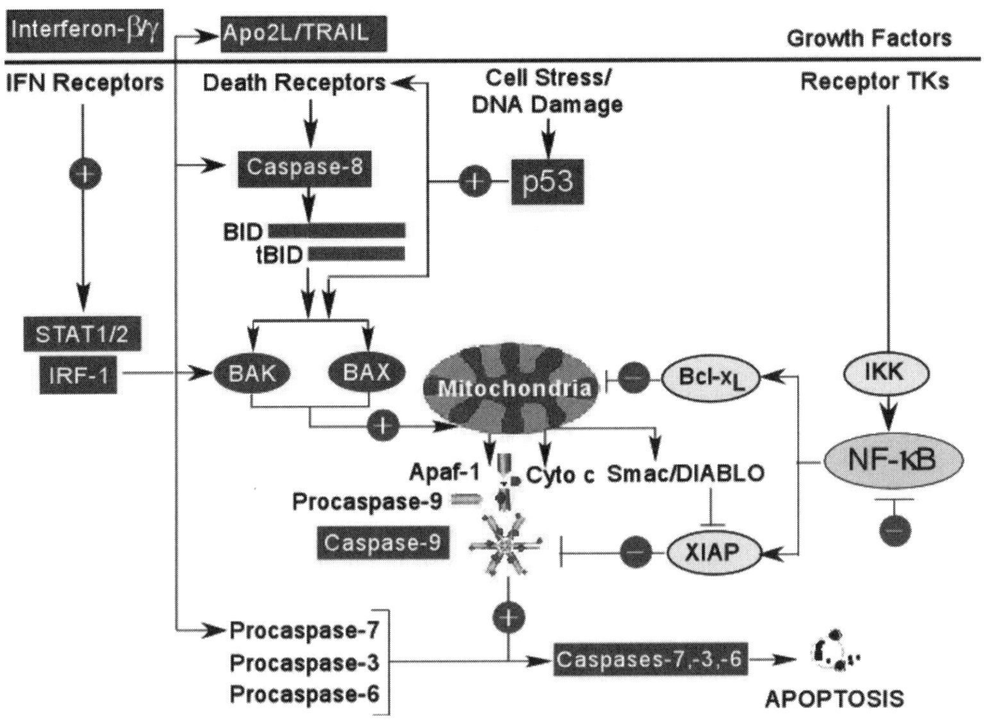

Fig. 1. Schematic representation of the molecular mechanisms and regulation of death receptor-induced apoptosis by NF-κB and interferon-signaling pathways. Ligand-induced trimerization of death receptors facilitates binding of the adaptor protein FADD/MORT1 through homotypic interactions between their death domains. FADD-dependent recruitment of multiple procaspase-8 molecules to the receptor FADD scaffold results in autocatalytic cleavage and cross-activation. Caspase-8 triggers proteolytic activation of caspase-3. Caspase-8 also cleaves and activates BID. The active truncated form of BID (tBID) translocates to the outer mitochondrial membrane, where it binds BAX or BAK. tBID-induced homoligomerization of BAX or BAK leads to mitochondrial disruption and release of pro-death cofactors (cytochrome c, Smac/DIABLO). The interaction of cytochrome c with Apaf-1 results in a nucleotide-dependent conformational change that allows binding and transactivation of procaspase-9. Caspase-9 activates downstream caspases (caspase-3 and caspase-7), thereby promoting apoptosis.

The death receptor-induced signaling pathway is regulated at multiple levels: (1) Decoy receptors interfere with the interaction of death ligands with their cognate death receptors. DcR1/TRAIL-R3 and DcR2/TRAIL-R4 compete with TRAIL-R1/TRAIL-R2 for Apo2L/TRAIL; DcR3 binds to CD95L and competitively inhibits the interaction of CD95 with CD95L. (2) The recruitment and activation of caspase-8 is inhibited by FLICE-inhibitory proteins (FLIPs). (3) Sequestration of tBID by the Bcl-2 homolog Bcl-x_L curtails its ability to promote the allosteric activation of BAX or BAK. (4) Inhibitor of apoptosis proteins (IAPs) inhibit effector caspases (caspase-3, caspase-7, caspase-9, and caspase-6), until they are themselves sequestered by Smac/DIABLO.

Type I (α and β) and type II (γ) interferons engage specific membrane receptors, which, in turn, bind and activate the Janus kinases (JAKs) and the signal transducers and activators of transcription (STATs). STAT1 homodimers, STAT1-2 heterodimers, and members of the interferon regulatory factor (IRF) family, such as IRF-1, promote death receptor–induced apoptosis by inducing death receptors and ligands, as well as expression of components of death receptor signaling pathways (caspases 8, 10, 7, 1, 3, 4, and BAK). In contrast, death receptor signaling is inhibited by NF-κB-mediated expression of multiple anti-apoptotic proteins that interrupt different steps along the death receptor signaling pathway (c-FLIP, Bcl-x_L, and members of the IAP family [c-IAP1, c-IAP2, XIAP]).

Formation of the Death-Inducing Signaling Complex—Activation of the Initiator Caspase-8/FLICE and/or Caspase-10

Death receptors are type I transmembrane proteins containing cytoplasmic sequences, termed *death domains*, that are essential for transduction of the apoptotic signal *(5,33)*. The oligomerization of death receptors by engagement of their cognate ligands results in the rapid assembly of a membrane-bound death-inducing signaling complex (DISC) *(34)*. Ligand-induced trimerization of the CD95/Fas/Apo1 receptor facilitates binding of the adaptor protein FADD (Fas-associated death domain protein; also known as mediator of receptor-induced toxicity [MORT1]) *(35,36)* through homotypic interactions between their death domains *(4,5,33)*. Receptor-bound FADD molecules form higher-order oligomers, or "fibers" *(37)*. FADD also carries a so-called death-effector domain (DED), which in turn, interacts with the analogous DED motifs found in the N-terminal region of the zymogen form of caspase-8 (procaspase-8; also called FLICE or MACH) *(38–40)*. FADD-dependent recruitment and aggregation of multiple procaspase-8 molecules to the receptor/FADD scaffold results in autocatalytic cleavage and cross-activation by induced proximity, thereby releasing active caspase-8 into the cytoplasm *(41–43)*.

Other death receptors activate caspase-8 in a fashion analogous to that of CD95. While death receptors for Apo2L/TRAIL (TRAIL-R1/DR4 and TRAIL-R2/DR5) directly bind FADD, TNF-α-bound TNFR1 binds the adapter molecule TNFR1-associated death-domain protein (TRADD), which in turn recruits FADD to the receptor complex *(44)*. Experiments with FADD gene-knockout mice *(45)* or transgenic mice expressing a dominant-negative mutant of FADD (FADD-DN) in T-cells *(46,47)* have demonstrated that FADD is essential for induction of apoptosis by CD95/Fas, TNFR1, and DR3. However, a similar obligatory role of FADD in apoptosis signaling by Apo2L/TRAIL or its death receptors has not been uniformly observed. Cells from FADD-deficient mice remain susceptible to TRAIL-R1/DR4-induced apoptosis *(48)*, and ectopic expression of FADD-DN failed to block induction of apoptosis by either Apo2L/TRAIL or overexpression of either TRAIL-R1/DR4 or TRAIL-R2/DR5 *(14,15)*. Whereas these studies suggest the existence of a FADD-independent mechanism by which Apo2L/TRAIL activates caspase-8 (perhaps through another adaptor), other conflicting observations indicate that TRAIL-R1/DR4- or TRAIL-R2/DR5-induced apoptosis can be inhibited by transfection of FADD-DN *(16)*. The physiological role of FADD is further supported by Apo2L/TRAIL-dependent recruitment of FADD and caspase-8 to TRAIL-R1/DR4 and TRAIL-R2/DR5 *(49)*. Regardless of the specific mechanism employed to activate caspase-8, experiments with embryonic fibroblasts from caspase-8-deficient mice confirm that caspase-8 is essential for initiation of apoptosis by CD95/Fas, TNFR1, DR3, DR4, and DR5 *(50)*.

In addition to caspase-8, death receptors can also induce recruitment and activation of the structurally related protein caspase-10. In cells with endogenous expression of both caspase-8 and caspase-10, CD95L and Apo2L/TRAIL can recruit either protein to their DISC, where both enzymes are proteolytically activated with similar kinetics *(51)*. Caspase-10 recruitment and cleavage requires the adaptor FADD/MORT1 and DISC assembly. Cells expressing either caspase-8 or caspase-10 can undergo ligand-induced apoptosis, indicating that each caspase can initiate apoptosis independently of the other *(51)*. Thus, apoptosis signaling by death receptors involves not only caspase-8 but also caspase-10, and both caspases may have equally important roles in apoptosis initiation. However, caspase-8 plays an obligatory role in death receptor-induced apoptosis of cell types that do not express caspase-10, such as many cancer cells *(51)*.

Caspase-8-Mediated Activation of Downstream Effector Caspases

In some cell types (termed type I), robust activation of caspase-8 by formation of the DISC results in the direct cleavage and activation of the downstream effector caspase-3, which in turn, cleaves other caspases (such as caspase-6) and vital substrates, leading to the terminal events of apoptosis *(52)*. Such cells can undergo apoptosis via death receptor-induced activation of the caspase cascade independently of the mitochondria. However, experiments with caspase-3 knockout mice indicate that while caspase-3 may serve an important role in internucleosomal DNA fragmentation, it is not required for CD95- or TNF-induced apoptosis *(53)*.

Caspase-8 cleaves and activates BID (p22), a "BH-3 domain only" prodeath member of the Bcl-2 family *(54–58)*. The active truncated form of BID (tBID; p15) translocates to the outer mitochondrial membrane, where it binds and homo-oligomerizes BAX or BAK, two multidomain proapoptotic members of the Bcl-2 family *(59,60)*. tBID-induced homo-oligomerization of BAX or BAK results in an allosteric conformational change that leads to mitochondrial disruption and release of a cocktail of prodeath cofactors (such as cytochrome c, Smac/DIABLO) into the cytoplasm *(56,57)*. The interaction of the released cytochrome c with Apaf-1 results in a nucleotide-dependent conformational change that allows binding of procaspase-9 through N-terminal caspase recruitment domains (CARD) present on both molecules *(61)*. The formation of the procaspase-9/Apaf-1/cytochrome c complex (also called the *apoptosome*) promotes the transcatalytic cleavage and scaffold-mediated transactivation of caspase-9 *(62,63)*. Caspase-9 activates further downstream caspases such as caspase-3 and caspase-7, thereby amplifying the caspase cascade and promoting apoptosis *(64)*. Therefore, BID represents a mechanistic link between death receptor-induced activation of caspase-8 (the extrinsic pathway) and the mitochondrial activation of caspase 9 and 3 (the intrinsic or mitochondrial pathway) *(58)*.

Caspase-8-induced cleavage of BID is instrumental for death receptor-induced apoptosis in certain cell types (termed type II) that show weak DISC formation and therefore depend upon mitochondrial activation of caspase-9 to amplify the caspase cascade *(52)*. Studies with BID-deficient mice indicate that BID is required for CD95-induced apoptosis in hepatocytes, but not in thymocytes or fibroblasts *(65)*. Studies of BAX-deficient, BAK-deficient, or BAX/BAK-deficient mice suggest that BAX and BAK play essential yet mutually redundant roles for death receptor-mediated apoptosis in hepatocytes, but are not required for CD95-induced death of thymocytes or fibroblasts *(66,67)*. While $BAX^{-/-}/BAK^{-/-}$ hepatocytes resist CD95-induced apoptosis, hepatocytes from either $BAX^{-/-}$ or $BAK^{-/-}$ mice remain sensitive to death receptor-induced apoptosis. In contrast, recent studies using colon carcinoma lines that have wild-type BAX and their isogenic BAX-deficient sister clones have demonstrated that BAX may be required for death receptor-induced apoptosis in cancer cells *(68–71)*. These reports indicate that although BAX is dispensable for apical death receptor signals, including activation of caspase-8 and cleavage of BID, it is necessary for mitochondrial activation of caspase-9 and induction of apoptosis in response to Apo2L/TRAIL, CD95/Fas, or TNF-α *(68,69)*. These data suggest that the basal expression of BAK in these cells cannot substitute for BAX in mediating death receptor-induced apoptosis of tumor cells. However, upregulation of BAK expression by exposure to chemotherapeutic agents (e.g., irinotecan) or interferon (IFN)-β/γ, is associated with sensitization of $BAX^{-/-}$ cancer cells to death receptor-induced apoptosis *(69)*. Therefore, tBID may employ BAX or BAK for mitochondrial activation of apoptosis in a cell type- and death signal-specific manner.

Since loss of BAX and BAK confers resistance to death receptor-induced apoptosis, mitochondrial disruption appears to be critical for induction of apoptosis in type II cells. However, activation of the caspase-9/Apaf1 complex and caspase-3 is not the only mechanism by which mitochondrial disruption results in apoptosis *(72)*. Absence of these downstream effectors provides only transient protection from tBID-induced apoptosis. Cells from caspase-$9^{-/-}$, Apaf$^{-/-}$, or caspase-$3^{-/-}$ mice remain viable for 24 h after retroviral expression of tBID, but are killed after 48 h *(72)*. In line with these observations, cells from caspase-$9^{-/-}$ *(73,74)*, Apaf$^{-/-}$ *(75,76)*, or caspase-$3^{-/-}$ *(53,77)* mice remain susceptible to CD95-induced apoptosis. One possible mechanism by which tBID-mediated mitochondrial depolarization can promote death in the absence of either cyto c/Apaf-1/caspase-9 or caspase-3 may involve the activation of redundant effector caspases via release of Smac/DIABLO (second mitochondria-derived activator of caspase). Smac/DIABLO promotes caspase activation by binding and antagonizing members of the inhibitor of apoptosis (IAP) family of proteins *(78,79)*. The human IAP family is comprised of six members, which inhibit the effector caspases 9, 3, and 7 *(64,80,81)*. The mitochondrial release of Smac/DIABLO into the cytoplasm via the caspase-8-BID-BAX/BAK pathway may sequester IAPs and allow activation of multiple effector caspases. The simultaneous activation of multiple redundant effector caspases may explain why deficiency of any single caspase (caspase-9 or caspase-3) is insufficient to block death receptor-induced apoptosis. It is also possible that irreversible damage to the mitochondria may itself be sufficient to induce apoptosis in a caspase-independent manner.

While these observations indicate that mitochondrial disruption via the BID-BAX/BAK pathway is essential for death receptor-induced apoptosis of certain cell types (hepatocytes, cancer cells), embryonic fibroblasts and thymocytes from BID-deficient or BAX/BAK double knockout (DKO) mice remain sensitive to CD95/Fas-induced apoptosis *(66,67)*. The precise reasons for the differential requirement of the cross-talk between the extrinsic and intrinsic pathways in type I and type II cells have yet to be elucidated. These may involve biochemical differences at the receptor level and/or differences in the expression of initiator caspases and/or antiapoptotic proteins that determine the threshold that must be crossed for death receptors to activate downstream caspases.

Potentiation of Death Receptor-Induced Apoptosis by Apoptosis Signal Regulating Kinase (ASK1) and c-Jun Amino Terminal Kinase (JNK)

While there is overwhelming evidence that confirms the requirement of FADD/caspase-8-mediated signaling pathways in death receptor-induced apoptosis, other putative death receptor signaling pathways have also been described. Apoptosis signal-regulating ASK1 is a mammalian MAPKKK that activates SEK1 (or MKK4), which in turn activates stress-activated protein kinase (SAPK, also known as JNK—c-Jun amino-terminal kinase). Overexpression of ASK1 induces apoptotic cell death, and ASK1 is activated in cells treated with TNF-α; TNF-α-induced apoptosis is inhibited by a catalytically inactive form of ASK1 *(82)*. These observations suggest that ASK1 may be a key element in the mechanism of stress- and cytokine-induced apoptosis. ASK1 leads to activation of JNK. However, the role of JNK activation in TNF-α-induced apoptosis is less clear. Experiments using JNK activators or dominant-negative forms of the JNK substrate c-Jun suggest a proapoptotic role of JNK in TNF-α-induced death *(83)*. However, JNK-deficient mouse fibroblasts remain sensitive to TNF-α- or CD95L-induced apoptosis *(84)*. Therefore JNK activation may potentiate death receptor-induced apoptosis, but is not obligatory for this process.

REGULATION OF DEATH RECEPTOR-INDUCED APOPTOSIS

Death receptors play an instrumental role in the physiologic induction of apoptosis during development and tissue turnover in adult animals. However, the unscheduled activation of death receptor-induced signals could lead to inadvertent caspase activation, with devastating consequences for the organism. In order to direct the "instructive" apoptosis of cells without sustaining uncontrolled cell death, death receptor-induced signaling is tightly regulated at multiple levels (Fig. 1). These regulatory mechanisms are described below.

Expression of Death and Decoy Receptors

At the most apical level, death receptor–ligand interactions may be regulated by the tissue-specific or inducible expression of death receptors or their respective ligands. TNFR1 is expressed ubiquitously, while its ligand (TNF) is expressed mainly by activated T-cells and macrophages *(3)*. Likewise, CD95/Fas is widely expressed and its cell-surface expression is elevated by immune activation of lymphocytes or in response to cytokines such as IFNs, TNF, and CD40 ligand *(85,86)*. Expression of CD95 ligand (CD95L) is however restricted to cytotoxic T-cells, NK cells, and antigen-presenting cells (APCs) *(87)*.

Akin to TNFR1 and CD95, the death receptors for Apo2L/TRAIL (DR4/TRAIL-R1 and DR5/TRAIL-R2) are broadly expressed in most organ systems *(2,88)*. However, unlike the restricted pattern of TNF and CD95L expression in immune activated T-cells and APCs, Apo2L/TRAIL mRNA is expressed constitutively in many tissues and transcript levels increase upon stimulation in peripheral blood T-cells *(13,89,90)*. Since several tissues constitutively express both Apo2L and its death receptors, normal cells must employ mechanisms to protect themselves from autocrine or paracrine Apo2L-DR4/DR5 interactions. One such line of defense is provided by expression of a set of decoy receptors (DcRs). DcR1 (also called TRAIL-R3, TRID, or LIT) is a glycosyl phosphatidylinositol (GPI)-anchored cell-surface protein that is structurally related to DR4 and DR5, but lacks a cytoplasmic tail *(12,15,91–94)*. DcR2 (also called TRAIL-R4 or TRUNDD) also resembles DR4 and DR5, but has a truncated cytoplasmic death domain that is only a third as long as that of functional death domains that are capable of transducing apoptotic signals *(95–97)*. The extracellular domains of DcR1 and DcR2 compete with DR4 and DR5 for binding to Apo2L/TRAIL, but cannot initiate death signals in response to ligand engagement. Transfection of Apo2L-sensitive cells with either DcR1 or DcR2 substantially reduces their sensitivity to Apo2L-induced apoptosis. Deletion of the truncated cytoplasmic region of DcR2 does not affect its ability to protect cells from Apo2L-induced death. Enzymatic cleavage of the GPI anchor also results in the sensitization of DcR1-expressing cells to Apo2L-induced apoptosis. These observations indicate that DcR1 and DcR2 may protect normal cells from Apo2L by acting as decoys that compete with TRAIL-R1/TRAIL-R2 for their shared ligand. The expression of decoy receptors provides a potential molecular basis for the relative resistance of normal cells to TRAIL/Apo2L-induced death. In support of this notion, resting peripheral T-cells (which resist Apo2L) exhibit an elevation of DR5 *(13)* and concomitant reduction of DcR1 levels *(94)* when they acquire an Apo2L-sensitive phenotype upon activation by interleukin-2 *(89)*. However, the level of decoy receptors on many tumor cell lines does not always correlate with resistance to Apo2L-induced death *(98)*. Therefore, it is likely that the susceptibility of cells to Apo2L-induced apoptosis must involve additional regulatory mechanisms beyond the ratio of death and decoy receptors.

A third decoy receptor, DcR3, is a secreted soluble protein the binds to CD95L *(99)*. DcR3 competitively inhibits the interaction of CD95 with CD95L, and overexpression of DcR3 inhibits CD95-induced apoptosis *(99)*. DcR3 mRNA is expressed in the spleen, colon, and lung. While its physiologic role remains unclear, the frequent amplification of the DcR3 gene in primary lung and colon cancers may protect tumor cells from CD95L-induced death.

Inhibition of Death Domain Signaling by Silencer of Death Domains (SODD)

The death domains of death receptors (TNFR1, CD95, DR3, DR4, and DR5) can self-associate and bind other death domain-containing proteins. Overexpression of death domain receptors may lead to ligand-independent receptor aggregation and cell death. However, cells are protected from such spontaneous ligand-independent signaling by death receptors via expression of an approx 60-kilodalton protein termed silencer of death domains (SODD) *(100)*. SODD associates with the death domains of TNFR1 and inhibits the intrinsic self-aggregation of the death domain *(100)*. This inhibition is lost by triggering the release of SODD from the death domain in response to cross-linkage of TNFR1 with TNF-α. This allows ligand-dependent recruitment of adapter proteins to form an active signaling complex. However, the duration of TNF signaling is controlled by the rapid dissociation of signaling proteins from TNFR1 and reformation of the TNFR1-SODD complex *(100)*. While SODD interacts with TNFR1 and DR3, other SODD-related proteins may play a similar role in preventing ligand-independent signaling by CD95, DR4, or DR5.

Regulation of Caspase-8 by FLICE-Inhibitory Proteins (FLIPs)

The recruitment and activation of caspases by death receptor engagement can be inhibited by FLICE-inhibitory protein (FLIP; also called I-FLICE, CASH, CLARP, MRIT, or usurpin) *(101–110)*. FLIP contains DEDs that bind to the DED of FADD and the prodomains of procaspases 8 and 10, thereby inhibiting their recruitment to the CD95-FADD or TNFR1-induced activation complex *(105–107,109)*. Enforced expression of v-FLIP (found in γ-herpes and pox viruses) inhibits apoptosis induced by CD95, TNFR1, DR3, and DR4/TRAIL-R1 *(101)*. The equine herpes II virus E8 protein and molluscum contagiosum MC159 and MC160 also contain DEDs homologous to those of procaspase-8, and inhibit its recruitment to the death receptor signaling complex *(103)*.

Multiple spice variants of the human homologs of FLIP have been identified. The longer, more abundant form, $FLIP_L$, has two DEDs and a caspase-like C-terminal domain, but lacks the catalytic cysteine and histidine residues that contribute to substrate binding. The shorter splice variant, $FLIP_S$, consists only of the two DEDs. The effects of cellular FLIPs appear to vary depending on the cellular context. Enforced expression of FLIP (the long splice variant) has an apparently paradoxical proapoptotic effect, possibly mediated by the aggregation of procaspase-8. However, experiments with c-FLIP-deficient mice support an antiapoptotic role of c-FLIP that is analogous to its viral counterparts. Embryonic fibroblasts from c-FLIP-deficient mice are hypersensitive to TNF-α- or CD95/Fas-induced apoptosis *(111)*. Akin to v-FLIP, c-FLIP appears to function as a physiologic inhibitor of death receptor-induced apoptosis via homotypic DED-mediated interactions with FADD and procaspase-8 *(105,107)*. c-FLIP also interacts with TNFR-associated factor (TRAF)2 and receptor-interacting protein (RIP), which are responsible for TNFR1-induced activation of NF-κB and JNK. However, c-FLIP-deficient cells do not exhibit any change in TNF-α-induced activation of NF-κB *(111)*. Conversely, NF-κB activation is required for TNF-α-induced expression of c-FLIP *(112)*. These observations indicate that NF-κB-induced expression of c-FLIP protects cells from death receptor-induced apoptosis by preventing initiation of the caspase cascade.

Regulation of BID Cleavage and Function

Caspase-8-induced cleavage of BID is required for mitochondrial amplification of downstream caspases in response to death receptor engagement in type II cells. Therefore, regulation of BID cleavage or activity is a mechanism of controlling death receptor-induced apoptosis in type II cells. These regulatory mechanisms are described below.

Regulation of BID Phosphorylation and Cleavage by Casein Kinases I and II

BID is cleaved by caspase-8 at Asp 59, which resides in a large flexible loop between the second and third α helices *(55,56)*. This cleavage site is located between the Thr and Ser residues that are phosphorylated by casein kinases I and II (CKI and CKII) *(113)*. CKI exists as monomers of seven isoforms encoded by distinct genes (α, β, γ1, γ2, γ3, Δ, and ε) *(114)*. CKII is an evolutionarily conserved holoenzyme composed of two catalytic α (and/or α') subunits and two regulatory β subunits *(114)*. Phosphorylation of BID by CKI and CKII has been reported to render BID resistant to caspase-8-mediated cleavage *(113)*. Conversely, a mutant of BID that cannot be phosphorylated at these residues is apparently more sensitive to caspase-8-induced cleavage and more effective than wild-type BID in promoting apoptosis. Consistent with these observations, activation of CKI and CKII reportedly delays CD95/Fas-induced apoptosis, whereas CK inhibitors potentiate death receptor-induced apoptosis *(113)*. While these observations suggest that the protection conferred by CKs is mediated by phosphorylation of BID, CKs may also activate NF-κB-mediated expression of survival proteins that regulate the caspase-8-BID-BAX/BAK death pathway.

Sequestration of BID by Bcl-x_L—Competition With BAX or BAK

BH-3 domain-only members of the Bcl-2 family, such as BID, absolutely require multidomain members of the Bcl-2 family (BAX, BAK) to induce apoptosis. Antiapoptotic members of the Bcl-2 family, such as Bcl-x_L, heterodimerize with BAX or BAK, as well as BID *(72)*. While mutants of Bcl-x_L that cannot bind either BAX or BAK (bearing F131V or D133A substitutions) remain capable of protecting cells from death receptor-induced apoptosis, Bcl-x_L mutants that fail to bind BID (bearing G138E, R139L, and I140N substitutions) are unable to inhibit apoptosis *(72)*. These observations support a model in which antiapoptotic Bcl-2 family members, such as Bcl-x_L, sequester tBID in stable mitochondrial complexes, thereby curtailing its ability to promote the allosteric activation of BAX or BAK. In this scenario, proapoptotic multidomain members (BAX,

BAK) compete with antiapoptotic members (Bcl-2, Bcl-x_L) for binding to tBID to regulate the mitochondrial disruption and efflux required for the terminal events of apoptosis.

IAPs—Sequestration of Smac/DIABLO and Inhibition of Caspases

Caspases are directly regulated by interactions with IAPs. At least five mammalian homologs of the baculovirus IAP have been identified. Four of these (c-IAP1, c-IAP2, XIAP, and NAIP) consist of an N-terminal domain containing multiple copies of a so-called baculovirus IAP repeat (BIR) motif *(115)*, and a C-terminal zinc-containing protein-protein interaction domain (RING finger) *(116)*. The fifth member (Survivin) contains only the BIR domain. XIAP (X chromosome linked IAP; also known as hILP), c-IAP1, and c-IAP2 (but not NAIP) directly bind and inhibit effector caspases, such as caspase-3 and caspase-7 *(80,117)*. In addition, they also prevent activation of procaspase-9 and procaspase-6 by upstream signals *(64)*. XIAP inhibits caspase-3 and caspase-7 via its second BIR domain and BH2-terminal linker *(118)*, and prevents activation of procaspase-9 through a region containing its third BIR domain (BIR3) *(119)*. The BIR2 region facilitates caspase-binding, and the NH2-terminal linker directly blocks the catalytic cleft of caspase-3 and caspase-7 *(108,120,121)*. Consistent with its ability to inhibit multiple effector caspases, overexpression of XIAP can inhibit TNF-α- or Apo2L/TRAIL-induced apoptosis *(122)*. While these direct interactions with caspases may be responsible for the antiapoptotic effects of IAPs, c-IAP1 and c-IAP2 also interact with the TNFR1-associated proteins, TRAF1 and TRAF2 via their BIR domains *(123)*. Therefore, although cIAPs do not directly interact with caspase-8, it is possible their recruitment to the TNFR1 signaling complex via an interaction with TRAF2 may regulate caspase-8 activation and/or TRAF-dependent signaling. Consistent with this scenario, expression of c-IAP1 or c-IAP2 alone was not sufficient to reduce cellular sensitivity to TNF-α-induced death; however, the expression of both c-IAP1 and c-IAP2, coupled with TRAF1 and TRAF2, suppresses TNF-α-induced apoptosis *(124)*.

The basal expression of mammalian IAPs vary in different cell types in response to cytokines, such as TNF-α. As shall be discussed below, TNF-α-induced expression of c-IAP1, c-IAP2, and XIAP is dependent upon the NF-κB transcription factor *(124,125)*. In these physiologic situations, IAPs may serve to keep caspases in check until they are themselves sequestered and antagonized by the mitochondrial efflux of Smac/DIABLO in response to death signals. However, the constitutively high expression of IAPs in many different types of tumor cells may render such cells abnormally resistant to death receptor-induced apoptosis *(126)*.

DYNAMIC BALANCE BETWEEN DEATH RECEPTOR SIGNALS AND APOPTOSIS INHIBITORS

The activation of caspases by death receptor-induced signals is held in check by the antiapoptotic proteins described under the subheading "Regulation of Death Receptor-Induced Apoptosis." While this serves to prevent unscheduled or uncontrolled cell death, the induction of apoptosis in response to physiologic death signals requires mechanisms to circumvent or overcome these antiapoptotic proteins. Without such mechanisms, the failure of death receptor-induced apoptosis would disrupt homeostasis and result in immune and neoplastic disorders. The dynamic balance between the antagonistic functions of death receptor signals and antiapoptotic proteins ensures that death receptor-induced apoptosis is allowed to proceed in a signal-dependent, scheduled, and controlled fashion. The relative expression of death-signaling proteins and the survival proteins that counteract their activity is, in turn, governed by specific transcription factors. While the NF-κB/Rel family induces survival proteins that hold death receptor signals in check, this balance is tipped in favor of instructive apoptosis via induction of death receptors/ligands/ signaling proteins by IFN-responsive transcription factors and the p53 tumor suppressor. The induction of cell death is further augmented via caspase-mediated proteolysis of many of the key proteins that inhibit death receptor-induced apoptosis.

Inhibition of Death Receptor-Induced Apoptosis by NF-κB

While each of the regulatory mechanism(s) described under the subheading "Regulation of Death Receptor-Induced Apoptosis" serve to interrupt specific steps along the death receptor-induced signaling pathway, the master regulator responsible for orchestrating the coordinated control of death receptor-induced apoptosis is NF-κB, a family of heterodimeric transcription factors (Rel proteins) that plays an important role in determining lymphocyte survival during immune, inflammatory, and stress responses *(127–136)*. Mammals express five Rel proteins that belong to two classes *(137,138)*. Members of one group (RelA, c-Rel, and RelB) are synthesized as mature proteins, while the other (encoded by *NFkb1* and *NFkb2*) includes precursor proteins (p105 and p100, respectively) that undergo proteolysis to yield their mature products (p50 and p52 NF-κB proteins).

NF-κB dimers containing RelA or c-Rel are held in an inactive cytoplasmic complex with inhibitory proteins, the IκBs. Phosphorylation of IκBs at two critical serine residues (Ser^{32} and Ser^{36} in IκBα, Ser^{19} and Ser^{23} in IκBβ) in their N-terminal regulatory domain by the IKK complex targets them for rapid ubiquitin-mediated proteasomal degradation *(137)*. IKK is a multisubunit protein kinase consisting of two catalytic subunits, IKKα and IKKβ, which phosphorylate IκB, and a regulatory subunit, IKKγ (also called NEMO, NF-κB essential modifier/modulator, or IKKAP1), which is required for activation of IKKα/IKKβ heterodimers in response to proinflammatory cytokines, such as TNF-α and interleukin (IL)-1. The C-terminus of IKKγ subunit serves as a docking site for upstream signals, and the N-terminal half of IKKγ (minus the first 100 amino acids) binds to IKKβ. This results in phosphorylation of specific conserved serine residues (S177 and S181) within the T-loop (activation domain) in the catalytic domain of IKKβ. Activation of the canonical NF-κB pathway involving degradation of IκB is mostly dependent on the IKKβ subunit, and is essential for innate immunity *(132,139–141)*. A second pathway is involved in activation of the NF-κB dimer between RelB and p52 *(142)*. RelB is held in an inactive cytoplasmic complex by NF-κB2p100 until IKKα-dependent degradation of the IκB-like COOH-terminus of p100 allows the release and nuclear translocation of the active RelB/p52 dimer *(142)*. The activation of the RelB/p52 dimer by proteolytic processing is important for lymphoid organ development and the adaptive immune response *(143)*. In addition to the release and nuclear translocation of the dimer, transcriptional induction of target genes by NF-κB requires phosphorylation of Rel proteins by serine/ threonine kinases, such as casein kinase II and Akt *(144–147)*.

Role of NF-κB in Protection of Cells From Death Receptor-Induced Apoptosis

Targeted disruption of the RelA subunit of NF-κB or either IKKβ or IKKγ/NEMO results in embryonic death of mice as a result of massive hepatic (liver) apoptosis *(139,148,149)*. $RelA^{-/-}$ fibroblasts, unlike their wild-type ($RelA^{+/+}$) counterparts, exhibit a profound sensitivity to TNF-α-induced apoptosis *(133)*. Likewise, IKKβ$^{-/-}$ fibroblasts, or cells stably transfected with phosphorylation mutants of IκBα fail to activate NF-κB and display increased sensitivity to TNF-α-induced death *(132,135,141)*. These observations demonstrate an important role of NF-κB in protecting cells from death receptor-induced apoptosis.

Engagement of TNFR1 by TNF leads to the recruitment of the adapter protein TRADD to the clustered death domains of the trimerized receptors. TRADD, in turn, serves as a platform for the docking of multiple signaling molecules to the activated receptor complex. As discussed earlier, TNF-induced apoptosis is triggered by recruitment of the adapter molecule FADD to the TNFR1-TRADD complex. Therefore, the apoptotic signaling pathways triggered by different members of the death receptor family (TNFR1, CD95/Fas, and TRAIL-R1/R-2) are all initiated by ligand-induced recruitment of FADD and FADD-mediated activation of caspase-8. While they share a common death-signaling pathway, these receptors exhibit a differential ability to activate NF-κB. While FasL is unable to activate NF-κB, TNF-α-induces activation of the transcription factors, NF-κB and JNK/AP1, via recruitment of receptor-interacting protein (RIP) and (TRAF2) to the receptor complex. TRAF2 and RIP activate the NF-κB-inducing kinase (NIK), which in turn activates the IKK and IKKβ-dependent activation of NF-κB *(150–152)*. TRAF2 and RIP also stimulate JNK/AP-1 via activation of apoptosis signal regulating kinase (ASK)1 *(153)*. Cells from TRAF2 gene knockout mice or transgenic mice expressing a dominant-negative TRAF2 mutant fail to activate JNK in response to TNF, but have only slight defects in TNF-induced activation of NF-κB *(154,155)*. In contrast, RIP-deficient cells remain capable of activating JNK but lack the ability to activate NF-κB in response to TNF *(150)*. Therefore, RIP is essential for TNF-induced activation of NF-κB while TRAF2 is required for signaling the activation of JNK. In addition to inducing expression of diverse proinflammatory and immunomodulatory genes, NF-κB promotes the expression of genes that protect cells from TNF-induced apoptosis (discussed in the next section). Because the proapoptotic activity of TNF-α is opposed by the concurrent expression of antiapoptotic NF-κB target genes, the ability of TNF-α to induce apoptosis requires the inhibition of NF-κB. The differential ability to activate NF-κB may explain why TNF-α, unlike FasL, rarely triggers apoptosis unless new protein synthesis is simultaneously blocked *(156)*.

In addition to protecting cells from the latent death-signaling arm of TNFR1, TNF-α-induced activation of NF-κB promotes the expression of a host of proinflammatory and immunomodulatory genes that mediate the biological function of this cytokine. In the absence of the protection conferred by NF-κB, TNF-α loses its native function in the immune response, and instead acquires a proapoptotic role. The mid-gestational lethality of RelA$^{-/-}$, IKKβ$^{-/-}$, or IKKγ$^{-/-}$ mice results from the extensive hepatocyte apoptosis induced by the production of TNF-α by hematopoietic progenitors that are resident in the fetal liver. The massive liver apoptosis resulting from embryonic deficiency of RelA is completely reversed by the concurrent deficiency of TNFR1 or TNF-α in double knockout mice *(129,157,158)*. NF-κB also protects lymphoid cells from death receptor-induced apoptosis during the immune response *(159)*. Activation of NF-κB by co-stimulation of lymphocytes mediates cell survival and clonal proliferation, while inhibition of NF-κB by IκB mutants promotes activation-induced apoptosis of T-cells, and loss of CD8^{+} T-cells in the thymus. As such, NF-κB-mediated protection of cells from death receptor-induced apoptosis plays an instrumental role in regulating the immune response. As discussed later, the constitutive activation of NF-κB by diverse growth factors, cytokines, or genetic aberrations also protect tumor cells from Apo2L/TRAIL; conversely, such tumors may be sensitized to Apo2L/TRAIL by agents that inhibit NF-κB.

Molecular Mechanisms by Which NF-κB Regulates Death Receptor-Induced Apoptosis

NF-κB is a critical determinant of the expression of genes that modulate death receptor-induced apoptosis. NF-κB promotes the expression of a number of survival factors, including c-FLIP, members of the IAP family (c-IAP1, c-IAP2, XIAP), TRAF1 and TRAF2, and the Bcl-2 homologs, A1 (also known as Bfl-1) and Bcl-x_L. As discussed above, these proteins serve to interrupt different steps along the death receptor signaling pathway. By inducing the concurrent expression of multiple antiapoptotic proteins, NF-κB exerts a multipronged inhibition of death receptor signals (Fig. 1).

c-FLIP is an NF-κB-inducible protein (encoded by *Cflar*) that prevents death receptor-induced activation of the initiator procaspase-8 *(105,111)*. NF-κB activation is required for TNF-α-induced expression of c-FLIP *(112)*. Although TNF-α-induced induction of c-FLIP is repressed by a degradation-resistant mutant of IκBα, c-FLIP can still be induced by TNF-α in RelA$^{-/-}$ cells *(111)*. Therefore, the identity of the NF-κB dimer responsible for promoting c-FLIP expression remains unknown.

The promoter of the *cIap2* gene contains two functional κB sites *(160)*. Induction of *c-Iap2* by TNF-α is blocked by introduction of a phosphorylation mutant form of IκBα that resists IKK-induced degradation *(124)*. Akin to c-IAP2, c-IAP1 and XIAP are also NF-κB-induced proteins that block the activation of caspases (-3, -7, and -9) by death receptors *(161)*. cIAPs cannot directly interact with procaspase-8, and expression of either protein alone is not sufficient to protect cells from TNF-α-induced death *(124)*. Therefore, the recruitment of cIAPs to the TNFR1 signaling complex via interactions with TRAF2 may be required for inhibition of caspase-8 and proximal blockade of the death signal *(124,162)*. TRAF1 and TRAF2 are also NF-κB-inducible genes, which, along with c-IAP1 and c-IAP2, suppress TNF-α-induced activation of caspase-8. Since TRAF2 also serves as an adaptor that augments TNF-α-induced activation of NF-κB, TRAF2 and NF-κB may participate in a positive feedback loop to prevent TNF-α-induced apoptosis. Consistent with this notion, cells from TRAF2$^{-/-}$ mice are partially defective in TNF-α-induced NF-κB activation and exhibit exaggerated sensitivity to TNF-α-induced apoptosis *(154,155)*. Akin to cIAPs, XIAP serves to protect cells from Apo2L/TRAIL-induced apoptosis until it is sequestered and antagonized by the mitochondrial efflux of Smac/DIABLO in response to death signals. The prototypic antiapoptotic member of the Bcl-2 family, Bcl-x_L, contains a κB DNA site (TTTACTGCCC; 298/+22) in its promoter *(163)*. The Rel-dependent induction of Bcl-x_L in response to TNF-α is sufficient to protect cells carrying a degradation-resistant form of IκB from TNF-α-induced death *(163)*. Likewise, NF-κB-dependent expression of Bcl-x_L in response to co-stimulatory signals (CD40-CD40L or CD28-B7 interactions) serves to protects B- or T-lymphocytes from CD95/Fas- or Apo2L/TRAIL-induced apoptosis *(163,164)* .

Bfl-1/A1 is a hematopoietic-specific Bcl-2 homolog that contains a functional κB site in its promoter and is induced in an NF-κB-dependent fashion in response to TNF-α *(165)*. Overexpression of A1 partially protects Rel-deficient cells from TNF-α-induced apoptosis *(165)*. Since $A1^{-/-}$ mice exhibit only increased neutrophil apoptosis, it is likely that A1 is dispensable for the antiapoptotic function of NF-κB in all other tissue types *(166)*.

NF-κB may also protect cells from death receptor-induced apoptosis by attenuating expression of the proapoptotic protein BAX *(167)*. In certain cell types, inhibition of NF-κB by a degradation-resistant mutant of IκBα results in increased *Bax* promoter activity and expression of BAX. Although the *Bax* promoter has a κB site that binds Rel proteins, it is not required for NF-κB-mediated inhibition of BAX expression. Therefore, NF-κB may increase BAX expression via an indirect mechanism. One possibility is that NF-κB may repress stimulation of the *Bax* promoter by interfering with the function of the *p53* tumor suppressor gene. While the precise molecular mechanism remains unclear, the reduced expression of BAX may contribute to the resistance of cells with constitutive activation of NF-κB to death receptor-induced apoptosis. As discussed earlier, targeted loss of the *Bax* gene renders cancer cells resistant to CD95L, TNF-α, and Apo2L/TRAIL-induced apoptosis *(68–70)*. Since NF-κB is constitutively activated by diverse genetic aberrations in human cancers, NF-κB-mediated repression of BAX may play a role in protecting tumor cells from death receptor–ligand interactions *(68)*.

Finally, NF-κB also induces expression of a JNK inhibitor *(168–170)*. TNF-α-induced activation of JNK occurs transiently in normal cells but is increased and prolonged in IKKβ- or RelA-deficient cells *(168)*. Although the identity of the NF-κB-induced JNK inhibitor remains unclear, the identified candidates include XIAP and the GADD45β protein *(168,169)*. Ectopic expression of GADD45β abrogates TNF-α-induced activation of JNK and rescues $RelA^{-/-}$ cells from TNF-α-induced apoptosis. Although the suppression of JNK may contribute to the antiapoptotic function of NF-κB, JNK is not an essential mediator of death receptor-induced apoptosis.

These observations suggest that NF-κB inhibits death receptor-induced apoptosis by concomitant induction of multiple survival genes as well as repression or inactivation of proapoptotic genes.

Sensitization of Cells to Death Receptor-Induced Apoptosis by IFNs (JAKs/STATs and Interferon Regulatory Factors [IRFs])

The IFN family of cytokines plays an instrumental role in antiviral, immunomodulatory, and antitumor responses *(171)*. Type I (α and β) and type II (γ) IFNs engage specific membrane receptors, which, in turn, bind and activate the Janus kinases (JAKs) and the signal transducers and activators of transcription (STATs) via phosphorylation of specific tyrosine residues *(172)*. Four mammalian JAKs and seven STATs have been identified *(173)*. Following their activation by JAKs, STATs form homo- or heterodimers via phosphotyrosine-Src homology region 2 (SH2) interactions. STAT dimers drive gene expression by binding gamma-activated sequence (GAS) elements in target genes. STAT1 homodimers and STAT1-2 heterodimers also bind p48, a member of the interferon regulatory factor (IRF) family, to form trimers (e.g., the STAT1-2-p48 trimer, termed IFN-stimulated gene factor 3 [ISGF3]) that bind IFN-stimulated regulatory elements (ISREs) and drive the expression of most IFNα/β- and a few IFN-γ-stimulated target genes. Nearly all cell types express IFN-γ receptors, which mediate IFN-γ-dependent recruitment and activation of STAT1 homodimers. Cells from mice with targeted disruption of STAT1 are incapable of responding to IFN-γ (and in many cases to IFN-α/β), display diminished steady-state levels of procaspases, and are less sensitive to various apoptotic signals *(174)*. Another IFN-responsive transcription factor, IFN regulatory factor (IRF)-1, also promotes caspase gene expression and apoptosis *(175)*. While DNA damage-induced apoptosis of resting T-cells and thymocytes is dependent on the function of the *p53* tumor suppressor gene, IRF-1 mediates p53-independent death of activated T-cells in response to DNA damage *(175)*. While p53 upregulates BAX, IFN-γ induces p53-independent IRF-1-mediated expression of BAK, another proapoptotic member of the Bcl-2 family *(176)*. These findings suggest that the STAT1/IRF-1 pathway is involved in IFN-mediated sensitization of cells to apoptosis (Fig. 1).

IFNs (β- and γ) increase the sensitivity of various tumor cell lines to apoptosis in response to TNF-α, CD95L, or Apo2L/TRAIL. The molecular mechanisms by which IFNs promote death receptor-induced apoptosis include the induction of death receptors and ligands, as well as expression of components of death receptor signaling pathways. IFN-γ induces expression of death receptors (CD95, TNFR1, and TRAIL-R2/DR5) and dramatically enhances expression of several procaspases, including caspase-8, caspase-10, and caspase-7 *(176)*. IFN-γ also induces less significant increases in levels of caspase-1, caspase-3, and caspase-4. In addition, IFN-γ induces expression of BAK *(176)*. Akin to IFN-γ, IFN-β promotes expression of caspases 8 and 7, and sensitizes cells to TNF-, CD95L-, or Apo2L/TRAIL-induced apoptosis. IFN-β also induces expression of Apo2L/TRAIL, and conversely, Apo2L/TRAIL induces IFN-β and IFN-responsive genes *(177)*. IFN-β also induces X-linked inhibitor of apoptosis-associated factor-1 (XAF1), a XIAP-interacting proapoptotic protein that augments Apo2L/TRAIL-induced apoptosis *(178)*. The molecular cross-talk and functional synergy between Apo2L/TRAIL and IFNs indicate that tumor cells may be sensitized to CD95L- or Apo2L/TRAIL-induced apoptosis by pretreatment with IFNs. Indeed, even BAX-deficient or p53-deficient cancer cells are rendered susceptible to CD95L- or Apo2L/TRAIL-induced apoptosis by IFN-induced upregulation of caspase-8 and BAK (Ravi, R., and Bedi, A; unpublished observations). The ability of IFNs to prime cells for death ligand-induced apoptosis is important for the antiviral and antitumor function of CD8+ or CD4+ T-cells and NK cells *(179–186)*.

Augmentation of Death Receptor Signaling by Caspase-Mediated Cleavage of Antiapoptotic Proteins

Because immune activation and clonal lymphoid expansion must be followed by cellular demise to preserve homeostasis, the immune system must employ molecular mechanisms to couple immune activation (and expression of survival proteins) with the induction of death receptors that mediate the decay of the immune response. Cell-surface expression of CD95/Fas is elevated by immune activation of lymphocytes or in response to cytokines such as IFN-γ, TNF, and CD40 ligand (CD40L) *(86,187)*. Likewise, immune activation of lymphocytes results in an elevation of DR5 *(13)* and concomitant reduction of DcR1 levels *(94)*. Once the induced death receptors are engaged, their signaling is amplified by caspase-induced proteolytic cleavage of several key antiapoptotic proteins, including NF-κB and NF-κB-induced survival proteins. The proteins targeted by caspases and the functional effects of their cleavage are described below.

Inactivation of NF-κB by Caspase-Mediated Proteolysis—Loss of Survival Gene Expression

The proteins responsible for mediating TNF-α-induced activation of NF-κB are themselves substrates of caspases. Caspase-8-mediated cleavage of RIP at Asp^{32} destroys its ability to activate IKK *(188)*. In addition to inhibiting NF-κB activation, the NH_2-terminal-deficient fragment (RIPc) generated by such cleavage promotes the assembly of the TNFR1-TRADD-FADD complex and potentiates TNF-α-induced apoptosis *(188)*. Proteolysis of TRAF1 and TRAF2 also results in increased sensitivity to death receptor-induced apoptosis *(189–191)*. Caspase-8-mediated cleavage of TRAF1 at Asp^{163} during TNF-α- or CD95L-induced apoptosis generates a COOH-terminal fragment that inhibits TRAF2- or TNFR1-mediated activation of NF-κB *(191)*. Since the truncated protein contains a TRAF domain, it may act as a dominant-negative inhibitor of interactions of TRAF1 with either TRAF2 or cIAPs *(192)*.

IKKβ, the catalytic subunit responsible for the canonical pathway of NF-κB activation, is itself inactivated by caspase-3-mediated proteolysis (at Asp^{78}, Asp^{214}, Asp^{373}, and Asp^{546}) during TNF-α- or CD95-induced apoptosis *(193)*. Expression of the IKKβ(1-546) fragment inhibits endogenous IKK and sensitizes cells to TNF-α-induced apoptosis *(193)*. Conversely, overexpression of a caspase-resistant mutant of IKKβ promotes the sustained activation of NF-κB and prevents TNF-α-induced apoptosis. Therefore, caspase-mediated cleavage of IKKβ may be a mechanism by which caspases terminate the activation of NF-κB and remove the key obstacle to their own activity. Caspases may also achieve this end by proteolytic removal of the NH_2-terminal domain (containing the Ser^{32} and Ser^{36} phosphorylation residues) of IκBα, thereby generating a IκB fragment that is resistant to TNF-α-induced degradation and functions as a super-repressor of NF-κB activation *(194,195)*.

While caspases may prevent activation of NF-κB via proteolytic inactivation of the upstream signals (described above), ligation of death receptors can directly induce caspase-mediated cleavage of RelA *(196)*. The truncation of the transactivation domain generates a transcriptionally inactive dominant-negative fragment of RelA that serves as an efficient proapoptotic feedback mechanism between caspase activation and NF-κB inactivation *(197)*.

These observations suggest that the protection conferred by NF-κB against death receptor-induced apoptosis may be eliminated by caspase-mediated proteolysis of the RIP/TRAF-IKK-IκBα-RelA pathway, thereby tilting the dynamic balance between death receptors and NF-κB-induced survival proteins in favor of cell death. The direct cleavage of RelA ensures the irreversible loss of NF-κB activity, resulting in the rapid amplification of caspase activity and inevitable cell death.

Caspase-Mediated Cleavage of Bcl-2, Bcl-x_L, and IAPs—Amplification of Caspase Activity

Many of the key antiapoptotic proteins that inhibit caspases, are themselves targets of caspases. Antiapoptotic members of the Bcl-2 family (Bcl-2, Bcl-x_L) compete with proapoptotic multidomain members (BAX, BAK) for binding to tBID. As such, Bcl-2 and Bcl-x_L inhibit tBID-mediated activation of BAX/BAK, thereby limiting mitochondrial disruption. However, both Bcl-2 and Bcl-x_L are themselves substrates for caspases. The loop domain of Bcl-2 is cleaved at Asp^{34} by caspase-3 in vitro, in cells overexpressing caspase-3, and during induction of apoptosis by death receptors (CD95/Fas, TRAIL-R1/R2) *(164,198)*. Death receptor-induced caspase-mediated proteolytic cleavage of Bcl-2 inactivates its survival function by removal of the BH4 domain. The carboxy-terminal Bcl-2 cleavage product, which retains the BH3 homology and transmembrane regions, behaves as a BAX-like death effector and potentiates apoptosis *(198)*. Cleavage of Bcl-2 contributes to amplification of the caspase cascade, and cleavage-resistant mutants of Bcl-2 confer increased protection against apoptosis. Akin to Bcl-2, Bcl-x_L is cleaved by caspases during induction of apoptosis by diverse stressful stimuli *(199,200)*. Likewise, proteolytic cleavage converts Bcl-x_L into two prodeath fragments. However, it is not yet known whether Bcl-x_L is cleaved during death receptor-induced apoptosis or whether cleavage-resistant mutants of Bcl-x_L offer better protection against death receptor-induced apoptosis. Akin to Bcl-2 family members, both c-IAP1 and XIAP are also caspase substrates *(119,201)*. Overexpression of the caspase-induced cleavage product of c-IAP1 induces apoptosis *(201)*. Likewise, caspase-induced cleavage of XIAP at Asp^{24} generates a COOH-terminal fragment that potentiates CD95-induced apoptosis *(119)*. These observations suggest that caspase-induced proteolysis of critical survival proteins may serve to rapidly amplify the caspase cascade, thereby potentiating death receptor-induced apoptosis.

DEATH RECEPTOR-INDUCED APOPTOSIS OF TUMOR CELLS

Role of Death Receptors/Ligands in Tumor Surveillance

Induction of Cell Death by Cytotoxic T-Cells and NK Cells

Mature $CD8^+$ T-lymphocytes (cytotoxic T-lymphocytes; CTLs) and natural killer (NK) cells are effectors of innate and adaptive immune responses against intracellular pathogens, cancer cells, or transplanted tissues. CTLs and NK cells induce apoptosis of these targets by two major mechanisms. One mechanism involves ligation of CD95 on target cells by FasL expressed on CTLs *(87)*. The second mechanism involves calcium-dependent exocytosis of CTL-derived granule proteins, perforin, and granzymes *(202,203)*. Perforin facilitates the delivery of granzyme B into target cells via an as yet obscure mechanism that does not require plasma membrane pore formation *(204,205)*. Granzyme B, the prototypic member of this family of serine proteases, induces cleavage and activation of multiple caspases, including caspase-3, -6, -7, -8, -9, and -10 *(206)*. Granzyme B also cleaves BID at a site distinct from that targeted by caspase-8 *(207)*. Akin to tBID (generated by caspase-8), the truncated BID generated by granzyme B (gtBID) translocates to the mitochondrial membrane and promotes the release of mitochondrial death factors via BAX or BAK *(207–209)*. Since granzyme B and CD95L can both activate the BID-BAX/BAK death-signaling pathway, they provide independent mechanisms of inducing target cell apoptosis. Accordingly, cells deficient in CD95 or overexpressing c-FLIP remain susceptible to CTL-induced death *(210)*. It will be important to determine whether interruption of a distal step of the death-signaling pathway shared by CD95L and granzyme B (such as loss of BAX/BAK or overexpression of Bcl-x_L) reduces CTL-induced death of type II target cells that require cross-talk between the extrinsic and intrinsic pathways to undergo apoptosis. Such genetic impediments to CTL-induced death may be an important mechanism by which tumor cells could evade immune surveillance.

Death receptor–ligand interactions may serve a critical physiologic function in tumor surveillance *(211)*. NK cells play a pivotal role in the control of tumor metastasis *(212,213)*. Freshly isolated murine liver NK cells, but not natural killer T-cells or ordinary T-cells, constitutively express cell-surface Apo2L/TRAIL, which, together with perforin and Fas ligand (FasL), mediate NK cell-dependent suppression of experimental liver metastasis of tumor cells *(214)*. Administration of neutralizing monoclonal antibodies against either Apo2L/TRAIL or FasL significantly increases hepatic metastases of several tumor cell lines. While inhibition of perforin-mediated killing also inhibits NK-mediated cytotoxicity *(215)*, complete inhibition is achieved only with the combination of anti-TRAIL and anti-FasL antagonistic antibodies *(214)*. Endogenously produced IFN-γ plays a critical role in inducing Apo2L/TRAIL expression in NK cells and T-cells *(180)*. These findings suggest that Apo2L/TRAIL and FasL may contribute to the natural suppression of tumors by NK cells. Expression of FasL in cells other than NK cells might also contribute to tumor suppression *(216)*.

Establishment of Zones of Immune Privilege

Immune-privileged sites such as the eye, brain, and testes may evade damage by constitutively expressing CD95L to counterattack and eliminate CD95-expressing infiltrating lymphocytes *(217)*. Some reports suggest that expression of CD95L by certain types of cancer cells may protect such tumors from immune surveillance. While ectopic expression of FasL by gene transfer can confer immune privilege on some tissues, it can also induce a granulocytic infiltrate and increased rejection in tissue transplants. The role of CD95L-CD95 interactions in the creation of zones of immune privilege in tumors or tissue allografts in vivo remains debatable *(217)*.

Involvement of Death Receptors in Response of Tumor Cells to Anticancer Therapy

The response of cancer cells to chemotherapeutic agents and γ-radiation involves induction of apoptosis in response to the inflicted cellular damage *(218)*. The ability of anticancer agents to induce tumor cell apoptosis is influenced by a host of oncogenes and tumor suppressor genes that regulate cell-cycle checkpoints and death-signaling pathways. The *p53* tumor suppressor gene is a key determinant of these responses *(219,220)*. Phosphorylation-induced stabilization of p53 in response to cellular damage plays a pivotal role in mediating cell-cycle arrest as well as apoptosis. The particular response elicited by p53 depends on the cell type and context, as well as the presence of co-existing genetic aberrations. The induction of apoptosis by p53 involves multiple and apparently redundant mechanisms *(221)*. p53 can directly activate the mitochondrial death pathway by inducing the expression of specific target genes, such as *Noxa (222)*, *PUMA (223)*, *BAX (224)*, or *BAK (225,226)*. p53 may also promote cell death by inhibiting the transcriptional activity of NF-κB *(227–229)*, thereby repressing NF-κB-dependent expression of a host of survival genes. These observations indicate that p53-induced death is mediated by multiple redundant pathways leading to mitochondrial activation of Apaf-1/caspase-9. In support of this notion, cells from caspase-$9^{-/-}$ mice are highly resistant to chemotherapeutic drugs and irradiation *(73)*. Accordingly, inhibition of this mitochondrial pathway by overexpression of Bcl-2 *(230)* or inactivation of *Bax (231)* can also render tumor cells resistant to anticancer drugs or γ-radiation.

DNA damage also promotes the expression of death receptors CD95 *(232)* and DR5/TRAIL-R2 *(233)*. Although p53 promotes their DNA damage-induced expression, death receptors are not essential for DNA damage-induced apoptosis. Cells from CD95-deficient (*lpr*), CD95L-deficient (*gld*), FADD$^{-/-}$, or caspase-8$^{-/-}$ mice are resistant to death receptor-induced signals, but remain sensitive to chemotherapy and irradiation-induced apoptosis *(234–236)*. Likewise, overexpression of FLIP prevents tumor cell apoptosis by death receptors, but not by chemotherapeutic agents or γ-radiation *(210)*. Conversely, cells from *p53*$^{-/-}$ mice resist DNA damage-induced apoptosis, but remain normally susceptible to CD95-induced death, and p53-deficient tumor cells can be killed with CD95L or Apo2L/TRAIL *(164,234)*. These findings indicate that the death receptor- and DNA damage/stress-induced signaling pathways can operate independently until they converge at the level of mitochondrial disruption.

Although death receptors play contributory, yet dispensable, roles in the response to conventional chemotherapy or irradiation, death receptor–ligand interactions may be instrumental for the action of cancer immunotherapy or specific anticancer agents. As discussed earlier, death receptor-induced signals may be a key component of the antitumor effects of interferons. Likewise, all-trans-retinoic acid (ATRA) induces acute promyelocytic leukemia (APL) differentiation followed by postmaturation apoptosis through induction of Apo2L/TRAIL *(237)*.

Targeting Death Receptors for Treatment of Cancers

Genetic aberrations that render cells resistant to diverse chemotherapeutic agents or ionizing radiation, such as loss of the *p53* tumor suppressor gene or overexpression of Bcl-2, underlie the observed resistance of human cancers to conventional anticancer therapy *(238)*. Identifying approaches to induce apoptosis in tumors that harbor such genetic impediments could lead to effective therapeutic interventions against resistant human cancers. Since death receptors provide an alternative mechanism of activating caspases and triggering cell death, ligand- or antibody-induced engagement of death receptors may be an attractive strategy for anticancer therapy. However, the clinical utility and therapeutic ratio of this approach depends on the differential sensitivity of tumor cells and normal tissues to each agent and/or the ability to target delivery of death ligands/antibodies to tumor cells. Although TNF-α and CD95L can induce apoptosis of several types of tumor cells in vitro, their clinical application in cancer therapy is hindered by the serious toxicity of these ligands in vivo. Systemic administration of TNF-α causes a serious inflammatory septic shock-like syndrome that is induced by NF-κB-mediated expression of proinflammatory genes in macrophages and T-cells. Systemic administration of FasL or agonistic antibodies against CD95 causes lethal hepatic apoptosis. In contrast to these ligands, Apo2L/TRAIL holds enormous promise for anticancer therapy.

A broad spectrum of human cancer cell lines express death receptors for Apo2L/TRAIL (TRAIL-R1/DR4 and TRAIL-R2/DR5) and exhibit variable sensitivity to Apo2L/TRAIL-induced apoptosis *(239)*. Although Bcl-2 protects cells from diverse cytotoxic insults, Bcl-2 overexpression does not confer significant protection against induction of apoptosis by Apo2L/TRAIL *(164)*. Likewise, tumor cells that resist DNA damage-induced apoptosis by virtue of loss of p53 remain susceptible to induction of apoptosis by Apo2L/TRAIL. Cancer cells with wild-type p53 (p53$^{+/+}$), and their isogenic p53$^{-/-}$ derivatives generated by deletion of p53 via targeted homologous recombination, are equally sensitive to Apo2L/TRAIL-induced apoptosis *(68)*. The tumoricidal activity of Apo2L/TRAIL in vivo has been confirmed in preclinical animal models (athymic nude or SCID mice) carrying human tumor xenografts without any evidence of toxicity to normal tissues *(239–241)*. Apo2L/TRAIL prevented the growth of evolving breast or colon or glial cancers after xenotransplantation and decreased the size of established tumors. More importantly, systemic treatment with Apo2L/TRAIL significantly improved the survival of tumor-bearing animals without any deleterious effects on normal tissues. Likewise, monoclonal antibodies that engage the human Apo2L/TRAIL receptors, DR4 and DR5, also demonstrate potent antitumor activity without any evidence of toxicity *(242,243)*.

An especially encouraging feature of Apo2L/TRAIL or agonistic antibodies against death receptors for Apo2L/TRAIL is that they induce apoptosis of tumor cells while sparing normal tissues. While TRAIL-R1 and TRAIL-R2 are broadly expressed in most organ systems, normal cells frequently express two additional TRAIL receptors, TRAIL-R3 (TRID or DcR1) and TRAIL-R4 (TRUNDD or DcR2), which serve as decoys and confer protection against Apo2L/TRAIL-induced death. The expression of decoy receptors provides a potential molecular basis for the relative resistance of normal cells to Apo2L/TRAIL-induced death *(244)*. Other studies indicate that high levels of FLIP may protect normal cells from death receptor-induced apoptosis *(245)*. Regardless of the specific mechanism(s) involved, the differential sensitivity of tumor cells and normal tissues to Apo2L/TRAIL-induced cytotoxicity makes this ligand a promising investigational anticancer agent. One potential concern was raised by the reported ability of a polyhistidine-tagged recombinant version of human Apo2L/TRAIL (Apo2L/TRAIL.His) to induce apoptosis in vitro in isolated human hepatocytes *(246)*. This concern was alleviated by subsequent studies using a Zn-bound homotrimeric version of human Apo2L/TRAIL that lacks exogenous sequence tags (Apo2L/TRAIL.0), which has been developed as a candidate for human clinical trials *(247)*. These studies demonstrated that Apo2L/TRAIL retains potent antitumor activity but is nontoxic to human or nonhuman primate hepatocytes in vitro. Moreover, intravenous administration of Apo2L/TRAIL in cynomolgus monkeys or chimpanzees was well tolerated with no evidence of changes in liver enzyme activities, bilirubin, serum albumin, coagulation parameters, or liver histology *(247)*.

Sensitization of Tumor Cells to Death Receptor-Induced Apoptosis

Although Apo2L/TRAIL can induce apoptosis independently of p53 or Bcl-2, cancer cell lines exhibit a wide heterogeneity in their sensitivity to Apo2L/TRAIL in vitro, and certain lines are resistant to this ligand *(239)*. As might be appreciated from the earlier discussion of the molecular determinants and regulators of death receptor-induced apoptosis, cancer cells may evade Apo2L/TRAIL-mediated apoptosis by mutational inactivation of death-signaling genes or aberrant expression of proteins that block death-signaling pathways. *Bax* is a frequent target of mutational inactivation in human cancers that harbor mutations in genes that govern DNA mismatch repair (MMR) (approx 15% of human colon, endometrial, and gastric carcinomas). More than 50% of MMR-deficient colon adenocarcinomas contain somatic frameshift mutations in an unstable tract of eight deoxyguanosines in the third coding exon (spanning codons 38-41 [$(G)_8$]) within Bax *(248)*. In addition, a similar frameshift mutation results from loss of a G residue from a repetitive sequence in the second exon *(69)*. MMR-deficient human colon carcinoma cells are rendered completely resistant to Apo2L/TRAIL by inactivation of *Bax (68–70)*. While both $Bax^{+/-}$ and $Bax^{-/-}$ sister clones activated apical death receptor signals, including activation of caspase-8 and cleavage of BID, Apo2L/TRAIL could not induce mitochondrial disruption or cell death in $Bax^{-/-}$ tumor cells. These data suggest that the basal expression of BAK in tumor cells may not be sufficient to substitute for BAX in mediating death receptor-induced apoptosis. In addition to loss of BAX, cancer cells may also evade Apo2L/TRAIL-induced death by overexpression of FLIP, Bcl-x_L, or XIAP *(71)*. As FLIP, Bcl-x_L, and XIAP are all NF-κB-inducible proteins, this mechanism of resistance may operate in cancers that have constitutively high NF-κB activity *(164)*.

Insights into the molecular control of death receptor expression and signaling suggest that cancers may be sensitized to Apo2L/TRAIL-induced death by the following approaches:

1. *Chemotherapeutic anticancer agents or ionizing radiation*: Because death receptor- and DNA damage/stress-induced pathways may operate independently to effect mitochondrial disruption, the simultaneous delivery of both signals may have synergistic cytotoxicity. Moreover, conventional chemotherapeutic agents may also potentiate Apo2L/TRAIL-induced tumor cell death by upregulating p53, and elevating expression of DR5/TRAIL-R2, BAX, and BAK *(69)*. Several studies have demonstrated that tumor cells are sensitized to Apo2L/TRAIL-induced apoptosis by diverse chemotherapeutic agents or ionizing radiation.
2. *Interferons*: Tumor cells, including those with p53 or BAX deficiency, are sensitized to Apo2L/TRAIL-induced apoptosis by IFN-induced upregulation of death receptors, Apo2L/TRAIL, caspase-8, and BAK. Several studies have demonstrated that pre-treatment with IFN-γ or -β can augment Apo2L/TRAIL-induced death of diverse tumor cell types.
3. *NF-κB inhibitors*: Since NF-κB is frequently activated by diverse genetic aberrations, growth factors, cytokines, viral proteins, costimulatory interactions, and stressful stimuli in diverse cancer types, it may be a common denominator of the resistance of many human cancers to Apo2L/TRAIL. Tumor cells are sensitized to Apo2L/TRAIL-induced apoptosis by inhibition of NF-κB *(68)*. NF-κB inhibition may be achieved by the following approaches: (a) IKKβ inhibitors, which prevent the phosphorylation of IκBs; (b) proteasomal inhibitors, which prevent the ubiquitin-mediated degradation of IκB and processing of p105. Each of these agents has been shown to augment Apo2L/TRAIL-induced death of diverse cancer cell lines.

Although the combination of Apo2L/TRAIL with conventional chemotherapeutic agents, NF-κB inhibitors, and/or interferons may exert synergistic antitumor effects, additional studies are required to evaluate and optimize the safety and therapeutic ratio of such regimens in vivo.

CONCLUSION

As our knowledge of death receptors and their signaling pathways has grown, so too has our appreciation of the key molecular mechanisms that regulate their activity. It is now evident that evolution has designed an intricate molecular circuitry that maintains a dynamic balance between death receptor-induced signals and antiapoptotic proteins. The stringent regulation of death receptor-induced apoptosis enables signal-dependent induction of physiologic cell death while protecting the organism from the devastating consequences of unscheduled or uncontrolled apoptosis. Insights into the molecular regulation of cell death have opened exciting avenues for therapeutic interventions against cancer cells that resist conventional therapy. The challenge before us is to design innovative anticancer therapeutic strategies that counteract these defects by targeting death receptors or their regulatory pathways without incurring prohibitive toxicity from such combinatorial regimens.

ACKNOWLEDGMENTS

Work in our laboratories is supported by the National Institutes of Health (National Cancer Institute), the U.S. Army Medical Research and Materiel Command—Department of Defense, the Passano Foundation, the Valvano Foundation for Cancer Research, the Mary Kay Ash Charitable Foundation, the Susan G. Komen Breast Cancer Foundation, and the Virginia and D.K. Ludwig Fund for Cancer Research. We thank our colleagues for their insights, stimulating discussions, and contributions, and apologize to those scientists whose work we have either inadvertently failed to mention or cited indirectly through reviews.

REFERENCES

1. Hengartner MO. The biochemistry of apoptosis. Nature 2000;407(6805):770–776.
2. Ashkenazi A, Dixit VM. Death receptors: signaling and modulation. Science 1998;281(5381):1305–1308.
3. Smith CA, Farrah T, Goodwin RG. The TNF receptor superfamily of cellular and viral proteins: activation, costimulation, and death. Cell 1994;76(6):959–962.
4. Brakebusch C, Nophar Y, Kemper O, Engelmann H, Wallach D. Cytoplasmic truncation of the p55 tumour necrosis factor (TNF) receptor abolishes signalling, but not induced shedding of the receptor. EMBO J 1992;11(3):943–950.
5. Itoh N, Nagata S. A novel protein domain required for apoptosis. Mutational analysis of human Fas antigen. J Biol Chem 1993;268(15):10932–10937.
6. Nagata S. Apoptosis by death factor. Cell 1997;88(3):355–365.
7. Chinnaiyan AM, O'Rourke K, Yu GL, et al. Signal transduction by DR3, a death domain-containing receptor related to TNFR-1 and CD95. Science 1996;274(5289):990–992.
8. Marsters SA, Sheridan JP, Donahue CJ, et al. Apo-3, a new member of the tumor necrosis factor receptor family, contains a death domain and activates apoptosis and NF-kappa B. Curr Biol 1996; 6(12):1669–1676.
9. Kitson J, Raven T, Jiang YP, et al. A death-domain-containing receptor that mediates apoptosis. Nature 1996;384(6607):372–375.
10. Bodmer JL, Burns K, Schneider P, et al. TRAMP, a novel apoptosis-mediating receptor with sequence homology to tumor necrosis factor receptor 1 and Fas(Apo-1/CD95). Immunity 1997;6(1):79–88.
11. Screaton GR, Xu XN, Olsen AL, et al. LARD: a new lymphoid-specific death domain containing receptor regulated by alternative pre-mRNA splicing. Proc Natl Acad Sci USA 1997;94(9):4615–4619.
12. Pan G, O'Rourke K, Chinnaiyan AM, et al. The receptor for the cytotoxic ligand TRAIL. Science 1997;276(5309):111–113.
13. Screaton GR, Mongkolsapaya J, Xu XN, Cowper AE, McMichael AJ, Bell JI. TRICK2, a new alternatively spliced receptor that transduces the cytotoxic signal from TRAIL. Curr Biol 1997;7(9):693–696.
14. Pan G, Ni J, Wei YF, Yu G, Gentz R, Dixit VM. An antagonist decoy receptor and a death domain-containing receptor for TRAIL. Science 1997;277(5327):815–818.
15. Sheridan JP, Marsters SA, Pitti RM, et al. Control of TRAIL-induced apoptosis by a family of signaling and decoy receptors. Science 1997;277(5327):818–821.
16. Walczak H, Degli-Esposti MA, Johnson RS, et al. TRAIL-R2: a novel apoptosis-mediating receptor for TRAIL. EMBO J 1997;16(17):5386–5397.
17. Wu GS, Burns TF, McDonald ER, III, et al. KILLER/DR5 is a DNA damage-inducible p53-regulated death receptor gene. Nat Genet 1997;17(2):141–143.

18. Pan G, Bauer JH, Haridas V, et al. Identification and functional characterization of DR6, a novel death domain-containing TNF receptor. FEBS Lett 1998;431(3):351–356.
19. Marsters SA, Sheridan JP, Pitti RM, Brush J, Goddard A, Ashkenazi A. Identification of a ligand for the death-domain-containing receptor Apo3. Curr Biol 1998;8(9):525–528.
20. Chicheportiche Y, Bourdon PR, Xu H, et al. TWEAK, a new secreted ligand in the tumor necrosis factor family that weakly induces apoptosis. J Biol Chem 1997;272(51):32,401–32,410.
21. Pitti RM, Marsters SA, Ruppert S, Donahue CJ, Moore A, Ashkenazi A. Induction of apoptosis by Apo-2 ligand, a new member of the tumor necrosis factor cytokine family. J Biol Chem 1996;271(22): 12,687–12,690.
22. Wiley SR, Schooley K, Smolak PJ, et al. Identification and characterization of a new member of the TNF family that induces apoptosis. Immunity 1995;3(6):673–682.
23. Earnshaw WC, Martins LM, Kaufmann SH. Mammalian caspases: structure, activation, substrates, and functions during apoptosis. Annu Rev Biochem 1999;68:383–424.
24. Thornberry NA, Rano TA, Peterson EP, et al. A combinatorial approach defines specificities of members of the caspase family and granzyme B. Functional relationships established for key mediators of apoptosis. J Biol Chem 1997;272(29):17,907–17,911.
25. Rao L, Perez D, White E. Lamin proteolysis facilitates nuclear events during apoptosis. J Cell Biol 1996;135(6 Pt 1):1441–1455.
26. Buendia B, Santa-Maria A, Courvalin JC. Caspase-dependent proteolysis of integral and peripheral proteins of nuclear membranes and nuclear pore complex proteins during apoptosis. J Cell Sci 1999;112(Pt 11):1743–1753.
27. Rudel T, Bokoch GM. Membrane and morphological changes in apoptotic cells regulated by caspase-mediated activation of PAK2. Science 1997;276(5318):1571–1574.
28. Coleman ML, Sahai EA, Yeo M, Bosch M, Dewar A, Olson MF. Membrane blebbing during apoptosis results from caspase-mediated activation of ROCK I. Nat Cell Biol 2001;3(4):339–345.
29. Sebbagh M, Renvoize C, Hamelin J, Riche N, Bertoglio J, Breard J. Caspase-3-mediated cleavage of ROCK I induces MLC phosphorylation and apoptotic membrane blebbing. Nat Cell Biol 2001; 3(4):346–352.
30. Liu X, Zou H, Slaughter C, Wang X. DFF, a heterodimeric protein that functions downstream of caspase-3 to trigger DNA fragmentation during apoptosis. Cell 1997;89(2):175–184.
31. Enari M, Sakahira H, Yokoyama H, Okawa K, Iwamatsu A, Nagata S. A caspase-activated DNase that degrades DNA during apoptosis, and its inhibitor ICAD. Nature 1998;391(6662):43–50.
32. Sakahira H, Enari M, Nagata S. Cleavage of CAD inhibitor in CAD activation and DNA degradation during apoptosis. Nature 1998;391(6662):96–99.
33. Tartaglia LA, Ayres TM, Wong GH, Goeddel DV. A novel domain within the 55 kd TNF receptor signals cell death. Cell 1993;74(5):845–853.
34. Kischkel FC, Hellbardt S, Behrmann I, et al. Cytotoxicity-dependent APO-1 (Fas/CD95)-associated proteins form a death-inducing signaling complex (DISC) with the receptor. EMBO J 1995;14(22): 5579–5588.
35. Chinnaiyan AM, O'Rourke K, Tewari M, Dixit VM. FADD, a novel death domain-containing protein, interacts with the death domain of Fas and initiates apoptosis. Cell 1995;81(4):505–512.
36. Boldin MP, Varfolomeev EE, Pancer Z, Mett IL, Camonis JH, Wallach D. A novel protein that interacts with the death domain of Fas/APO1 contains a sequence motif related to the death domain. J Biol Chem 1995;270(14):7795–7798.
37. Siegel RM, Martin DA, Zheng L, et al. Death-effector filaments: novel cytoplasmic structures that recruit caspases and trigger apoptosis. J Cell Biol 1998;141(5):1243–1253.
38. Boldin MP, Goncharov TM, Goltsev YV, Wallach D. Involvement of MACH, a novel MORT1/FADD-interacting protease, in Fas/APO-1- and TNF receptor-induced cell death. Cell 1996;85(6):803–815.
39. Muzio M, Chinnaiyan AM, Kischkel FC, et al. FLICE, a novel FADD-homologous ICE/CED-3-like protease, is recruited to the CD95 (Fas/APO-1) death-inducing signaling complex. Cell 1996;85(6): 817–827.
40. Medema JP, Scaffidi C, Kischkel FC, et al. FLICE is activated by association with the CD95 death-inducing signaling complex (DISC). EMBO J 1997;16(10):2794–2804.
41. Yang X, Chang HY, Baltimore D. Autoproteolytic activation of pro-caspases by oligomerization. Mol Cell 1998;1(2):319–325.
42. Martin DA, Siegel RM, Zheng L, Lenardo MJ. Membrane oligomerization and cleavage activates the caspase-8 (FLICE/MACHalpha1) death signal. J Biol Chem 1998;273(8):4345–4349.

43. Muzio M, Stockwell BR, Stennicke HR, Salvesen GS, Dixit VM. An induced proximity model for caspase-8 activation. J Biol Chem 1998;273(5):2926–2930.
44. Hsu H, Shu HB, Pan MG, Goeddel DV. TRADD-TRAF2 and TRADD-FADD interactions define two distinct TNF receptor 1 signal transduction pathways. Cell 1996;84(2):299–308.
45. Zhang J, Cado D, Chen A, Kabra NH, Winoto A. Fas-mediated apoptosis and activation-induced T-cell proliferation are defective in mice lacking FADD/Mort1. Nature 1998;392(6673):296–300.
46. Newton K, Harris AW, Bath ML, Smith KG, Strasser A. A dominant interfering mutant of FADD/MORT1 enhances deletion of autoreactive thymocytes and inhibits proliferation of mature T lymphocytes. EMBO J 1998;17(3):706–718.
47. Zornig M, Hueber AO, Evan G. p53-dependent impairment of T-cell proliferation in FADD dominant-negative transgenic mice. Curr Biol 1998;8(8):467–470.
48. Yeh WC, Pompa JL, McCurrach ME, et al. FADD: essential for embryo development and signaling from some, but not all, inducers of apoptosis. Science 1998;279(5358):1954–1958.
49. Kischkel FC, Lawrence DA, Chuntharapai A, Schow P, Kim KJ, Ashkenazi A. Apo2L/TRAIL-dependent recruitment of endogenous FADD and caspase-8 to death receptors 4 and 5. Immunity 2000;12(6):611–620.
50. Varfolomeev EE, Schuchmann M, Luria V, et al. Targeted disruption of the mouse Caspase 8 gene ablates cell death induction by the TNF receptors, Fas/Apo1, and DR3 and is lethal prenatally. Immunity 1998;9(2):267–276.
51. Kischkel FC, Lawrence DA, Tinel A, et al. Death receptor recruitment of endogenous caspase-10 and apoptosis initiation in the absence of caspase-8. J Biol Chem 2001;276(49):46,639–46,646.
52. Scaffidi C, Fulda S, Srinivasan A, et al. Two CD95 (APO-1/Fas) signaling pathways. EMBO J 1998;17(6):1675–1687.
53. Woo M, Hakem R, Soengas MS, et al. Essential contribution of caspase 3/CPP32 to apoptosis and its associated nuclear changes. Genes Dev 1998;12(6):806–819.
54. Wang K, Yin XM, Chao DT, Milliman CL, Korsmeyer SJ. BID: a novel BH3 domain-only death agonist. Genes Dev 1996;10(22):2859–2869.
55. Luo X, Budihardjo I, Zou H, Slaughter C, Wang X. Bid, a Bcl2 interacting protein, mediates cytochrome c release from mitochondria in response to activation of cell surface death receptors. Cell 1998;94(4):481–490.
56. Li H, Zhu H, Xu CJ, Yuan J. Cleavage of BID by caspase 8 mediates the mitochondrial damage in the Fas pathway of apoptosis. Cell 1998;94(4):491–501.
57. Gross A, Yin XM, Wang K, et al. Caspase cleaved BID targets mitochondria and is required for cytochrome c release, while BCL-XL prevents this release but not tumor necrosis factor-R1/Fas death. J Biol Chem 1999;274(2):1156–1163.
58. Roy S, Nicholson DW. Cross-talk in cell death signaling. J Exp Med 2000;192(8):F21-F25.
59. Eskes R, Desagher S, Antonsson B, Martinou JC. Bid induces the oligomerization and insertion of Bax into the outer mitochondrial membrane. Mol Cell Biol 2000;20(3):929–935.
60. Wei MC, Lindsten T, Mootha VK, et al. tBID, a membrane-targeted death ligand, oligomerizes BAK to release cytochrome c. Genes Dev 2000;14(16):2060–2071.
61. Vaux DL. CED-4—the third horseman of apoptosis. Cell 1997;90(3):389–390.
62. Stennicke HR, Deveraux QL, Humke EW, Reed JC, Dixit VM, Salvesen GS. Caspase-9 can be activated without proteolytic processing. J Biol Chem 1999;274(13):8359–8362.
63. Srinivasula SM, Ahmad M, Fernandes-Alnemri T, Alnemri ES. Autoactivation of procaspase-9 by Apaf-1-mediated oligomerization. Mol Cell 1998;1(7):949–957.
64. Deveraux QL, Roy N, Stennicke HR, et al. IAPs block apoptotic events induced by caspase-8 and cytochrome c by direct inhibition of distinct caspases. EMBO J 1998;17(8):2215–2223.
65. Yin XM, Wang K, Gross A, et al. Bid-deficient mice are resistant to Fas-induced hepatocellular apoptosis. Nature 1999;400(6747):886–891.
66. Lindsten T, Ross AJ, King A, et al. The combined functions of proapoptotic Bcl-2 family members bak and bax are essential for normal development of multiple tissues. Mol Cell 2000;6(6):1389–1399.
67. Wei MC, Zong WX, Cheng EH, et al. Proapoptotic BAX and BAK: a requisite gateway to mitochondrial dysfunction and death. Science 2001;292(5517):727–730.
68. Ravi R, Bedi A. Requirement of BAX for TRAIL/Apo2L-induced apoptosis of colorectal cancers: synergism with sulindac-mediated inhibition of Bcl-x(L). Cancer Res 2002;62(6):1583–1587.
69. LeBlanc H, Lawrence D, Varfolomeev E, et al. Tumor-cell resistance to death receptor-induced apoptosis through mutational inactivation of the proapoptotic Bcl-2 homolog Bax. Nat Med 2002;8(3):274–281.

70. Deng Y, Lin Y, Wu X. TRAIL-induced apoptosis requires Bax-dependent mitochondrial release of Smac/DIABLO. Genes Dev 2002;16(1):33–45.
71. Burns TF, el Deiry WS. Identification of inhibitors of TRAIL-induced death (ITIDs) in the TRAIL-sensitive colon carcinoma cell line SW480 using a genetic approach. J Biol Chem 2001;276(41):37,879–37,886.
72. Cheng EH, Wei MC, Weiler S, et al. BCL-2, BCL-X(L) sequester BH3 domain-only molecules preventing BAX- and BAK-mediated mitochondrial apoptosis. Mol Cell 2001;8(3):705–711.
73. Kuida K, Haydar TF, Kuan CY, et al. Reduced apoptosis and cytochrome c-mediated caspase activation in mice lacking caspase 9. Cell 1998;94(3):325–337.
74. Hakem R, Hakem A, Duncan GS, et al. Differential requirement for caspase 9 in apoptotic pathways in vivo. Cell 1998;94(3):339–352.
75. Yoshida H, Kong YY, Yoshida R, et al. Apaf1 is required for mitochondrial pathways of apoptosis and brain development. Cell 1998;94(6):739–750.
76. Cecconi F, Alvarez-Bolado G, Meyer BI, Roth KA, Gruss P. Apaf1 (CED-4 homolog) regulates programmed cell death in mammalian development. Cell 1998;94(6):727–737.
77. Kuida K, Zheng TS, Na S, et al. Decreased apoptosis in the brain and premature lethality in CPP32-deficient mice. Nature 1996;384(6607):368–372.
78. Du C, Fang M, Li Y, Li L, Wang X. Smac, a mitochondrial protein that promotes cytochrome c-dependent caspase activation by eliminating IAP inhibition. Cell 2000;102(1):33–42.
79. Verhagen AM, Ekert PG, Pakusch M, et al. Identification of DIABLO, a mammalian protein that promotes apoptosis by binding to and antagonizing IAP proteins. Cell 2000;102(1):43–53.
80. Deveraux QL, Takahashi R, Salvesen GS, Reed JC. X-linked IAP is a direct inhibitor of cell-death proteases. Nature 1997;388(6639):300–304.
81. Goyal L. Cell death inhibition: keeping caspases in check. Cell 2001;104(6):805–808.
82. Ichijo H, Nishida E, Irie K, et al. Induction of apoptosis by ASK1, a mammalian MAPKKK that activates SAPK/JNK and p38 signaling pathways. Science 1997;275(5296):90–94.
83. Verheij M, Bose R, Lin XH, et al. Requirement for ceramide-initiated SAPK/JNK signalling in stress-induced apoptosis. Nature 1996;380(6569):75–79.
84. Tournier C, Hess P, Yang DD, et al. Requirement of JNK for stress-induced activation of the cytochrome c-mediated death pathway. Science 2000;288(5467):870–874.
85. Krammer PH. CD95's deadly mission in the immune system. Nature 2000;407(6805):789–795.
86. Leithauser F, Dhein J, Mechtersheimer G, et al. Constitutive and induced expression of APO-1, a new member of the nerve growth factor/tumor necrosis factor receptor superfamily, in normal and neoplastic cells. Lab Invest 1993;69(4):415–429.
87. Li JH, Rosen D, Ronen D, et al. The regulation of CD95 ligand expression and function in CTL. J Immunol 1998;161(8):3943–3949.
88. Golstein P. Cell death: TRAIL and its receptors. Curr Biol 1997;7(12):R750–R753.
89. Martinez-Lorenzo MJ, Alava MA, Gamen S, et al. Involvement of APO2 ligand/TRAIL in activation-induced death of Jurkat and human peripheral blood T cells. Eur J Immunol 1998;28(9):2714–2725.
90. Jeremias I, Herr I, Boehler T, Debatin KM. TRAIL/Apo-2-ligand-induced apoptosis in human T cells. Eur J Immunol 1998;28(1):143–152.
91. MacFarlane M, Ahmad M, Srinivasula SM, Fernandes-Alnemri T, Cohen GM, Alnemri ES. Identification and molecular cloning of two novel receptors for the cytotoxic ligand TRAIL. J Biol Chem 1997;272(41):25,417–25,420.
92. Schneider P, Bodmer JL, Thome M, Hofmann K, Holler N, Tschopp J. Characterization of two receptors for TRAIL. FEBS Lett 1997;416(3):329–334.
93. Degli-Esposti MA, Smolak PJ, Walczak H, et al. Cloning and characterization of TRAIL-R3, a novel member of the emerging TRAIL receptor family. J Exp Med 1997;186(7):1165–1170.
94. Mongkolsapaya J, Cowper AE, Xu XN, et al. Lymphocyte inhibitor of TRAIL (TNF-related apoptosis-inducing ligand): a new receptor protecting lymphocytes from the death ligand TRAIL. J Immunol 1998;160(1):3–6.
95. Marsters SA, Sheridan JP, Pitti RM, et al. A novel receptor for Apo2L/TRAIL contains a truncated death domain. Curr Biol 1997;7(12):1003–1006.
96. Pan G, Ni J, Yu G, Wei YF, Dixit VM. TRUNDD, a new member of the TRAIL receptor family that antagonizes TRAIL signalling. FEBS Lett 1998;424(1–2):41–45.
97. Degli-Esposti MA, Dougall WC, Smolak PJ, Waugh JY, Smith CA, Goodwin RG. The novel receptor TRAIL-R4 induces NF-kappaB and protects against TRAIL-mediated apoptosis, yet retains an incomplete death domain. Immunity 1997;7(6):813–820.

98. Griffith TS, Lynch DH. TRAIL: a molecule with multiple receptors and control mechanisms. Curr Opin Immunol 1998;10(5):559–563.
99. Pitti RM, Marsters SA, Lawrence DA, et al. Genomic amplification of a decoy receptor for Fas ligand in lung and colon cancer. Nature 1998;396(6712):699–703.
100. Jiang Y, Woronicz JD, Liu W, Goeddel DV. Prevention of constitutive TNF receptor 1 signaling by silencer of death domains. Science 1999;283(5401):543–546.
101. Thome M, Schneider P, Hofmann K, et al. Viral FLICE-inhibitory proteins (FLIPs) prevent apoptosis induced by death receptors. Nature 1997;386(6624):517–521.
102. Hu S, Vincenz C, Buller M, Dixit VM. A novel family of viral death effector domain-containing molecules that inhibit both CD-95- and tumor necrosis factor receptor-1-induced apoptosis. J Biol Chem 1997;272(15):9621–9624.
103. Bertin J, Armstrong RC, Ottilie S, et al. Death effector domain-containing herpesvirus and poxvirus proteins inhibit both Fas- and TNFR1-induced apoptosis. Proc Natl Acad Sci USA 1997;94(4):1172–1176.
104. Inohara N, Koseki T, Hu Y, Chen S, Nunez G. CLARP, a death effector domain-containing protein interacts with caspase-8 and regulates apoptosis. Proc Natl Acad Sci USA 1997;94(20):10,717–10,722.
105. Irmler M, Thome M, Hahne M, et al. Inhibition of death receptor signals by cellular FLIP. Nature 1997;388(6638):190–195.
106. Goltsev YV, Kovalenko AV, Arnold E, Varfolomeev EE, Brodianskii VM, Wallach D. CASH, a novel caspase homologue with death effector domains. J Biol Chem 1997;272(32):19,641–19,644.
107. Srinivasula SM, Ahmad M, Ottilie S, et al. FLAME-1, a novel FADD-like anti-apoptotic molecule that regulates Fas/TNFR1-induced apoptosis. J Biol Chem 1997;272(30):18,542–18,545.
108. Chai J, Wu Q, Shiozaki E, Srinivasula SM, Alnemri ES, Shi Y. Crystal structure of a procaspase-7 zymogen: mechanisms of activation and substrate binding. Cell 2001;107(3):399–407.
109. Han DK, Chaudhary PM, Wright ME, et al. MRIT, a novel death-effector domain-containing protein, interacts with caspases and BclXL and initiates cell death. Proc Natl Acad Sci USA 1997;94(21): 11,333–11,338.
110. Rasper DM, Vaillancourt JP, Hadano S, et al. Cell death attenuation by "Usurpin," a mammalian DED-caspase homologue that precludes caspase-8 recruitment and activation by the CD-95 (Fas, APO-1) receptor complex. Cell Death Differ 1998;5(4):271–288.
111. Yeh WC, Itie A, Elia AJ, et al. Requirement for Casper (c-FLIP) in regulation of death receptor-induced apoptosis and embryonic development. Immunity 2000;12(6):633–642.
112. Kreuz S, Siegmund D, Scheurich P, Wajant H. NF-kappaB inducers upregulate cFLIP, a cycloheximide-sensitive inhibitor of death receptor signaling. Mol Cell Biol 2001;21(12):3964–3973.
113. Desagher S, Osen-Sand A, Montessuit S, et al. Phosphorylation of bid by casein kinases I and II regulates its cleavage by caspase 8. Mol Cell 2001;8(3):601–611.
114. Tuazon PT, Traugh JA. Casein kinase I and II—multipotential serine protein kinases: structure, function, and regulation. Adv Second Messenger Phosphoprotein Res 1991;23:123–164.
115. Birnbaum MJ, Clem RJ, Miller LK. An apoptosis-inhibiting gene from a nuclear polyhedrosis virus encoding a polypeptide with Cys/His sequence motifs. J Virol 1994;68(4):2521–2528.
116. Lovering R, Hanson IM, Borden KL, et al. Identification and preliminary characterization of a protein motif related to the zinc finger. Proc Natl Acad Sci USA 1993;90(6):2112–2116.
117. Roy N, Deveraux QL, Takahashi R, Salvesen GS, Reed JC. The c-IAP-1 and c-IAP-2 proteins are direct inhibitors of specific caspases. EMBO J 1997;16(23):6914–6925.
118. Takahashi R, Deveraux Q, Tamm I, et al. A single BIR domain of XIAP sufficient for inhibiting caspases. J Biol Chem 1998;273(14):7787–7790.
119. Deveraux QL, Leo E, Stennicke HR, Welsh K, Salvesen GS, Reed JC. Cleavage of human inhibitor of apoptosis protein XIAP results in fragments with distinct specificities for caspases. EMBO J 1999;18(19):5242–5251.
120. Huang Y, Park YC, Rich RL, Segal D, Myszka DG, Wu H. Structural basis of caspase inhibition by XIAP: differential roles of the linker versus the BIR domain. Cell 2001;104(5):781–790.
121. Riedl SJ, Renatus M, Schwarzenbacher R, et al. Structural basis for the inhibition of caspase-3 by XIAP. Cell 2001;104(5):791–800.
122. Stehlik C, de Martin R, Kumabashiri I, Schmid JA, Binder BR, Lipp J. Nuclear factor (NF)-kappaB-regulated X-chromosome-linked iap gene expression protects endothelial cells from tumor necrosis factor alpha-induced apoptosis. J Exp Med 1998;188(1):211–216.

123. Rothe M, Pan MG, Henzel WJ, Ayres TM, Goeddel DV. The TNFR2-TRAF signaling complex contains two novel proteins related to baculoviral inhibitor of apoptosis proteins. Cell 1995;83(7):1243–1252.
124. Wang CY, Mayo MW, Korneluk RG, Goeddel DV, Baldwin AS, Jr. NF-kappaB antiapoptosis: induction of TRAF1 and TRAF2 and c-IAP1 and c-IAP2 to suppress caspase-8 activation. Science 1998;281(5383):1680–1683.
125. Chu ZL, McKinsey TA, Liu L, Gentry JJ, Malim MH, Ballard DW. Suppression of tumor necrosis factor-induced cell death by inhibitor of apoptosis c-IAP2 is under NF-kappaB control. Proc Natl Acad Sci USA 1997;94(19):10,057–10,062.
126. Ambrosini G, Adida C, Altieri DC. A novel anti-apoptosis gene, survivin, expressed in cancer and lymphoma. Nat Med 1997;3(8):917–921.
127. Karin M, Lin A. NF-kappaB at the crossroads of life and death. Nat Immunol 2002;3(3):221–227.
128. Sha WC, Liou HC, Tuomanen EI, Baltimore D. Targeted disruption of the p50 subunit of NF-kappa B leads to multifocal defects in immune responses. Cell 1995;80(2):321–330.
129. Alcamo E, Mizgerd JP, Horwitz BH, et al. Targeted mutation of TNF receptor I rescues the RelA-deficient mouse and reveals a critical role for NF-kappa B in leukocyte recruitment. J Immunol 2001;167(3):1592–1600.
130. Franzoso G, Carlson L, Poljak L, et al. Mice deficient in nuclear factor (NF)-kappa B/p52 present with defects in humoral responses, germinal center reactions, and splenic microarchitecture. J Exp Med 1998;187(2):147–159.
131. Attar RM, Caamano J, Carrasco D, et al. Genetic approaches to study Rel/NF-kappa B/I kappa B function in mice. Semin Cancer Biol 1997;8(2):93–101.
132. Senftleben U, Li ZW, Baud V, Karin M. IKKbeta is essential for protecting T cells from TNFalpha-induced apoptosis. Immunity 2001;14(3):217–230.
133. Beg AA, Baltimore D. An essential role for NF-kappaB in preventing TNF-alpha-induced cell death. Science 1996;274(5288):782–784.
134. Wang CY, Mayo MW, Baldwin AS, Jr. TNF- and cancer therapy-induced apoptosis: potentiation by inhibition of NF-kappaB. Science 1996;274(5288):784–787.
135. Van Antwerp DJ, Martin SJ, Kafri T, Green DR, Verma IM. Suppression of TNF-alpha-induced apoptosis by NF-kappaB. Science 1996;274(5288):787–789.
136. Liu ZG, Hsu H, Goeddel DV, Karin M. Dissection of TNF receptor 1 effector functions: JNK activation is not linked to apoptosis while NF-kappaB activation prevents cell death. Cell 1996;87(3):565–576.
137. Karin M, Ben Neriah Y. Phosphorylation meets ubiquitination: the control of NF-[kappa]B activity. Annu Rev Immunol 2000;18:621–663.
138. Grimm S, Baeuerle PA. The inducible transcription factor NF-kappa B: structure-function relationship of its protein subunits. Biochem J 1993;290 (Pt 2):297–308.
139. Li Q, Van Antwerp D, Mercurio F, Lee KF, Verma IM. Severe liver degeneration in mice lacking the IkappaB kinase 2 gene. Science 1999;284(5412):321–325.
140. Delhase M, Hayakawa M, Chen Y, Karin M. Positive and negative regulation of IkappaB kinase activity through IKKbeta subunit phosphorylation. Science 1999;284(5412):309–313.
141. Li ZW, Chu W, Hu Y, et al. The IKKbeta subunit of IkappaB kinase (IKK) is essential for nuclear factor kappaB activation and prevention of apoptosis. J Exp Med 1999;189(11):1839–1845.
142. Solan NJ, Miyoshi H, Carmona EM, Bren GD, Paya CV. RelB cellular regulation and transcriptional activity are regulated by p100. J Biol Chem 2002;277(2):1405–1418.
143. Senftleben U, Cao Y, Xiao G, et al. Activation by IKKalpha of a second, evolutionary conserved, NF-kappa B signaling pathway. Science 2001;293(5534):1495–1499.
144. Wang D, Westerheide SD, Hanson JL, Baldwin AS, Jr. Tumor necrosis factor alpha-induced phosphorylation of RelA/p65 on Ser529 is controlled by casein kinase II. J Biol Chem 2000;275(42):32,592–32,597.
145. Zhong H, SuYang H, Erdjument-Bromage H, Tempst P, Ghosh S. The transcriptional activity of NF-kappaB is regulated by the IkappaB-associated PKAc subunit through a cyclic AMP-independent mechanism. Cell 1997;89(3):413–424.
146. Sizemore N, Leung S, Stark GR. Activation of phosphatidylinositol 3-kinase in response to interleukin-1 leads to phosphorylation and activation of the NF-kappaB p65/RelA subunit. Mol Cell Biol 1999;19(7):4798–4805.
147. Madrid LV, Wang CY, Guttridge DC, Schottelius AJ, Baldwin AS, Jr., Mayo MW. Akt suppresses apoptosis by stimulating the transactivation potential of the RelA/p65 subunit of NF-kappaB. Mol Cell Biol 2000;20(5):1626–1638.

148. Beg AA, Sha WC, Bronson RT, Ghosh S, Baltimore D. Embryonic lethality and liver degeneration in mice lacking the RelA component of NF-kappa B. Nature 1995;376(6536):167–170.
149. Rudolph D, Yeh WC, Wakeham A, et al. Severe liver degeneration and lack of NF-kappaB activation in NEMO/IKKgamma-deficient mice. Genes Dev 2000;14(7):854–862.
150. Kelliher MA, Grimm S, Ishida Y, Kuo F, Stanger BZ, Leder P. The death domain kinase RIP mediates the TNF-induced NF-kappaB signal. Immunity 1998;8(3):297–303.
151. Malinin NL, Boldin MP, Kovalenko AV, Wallach D. MAP3K-related kinase involved in NF-kappaB induction by TNF, CD95 and IL-1. Nature 1997;385(6616):540–544.
152. Scheidereit C. Signal transduction. Docking IkappaB kinases. Nature 1998;395(6699):225–226.
153. Nishitoh H, Saitoh M, Mochida Y, et al. ASK1 is essential for JNK/SAPK activation by TRAF2. Mol Cell 1998;2(3):389–395.
154. Lee SY, Reichlin A, Santana A, Sokol KA, Nussenzweig MC, Choi Y. TRAF2 is essential for JNK but not NF-kappaB activation and regulates lymphocyte proliferation and survival. Immunity 1997; 7(5):703–713.
155. Yeh WC, Shahinian A, Speiser D, et al. Early lethality, functional NF-kappaB activation, and increased sensitivity to TNF-induced cell death in TRAF2-deficient mice. Immunity 1997;7(5):715–725.
156. Baud V, Karin M. Signal transduction by tumor necrosis factor and its relatives. Trends Cell Biol 2001;11(9):372–377.
157. Rosenfeld ME, Prichard L, Shiojiri N, Fausto N. Prevention of hepatic apoptosis and embryonic lethality in RelA/TNFR-1 double knockout mice. Am J Pathol 2000;156(3):997–1007.
158. Doi TS, Marino MW, Takahashi T, et al. Absence of tumor necrosis factor rescues RelA-deficient mice from embryonic lethality. Proc Natl Acad Sci USA 1999;96(6):2994–2999.
159. Van Parijs L, Ibraghimov A, Abbas AK. The roles of costimulation and Fas in T cell apoptosis and peripheral tolerance. Immunity 1996;4(3):321–328.
160. Hong SY, Yoon WH, Park JH, Kang SG, Ahn JH, Lee TH. Involvement of two NF-kappa B binding elements in tumor necrosis factor alpha -, CD40-, and Epstein-Barr virus latent membrane protein 1-mediated induction of the cellular inhibitor of apoptosis protein 2 gene. J Biol Chem 2000;275(24): 18,022–18,028.
161. Liston P, Roy N, Tamai K, et al. Suppression of apoptosis in mammalian cells by NAIP and a related family of IAP genes. Nature 1996;379(6563):349–353.
162. Shu HB, Takeuchi M, Goeddel DV. The tumor necrosis factor receptor 2 signal transducers TRAF2 and c-IAP1 are components of the tumor necrosis factor receptor 1 signaling complex. Proc Natl Acad Sci USA 1996;93(24):13,973–13,978.
163. Chen C, Edelstein LC, Gelinas C. The Rel/NF-kappaB family directly activates expression of the apoptosis inhibitor Bcl-x(L). Mol Cell Biol 2000;20(8):2687–2695.
164. Ravi R, Bedi GC, Engstrom LW, et al. Regulation of death receptor expression and TRAIL/Apo2L-induced apoptosis by NF-kappaB. Nat Cell Biol 2001;3(4):409–416.
165. Zong WX, Edelstein LC, Chen C, Bash J, Gelinas C. The prosurvival Bcl-2 homolog Bfl-1/A1 is a direct transcriptional target of NF-kappaB that blocks TNFalpha-induced apoptosis. Genes Dev 1999;13(4):382–387.
166. Hamasaki A, Sendo F, Nakayama K, et al. Accelerated neutrophil apoptosis in mice lacking A1-a, a subtype of the bcl-2-related A1 gene. J Exp Med 1998;188(11):1985–1992.
167. Bentires-Alj M, Dejardin E, Viatour P, et al. Inhibition of the NF-kappa B transcription factor increases Bax expression in cancer cell lines. Oncogene 2001;20(22):2805–2813.
168. Tang G, Minemoto Y, Dibling B, et al. Inhibition of JNK activation through NF-kappaB target genes. Nature 2001;414(6861):313–317.
169. De Smaele E, Zazzeroni F, Papa S, et al. Induction of gadd45beta by NF-kappaB downregulates pro-apoptotic JNK signalling. Nature 2001;414(6861):308–313.
170. Javelaud D, Besancon F. NF-kappa B activation results in rapid inactivation of JNK in TNF alpha-treated Ewing sarcoma cells: a mechanism for the anti-apoptotic effect of NF-kappa B. Oncogene 2001;20(32):4365–4372.
171. Stark GR, Kerr IM, Williams BR, Silverman RH, Schreiber RD. How cells respond to interferons. Annu Rev Biochem 1998;67:227–264.
172. Darnell JE, Jr., Kerr IM, Stark GR. Jak-STAT pathways and transcriptional activation in response to IFNs and other extracellular signaling proteins. Science 1994;264(5164):1415–1421.
173. Ihle JN. STATs: signal transducers and activators of transcription. Cell 1996;84(3):331–334.

174. Kumar A, Commane M, Flickinger TW, Horvath CM, Stark GR. Defective TNF-alpha-induced apoptosis in STAT1-null cells due to low constitutive levels of caspases. Science 1997;278(5343):1630–1632.
175. Tamura T, Ishihara M, Lamphier MS, et al. An IRF-1-dependent pathway of DNA damage-induced apoptosis in mitogen-activated T lymphocytes. Nature 1995;376(6541):596–599.
176. Ossina NK, Cannas A, Powers VC, et al. Interferon-gamma modulates a p53-independent apoptotic pathway and apoptosis-related gene expression. J Biol Chem 1997;272(26):16,351–16,357.
177. Kumar-Sinha C, Varambally S, Sreekumar A, Chinnaiyan AM. Molecular cross-talk between the TRAIL and interferon signaling pathways. J Biol Chem 2002;277(1):575–585.
178. Leaman DW, Chawla-Sarkar M, Vyas K, et al. Identification of X-linked inhibitor of apoptosis-associated factor-1 as an interferon-stimulated gene that augments TRAIL Apo2L-induced apoptosis. J Biol Chem 2002;277(32):28,504–28,511.
179. Dorothee G, Vergnon I, Menez J, et al. Tumor-infiltrating CD4+ T lymphocytes express APO2 ligand (APO2L)/TRAIL upon specific stimulation with autologous lung carcinoma cells: role of IFN-alpha on APO2L/TRAIL expression and -mediated cytotoxicity. J Immunol 2002;169(2):809–817.
180. Kayagaki N, Yamaguchi N, Nakayama M, Eto H, Okumura K, Yagita H. Type I interferons (IFNs) regulate tumor necrosis factor-related apoptosis-inducing ligand (TRAIL) expression on human T cells: a novel mechanism for the antitumor effects of type I IFNs. J Exp Med 1999;189(9):1451–1460.
181. Lee JK, Sayers TJ, Brooks AD, et al. IFN-gamma-dependent delay of in vivo tumor progression by Fas overexpression on murine renal cancer cells. J Immunol 2000;164(1):231–239.
182. Oshima K, Yanase N, Ibukiyama C, et al. Involvement of TRAIL/TRAIL-R interaction in IFN-alpha-induced apoptosis of Daudi B lymphoma cells. Cytokine 2001;14(4):193–201.
183. Sedger LM, Shows DM, Blanton RA, et al. IFN-gamma mediates a novel antiviral activity through dynamic modulation of TRAIL and TRAIL receptor expression. J Immunol 1999;163(2):920–926.
184. Smyth MJ, Hayakawa Y, Takeda K, Yagita H. New aspects of natural-killer-cell surveillance and therapy of cancer. Nat Rev Cancer 2002;2(11):850–861.
185. Takeda K, Smyth MJ, Cretney E, et al. Involvement of tumor necrosis factor-related apoptosis-inducing ligand in NK cell-mediated and IFN-gamma-dependent suppression of subcutaneous tumor growth. Cell Immunol 2001;214(2):194–200.
186. Takeda K, Smyth MJ, Cretney E, et al. Critical role for tumor necrosis factor-related apoptosis-inducing ligand in immune surveillance against tumor development. J Exp Med 2002;195(2):161–169.
187. Krammer PH. CD95's deadly mission in the immune system. Nature 2000;407(6805):789–795.
188. Lin Y, Devin A, Rodriguez Y, Liu ZG. Cleavage of the death domain kinase RIP by caspase-8 prompts TNF-induced apoptosis. Genes Dev 1999;13(19):2514–2526.
189. Duckett CS, Thompson CB. CD30-dependent degradation of TRAF2: implications for negative regulation of TRAF signaling and the control of cell survival. Genes Dev 1997;11(21):2810–2821.
190. Arch RH, Gedrich RW, Thompson CB. Translocation of TRAF proteins regulates apoptotic threshold of cells. Biochem Biophys Res Commun 2000;272(3):936–945.
191. Leo E, Deveraux QL, Buchholtz C, et al. TRAF1 is a substrate of caspases activated during tumor necrosis factor receptor-alpha-induced apoptosis. J Biol Chem 2001;276(11):8087–8093.
192. Schwenzer R, Siemienski K, Liptay S, et al. The human tumor necrosis factor (TNF) receptor-associated factor 1 gene (TRAF1) is up-regulated by cytokines of the TNF ligand family and modulates TNF-induced activation of NF-kappaB and c-Jun N-terminal kinase. J Biol Chem 1999;274(27):19,368–19,374.
193. Tang G, Yang J, Minemoto Y, Lin A. Blocking caspase-3-mediated proteolysis of IKKbeta suppresses TNF-alpha-induced apoptosis. Mol Cell 2001;8(5):1005–1016.
194. Reuther JY, Baldwin AS, Jr. Apoptosis promotes a caspase-induced amino-terminal truncation of IkappaBalpha that functions as a stable inhibitor of NF-kappaB. J Biol Chem 1999;274(29):20,664–20,670.
195. Barkett M, Xue D, Horvitz HR, Gilmore TD. Phosphorylation of IkappaB-alpha inhibits its cleavage by caspase CPP32 in vitro. J Biol Chem 1997;272(47):29,419–29,422.
196. Ravi R, Bedi A, Fuchs EJ, Bedi A. CD95 (Fas)-induced caspase-mediated proteolysis of NF-kappaB. Cancer Res 1998;58(5):882–886.
197. Levkau B, Scatena M, Giachelli CM, Ross R, Raines EW. Apoptosis overrides survival signals through a caspase-mediated dominant-negative NF-kappa B loop. Nat Cell Biol 1999;1(4):227–233.
198. Cheng EH, Kirsch DG, Clem RJ, et al. Conversion of Bcl-2 to a Bax-like death effector by caspases. Science 1997;278(5345):1966–1968.
199. Clem RJ, Cheng EH, Karp CL, et al. Modulation of cell death by Bcl-XL through caspase interaction. Proc Natl Acad Sci USA 1998;95(2):554–559.

200. Fujita N, Nagahashi A, Nagashima K, Rokudai S, Tsuruo T. Acceleration of apoptotic cell death after the cleavage of Bcl-XL protein by caspase-3-like proteases. Oncogene 1998;17(10):1295–1304.
201. Clem RJ, Sheu TT, Richter BW, et al. c-IAP1 is cleaved by caspases to produce a proapoptotic C-terminal fragment. J Biol Chem 2001;276(10):7602–7608.
202. Heusel JW, Wesselschmidt RL, Shresta S, Russell JH, Ley TJ. Cytotoxic lymphocytes require granzyme B for the rapid induction of DNA fragmentation and apoptosis in allogeneic target cells. Cell 1994;76(6):977–987.
203. Shresta S, MacIvor DM, Heusel JW, Russell JH, Ley TJ. Natural killer and lymphokine-activated killer cells require granzyme B for the rapid induction of apoptosis in susceptible target cells. Proc Natl Acad Sci USA 1995;92(12):5679–5683.
204. Shi L, Mai S, Israels S, Browne K, Trapani JA, Greenberg AH. Granzyme B (GraB) autonomously crosses the cell membrane and perforin initiates apoptosis and GraB nuclear localization. J Exp Med 1997;185(5):855–866.
205. Metkar SS, Wang B, Aguilar-Santelises M, et al. Cytotoxic cell granule-mediated apoptosis: perforin delivers granzyme B-serglycin complexes into target cells without plasma membrane pore formation. Immunity 2002;16(3):417–428.
206. MacDonald G, Shi L, Vande VC, Lieberman J, Greenberg AH. Mitochondria-dependent and -independent regulation of granzyme B-induced apoptosis. J Exp Med 1999;189(1):131–144.
207. Alimonti JB, Shi L, Baijal PK, Greenberg AH. Granzyme B induces BID-mediated cytochrome c release and mitochondrial permeability transition. J Biol Chem 2001;276(10):6974–6982.
208. Wang GQ, Wieckowski E, Goldstein LA, et al. Resistance to granzyme B-mediated cytochrome c release in Bak-deficient cells. J Exp Med 2001;194(9):1325–1337.
209. Heibein JA, Goping IS, Barry M, et al. Granzyme B-mediated cytochrome c release is regulated by the Bcl-2 family members bid and Bax. J Exp Med 2000;192(10):1391–1402.
210. Kataoka T, Schroter M, Hahne M, et al. FLIP prevents apoptosis induced by death receptors but not by perforin/granzyme B, chemotherapeutic drugs, and gamma irradiation. J Immunol 1998;161(8): 3936–3942.
211. Kashii Y, Giorda R, Herberman RB, Whiteside TL, Vujanovic NL. Constitutive expression and role of the TNF family ligands in apoptotic killing of tumor cells by human NK cells. J Immunol 1999;163(10):5358–5366.
212. Talmadge JE, Meyers KM, Prieur DJ, Starkey JR. Role of NK cells in tumour growth and metastasis in beige mice. Nature 1980;284(5757):622–624.
213. Karre K, Ljunggren HG, Piontek G, Kiessling R. Selective rejection of H-2-deficient lymphoma variants suggests alternative immune defence strategy. Nature 1986;319(6055):675–678.
214. Takeda K, Hayakawa Y, Smyth MJ, et al. Involvement of tumor necrosis factor-related apoptosis-inducing ligand in surveillance of tumor metastasis by liver natural killer cells. Nat Med 2001;7(1): 94–100.
215. Smyth MJ, Thia KY, Cretney E, et al. Perforin is a major contributor to NK cell control of tumor metastasis. J Immunol 1999;162(11):6658–6662.
216. Owen-Schaub LB, van Golen KL, Hill LL, Price JE. Fas and Fas ligand interactions suppress melanoma lung metastasis. J Exp Med 1998;188(9):1717–1723.
217. Green DR, Ferguson TA. The role of Fas ligand in immune privilege. Nat Rev Mol Cell Biol 2001;2(12):917–924.
218. Rich T, Allen RL, Wyllie AH. Defying death after DNA damage. Nature 2000;407(6805):777–783.
219. el Deiry WS. Regulation of p53 downstream genes. Semin Cancer Biol 1998;8(5):345–357.
220. Kirsch DG, Kastan MB. Tumor-suppressor p53: implications for tumor development and prognosis. J Clin Oncol 1998;16(9):3158–3168.
221. Schuler M, Green DR. Mechanisms of p53-dependent apoptosis. Biochem Soc Trans 2001;29(Pt 6):684–688.
222. Oda E, Ohki R, Murasawa H, et al. Noxa, a BH3-only member of the Bcl-2 family and candidate mediator of p53-induced apoptosis. Science 2000;288(5468):1053–1058.
223. Nakano K, Vousden KH. PUMA, a novel proapoptotic gene, is induced by p53. Mol Cell 2001;7(3):683–694.
224. Miyashita T, Reed JC. Tumor suppressor p53 is a direct transcriptional activator of the human bax gene. Cell 1995;80(2):293–299.
225. Pearson AS, Spitz FR, Swisher SG, et al. Up-regulation of the proapoptotic mediators Bax and Bak after adenovirus-mediated p53 gene transfer in lung cancer cells. Clin Cancer Res 2000;6(3):887–890.

226. Pohl U, Wagenknecht B, Naumann U, Weller M. p53 enhances BAK and CD95 expression in human malignant glioma cells but does not enhance CD95L-induced apoptosis. Cell Physiol Biochem 1999;9(1):29–37.
227. Ravi R, Mookerjee B, van Hensbergen Y, et al. p53-mediated repression of nuclear factor-kappaB RelA via the transcriptional integrator p300. Cancer Res 1998;58(20):4531–4536.
228. Webster GA, Perkins ND. Transcriptional cross talk between NF-kappaB and p53. Mol Cell Biol 1999;19(5):3485–3495.
229. Wadgaonkar R, Phelps KM, Haque Z, Williams AJ, Silverman ES, Collins T. CREB-binding protein is a nuclear integrator of nuclear factor-kappaB and p53 signaling. J Biol Chem 1999;274(4):1879–1882.
230. Strasser A, Harris AW, Jacks T, Cory S. DNA damage can induce apoptosis in proliferating lymphoid cells via p53-independent mechanisms inhibitable by Bcl-2. Cell 1994;79(2):329–339.
231. Zhang L, Yu J, Park BH, Kinzler KW, Vogelstein B. Role of BAX in the apoptotic response to anticancer agents. Science 2000;290(5493):989–992.
232. Muller M, Wilder S, Bannasch D, et al. p53 activates the CD95 (APO-1/Fas) gene in response to DNA damage by anticancer drugs. J Exp Med 1998;188(11):2033–2045.
233. Wu GS, Burns TF, McDonald ER, III, et al. KILLER/DR5 is a DNA damage-inducible p53-regulated death receptor gene. Nat Genet 1997;17(2):141–143.
234. Fuchs EJ, McKenna KA, Bedi A. p53-dependent DNA damage-induced apoptosis requires Fas/APO-1-independent activation of CPP32beta. Cancer Res 1997;57(13):2550–2554.
235. Eischen CM, Kottke TJ, Martins LM, et al. Comparison of apoptosis in wild-type and Fas-resistant cells: chemotherapy-induced apoptosis is not dependent on Fas/Fas ligand interactions. Blood 1997;90(3):935–943.
236. Newton K, Strasser A. Ionizing radiation and chemotherapeutic drugs induce apoptosis in lymphocytes in the absence of Fas or FADD/MORT1 signaling. Implications for cancer therapy. J Exp Med 2000;191(1):195–200.
237. Altucci L, Rossin A, Raffelsberger W, Reitmair A, Chomienne C, Gronemeyer H. Retinoic acid-induced apoptosis in leukemia cells is mediated by paracrine action of tumor-selective death ligand TRAIL. Nat Med 2001;7(6):680–686.
238. Kaufmann SH, Earnshaw WC. Induction of apoptosis by cancer chemotherapy. Exp Cell Res 2000;256(1):42–49.
239. Ashkenazi A, Pai RC, Fong S, et al. Safety and antitumor activity of recombinant soluble Apo2 ligand. J Clin Invest 1999;104(2):155–162.
240. Walczak H, Miller RE, Ariail K, et al. Tumoricidal activity of tumor necrosis factor-related apoptosis-inducing ligand in vivo. Nat Med 1999;5(2):157–163.
241. Roth W, Isenmann S, Naumann U, et al. Locoregional Apo2L/TRAIL eradicates intracranial human malignant glioma xenografts in athymic mice in the absence of neurotoxicity. Biochem Biophys Res Commun 1999;265(2):479–483. 242. Chuntharapai A, Dodge K, Grimmer K, et al. Isotype-dependent inhibition of tumor growth in vivo by monoclonal antibodies to death receptor 4. J Immunol 2001;166(8):4891–4898.
243. Ichikawa K, Liu W, Zhao L, et al. Tumoricidal activity of a novel anti-human DR5 monoclonal antibody without hepatocyte cytotoxicity. Nat Med 2001;7(8):954–960.
244. Marsters SA, Pitti RA, Sheridan JP, Ashkenazi A. Control of apoptosis signaling by Apo2 ligand. Recent Prog Horm Res 1999;54:225–234.
245. Kim K, Fisher MJ, Xu SQ, el Deiry WS. Molecular determinants of response to TRAIL in killing of normal and cancer cells. Clin Cancer Res 2000;6(2):335–346.
246. Jo M, Kim TH, Seol DW, et al. Apoptosis induced in normal human hepatocytes by tumor necrosis factor-related apoptosis-inducing ligand. Nat Med 2000;6(5):564–567.
247. Lawrence D, Shahrokh Z, Marsters S, et al. Differential hepatocyte toxicity of recombinant Apo2L/TRAIL versions. Nat Med 2001;7(4):383–385.
248. Rampino N, Yamamoto H, Ionov Y, et al. Somatic frameshift mutations in the BAX gene in colon cancers of the microsatellite mutator phenotype. Science 1997;275(5302):967–969.

15 TRAIL in Cancer Therapy

Mahaveer Swaroop Bhojani, PhD,
Brian D. Ross, PhD,
and Alnawaz Rehemtulla, PhD

SUMMARY

Death receptors and their ligands have recently garnered much attention for therapeutic intervention of tumor progression. In clinical oncology, tumor necrosis factor-related apoptosis-inducing ligand (TRAIL) and its receptors are the most prominent duos in the death-receptor-ligand guild for their ability to specifically eliminate cancer cells without any deleterious effect on normal cells. Although in recent years five TRAIL receptors have been identified and a number of checkpoints involved in the TRAIL pathway are known, a well defined signaling pathway remains elusive and appears to be very complex. In spite of TRAIL possessing a high therapeutic index, some tumor cells evade TRAIL-mediated cell death by utilizing a plethora of different regulators, such as cellular FLICE- inhibitory protein (c-FLIP), caspase-8, NF-κB, Akt, and/or decoy receptors, which either stall or shunt death signaling by mechanisms that remain poorly understood. Interestingly, a number of recent reports suggest that a key to the success of TRAIL in cancer therapy is to use it in conjunction with chemo- or radiotherapy. Such a concept of combination therapy is gaining ground in eliminating tumors that are refractory to treatment with TRAIL, ionizing radiation, or chemotherapeutic agents alone. Results from preclinical studies on TRAIL have been very promising for cancer treatment; however, outcome from phase I/II clinical trials is eagerly awaited to assess its safety. Time will show whether TRAIL will be the foremost weapon in the clinical oncologist's arsenal to eradicate tumors.

DEATH RECEPTORS AND THEIR LIGANDS

Apoptosis is a genetically regulated physiological form of cell death that plays an important role in the removal of unwanted cells from most multicellular organisms *(1)*. It occurs in a variety of physiological processes, including embryonic development, tissue remodeling, immune regulation, and tumor regression, and in a variety pathological states, which include tumor growth, myocardial infarction, and neurodegenerative disorders *(2)*. Such forms of cell death culminate in a characteristic cellular morphology,

From: *Cancer Drug Discovery and Development: Death Receptors in Cancer Therapy*
Edited by: W. S. El-Deiry © Humana Press Inc., Totowa, NJ

which includes compaction of the cell, chromatin condensation, internucleosomal DNA degradation, membrane blebbing, and fragmentation of the cell into the apoptotic bodies *(1)* These key morphological alterations are brought about by activation of a family of intracellular proteases, collectively known as caspases—cysteine proteases with specificity for aspartic acid residues *(3)*. In the active state, caspases are dimeric and composed of two identical large subunits and two identical small subunits *(4)*. Targets for executioner caspases include various key cellular substrates, which when degraded signal the demise of the cells. It is interesting that a variety of different stimuli culminate in the activation of the same executioner caspases. These stimuli include environmental stress, cytotoxic agents, absence of growth factors, and activation of death receptors upon binding of their ligands.

The death receptors, as the name suggests, are cell-surface proteins with the potential to transmit a death message generated on the outside of the cell, by the binding of the death ligands to the apoptotic signaling machinery located inside the cell. There are seven known human death receptors: Fas (Apo-1, CD95), tumor necrosis factor receptor (TNFR)1 (p55-TNFR, CD120a), death receptor (DR)3 (WSL-1, APo-3, TRAMP, LARD), DR4 (TRAIL-R1), DR5 (TRAIL-R2, TRICK-2, KILLER), DR6, and EDA-R; each harbors a death domain (DD) at the cytoplasmic tail that couples the receptor to the caspase cascade essential for the induction of apoptosis *(5)* (*see also* Fig. 1). All known death receptors belong to the TNFR superfamily, and their ligands to the tumor necrosis factor (TNF) superfamily. Although Fas signaling remains the most extensively scrutinized death receptor signaling pathway, where the molecular mechanisms seem to be completely elucidated (reviewed in refs. *5–7*), investigating TRAIL and transduction of apoptotic signal by its cognate death receptors has been the most exciting exploration in oncology, since TRAIL possesses unique cytotoxic capability directed against a wide range of tumor cells but not normal cells *(5)*.

TRAIL and Its Receptors

TRAIL was discovered using a bioinformatics approach, where an expressed sequence tag database was screened for a characteristic TNF sequence motif, which lead to cloning of full-length TRAIL cDNA. Since it had sequence homology to the FAS/APO1 ligand (23% identity) and TNF (19% identity), the newly discovered protein was named APO2 ligand (APO2L) or TRAIL *(8,9)*. Investigation of TRAIL function revealed that it induces cell death in a wide variety of transformed cell lines, even those that were inherently resistant to high levels of chemotherapeutic drugs *(5,8,9)*. TRAIL is a type II transmembrane protein with a metalloprotease-susceptible exposed carboxyterminal region lying on the extracellular space *(10)*. Recombinant soluble TRAIL, which constitutes the extracellular portion, was sufficient for exerting its cytotoxic effect *(8,9,11,12)*. The biologically active form of TRAIL is a trimer that is stabilized by a zinc ion interacting with a cysteine residue at position 230 of each subunit *(13–15)*.

TRAIL induces apoptosis within the target cell by interacting with specific cell-surface receptors (Fig. 1). To date, five receptors that can bind TRAIL have been identified. Death receptor-4 (DR4, TRAIL-R1) and death receptor-5 (DR5, KILLER,TRAIL-R2,TRICK2) are type I transmembrane proteins containing two cysteine-rich extracellular ligand-binding domains and a cytoplasmic death domain, a region of approx 80 amino acids required for transmitting a cytotoxic signal *(16–21)*. In contrast, the other

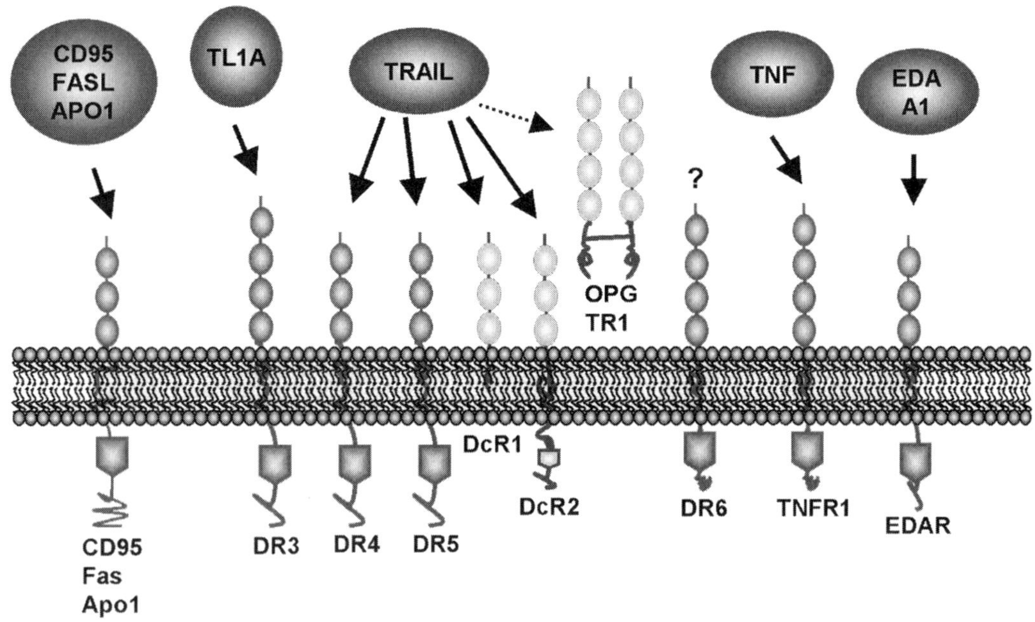

Fig. 1. Death receptors and their cognate ligands. The transmembrane ligands are labeled at top. The death receptors are the darker shaded ovals. Small circles and pentagons stand for the cysteine-rich domains and cytoplasmic death domains respectively. Arrows with solid lines symbolize strong binding, while dashed lines correspond to low-affinity binding between ligand and cognate receptor. The cognate ligand of DR6 is yet to be identified.

three receptors do not have a functional death domain and may act as decoy receptors *(16,17,19,20)*. Decoy receptor-1 (DcR1, TRID, TRAIL-R3), which lacks a death domain, and decoy receptor-2 (DcR2, TRUNDD, TRAIL-R4), which contains a truncated death domain, do not transduce apoptogenic signals. However, both decoy receptors (DcR1 and DcR2) and death receptors (DR4 and DR5) possess comparable affinity for binding to TRAIL. The third decoy receptor, osteoprotegerin (OPG), which was initially identified as a receptor for RANKL/OPGL, is a weak soluble receptor for TRAIL. Biological significance of OPG as a receptor for TRAIL remains to be elucidated *(22)*.

TRAIL and Apoptosis

The key feature of cell-death signaling is the activation of caspases, which may be achieved through two principle routes—the extrinsic and intrinsic death pathways *(*Fig. 2 and refs. *4,5)*. Death receptors use the extrinsic signaling pathway to convey the death cues to the cells, while the chemotherapeutic agents trigger the intrinsic pathway to apoptosis *(5)*. Increasing evidence suggests a cross-talk between the two pathways (*see* Fig. 2, next section, and the section on combination therapy).

The Extrinsic Pathway

The cell-extrinsic pathway utilizes the engagement of cell-surface death receptors by their ligands in initiating apoptosis *(5,23)*. Upon ligation of death receptors by their respective ligands, adaptor proteins such as FADD are recruited to the cytoplasmic tail

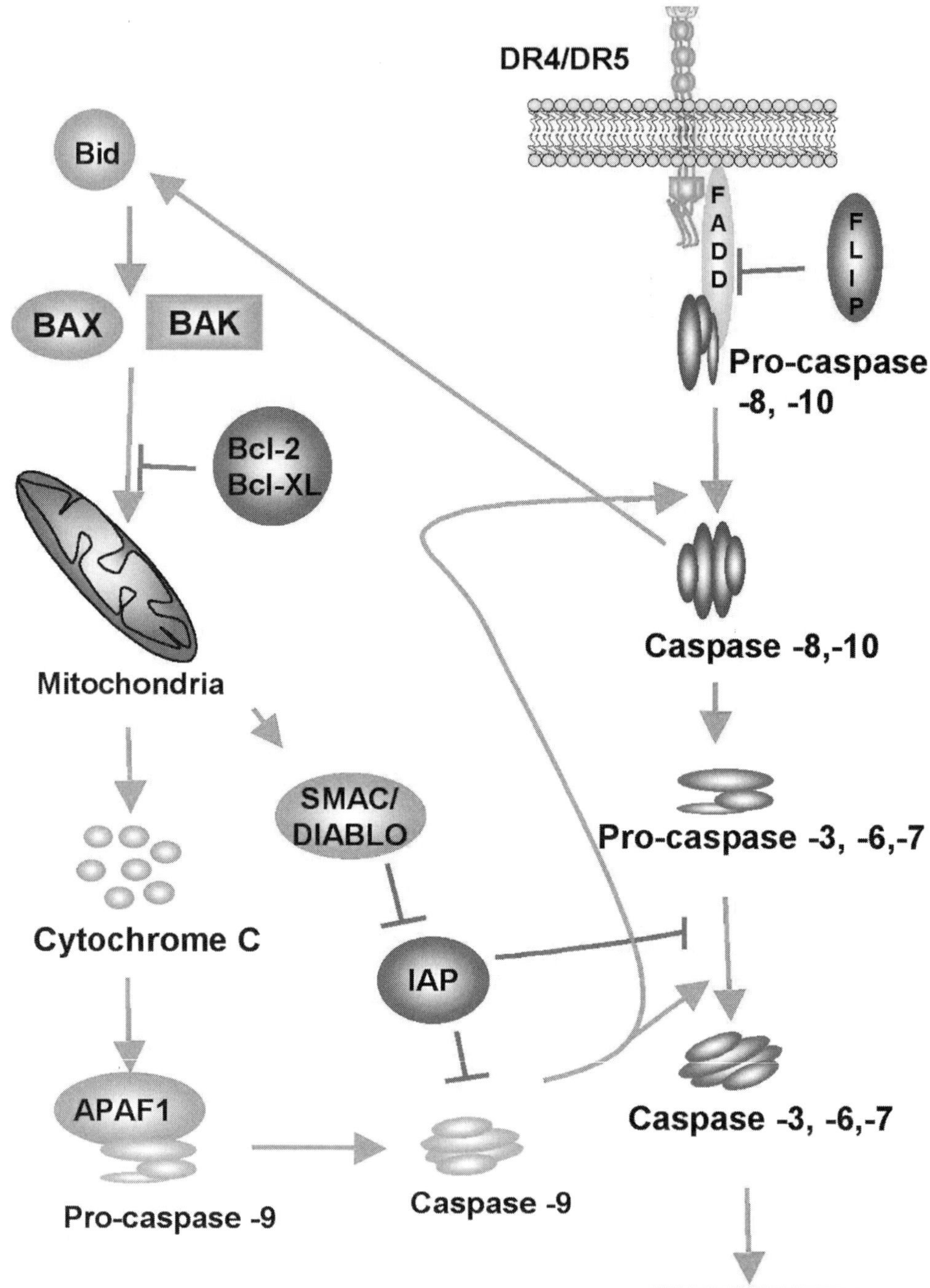

Fig. 2. Apoptotic pathway. Caspase activation and subsequent induction of apoptosis occur by two major pathways: the extrinsic and the intrinsic pathway. See text for further details.

of the receptor, which in turn recruit procaspases 8 and 10, leading to the assembly of the death-inducing signaling complex (DISC) *(24–26)*. By virtue of being brought into proximity with one another, procaspases 8 and 10 autocatalytically bring about their own activation *(3)*. Once active, these caspases consecutively activate the same set of executioner caspases (caspase-3, -6, and -7) that are activated by caspase-9 via the cell-intrinsic pathway *(5)*. This apoptogenic caspase machinery triggered by the cell-extrinsic pathway is independent of p53 status and is unaffected by Bcl-2 or Bcl-xL *(23)*. The prime negative regulator of TRAIL-induced apoptosis may be c-FLIP, which prevents apoptosis by blocking the assembly of DISC *(27–29,79)*.

The Intrinsic Pathway

The other route to activation of cell death is the cell-intrinsic, or mitochondrial, pathway (Fig. 2). This pathway is activated by cytotoxic agents, severe cell distress akin to DNA damage, defective cell cycle, detachment from the extracellular matrix, hypoxia, and loss of survival factors *(30)*. This pathway is triggered by the pro-apoptotic members of the *BCL2* superfamily, initially by a subset called the "BH3-only subfamily," which includes Bid, Bim, Harikari, and Noxa *(23,31)*. These proteins engage another set of proapoptotic Bcl-2 members, the Bax subfamily (which includes Bax, Bak, and probably Bok), loosely residing on the mitochondrial outer membranes or in the cytosol *(23)*. This interaction causes the latter to oligomerize and insert into the mitochondrial membrane, resulting in release of the key apoptogenic factors cytochrome c and Smac/DIABLO *(32,33)*. Within the cytosol, cytochrome *c* binds the adaptor APAF1, forming an apoptosome that recruits and activates the apoptosis-initiating protease caspase-9 *(34)*. Functional caspase-9 sets the momentum for activation of the executioner proteases caspase-3, -6, and -7 *(3)*. On the other hand, Smac/DIABLO exerts its role in supplementing apoptosis by binding to inhibitors of apoptosis (IAPs) and thereby preventing IAPs from attenuating caspase activation *(32,33,35)*. Funtional p53 appears to be a general requirement for engaging this death pathway *(23)*. DNA damage caused by most chemo- and radiotherapy triggers apoptosis in tumor cells by activating the intrinsic pathway. However, cells harboring non-functional p53 continue to proliferate and sidestep apoptosis, despite genotoxic stress induced by chemotherapy or irradiation *(23)*.

The Cross-Talk

Growing evidence suggests that the drug-induced intrinsic pathway and the death receptor-activated extrinsic pathway overlap during activation of cell death, and such convergence may be either at sharing of death receptors, caspase signaling cascade, upstream or downstream of mitochondrial signaling, or at the level of p53 or NF-κB signaling *(5,36)*. For example, certain DNA-damaging agents may activate both apoptotic pathways, such that blocking of either receptor pathway by overexpression of dominant-negative FADD or of the mitochondrial pathway by Bcl-xL only partially inhibited apoptosis *(37)*. Death receptors activate the cell-intrinsic pathway by caspase-8-mediated cleavage of BID, which interacts with BAX and BAK to induce release of cytochrome c and Smac/DIABLO, leading to increased activation of caspase-9 and -3 (Fig. 2 and ref. *38)*. Additionally, transcriptional upregulation of Fas and DR5 is reported to occur in response to DNA damage, via either a p53-independent or -dependent pathway *(39)*. Up-regulation increases the sensitivity of death receptor signals to their ligands. Furthermore, mismatch-repair-deficient tumors can acquire resistance to TRAIL by mutational inactivation of BAX, and such cells may be sensitized to TRAIL by pre-exposure to chemotherapeutic agents that lead to up-regulation of DR5 and BAK *(40)*. Thus the different death stimuli based on the target cell may use either of the signaling pathways or both, and such understanding is of immense importance in developing rationally designed therapy for human malignancies.

Biological Role of TRAIL and Its Receptors

The physiological function of TRAIL remains to be understood, but its main biological activity appears to be induction of apoptosis. TRAIL gene-knockout mice were more susceptible to experimental and spontaneous tumor metastasis, indicating that TRAIL has a crucial physiological role in antitumor surveillance by immune cells *(41)*. Alternately, experiments with mice in which the TRAIL activity was blocked by administration of neutralizing antibodies, incriminate TRAIL in interferon γ-dependent suppression of tumors by NK cells *(42)*. This is further corroborated by the observation that not only do activated NK cells, monocytes, and $CD4^+$ or $CD8^+$ T-cells express TRAIL, but they use it to trigger apoptosis in tumor targets *(43–50)*. TRAIL has been implicated in apoptogenic activity of type I interferon in renal cell carcinoma and multiple myleomas *(51,52)*. Furthermore, up-regulation of TRAIL is observed when cells are infected with reovirus or herpes virus, suggesting that virus-infected cells are eliminated using the TRAIL pathway *(53,54)*. These results suggest an important yet partially understood role for TRAIL in immune surveillance (suppressing tumor initiation, progression, and viral propagation).

TRAIL AND CANCER THERAPY

Most of the excitement with TRAIL as a promising therapeutic agent for treatment of malignancies is due to its ability to exert its cytotoxic effects on cancerous cells without any harm to normal cells *(5,55,56)*. Recombinant soluble TRAIL induces apoptosis within 4 to 8 h in a number of transformed cell lines derived from leukemia, multiple myeloma, neuroblastoma, and cancers of the colon, lung, breast, prostate, pancreas, kidney, central nervous system, and thyroid. Mice bearing solid tumors, when injected with soluble TRAIL, showed increased tumor cell apoptosis, suppressed tumor progression, and improved survival without any normal-tissue toxicity *(11,12,57–62)*. Administration of TRAIL to mice transplanted with human tumor xenografts derived from colon carcinoma, breast cancer, mammary adenocarcinoma, multiple myeloma, or malignant glioma, exerted marked antitumor activity without systemic toxicity *(10,12,63–66)*. TRAIL was also shown to inhibit growth of evolving tumors immediately after xenograft implantation, as well as in established tumors. Additionally, agonistic antibodies to DR5, whose binding to the receptor would imitate binding of TRAIL, were shown to induce apoptosis in human astroglioma cells and liver cancer cells *(67,68)*. Moreover, the fact that p53 status does not correlate with TRAIL sensitivity raises an optimistic view of TRAIL as an anticancer agent, as nearly 50% of human tumors show mutation in p53.

As an alternate to administration of soluble TRAIL, adenoviral gene therapy vehicles for TRAIL have been utilized with promising results both in vitro and in small experimental animals *(69–72)*. Prolonged survival of nude mice bearing ovarian cancer xenografts have been reported upon administration of adenoviral vectors harboring the TRAIL gene

(72). Therapeutic efficacy of TRAIL gene therapy has also been demonstrated with colon cancer, prostrate tumors, glioblastoma, breast cancer, and hepatocellular carcinoma *(71,73–76)*. Taken together, these results indicate substantial promise for TRAIL in the treatment of human cancers.

Warning bells were recently heard when normal human hepatocytes, brain cells, and keratinocytes were shown to be sensitive to TRAIL, which suggested a potential for systemic toxicity if TRAIL were to be used for clinical trials *(77–79)*. However, reassessment of these results suggests that TRAIL toxicity in hepatocytes and keratinocytes depended on the form and source of the recombinant TRAIL used *(80,81)*. For example, hepatotoxicity was observed with polyhistidine-tagged soluble TRAIL, and keratinocytes were sensitive to both the soluble version of the ligand, which contained a trimerizing leucine zipper, and polyhistidine-tagged TRAIL. However, when non-tagged soluble TRAIL was used, toxicity in hepatocytes and keratinocytes was not observed *(80,81)*. Furthermore, in preclinical trials in cynomolgus monkeys and chimpanzees, intravenous administration of non-tagged TRAIL was well tolerated, with no harmful symptoms in either laboratory parameters or organ histology *(80)*. Similarly, non-tagged TRAIL was well tolerated by normal human keratinocytes *(81)*. These results rebuild the enthusiasm of clinical oncologists for TRAIL as a potent cancer therapeutic. However, further studies are needed to evaluate toxicity and potential species-specific effects.

TUMOR RESISTANCE TO APOPTOSIS IN THE DEATH RECEPTOR SIGNALING PATHWAY

A major impediment for the clinical use of TRAIL is that there are a number of tumor cell lines resistant to TRAIL-mediated cell death (Table 1). Although mechanisms underlying such resistance are not fully understood, there is distinct delineation between resistance observed in normal and tumor cells *(5,23,55)*. Several factors have been proposed to impose resistance to TRAIL. For example, relative abundance and access of death and decoy receptors, relative activities of caspase-8 and -10, FLIP, and activity of phosphatidylinositol 3' kinase/Akt pathway ultimately determine sensitivity of cells to TRAIL. Additionally, tissue- and species-specific responses compound the understanding of factors involved in TRAIL-mediated apoptosis *(55)*.

Multiple Receptor Interactions for Tumor Proliferation

In the context of multiple receptors for TRAIL, some capable of triggering apoptosis while others abrogate TRAIL activity, resistance could be due to increased levels of DcR1 and DcR2 and decreased levels of proapoptotic DR4 and DR5. However, in the majority of normal and tumor cell lines, no decipherable correlation was observed between different types of TRAIL receptor expression and TRAIL susceptibility *(28,60,79,82–85)*. Such results suggest that subcellular distribution of death and decoy receptors and their reorganization upon treatment with TRAIL could play a key role. In melanoma cells, upon addition of TRAIL, reorganization of death receptors between different sub-cellular compartments and the cell surface is observed *(86,87)*. Relocation of decoy receptors DcR1 and DcR2 to the cell surface from the nucleus and down-regulation of cell-surface expression of DR5 were also observed in the same system *(87)*.

Table 1
Mechanisms of Synergy Between TRAIL and Cytotoxic Agent

1. Upregulation of death receptors by cytotoxic agents

Cytotoxic agent	*Death receptor upregulated*	*Tumor cell type (reference)*
Ara-C Doxorubicin Etoposide	DR5	Acute leukemia *(85)*
Etoposide	DR4 and DR5	Breast carcinoma *(128)*
Ionizing radiation	DR5	Breast carcinoma *(113)*
Etoposide CDDP	DR5	Glioma *(122)*
Topotecan	DR5	Renal cell carcinoma *(114)*
Retinoid CD437	DR4 and DR5	Lung and lung cancer *(129)*
Ionizing radiation	DR4	Erythroleukemia *(130)*
Adriamycin Etoposide	DR5	Multiple myeloma *(131)*
Adriamycin Cisplatin Etoposide	DR4 and DR5	Osteogenic sarcoma *(132)*
Doxorubicin cisplatin	DR5	Glioma *(133)*

2. Modulation of proteins involved in apoptosis by cytotoxic agents

Cytotoxic agents used in conjunction with TRAIL	*Targeted apoptotic protein*	*Tumor cell type (reference)*
Actinomycin D	Downregulation of Bcl-xL	AIDS–Kaposi's sarcoma *(134)*
Actinomycin D	Downregulation of FLIP	Melanoma *(28)*
5-FU Doxorubicin	Increased capsase-3 activity	Breast carcinoma *(58)*
Retinoid CD437	Increased Bid cleavage	Lung cancer *(129)*
Sodium butyrate Actinomycin D Cycloheximide	Downregulation of FLIP Increased caspase-3 activity	Colon carinoma *(29,135)*
Cisplatin Doxorubicin	Activation of caspase-8	Colon carcinoma *(117)*
Cisplatin Carboplatin	Upregulation of Bax	Bladder cancer *(59)*
Nitroprusside	Augmentation by intrinsic pathway	Colon carcinoma *(136)*
5'-aza-2'deoxycytidine	Demethylation of caspase-8 promoter and up-regulation of caspase-8	Neuroblastoma *(107,108)*

continued

2. Modulation of proteins involved in apoptosis by cytotoxic agents (continued)

Cytotoxic agents used in conjunction with TRAIL	*Targeted apoptotic protein*	*Tumor cell type (reference)*
Actinomycin	Downregulation of FLIP	Pancreatic cancer *(137)*
Smac agonist	Bypassing Bcl-3 block	Glioma *(138)*
5-FU	Upregulation of Bax and p53	Renal cell carcinoma *(139)*
Doxoruicin Epirubicin Pirarubicin Amrubicin	Activation of caspase cascade	Prostrate cancer *(140)*
Doxorubicin 5-FU	Increased FADD and procaspase-8 recruitment to DISC	Colon carcinoma *(141)*

3. Other examples of synergy between TRAIL and cytotoxic agents

Cytotoxic agent used in conjunction with TRAIL	*Tumor cell type (reference)*
Ionizing radiation	Acute leukemia *(142)*
Adriamycin Epirubicin Pirarubicin	Bladder cancer *(59)*
Proteasome inhibitors	Ewing's sarcoma *(143)*
Cycloheximide	Glioma *(144)*
Actinomycin D Doxorubicin Campothecin	Hepatocellular carcinoma *(116)*
Cisplatin Doxorubicin Paclitaxel	Ovarian cancer *(112)*
Proteasome inhibitors	Promonocytic leukemia *(145)*
Actinomycin D Gemcitabine	Prostrate cancer *(146)*
Cisplatin Doxorubicin Etoposide	Prostrate cancer *(123)*
Cycloheximide	Thyroid cancer *(147)*

FLIP

Abundant expression of an inhibitor of death receptor signaling, namely c-FLIP, has been shown to confer resistance to tumor cells *(28,88)*. Analysis of the expression pattern of FLIP and relative resistance/susceptibility to TRAIL in melanoma, glioma, and colon carcinoma revealed that expression of FLIP was highest in cells that were resistant to TRAIL *(28,89,90)*. Such resistant cells could be converted to TRAIL-susceptible cells when treated with protein-synthesis inhibitors or chemotherapeutic drugs that interfere with expression of FLIP *(28,91–94)*. These observations suggest that the balance of expression of DISC components may play a key role in transduction of the death signal. Interestingly, injection of cells overexpressing FLIP in mice consistently resulted in tumors, while cells with little or no FLIP were rejected in the majority of mice, suggesting that not only does FLIP make tumors more resistant to TRAIL-mediated cell death, but that it is also involved in the evasion by these tumors from the host immune system *(94a)*. Thus, understanding the mechanism underlying the action of DISC components and clinical intervention using targeted drug therapy at this early stage of apoptosis is critical for efficacious cancer therapy.

Akt

An equilibrium between anti- and proapoptotic signals could also play a key role in dictating the outcome of an apoptogenic trigger by a death ligand. For example, some prostate cancer cells express constitutively active Akt/protein kinase B due to the loss of lipid phosphatase gene PTEN, a negative regulator of PI-3 kinase *(95–97)*. TRAIL sensitivity of these cells was dependent on the level of Akt; cells expressing the highest level of Akt were the most resistant, and such resistance could be reversed by treating with a PI-3 kinase inhibitor such as wortmannin and LY294002 *(98–100)*. Recently, additional examples of a correlation between Akt activity and resistance to TRAIL signaling have been reported in human colon cancer cells, multiple myeloma, thyroid carcinoma, and non-small-cell lung cancer cells *(91,101–103)*. These observations suggest that modulation of Akt activity, by genetic or pharmacological intervention, may be important in effective killing of these cancer cells by TRAIL.

Caspase-8

Analysis of the native DISC components suggests that caspase-8 is a key player in early TRAIL-mediated signaling for apoptosis. On the other hand, caspase-10, though recruited to the DISC, is dispensable for induction of apoptosis *(3,104,105)*. However, dendritic cells harboring a mutant caspase-10 are refractory to TRAIL-induced cell death, suggesting that catalytically inactive mutant caspase-10 may act as a nonreleasable substrate trap for caspase-8 *(104)*. Alternatively, as observed in certain neuroblastomas, caspase-8 is downregulated by hypermethylation of its promoter, leading to a decreased response to TRAIL-induced cell death *(106)*. However, treatment of neuroblastoma cells with aza-2'-deoxycytidine restores mRNA expression of caspase-8 and TRAIL susceptibility *(107–110)*.

COMBINATION THERAPY

In an effort to overcome the fact that many human tumors cells are resistant to TRAIL, the concept of combination therapy was envisaged. This was based on the idea that pretreatment of tumor cells with a radio- or chemotherapeutic agent would sensitize them to TRAIL.

A number of studies have shown cooperation between chemotherapeutic drugs or radiation and TRAIL in inducing cell death in malignant mesothelioma, ovarian, prostate, bladder, renal, pancreatic, glial, and breast cells *(58,59,111–118)*. The molecular basis behind such synergy is being actively investigated, and a number of different mechanisms have been suggested. A list of possible mechanisms of synergy observed between various cytotoxic agents and TRAIL in different tumor cell types has been listed in Table 1.

First, chemotherapeutic drugs or radiation could trigger an apoptotic pathway that may be different than one exploited by TRAIL, to thus transduce a more potent pro-apoptotic signal. For example, Bcl-2 localized to mitochondria or endoplasmic reticulum inhibits apoptosis induced by DNA damage but is unable to confer similar resistance to TRAIL-induced cell death *(119)* Thus, dual treatment could lead to simultaneous activation of distinct apoptotic pathways, resulting in better killing of tumor cells. However, chemotherapeutic drugs have diverse cellular targets, which include RNA, DNA, topoisomerase I or II, kinases, microtubules, or the plasma membrane. The mechanism by which these drugs trigger apoptosis remains to be understood. Such knowledge would aid in choosing effective combination therapy to eliminate drug-resistant cells.

DNA damage has been reported to up-regulate DR5 transcription in human cancer cells *(113,115,120,121)*. By monitoring tumor therapy by noninvasive diffusion-weighted MRI, we have previously shown that TRAIL works in concert with radiation to eradicate breast cancer tumors, and that such synergy is mediated by up-regulation of the DR5 receptor *(113)*. Similar synergy between DNA-damaging drugs like cisplatin (CDDP) or etoposide and TRAIL was also observed in gliomas *(122,123)*. Using such combination therapy, normal tissue toxicity of the DNA-damaging drugs could be overcome using sublethal doses, which do not kill the normal cells but cause up-regulation of the DR5 in tumor cells. Addition of TRAIL to such tumors would systemically eliminate them. However, DR5 upregulation by DNA-damaging drugs was observed to be dependent on the tumor suppressor gene p53, thus limiting the use of such combination therapy, as the majority of cancer cells display p53 mutations *(113,121,124)*. On the contrary, recent studies demarcate the link between p53 and upregulation of DR5 expression in a number of tumor cell lines *(125)*. The other TRAIL death receptor, DR4, was recently shown to be upregulated upon DNA damage *(126)*. Interestingly, some reports indicate that such TRAIL and DNA-damaging agent synergy could be independent of DR4 and DR5 upregulation, suggesting that other mechanisms may prevail for a concerted effect *(127)*. Taken together, the combination therapy using TRAIL and DNA-damaging agents may be a safe therapeutic strategy for human malignancies, including TRAIL-resistant cancers.

ACKNOWLEDGMENTS

We thank Laura Griffin and Bharathi Laxman for critical reading of the manuscript. This work was supported by NIH/NCI P50CA01014 (BDR and AR) and NIH/NCI P01CA85878 (BDF and AR).

REFERENCES

1. Wyllie AH, Kerr JF, Currie AR. Cell death: the significance of apoptosis. Int Rev Cytol 1980;68:251–306.
2. Strasser A, O'Connor L, Dixit VM. Apoptosis signaling. Annu Rev Biochem 2000;69:217–245.
3. Shi Y. Mechanisms of caspase activation and inhibition during apoptosis. Mol Cell 2002;9:459–470.
4. Kaufmann SH, Gores GJ. Apoptosis in cancer: cause and cure. Bioessays 2000;22:1007–1017.
5. Ashkenazi A. Targeting death and decoy receptors of the tumour-necrosis factor superfamily. Nat Rev Cancer 2002;2:420–430.

6. Siegel RM, Chan FK, Chun HJ, Lenardo MJ. The multifaceted role of Fas signaling in immune cell homeostasis and autoimmunity. Nat Immunol 2000;1:469–474.
7. Krammer PH. CD95's deadly mission in the immune system. Nature 2000;407:789–795.
8. Wiley SR, Schooley K, Smolak PJ, et al. Identification and characterization of a new member of the TNF family that induces apoptosis. Immunity 1995;3:673–682.
9. Pitti RM, Marsters SA, Ruppert S, Donahue CJ, Moore A, Ashkenazi A. Induction of apoptosis by Apo-2 ligand, a new member of the tumor necrosis factor cytokine family. J Biol Chem 1996;271:12687–2690.
10. Ashkenazi A, Dixit VM. Apoptosis control by death and decoy receptors. Curr Opin Cell Biol 1999;11:255–260.
11. Ashkenazi A, Pai RC, Fong S, et al. Safety and antitumor activity of recombinant soluble Apo2 ligand. J Clin Invest 1999;104:155–162.
12. Walczak H, Miller RE, Ariail K, et al. Tumoricidal activity of tumor necrosis factor–related apoptosis-inducing ligand in vivo. Nat Med 1999;5:157–163.
13. Hymowitz SG, O'Connell MP, Ultsch MH, et al. A unique zinc-binding site revealed by a high-resolution X-ray structure of homotrimeric Apo2L/TRAIL. Biochemistry 2000;39:633–640.
14. Hymowitz SG, Christinger HW, Fuh G, et al. Triggering cell death: the crystal structure of Apo2L/TRAIL in a complex with death receptor 5. Mol Cell 1999;4:563–571.
15. Bodmer JL, Meier P, Tschopp J, Schneider P. Cysteine 230 is essential for the structure and activity of the cytotoxic ligand TRAIL. J Biol Chem 2000;275:20,632–20,637.
16. Sheridan JP, Marsters SA, Pitti RM, et al. Control of TRAIL-induced apoptosis by a family of signaling and decoy receptors. Science 1997;277:818–821.
17. Pan G, Ni J, Wei YF, Yu G, Gentz R, Dixit VM. An antagonist decoy receptor and a death domain-containing receptor for TRAIL. Science 1997;277:815–818.
18. Walczak H, Degli-Esposti MA, Johnson RS, et al. TRAIL-R2: a novel apoptosis-mediating receptor for TRAIL. Embo J 1997;16:5386–5397.
19. Degli-Esposti MA, Dougall WC, Smolak PJ, Waugh JY, Smith CA, Goodwin RG. The novel receptor TRAIL-R4 induces NF-kappaB and protects against TRAIL-mediated apoptosis, yet retains an incomplete death domain. Immunity 1997;7:813–820.
20. Degli-Esposti MA, Smolak PJ, Walczak H, et al. Cloning and characterization of TRAIL-R3, a novel member of the emerging TRAIL receptor family. J Exp Med 1997;186:1165–1170.
21. Pan G, O'Rourke K, Chinnaiyan AM, et al. The receptor for the cytotoxic ligand TRAIL. Science 1997;276:111–113.
22. Emery JG, McDonnell P, Burke MB, et al. Osteoprotegerin is a receptor for the cytotoxic ligand TRAIL. J Biol Chem 1998;273:14,363–14,367.
23. Igney FH, Krammer PH. Death and anti-death: tumour resistance to apoptosis. Nat Rev Cancer 2002;2:277–288.
24. Kischkel FC, Hellbardt S, Behrmann I, et al. Cytotoxicity-dependent APO-1 (Fas/CD95)-associated proteins form a death-inducing signaling complex (DISC) with the receptor. Embo J 1995;14:5579–5588.
25. Kischkel FC, Lawrence DA, Tinel A, et al. Death receptor recruitment of endogenous caspase-10 and apoptosis initiation in the absence of caspase-8. J Biol Chem 2001;276:46,639–46,646.
26. Muzio M, Chinnaiyan AM, Kischkel FC, et al. FLICE, a novel FADD-homologous ICE/CED-3-like protease, is recruited to the CD95 (Fas/APO-1) death-inducing signaling complex. Cell 1996;85:817–827.
27. Krueger A, Baumann S, Krammer PH, Kirchhoff S. FLICE-inhibitory proteins: regulators of death receptor-mediated apoptosis. Mol Cell Biol 2001;21:8247–8254.
28. Griffith TS, Chin WA, Jackson GC, Lynch DH, Kubin MZ. Intracellular regulation of TRAIL-induced apoptosis in human melanoma cells. J Immunol 1998;161:2833–2840.
29. Hernandez A, Wang QD, Schwartz SA, Evers BM. Sensitization of human colon cancer cells to TRAIL-mediated apoptosis. J Gastrointest Surg 2001;5:56–65.
30. Green DR, Reed JC. Mitochondria and apoptosis. Science 1998;281:1309–1312.
31. Gross A, McDonnell JM, Korsmeyer SJ. BCL-2 family members and the mitochondria in apoptosis. Genes Dev 1999;13:1899–1911.
32. Verhagen AM, Ekert PG, Pakusch M, et al. Identification of DIABLO, a mammalian protein that promotes apoptosis by binding to and antagonizing IAP proteins. Cell 2000;102:43–53.
33. Du C, Fang M, Li Y, Li L, Wang X. Smac, a mitochondrial protein that promotes cytochrome c-dependent caspase activation by eliminating IAP inhibition. Cell 2000;102:33–42.

34. Zou H, Li Y, Liu X, Wang X. An APAF-1.cytochrome c multimeric complex is a functional apoptosome that activates procaspase-9. J Biol Chem 1999;274:11,549–11,556.
35. Ekert PG, Silke J, Hawkins CJ, Verhagen AM, Vaux DL. DIABLO promotes apoptosis by removing MIHA/XIAP from processed caspase 9. J Cell Biol 2001;152:483–490.
36. Petak I, Houghton JA. Shared pathways: death receptors and cytotoxic drugs in cancer therapy. Pathol Oncol Res 2001;7:95–106.
37. Fulda S, Meyer E, Friesen C, Susin SA, Kroemer G, Debatin KM. Cell type specific involvement of death receptor and mitochondrial pathways in drug-induced apoptosis. Oncogene 2001;20:1063–1075.
38. Korsmeyer SJ, Wei MC, Saito M, Weiler S, Oh KJ, Schlesinger PH. Pro-apoptotic cascade activates BID, which oligomerizes BAK or BAX into pores that result in the release of cytochrome c. Cell Death Differ 2000;7:1166–1173.
39. El-Deiry WS. Insights into cancer therapeutic design based on p53 and TRAIL receptor signaling. Cell Death Differ 2001;8:1066–1075.
40. LeBlanc H, Lawrence D, Varfolomeev E, et al. Tumor-cell resistance to death receptor-induced apoptosis through mutational inactivation of the proapoptotic Bcl-2 homolog Bax. Nat Med 2002;8:274–281.
41. Cretney E, Takeda K, Yagita H, Glaccum M, Peschon JJ, Smyth MJ. Increased susceptibility to tumor initiation and metastasis in TNF-related apoptosis-inducing ligand-deficient mice. J Immunol 2002;168:1356–1361.
42. Takeda K, Smyth MJ, Cretney E, et al. Critical role for tumor necrosis factor–related apoptosis-inducing ligand in immune surveillance against tumor development. J Exp Med 2002;195:161–169.
43. Johnsen AC, Haux J, Steinkjer B, et al. Regulation of APO-2 ligand/trail expression in NK cells-involvement in NK cell-mediated cytotoxicity. Cytokine 1999;11:664–672.
44. Jeremias I, Herr I, Boehler T, Debatin KM. TRAIL/Apo-2-ligand-induced apoptosis in human T cells. Eur J Immunol 1998;28:143–152.
45. Thomas WD, Hersey P. TNF-related apoptosis-inducing ligand (TRAIL) induces apoptosis in Fas ligand-resistant melanoma cells and mediates CD4 T cell killing of target cells. J Immunol 1998;161:2195–2200.
46. Kayagaki N, Yamaguchi N, Nakayama M, et al. Expression and function of TNF-related apoptosis-inducing ligand on murine activated NK cells. J Immunol 1999;163:1906–1913.
47. Kayagaki N, Yamaguchi N, Nakayama M, et al. Involvement of TNF-related apoptosis-inducing ligand in human CD4+ T cell-mediated cytotoxicity. J Immunol 1999;162:2639–2647.
48. Martinez-Lorenzo MJ, Alava MA, Gamen S, et al. Involvement of APO2 ligand/TRAIL in activation-induced death of Jurkat and human peripheral blood T cells. Eur J Immunol 1998;28:2714–2725.
49. Mariani SM, Krammer PH. Surface expression of TRAIL/Apo-2 ligand in activated mouse T and B cells. Eur J Immunol 1998;28:1492–1498.
50. Griffith TS, Wiley SR, Kubin MZ, Sedger LM, Maliszewski CR, Fanger NA. Monocyte-mediated tumoricidal activity via the tumor necrosis factor-related cytokine, TRAIL. J Exp Med 1999;189: 1343–1354.
51. Kayagaki N, Yamaguchi N, Nakayama M, Eto H, Okumura K, Yagita H. Type I interferons (IFNs) regulate tumor necrosis factor-related apoptosis-inducing ligand (TRAIL) expression on human T cells: A novel mechanism for the antitumor effects of type I IFNs. J Exp Med 1999;189:1451–1460.
52. Chen Q, Gong B, Mahmoud-Ahmed AS, et al. Apo2L/TRAIL and Bcl-2-related proteins regulate type I interferon-induced apoptosis in multiple myeloma. Blood 2001;98:2183–2192.
53. Clarke P, Meintzer SM, Widmann C, Johnson GL, Tyler KL. Reovirus infection activates JNK and the JNK-dependent transcription factor c-Jun. J Virol 2001;75:11,275–11,283.
54. Secchiero P, Mirandola P, Zella D, et al. Human herpesvirus 7 induces the functional up-regulation of tumor necrosis factor-related apoptosis-inducing ligand (TRAIL) coupled to TRAIL-R1 down-modulation in CD4(+) T cells. Blood 2001;98:2474–2481.
55. Held J, Schulze-Osthoff K. Potential and caveats of TRAIL in cancer therapy. Drug Resist Updat 2001;4:243–252.
56. Fricker J. On the TRAIL to a new cancer therapy. Mol Med Today 1999;5:374.
57. Rieger J, Naumann U, Glaser T, Ashkenazi A, Weller M. APO2 ligand: a novel lethal weapon against malignant glioma? FEBS Lett 1998;427:124–128.
58. Keane MM, Ettenberg SA, Nau MM, Russell EK, Lipkowitz S. Chemotherapy augments TRAIL-induced apoptosis in breast cell lines. Cancer Res 1999;59:734–741.

59. Mizutani Y, Nakao M, Ogawa O, Yoshida O, Bonavida B, Miki T. Enhanced sensitivity of bladder cancer cells to tumor necrosis factor related apoptosis inducing ligand mediated apoptosis by cisplatin and carboplatin. J Urol 2001;165:263–270.
60. Mitsiades N, Poulaki V, Mitsiades C, Tsokos M. Ewing's sarcoma family tumors are sensitive to tumor necrosis factor-related apoptosis-inducing ligand and express death receptor 4 and death receptor 5. Cancer Res 2001;61:2704–2712.
61. Yu R, Mandlekar S, Ruben S, Ni J, Kong AN. Tumor necrosis factor-related apoptosis-inducing ligand-mediated apoptosis in androgen-independent prostate cancer cells. Cancer Res 2000;60:2384–2389.
62. Gazitt Y. TRAIL is a potent inducer of apoptosis in myeloma cells derived from multiple myeloma patients and is not cytotoxic to hematopoietic stem cells. Leukemia 1999;13:1817–1824.
63. Kelley SK, Harris LA, Xie D, et al. Preclinical studies to predict the disposition of Apo2L/tumor necrosis factor-related apoptosis-inducing ligand in humans: characterization of in vivo efficacy, pharmacokinetics, and safety. J Pharmacol Exp Ther 2001;299:31–38.
64. Mitsiades CS, Treon SP, Mitsiades N, et al. TRAIL/Apo2L ligand selectively induces apoptosis and overcomes drug resistance in multiple myeloma: therapeutic applications. Blood 2001;98:795–804.
65. Roth W, Isenmann S, Naumann U, et al. Locoregional Apo2L/TRAIL eradicates intracranial human malignant glioma xenografts in athymic mice in the absence of neurotoxicity. Biochem Biophys Res Commun 1999;265:479–483.
66. Pollack IF, Erff M, Ashkenazi A. Direct stimulation of apoptotic signaling by soluble Apo2l/tumor necrosis factor-related apoptosis-inducing ligand leads to selective killing of glioma cells. Clin Cancer Res 2001;7:1362–1369.
67. Ichikawa K, Liu W, Zhao L, et al. Tumoricidal activity of a novel anti-human DR5 monoclonal antibody without hepatocyte cytotoxicity. Nat Med 2001;7:954–960.
68. Choi C, Kutsch O, Park J, Zhou T, Seol DW, Benveniste EN. Tumor necrosis factor–related apoptosis-inducing ligand induces caspase-dependent interleukin-8 expression and apoptosis in human astroglioma cells. Mol Cell Biol 2002;22:724–736.
69. Griffith TS, Anderson RD, Davidson BL, Williams RD, Ratliff TL. Adenoviral-mediated transfer of the TNF-related apoptosis-inducing ligand/Apo-2 ligand gene induces tumor cell apoptosis. J Immunol 2000;165:2886–2894.
70. Kagawa S, He C, Gu J, et al. Antitumor activity and bystander effects of the tumor necrosis factor-related apoptosis-inducing ligand (TRAIL) gene. Cancer Res 2001;61:3330–3338.
71. Griffith TS, Broghammer EL. Suppression of tumor growth following intralesional therapy with TRAIL recombinant adenovirus. Mol Ther 2001;4:257–266.
72. Huang X, Lin T, Gu J, et al. Combined TRAIL and Bax gene therapy prolonged survival in mice with ovarian cancer xenograft. Gene Ther 2002;9:1379–1386.
73. Norris JS, Hyer ML, Voelkel-Johnson C, Lowe SL, Rubinchik S, Dong JY. The use of Fas Ligand, TRAIL and Bax in gene therapy of prostate cancer. Curr Gene Ther 2001;1:123–136.
74. Lee J, Hampl M, Albert P, Fine HA. Antitumor activity and prolonged expression from a TRAIL-expressing adenoviral vector. Neoplasia 2002;4:312–323.
75. Voelkel-Johnson C, King DL, Norris JS. Resistance of prostate cancer cells to soluble TNF-related apoptosis-inducing ligand (TRAIL/Apo2L) can be overcome by doxorubicin or adenoviral delivery of full-length TRAIL. Cancer Gene Ther 2002;9:164–172.
76. Yamashita Y, Shimada M, Tanaka S, Okamamoto M, Miyazaki J, Sugimachi K. Electroporation-mediated tumor necrosis factor–related apoptosis-inducing ligand (TRAIL)/Apo2L gene therapy for hepatocellular carcinoma. Hum Gene Ther 2002;13:275–286.
77. Nitsch R, Bechmann I, Deisz RA, et al. Human brain-cell death induced by tumour-necrosis-factor-related apoptosis-inducing ligand (TRAIL). Lancet 2000;356:827–828.
78. Jo M, Kim TH, Seol DW, et al. Apoptosis induced in normal human hepatocytes by tumor necrosis factor-related apoptosis-inducing ligand. Nat Med 2000;6:564–567.
79. Leverkus M, Neumann M, Mengling T, et al. Regulation of tumor necrosis factor-related apoptosis-inducing ligand sensitivity in primary and transformed human keratinocytes. Cancer Res 2000;60: 553–559.
80. Lawrence D, Shahrokh Z, Marsters S, et al. Differential hepatocyte toxicity of recombinant Apo2L/ TRAIL versions. Nat Med 2001;7:383–385.
81. Qin J, Chaturvedi V, Bonish B, Nickoloff BJ. Avoiding premature apoptosis of normal epidermal cells. Nat Med 2001;7:385–386.

82. Wuchter C, Krappmann D, Cai Z, et al. In vitro susceptibility to TRAIL-induced apoptosis of acute leukemia cells in the context of TRAIL receptor gene expression and constitutive NF-kappa B activity. Leukemia 2001;15:921–928.
83. Zhang XD, Franco A, Myers K, Gray C, Nguyen T, Hersey P. Relation of TNF-related apoptosis-inducing ligand (TRAIL) receptor and FLICE-inhibitory protein expression to TRAIL-induced apoptosis of melanoma. Cancer Res 1999;59:2747–2753.
84. Griffith TS, Rauch CT, Smolak PJ, et al. Functional analysis of TRAIL receptors using monoclonal antibodies. J Immunol 1999;162:2597–2605.
85. Wen J, Ramadevi N, Nguyen D, Perkins C, Worthington E, Bhalla K. Antileukemic drugs increase death receptor 5 levels and enhance Apo-2L-induced apoptosis of human acute leukemia cells. Blood 2000;96:3900–3906.
86. Zhang XD, Nguyen T, Thomas WD, Sanders JE, Hersey P. Mechanisms of resistance of normal cells to TRAIL induced apoptosis vary between different cell types. FEBS Lett 2000;482:193–199.
87. Zhang XD, Franco AV, Nguyen T, Gray CP, Hersey P. Differential localization and regulation of death and decoy receptors for TNF-related apoptosis-inducing ligand (TRAIL) in human melanoma cells. J Immunol 2000;164:3961–3970.
88. Irmler M, Thome M, Hahne M, et al. Inhibition of death receptor signals by cellular FLIP. Nature 1997;388:190–195.
89. Xiao C, Yang BF, Asadi N, Beguinot F, Hao C. Tumor necrosis factor-related apoptosis-inducing ligand-induced death-inducing signaling complex and its modulation by c-FLIP and PED/PEA-15 in glioma cells. J Biol Chem 2002;277:25,020–25,025.
90. Bin L, Li X, Xu LG, Shu HB. The short splice form of Casper/c-FLIP is a major cellular inhibitor of TRAIL-induced apoptosis. FEBS Lett 2002;510:37–40.
91. Poulaki V, Mitsiades CS, Kotoula V, et al. Regulation of Apo2L/tumor necrosis factor-related apoptosis-inducing ligand-induced apoptosis in thyroid carcinoma cells. Am J Pathol 2002;161:643–654.
92. Shin EC, Seong YR, Kim CH, et al. Human hepatocellular carcinoma cells resist to TRAIL-induced apoptosis, and the resistance is abolished by cisplatin. Exp Mol Med 2002;34:114–122.
93. Elnemr A, Ohta T, Yachie A, et al. Human pancreatic cancer cells disable function of Fas receptors at several levels in Fas signal transduction pathway. Int J Oncol 2001;18:311–316.
94. Tepper CG, Seldin MF. Modulation of caspase-8 and FLICE-inhibitory protein expression as a potential mechanism of Epstein-Barr virus tumorigenesis in Burkitt's lymphoma. Blood 1999;94:1727–737.
94a. Djerbi M, Screpanti V, Bogen B, Catrina A, Biberfeld P, Grandien A. The inhibitor of death receptor signaling, FLICE-inhibitory protein defines a new class of tumour progression factors. J Exp Med 1999;190:1025–1032.
95. Li J, Yen C, Liaw D, et al. PTEN, a putative protein tyrosine phosphatase gene mutated in human brain, breast, and prostate cancer. Science 1997;275:1943–1947.
96. Whang YE, Wu X, Suzuki H, et al. Inactivation of the tumor suppressor PTEN/MMAC1 in advanced human prostate cancer through loss of expression. Proc Natl Acad Sci USA 1998;95:5246–5250.
97. Vlietstra RJ, van Alewijk DC, Hermans KG, van Steenbrugge GJ, Trapman J. Frequent inactivation of PTEN in prostate cancer cell lines and xenografts. Cancer Res 1998;58:2720–2723.
98. Nesterov A, Lu X, Johnson M, Miller GJ, Ivashchenko Y, Kraft AS. Elevated AKT activity protects the prostate cancer cell line LNCaP from TRAIL-induced apoptosis. J Biol Chem 2001; 276:10,767–10,774.
99. Chen X, Thakkar H, Tyan F, et al. Constitutively active Akt is an important regulator of TRAIL sensitivity in prostate cancer. Oncogene 2001;20:6073–6083.
100. Thakkar H, Chen X, Tyan F, et al. Pro-survival function of Akt/protein kinase B in prostate cancer cells: relationship with trail resistance. J Biol Chem 2001;276:38,361–38,369.
101. Mitsiades CS, Mitsiades N, Poulaki V, et al. Activation of NF-kappaB and upregulation of intracellular anti-apoptotic proteins via the IGF-1/Akt signaling in human multiple myeloma cells: therapeutic implications. Oncogene 2002;21:5673–5683.
102. Wang Q, Wang X, Hernandez A, Hellmich MR, Gatalica Z, Evers BM. Regulation of trail expression by the PI3-KINASE/Akt/GSK-3 pathway in human colon cancer cells. J Biol Chem 2002;277: 36,602–36,610.
103. Kandasamy K, Srivastava RK. Role of the phosphatidylinositol 3'-kinase/PTEN/Akt kinase pathway in tumor necrosis factor-related apoptosis-inducing ligand-induced apoptosis in non-small cell lung cancer cells. Cancer Res 2002;62:4929–4937.

104. Wang J, Zheng L, Lobito A, et al. Inherited human caspase 10 mutations underlie defective lymphocyte and dendritic cell apoptosis in autoimmune lymphoproliferative syndrome type II. Cell 1999;98:47–58.
105. Sprick MR, Rieser E, Stahl H, Grosse-Wilde A, Weigand MA, Walczak H. Caspase-10 is recruited to and activated at the native TRAIL and CD95 death-inducing signalling complexes in a FADD-dependent manner but can not functionally substitute caspase-8. Embo J 2002;21:4520–4530.
106. Teitz T, Wei T, Valentine MB, et al. Caspase 8 is deleted or silenced preferentially in childhood neuroblastomas with amplification of MYCN. Nat Med 2000;6:529–535.
107. Hopkins-Donaldson S, Bodmer JL, Bourloud KB, Brognara CB, Tschopp J, Gross N. Loss of caspase-8 expression in highly malignant human neuroblastoma cells correlates with resistance to tumor necrosis factor-related apoptosis-inducing ligand-induced apoptosis. Cancer Res 2000;60:4315–4319.
108. Fulda S, Kufer MU, Meyer E, van Valen F, Dockhorn-Dworniczak B, Debatin KM. Sensitization for death receptor- or drug-induced apoptosis by re-expression of caspase-8 through demethylation or gene transfer. Oncogene 2001;20:5865–5877.
109. Eggert A, Grotzer MA, Zuzak TJ, et al. Resistance to tumor necrosis factor-related apoptosis-inducing ligand (TRAIL)-induced apoptosis in neuroblastoma cells correlates with a loss of caspase-8 expression. Cancer Res 2001;61:1314–1319.
110. Zuzak TJ, Steinhoff DF, Sutton LN, Phillips PC, Eggert A, Grotzer MA. Loss of caspase-8 mRNA expression is common in childhood primitive neuroectodermal brain tumour/medulloblastoma. Eur J Cancer 2002;38:83–91.
111. Gliniak B, Le T. Tumor necrosis factor-related apoptosis-inducing ligand's antitumor activity in vivo is enhanced by the chemotherapeutic agent CPT-11. Cancer Res 1999;59:6153–6158.
112. Cuello M, Ettenberg SA, Nau MM, Lipkowitz S. Synergistic induction of apoptosis by the combination of trail and chemotherapy in chemoresistant ovarian cancer cells. Gynecol Oncol 2001;81:380–390.
113. Chinnaiyan AM, Prasad U, Shankar S, et al. Combined effect of tumor necrosis factor-related apoptosis-inducing ligand and ionizing radiation in breast cancer therapy. Proc Natl Acad Sci USA 2000;97:1754–1759.
114. Dejosez M, Ramp U, Mahotka C, et al. Sensitivity to TRAIL/APO-2L-mediated apoptosis in human renal cell carcinomas and its enhancement by topotecan. Cell Death Differ 2000;7:1127–1136.
115. Gong B, Almasan A. Apo2 ligand/TNF-related apoptosis-inducing ligand and death receptor 5 mediate the apoptotic signaling induced by ionizing radiation in leukemic cells. Cancer Res 2000;60:5754–5760.
116. Yamanaka T, Shiraki K, Sugimoto K, et al. Chemotherapeutic agents augment TRAIL-induced apoptosis in human hepatocellular carcinoma cell lines. Hepatology 2000;32:482–490.
117. Lacour S, Hammann A, Wotawa A, Corcos L, Solary E, Dimanche-Boitrel MT. Anticancer agents sensitize tumor cells to tumor necrosis factor-related apoptosis-inducing ligand-mediated caspase-8 activation and apoptosis. Cancer Res 2001;61:1645–1651.
118. Liu W, Bodle E, Chen JY, Gao M, Rosen GD, Broaddus VC. Tumor necrosis factor–related apoptosis-inducing ligand and chemotherapy cooperate to induce apoptosis in mesothelioma cell lines. Am J Respir Cell Mol Biol 2001;25:111–118.
119. Rudner J, Lepple-Wienhues A, Budach W, et al. Wild-type, mitochondrial and ER-restricted Bcl-2 inhibit DNA damage-induced apoptosis but do not affect death receptor-induced apoptosis. J Cell Sci 2001;114:4161–4172.
120. Sheikh MS, Burns TF, Huang Y, et al. p53-dependent and -independent regulation of the death receptor KILLER/DR5 gene expression in response to genotoxic stress and tumor necrosis factor alpha. Cancer Res 1998;58:1593–1598.
121. Wu GS, Burns TF, McDonald ER, 3rd, et al. KILLER/DR5 is a DNA damage–inducible p53-regulated death receptor gene. Nat Genet 1997;17:141–143.
122. Nagane M, Pan G, Weddle JJ, Dixit VM, Cavenee WK, Huang HJ. Increased death receptor 5 expression by chemotherapeutic agents in human gliomas causes synergistic cytotoxicity with tumor necrosis factor–related apoptosis-inducing ligand in vitro and in vivo. Cancer Res 2000;60:847–853.
123. Munshi A, McDonnell TJ, Meyn RE. Chemotherapeutic agents enhance TRAIL-induced apoptosis in prostate cancer cells. Cancer Chemother Pharmacol 2002;50:46–52.
124. Wu GS, Kim K, el-Deiry WS. KILLER/DR5, a novel DNA-damage inducible death receptor gene, links the p53-tumor suppressor to caspase activation and apoptotic death. Adv Exp Med Biol 2000;465:143–151.
125. Meng RD, El-Deiry WS. p53-independent upregulation of KILLER/DR5 TRAIL receptor expression by glucocorticoids and interferon-gamma. Exp Cell Res 2001;262:154–169.

126. Guan B, Yue P, Clayman GL, Sun SY. Evidence that the death receptor DR4 is a DNA damage-inducible, p53-regulated gene. J Cell Physiol 2001;188:98–105.
127. Rohn TA, Wagenknecht B, Roth W, et al. CCNU-dependent potentiation of TRAIL/Apo2L-induced apoptosis in human glioma cells is p53-independent but may involve enhanced cytochrome c release. Oncogene 2001;20:4128–4137.
128. Gibson SB, Oyer R, Spalding AC, Anderson SM, Johnson GL. Increased expression of death receptors 4 and 5 synergizes the apoptosis response to combined treatment with etoposide and TRAIL. Mol Cell Biol 2000;20:205–212.
129. Sun SY, Yue P, Hong WK, Lotan R. Augmentation of tumor necrosis factor-related apoptosis-inducing ligand (TRAIL)-induced apoptosis by the synthetic retinoid 6-[3-(1-adamantyl)-4-hydroxyphenyl]-2-naphthalene carboxylic acid (CD437) through up-regulation of TRAIL receptors in human lung cancer cells. Cancer Res 2000;60:7149–7155.
130. Di Pietro R, Secchiero P, Rana R, et al. Ionizing radiation sensitizes erythroleukemic cells but not normal erythroblasts to tumor necrosis factor-related apoptosis-inducing ligand (TRAIL)-mediated cytotoxicity by selective up-regulation of TRAIL-R1. Blood 2001;97:2596–2603.
131. Jazirehi AR, Ng CP, Gan XH, Schiller G, Bonavida B. Adriamycin sensitizes the adriamycin-resistant 8226/Dox40 human multiple myeloma cells to Apo2L/tumor necrosis factor-related apoptosis-inducing ligand-mediated (TRAIL) apoptosis. Clin Cancer Res 2001;7:3874–3883.
132. Evdokiou A, Bouralexis S, Atkins GJ, et al. Chemotherapeutic agents sensitize osteogenic sarcoma cells, but not normal human bone cells, to Apo2L/TRAIL-induced apoptosis. Int J Cancer 2002;99:491–504.
133. Arizono Y, Yoshikawa H, Naganuma H, Hamada Y, Nakajima Y, Tasaka K. A mechanism of resistance to TRAIL/Apo2L-induced apoptosis of newly established glioma cell line and sensitisation to TRAIL by genotoxic agents. Br J Cancer 2003;88:298–306.
134. Mori S, Murakami-Mori K, Jewett A, Nakamura S, Bonavida B. Resistance of AIDS-associated Kaposi's sarcoma cells to Fas-mediated apoptosis. Cancer Res 1996;56:1874–1879.
135. Hernandez A, Thomas R, Smith F, et al. Butyrate sensitizes human colon cancer cells to TRAIL-mediated apoptosis. Surgery 2001;130:265–272.
136. Lee YJ, Lee KH, Kim HR, et al. Sodium nitroprusside enhances TRAIL-induced apoptosis via a mitochondria-dependent pathway in human colorectal carcinoma CX-1 cells. Oncogene 2001;20:1476–1485.
137. Matsuzaki H, Schmied BM, Ulrich A, et al. Combination of tumor necrosis factor–related apoptosis-inducing ligand (TRAIL) and actinomycin D induces apoptosis even in TRAIL-resistant human pancreatic cancer cells. Clin Cancer Res 2001;7:407–414.
138. Fulda S, Wick W, Weller M, Debatin KM. Smac agonists sensitize for Apo2L/TRAIL- or anticancer drug-induced apoptosis and induce regression of malignant glioma in vivo. Nat Med 2002;8:808–815.
139. Mizutani Y, Nakanishi H, Yoshida O, Fukushima M, Bonavida B, Miki T. Potentiation of the sensitivity of renal cell carcinoma cells to TRAIL-mediated apoptosis by subtoxic concentrations of 5-fluorouracil. Eur J Cancer 2002;38:167–176.
140. Wu XX, Kakehi Y, Mizutani Y, et al. Doxorubicin enhances TRAIL-induced apoptosis in prostate cancer. Int J Oncol 2002;20:949–954.
141. Lacour S, Micheau O, Hammann A, et al. Chemotherapy enhances TNF-related apoptosis-inducing ligand DISC assembly in HT29 human colon cancer cells. Oncogene 2003;22:1807–1816.
142. Belka C, Schmid B, Marini P, et al. Sensitization of resistant lymphoma cells to irradiation-induced apoptosis by the death ligand TRAIL. Oncogene 2001;20:2190–2196.
143. Van Valen F, Fulda S, Truckenbrod B, et al. Apoptotic responsiveness of the Ewing's sarcoma family of tumours to tumour necrosis factor-related apoptosis-inducing ligand (TRAIL). Int J Cancer 2000;88:252–259.
144. Wu M, Das A, Tan Y, Zhu C, Cui T, Wong MC. Induction of apoptosis in glioma cell lines by TRAIL/Apo-2l. J Neurosci Res 2000;61:464–470.
145. Mlynarczuk I, Hoser G, Grzela T, et al. Augmented pro-apoptotic effects of TRAIL and proteasome inhibitor in human promonocytic leukemic U937 cells. Anticancer Res 2001;21:1237–1240.
146. Zisman A, Ng CP, Pantuck AJ, Bonavida B, Belldegrun AS. Actinomycin D and gemcitabine synergistically sensitize androgen-independent prostate cancer cells to Apo2L/TRAIL-mediated apoptosis. J Immunother 2001;24:459–471.
147. Ahmad M, Shi Y. TRAIL-induced apoptosis of thyroid cancer cells: potential for therapeutic intervention. Oncogene 2000;19:3363–3371.

16 Expression and Regulation of Death Receptors in Multiple Myeloma and Prostate Carcinoma

Subrata Ray, PhD, *John G. Hissong,* MD, PhD, *Marcela Oancea, and Alex Almasan,* PhD

SUMMARY

Several members of the tumor necrosis factor (TNF) gene superfamily induce apoptosis through engagement of their cognate death receptors (TNFR). To explore how their expression may be regulated, we used oligonucleotide arrays to determine TNFR gene expression using as a model multiple myeloma and prostate cancer cell lines. Expression levels for BCMA, HVEM, CD40, CD30, TACI, TNFR2, and Fas were considerably higher in multiple myeloma, pointing to their role in B-cell biology. Treatment with ionizing radiation led to increased levels of Fas, death receptor (DR)5, to a lesser extent decoy receptor (DcR)1 and DcR2, as well as BCMA, RANK, and ILA. Treatment with the topoisomerase I inhibitor CPT-11 led to increased expression of Fas, RANK, and DcR2, but not of BCMA or ILA, indicating a different transcriptional "signature" for ionizing radiation and chemotherapeutics. This increased expression level following genotoxic stress was prevented or attenuated in prostate cancer cells stably expressing a dominant-negative p53 mutant. Of the TNF family members, one that has received much attention recently is Apo2L/TRAIL (Apo2 ligand or TNF-related apoptosis-inducing ligand). Apo2L/TRAIL is unusual compared to any other cytokine, as it interacts with a complex system of receptors: two pro-apoptotic death receptors (DR4, DR5) and three anti-apoptotic decoy receptors (DcR1, DcR2, and osteoprotegerin [OPG]). This protein has generated tremendous excitement as a potential tumor-specific cancer therapeutic because, as a stable soluble trimer, it selectively induces apoptosis in many transformed cells but not in normal cells. We found that its expression can also be modulated by therapeutic agents.

From: *Cancer Drug Discovery and Development: Death Receptors in Cancer Therapy*
Edited by: W. S. El-Deiry © Humana Press Inc., Totowa, NJ

INTRODUCTION

Apoptosis induction in response to many DNA-damaging drugs usually requires the function of the tumor suppressor p53 *(1)*, which activates primarily the cell-intrinsic apoptotic signaling pathway *(2,3)*. In most human cancers, following tumor progression or as a result of clinical treatments, p53 is inactivated, resulting in resistance to further therapy. However, death receptors can trigger apoptosis independently of p53, and therefore their targeting might be a useful therapeutic strategy, particularly in cells in which the p53-response pathway has been inactivated, helping to circumvent resistance to chemo- and radiotherapy *(4,5)*. In those tumors that remain responsive to conventional therapy, death receptor activation in combination with radiation or chemotherapy might lead to synergistic apoptosis activation. In those tumors that no longer have a functional p53, death receptor targeting might help circumvent resistance to radio- or chemotherapy.

TNF-Related Ligands and Their Receptors

The nomenclature used for the tumor necrosis factor (TNF) receptors (TNFR) and their activating ligands is summarized in Table 1. The common designation for these ligands is TNFSF (TNF superfamily) with the receptors being designated as TNFRSF, followed by a specific number. Clearly not all TNF receptors (TNFR) are bona fide death receptors (DR), as many lack canonical death domains and have other important biological functions attributed to them, such as in immunity and cell proliferation. Still other TNFRs are incapable of signaling. TNFR1 and -2 were the first to be discovered. It was shown that there were two different proteins that serve as major receptors for TNF-α, one associated with myeloid cells and the other associated with epithelial cells *(6)*. These two distinct TNF-binding proteins bind TNF-α and TNF-β specifically and with high affinity. TNFR2 (TNF75; TNFRSF1B) is the larger of the two TNF receptors. It is present on many cell types, especially those of myeloid origin, and is strongly expressed on stimulated T- and B-lymphocytes. TNFR2 is the main TNF receptor found on circulating T-cells and is the major mediator of autoregulatory apoptosis in $CD8^+$ cells. TNFR2 may act with TNFR1 (TNF55, TNFRSF1A) to kill non-lymphoid cells *(5)*.

Each member of the TNFRSF binds at least one ligand; several receptors may bind the same ligand. For example, there are an unprecedented number of receptors (five) that bind Apo2L/TRAIL. Conversely, one receptor may bind several ligands. For example TNFR1 binds both TNF-α and LT-α, while LT-βR is shared by LIGHT and LT-β, even though HVEM binds selectively only LT-βR. TAC1 and BAFF are used as receptors for both BCMA and APRIL *(4)*.

Preassembly or self-association of cytokine receptor dimers (e.g., IL1R and EPOR) occurs via the same amino acid contacts that are critical for ligand binding. In contrast, TNFR1, TNFR2, and Fas self-assemble through a distinct functional domain in their extracellular domain, termed the preligand assembly domain (PLAD) *(7)*, in the absence of ligand *(8)*. Deletion of the PLAD results in monomeric presentation of TNFR1 or TNFR2. Flow cytometric analyses indicate that efficient TNF-α binding depends on receptor self-assembly. Other members of the TNF receptor superfamily, including the extracellular domains of Apo2L/TRAIL (TNFRSF10A), CD40 (TNFRSF5), and Fas (TNFRSF6), all self-associate but do not interact with heterologous receptors.

Table 1
TNF Receptor Genes: Nomenclature and Expression in Human Prostate Carcinoma and Multiple Myeloma Tumor Cells

Cell Line		*LNCaP*[a]	*C4-2*	*IM-9*			
Nomenclature	*Unigene*[b]	*Normal.*	*Normal.*	*Normal.*	*Common Name*	*Map*	*Ligand*
TNFRSF1A[c]	Hs.159	6.32	5.63	3.54	TNFR1, TR55, TR60	12p13.2	TNF, LT-α
TNFRSF1B	Hs.256278	1.04	0.84	4.52	TNFR2, TR75, TR80	1p36.3-2	TNF, LT-α
TNFSF3	Hs.1116	8.7	7.23	0.16	LTBR, LT-BETA-R	12p13	LT-α/β
TNFRSF4	Hs.129780	0.32	0.08	0.1	OX40, ACT35, CD134	1p36	OX40L, GP34
TNFRSF5	Hs.25648	2.46	3.59	14.48	CD40	20q12-13.2	CD40L
TNFRSF6	Hs.82359	0.5	0.59	3.02	Fas, APO1, CD95	10q24.1	FasL, CD95L
TNFRSF6	Hs.82359	0.52	0.42	2.64	Fas, APO1, CD95	10q24.1	FasL, CD95L
TNFRSF6	Hs.82359	0.04	0.28	1.23	Fas, APO1, CD95	10q24.1	FasL, CD95L
TNFRSF6	Hs.82359	0.18	0.11	1.75	Fas, APO1, CD95	10q24.1	FasL, CD95L
TNFRSF8	Hs.1314	0.33	0.19	1.9	CD30	1p36	CD30L
TNFRSF9	Hs.73895	0.16	0.32	0.07	ILA, 4-1BB, CD137	1p36	4-1BBL, LIGHT
TNFRSF10B	Hs.51233	9.02	12.38	6.67	KILLER/DR5, TRAIL-R2	8p22-p21	Apo2L/TRAIL
TNFRSF10C	Hs.119684	1.58	0.76	1.05	DcR1, TRAIL-R3, TRID	8p22-p21	Apo2L/TRAIL
TNFRSF10D	Hs.129844	1.88	0.97	1.32	DcR2,TRAILR4/TRUND	8p21	Apo2L/TRAIL
TNFRSF11A	Hs.114676	0.5	0.61	0.13	RANK, TRANCER	18q22.1	OPGL, RANKL
TNFRSF11B	Hs.129844	0.05	0.02	0.01	OPG, OCIF, TR1	8q24	APO2L, RANKL
TNFRSF12	Hs.180338	0.39	1.65	0.09	DR3, APO3, LARD	1p36.2	TL1A
TNFRSF12	Hs.180338	2.61	2.07	3.01	DR3,APO3, LARD	1p36.2	TL1A
TNFRSF12	Hs.180338	0.28	0.29	0.43	DR3, APO3, LARD	1p36.2	TL1A
TNFRSF12	Hs.180338	0.99	0.75	1.16	DR3, APO3, LARD	1p36.2	TL1A
TNFRSF13B	Hs.158341	2.59	2.56	9.04	TACI	17p11.2	APRIL, TWEAK
TNFRSF14	Hs.279899	2.18	2.1	6.24	HVEM, HVEA, TR2	1p36.3-2	LIGHT, LT-α
TNFRSF17[c]	Hs.2556	0.33	0.24	6.17	BCM, BCMA	16p13.1	BAFF, APRIL
TNFRSF21	Hs.159651	0.76	1.64	0.65	DR6	6p21.1-12.2	NA
EDAR	Hs.58346	0.72	0.43	NA	EDAR, EDA-A1R, DL	2q11-q13	EDA A1
XEDAR	Hs.302017	0.56	0.76	NA	XEDAR, EDA-A2R	Xq11.2	EDA A2
XEDAR	Hs.302017	0.4	0.78	NA	XEDAR, EDA-A2R	Xq11.2	EDA A2
ACTB	Hs.288061	219.22	212.76	245.44	β-actin	7p15-p12	None
GAPDH	Hs.169476	382.84	397.73	233.71	GAPDH	12p13	None

[a]LNCaP & C4-2 are androgen dependent and independent cells; the HGU95Av2-E arrays were used.
[b]Unigene Build Hs158 .
[c]Online Mendelian Inheritance in Man Online: http://www.ncbi.nlm.nih.gov/omim/

Signaling Through the TNFR Death Receptors

The Apo2L/TRAIL DISC

TNF, FasL, and Apo2L/TRAIL are the best studied cell-death ligands. Apo2L/TRAIL, which our laboratory has been mostly interested in, was originally identified and cloned based on sequence homology to the Fas/APO-1 ligand (FasL) and TNF *(9,10)*. Subsequently, four of its receptors were identified, as well as a fifth, soluble receptor more distantly related to the other four. Two of the receptors that bind Apo2L/TRAIL contain cytoplasmic death domains and signal apoptosis: death receptor 4 (DR4) *(11)* and DR5 *(12–20)*. The other three receptors appear to act as decoys.

Similar to FasL, Apo2L/TRAIL initiates apoptosis upon binding to its cognate death receptors by inducing the recruitment of specific cytoplasmic proteins to the intracellular death domain of the receptor, which form the death-inducing signaling complex (DISC) *(5,21)*. In untransfected cells, the Apo2L/TRAIL DISC is similar to that of FasL, with the adaptor protein Fas-associated death domain (FADD, also Mort-1; see chapter 5) and the apoptosis initiator caspase-8 being recruited to DR4 and/or DR5 shortly after addition of Apo2L/TRAIL *(22–24)*. Apo2L/TRAIL can trigger apoptosis independently through DR4 or DR5 *(22,23)*.

Nonsignaling Decoy Receptors

While some receptors are capable of signaling, others are not; these non-signaling receptors are called decoy receptors (DcR). Lack of DcR expression has been initially postulated to correlate with the increased Apo2L/TRAIL sensitivity of tumor cells. Apo2L/TRAIL binds with high affinity to two receptors, DcR1 *(11,12,17,25,26)* and DcR2 *(27–29)*, which are incapable of transmitting an apoptotic signal due to absent or incomplete death domains. Overexpression of these receptors protects cells from apoptosis induction by Apo2L/TRAIL, suggesting that they act as decoys, by sequestering the ligand from the signaling death receptors *(12,29)*. Many normal adult tissues express at least one of the DcRs *(12,27,29)*. However, recent examination of cancer cell lines and tumors failed to provide any correlations between DcR expression and Apo2L/TRAIL resistance. It is not clear how widespread the decoy receptor expression on the cell surface in tumor or normal cells is, or how these receptors modulate Apo2L/TRAIL signaling *(4)*.

Other decoys include DcR3, which binds FasL, TL1A, LIGHT, as well as OPG. The soluble TNFR family member OPG *(30–33)* was discovered first to bind the TNFSF member RANKL but later found to also bind Apo2L/TRAIL. However, a biological connection between OPG and Apo2L/TRAIL remains to be firmly established, as OPG has a low affinity for Apo2L/TRAIL at a physiological temperature *(33)*. Interestingly, a recent study suggests that cancer-derived OPG may be an important survival factor in hormone-resistant prostate cancer cells, as a strong negative correlation was observed between OPG levels and the capacity of Apo2L/TRAIL to induce apoptosis in prostate cancer cells that endogenously produced high levels of OPG *(32)*.

Signaling Through Nuclear Factor-κB (NF-κB)

NF-κB is potently and rapidly activated after TNF binding to TNFR1, generating a pro-survival signal that must be overcome in many cell lines to enable TNF to induce apoptosis *(34)*. NF-κB has been reported to induce expression of FLICE-inhibitory protein (FLIP), Bcl-XL, and XIAP, which are considered to be responsible for its protection against cell death. While Apo2L/TRAIL can also activate NF-κB, this stimulation is significantly attenuated and delayed as compared to that of TNF, and requires a high concentration of the ligand, suggesting that NF-κB induction by Apo2L/TRAIL may be a secondary, indirect event *(12)*. More on this topic can be found in chapter 14.

MATERIALS AND METHODS

Cells and Treatments

Multiple myeloma (MM) IM-9 cells were obtained from the American Type Culture Collection (ATCC). The LNCaP and derivative C4-2 human prostate cancer cells *(35)* were obtained from Dr. W. Heston (Cleveland Clinic). All cells were cultured in RPMI 1640 plus 10% FBS supplemented with antibiotics in a humidified atmosphere of 5% CO_2 and 95% air *(36,37)*.

IM-9 (2×10^5 cells/mL)*, C4-2, and derivative cells were irradiated to 10 Gy (^{137}Cs source; fixed dose rate of 2.8 Gy/min) *(2)*, or treated with CPT-11 (irinotecan hydrochloride; Pharmacia and Upjohn Co, Kalamazoo, MI) at a concentration of 100 ng/mL. Total RNA was isolated from cells at different time points post treatment using the TRIZOL reagent (Invitrogen, Carlsbad, CA). All chemicals, unless otherwise specified, were obtained from Sigma Chemical Co. (St. Louis, MO).

Affymetrix GeneChip Signal Preparation

Details for the sample preparation and microarray processing are available from Affymetrix (Santa Clara, CA). Briefly 15 μg of total RNA was isolated from all cells after various treatments and was converted to double-stranded cDNA (Superscript; Invitrogen) using a T7-oligo$(dT)_{24}$ primer and 1 μg purified ds cDNA was used to prepare biotinylated cRNA using the Bioarray High Yield kit (Enzo) according to the manufacturer's directions. After purification, biotinylated cRNA probes were fragmented to a sequence length of approx 50–100 nucleotides. About 10 μg of cRNA was hybridized to Affymetrix GeneChip arrays with constant rotation at 60 rpm for 16 h at 45°C, using either the HGU95Av2-E chip set, which contains probe sets for approx 60,000 cDNAs and ESTs, or the HGU95Av2 chip alone, which contains probe sets for approx 12,000 human cDNAs and ESTs. The chips were washed and stained by using the EukGE-WS2v4 protocol on an Affymetrix fluidics station. The stain included streptavidin-phycoerythrin (10 μg/mL; Molecular Probe) and biotinylated goat anti-streptavidin (3 μg/mL; Vector Laboratories). Chips were scanned with an HP argon-ion laser confocal microscope, with excitation at 488 nm and detection at 570 nm. The signal intensities from the hybridized cRNA were generated using Affymetrix's Microarray Suite 5.0 (MAS). Default values were used for all MAS expression analysis parameters.

Gene Expression Analysis

Data from MAS 5.0 was imported into GeneSpring 5.0.3 (Silicon Genetics). Each chip was normalized to the median expression level of all measured genes. Any remaining

---

*It has recently come to our attention that the IM-9 cells, although originating from a MM patient, may be Epstein–Barr virus-transformed B-lymphoblastoid cell line *(81)*.

negative values were then set equal to zero. Fold changes were calculated relative to the control dataset. Genes with an absolute fold change greater than 2.0 were considered up- or downregulated.

Blocking Apoptosis Signaling

C4-2 cells were transfected with pcDNA3-DR5Δ (residues 1 to 268) *(14)*, as described in *(36,37)*, or a retrovirus encoding a truncated nonfunctional p53 (GSE-56), acting as a dominant-negative mutant of p53 *(38)*. DR5Δ lacks the death domain and has been shown to function as a dominant-negative mutant, inactivating the function of the endogenous DR5 *(14)*. GSE-56 encodes a C-terminal portion of p53 (residues 275–368) and acts as an efficient inhibitor of p53 function by binding to the oligomerization domain of p53, resulting in accumulation of p53 in an inactive conformation and inhibition of p53 transactivation *(38)*. Both transfected cell lines were selected in the presence of G418 (Invitrogen).

Western Blotting

C4-2 cell lysates (50 μg in buffer containing 1% NP40, 20 m*M* HEPES, 4 m*M* EDTA, 1 m*M* phenylmethane-sulfonylfluoride, 50 μg/mL trypsin inhibitor, 5 m*M* benzamidine, and 1 μg/mL each aprotinin, leupeptin, and pepstatin) were separated by SDS-PAGE and electrotransferred onto nitrocellulose membranes (Schleicher and Schull, Keene, NH) *(39)*. Blots were blocked with 5% nonfat dry milk in 0.1% Tween-20 in PBS (PBST) for 1 h at room temperature, incubated overnight at 4°C with primary antibodies to DR5 (Alexis Biochemicals) and β-actin (Sigma), followed by incubation with secondary horseradish peroxidase-conjugated antibodies (Amersham Biosciences) for 1 h at 37°C. β-Actin was used as an internal standard for protein loading. Immunoreactive bands were visualized by ECL and subsequent exposure to hyperfilm (X-ray film, Eastman Kodak).

RESULTS AND DISCUSSION

Expression Levels of TNFR Family Members: Indicators of Biological Function?

Among the cDNAs and ESTs present on the HU95Av2 or HU95Av2-E GeneChip (Affymetrix) arrays, there were 20 TNFR family members present, with several being present in multiple copies. Further advances in DNA chip construction would add additional members of this family, their ligands, and adaptor molecules, thus making these types of global predictions on gene expression even more informative. We compared the expression levels of these receptors in prostate cancer (CaP: LNCaP and C4-2) and multiple myeloma (MM; IM-9) cells, and the results are illustrated in Table 1. Expression of two housekeeping genes, β-actin and GAPDH, are also shown as an independent indication for accuracy of the normalization method, based on the median value of all expression levels on the chip.

Constitutive expression levels for BCMA, HVEM, CD40, CD30, TAC1, TNFR2, and Fas were considerably higher in MM, as compared to CaP. These TNFR family members may be considered as key signaling molecules in B- and/or T-cells. For example, it is known that BCMA (B-cell maturation) is expressed in mature B-cells, but not in T-cells or monocytes. It promotes B-cell survival and plays a role in the regulation of humoral immunity.

BCMA activates NF-κB and c-Jun N-terminal kinase through association with TRAF1-3 or TRAF5-6. Interestingly, a disease association was found since a translocation was characterized in a patient with intestinal T-cell acute lymphoblastic leukemia (T-ALL), resulting in a rearrangement that involved BCMA and the interleukin (IL)-2 gene *(40)*. In a myeloma cell line, BCMA was reported to be primarily expressed in a perinuclear Golgi-like structure *(41)*. By transfection, it was demonstrated that in addition to the intracytoplasmic localization, BCMA is present on the cell surface *(42)*. As BCMA is lacking a death domain and its overexpression activates NF-κB and c-Jun N-terminal kinase, it is believed that upon binding of its corresponding ligand, BCMA transduces signals for cell survival and proliferation *(42)*. BAFF, the BCMA ligand, enhances B-cell survival in vitro and is a regulator of the peripheral B-cell population. Overexpression of BAFF in mice results in mature B-cell hyperplasia and symptoms of systemic lupus erythematosus (SLE) *(43)*. Likewise, some SLE patients have increased levels of BAFF in serum. Like APRIL, BAFF binds to both TACI and BCMA, both highly expressed in MM.

HVEM, CD40, and CD30 levels were also elevated in MM compared to CaP. By flow cytometric and RT-PCR analysis, it was previously shown that the expression of the HVEM ligand LIGHT (TNFSF14) is upregulated, whereas HVEM expression is downregulated after T-cell activation, particularly in CD8-positive cells *(44)*. CD40 is a cell-surface receptor that is expressed on the surface of all mature B-cells, most mature B-cell malignancies, and some early B-cell acute lymphocytic leukemias, but it is not expressed on plasma cells *(45)*. Interruption of CD40L-CD40 signaling by administration of an anti-CD40L antibody was found to limit experimental autoimmune diseases such as collagen-induced arthritis, lupus nephritis, acute or chronic graft-vs-host disease, multiple sclerosis, and thyroiditis *(46)*. Finally, CD30 is expressed by activated, but not by resting, B- or T-cells *(47)*. A variant of CD30 (CD30v) retains only the cytoplasmic region of the authentic CD30. CD30v expression was high in monocyte-oriented AMLs (FAB M4 and M5), B-cell chronic lymphocytic leukemia (B-CLL), and MM *(48)*. Taken together, the above reports indicate that expression of these receptors in MM may have an important biological significance.

Genotoxic Stress Control of TNFR Family Gene Expression

Genotoxic stress, such as treatment with ionizing radiation (IR) or chemotherapeutic agents, leads to increased expression of many genes. This may have an impact on cell-cycle control, in the case of cyclin E *(49,50)*, p21 *(51)*, or on apoptosis, in case of Bax *(2)*, DR5 *(20,36,52)*, or Apo2L/TRAIL *(36,37,53)* To better understand which genes are regulated following IR, we examined expression patterns following irradiation in prostate cancer (Buchsbaum, J., Gong, B., Hissong, J, Ray, S., Klein, E, Heston, W., Macklis, R.M., and Almasan, A., unpublished) or multiple myeloma (Oancea, M., Hissong, J.G., and Almasan, A., unpublished) cell lines. For this study, we analyzed levels of the TNFR superfamily genes following treatment with ionizing radiation or the topoisomerase I inhibitor CPT-11.

There was an increased expression of Fas, DR5, and to a lesser extent of DcR1 and DcR2, as previously reported *(20,36,54,55)*. Interestingly, we noted, in addition, increased levels of BCMA, RANK (receptor activator of NF-κB), and ILA (4-1BB) in both cell lines (Table 2). To our knowledge, genotoxic stress-regulated expression of these genes has

Table 2
Genotoxic Stress Response in Prostate Carcinoma C4-2 and Multiple Myeloma IM-9 Cells Exposed to Ionizing Radiation or CPT-11

Cell line		*C4-2*	*C4-2*	*C4-2*	*IM-9*	*IM-9*		
Time & treatment		*8 h[1] CPT-11*	*4 h 10 Gy*	*8 h 10 Gy*	*4 h 10 Gy*	*8 h 10 Gy*		
Nomenclature	*Unigene*	*Fold change*	*Fold change*	*Fold change*	*Fold change*	*Fold change*	*Change trend*	*Common name*
TNFRSF1A	Hs.159	1.10	0.91	1.05	1.15	1.36		TNFR1
TNFRSF1B	Hs.256278	0.74	1.04	0.84	0.57	0.59		TNFR2
TNFRSF3	Hs.1116	1.94	0.74	0.84	1.23	1.80		LTBR
TNFRSF4	Hs.129780	1.49	0.62	0.48	1.85	1.24		OX40
TNFRSF5	Hs.25648	1.18	0.97	1.26	0.55	0.77		CD40
TNFRSF6	Hs.82359	0.92	1.89	2.02	2.54	2.92	Up	Fas
TNFRSF6	Hs.82359	1.67	6.70	3.94	2.37	1.90	Up	Fas
TNFRSF6	Hs.82359	7.53	5.39	3.20	3.95	3.69	Up	Fas
TNFRSF6	Hs.82359	1.17	1.42	2.23	1.32	2.04	Up	Fas
TNFRSF8	Hs.1314	1.03	1.06	1.39	0.27	0.91		CD30
TNFRSF9	Hs.73895	1.46	3.39	1.93	2.89	1.35	Up[2]	ILA
TNFRSF10B	Hs.51233	0.65	2.20	1.51	1.09	2.27	Up	KILLER/DR5
TNFRSF10C	Hs.119684	1.33	0.93	1.14	1.00	1.98		DcR1
TNFRSF10D	Hs.129844	1.56	1.23	1.54	1.02	0.88		DcR2
TNFRSF11A	Hs.114676	2.97	0.69	2.00	4.43	2.26	Up[2]	RANK
TNFRSF11B	Hs.129844	2.01	1.62	1.44	5.09	2.73	Up[2]	OPG
TNFRSF12	Hs.180338	1.16	2.17	2.95	6.20	3.27		DR3
TNFRSF12	Hs.180338	1.00	0.93	0.91	1.13	1.14		DR3
TNFRSF12	Hs.180338	1.46	0.33	0.26	0.57	0.67		DR3
TNFRSF12	Hs.180338	7.13	0.88	0.67	0.84	0.21		DR3
TNFRSF13B	Hs.158341	0.77	1.09	1.24	0.74	0.98		TACI
TNFRSF14	Hs.279899	1.39	1.17	1.07	0.69	1.28		HVEM
TNFRSF17	Hs.2556	0.92	0.09	1.61	1.89	2.18	Up-M[3]	BCMA
TNFRSF21	Hs.159651	0.67	0.68	1.01	1.70	0.49		DR6
ACTB	Hs.288061	1.05	1.08	1.04	0.75	0.96		beta-actin
GAPDH	Hs.169476	1.05	1.12	1.24	0.99	1.10		GAPDH

[1]100 ng/mL CPT-11; [2] low basal expression levels; [3] UP-M, up only in MM.

not been previously reported, except for one publication on ILA *(56)*. CPT-11 treatment caused increased expression of Fas, RANK, and DcR2, but not of BCMA or ILA, indicating the different transcriptional signatures of ionizing radiation and various chemotherapeutic agents.

Changes in BCMA levels were more robust in MM (1.9- to 2.2-fold) with only a 1.6-fold change observed in CaP, at 8 h following IR. There was a slightly higher induction at 12 h (not shown) and 24 h, but p53DN expression in CaP did not seem to make a difference. However, constitutive levels of BCMA were quite low in CaP, so these preliminary observations need to be further confirmed. For OPG, it seemed to be a clear induction in both cell lines, however basal levels were extremely low (Table 1). The results with RANK were quite similar, except that RANK was clearly up-regulated by IR in IM-9 and C4-2 cells, and by CPT-11 in CaP.

There was an apparent two- to fourfold increase in the levels of ILA. ILA (4-1BB) is known to be expressed by activated T- and B-lymphocytes and monocytes. ILA inhibits proliferation of activated T-lymphocytes and induces programmed cell death *(57)*. Levels of ILA seem to be increased following irradiation in both cell lines, with DN-p53 having a consistent effect, except at 24 h. Again, mRNA levels were quite low in both cell lines, so these results have to be interpreted with caution. We obtained more limited data on EDAR and XEDAR, which were present only on HGU95B and HGU95C-D chips, respectively. Nevertheless, a 1.8- and 3.5-fold increase in levels of EDAR was noted at 6 and 24 h, respectively, following IR in C4-2 cells. These data indicate that modulation of receptor gene expression by genotoxic stress may have important biological consequences.

RANK-RANKL (OPGL): A Critical Signaling Pathway for Multiple Myeloma

MM is a hematologic malignancy characterized by accumulation of plasma cells in the bone marrow *(58)*. Bone destruction, caused by aberrant production and activation of osteoclasts, is a prominent feature of MM. OPGL (RANKL) binds to its functional receptor RANK (TNFRSF11A) to stimulate osteoclastogenesis. Osteotropic cytokines regulate this process by controlling bone marrow stromal expression of OPGL, with further control over osteoclastogenesis being maintained by regulated expression of OPG. In normal bone marrow, abundant stores of OPG in stroma, megakaryocytes, and myeloid cells provide a natural buffer against increased OPGL. MM disrupts these controls by increasing expression of OPGL and decreasing expression of the OPG decoy receptor. Concurrent deregulation of OPGL and OPG expression is found in bone-marrow biopsies from patients with MM but not in specimens from patients with non-MM hematologic malignancies. Addition of RANK-Fc virtually eliminates the formation of osteoclasts in co-cultures of MM with bone marrow and osteoblast/stromal cells. MM-induced bone destruction requires increased OPGL expression and is facilitated by a concurrent reduction in OPG, a natural decoy receptor for RANK-L. Administration of the OPGL antagonist RANK-Fc limits MM-induced osteoclastogenesis, development of bone disease, and MM tumor progression *(59)*. Within the hematological malignancy group, serum levels of OPG were significantly lower in patients with MM but were elevated in patients with Hodgkin's disease and non-Hodgkin's lymphoma *(60)*.

Myeloma stimulates osteoclastogenesis by triggering a coordinated increase in the levels of OPGL and decrease in its decoy receptor, OPG *(61)*. Immunohistochemistry and *in situ* hybridization studies of bone marrow specimens indicate that in vivo, deregulation of the OPGL-OPG cytokine axis occurs in myeloma, but not in the limited plasma-cell disorder monoclonal gammopathy of unknown significance or in nonmyeloma hematologic malignancies. In co-culture, myeloma cell lines stimulate expression of OPGL and inhibit expression of OPG by stromal cells. Osteoclastogenesis, the functional consequence of increased OPGL expression, is counteracted by addition of a recombinant OPGL inhibitor, RANK-Fc, to marrow/myeloma co-cultures. Myeloma-stroma interaction also has been postulated to support progression of the malignant clone. In the SCID-hu murine model of human myeloma, administration of RANK-Fc both prevents myeloma-induced bone destruction and interferes with myeloma progression. OPGL and OPG are thus key cytokines whose deregulation promotes bone destruction and supports myeloma growth *(61)*. Serum OPG levels are lower in patients with myeloma than in healthy individuals. Moreover, myeloma cells can bind, internalize, and degrade OPG, thereby providing a possible explanation for the lower levels of OPG in the bone marrow of patients with MM *(62)*.

p53-Dependent Regulation

The tumor suppressor p53, an important mediator of apoptosis in response to cell damage *(2)*, upregulates DR5, thereby sensitizing cells to Apo2L/TRAIL *(20)*. To determine the role of p53 in regulating TNFR family gene expression, we examined the response to radiation of C4-2 cells stably expressing a dominant-negative (DN) p53 mutant using Affymetrix GeneChips . It has been reported that several TNFR members may be, directly or indirectly, under transcriptional control of p53. It is known that expression of the KILLER/DR5 gene is induced by DNA-damaging agents in a p53-dependent manner. Moreover, KILLER/DR5 is also induced by wild-type p53 overexpression in the absence of DNA damage, with overexpression of KILLER/DR5 leading to apoptotic death of cancer cells *(20)*.

As expected, several well characterized p53-responsive genes, such as DR5 and Fas, were induced following IR, with this increased expression being abrogated by p53 ablation (Table 3). Indeed, Fas and DR5 were induced at 8 h following IR in both prostate and MM cells. Similar results were obtained for CPT-11 treatment, except that it took a longer time for DR5 upregulation. Moreover, stable expression of a dominant-negative p53 mutant completely blocked this activation at 6 and partially at 24 h. We also observed increased expression of DR4, similar to earlier reports. In fact, there was a more robust increase in the levels of DR4 compared to those of DR5 *(39)*. Moreover, there was a modest tissue-specific increase in expression levels of DcR1 and DcR2.

As changes in DR5 expression following CPT-11 treatment were modest, we next examined changes in protein levels. As shown in Fig. 1, there was a time-dependent increase in the levels of DR5, starting at 8 h and persisting for at least 12 h following treatment. This change was not significantly affected in cells stably expressing a dominant-negative mutant DR5 (DR5DNC4-2), which partially blocked apoptosis in these cells *(39)*. However, stable expression of p53DN effectively prevented any significant increase in DR5 levels.

Levels of RANK were upregulated by IR in MM and CaP cell lines as well as by CPT-11 in CaP. This increased expression was effectively prevented when p53 function was blocked. For OPG, although basal expression was very low, there was an apparent induction in both cell lines, with p53 possibly preventing any increase in gene expression. These data indicate that p53-dependent modulation by genotoxic stress of these receptors may have biological significance. A comprehensive analysis of the role of p53 in TNFR regulation is presented in Chapter 12.

Death Receptor Activation Through Ligand Regulation: Apo2L/TRAIL Activation

The best characterized cell-death ligands, TNF, FasL and more recently Apo2L/TRAIL, can also be regulated by a number of biological or physiological stimuli. We have

Table 3
Role of p53 in Radiation-Induced Gene Expression in Prostate Carcinoma C4-2 Cells

Cell line		*C4-2*	*P53DNC4-2*	*C4-2*	*P53DNC4-2*		
Time		*6 h*	*6 h*	*24 h*	*24 h*		
Nomenclature	*Unigene*	*Fold change*	*Fold change*	*Fold change*	*Fold change*	*P53 response*	*Common name*
TNFRSF1A	Hs.159	1.00	0.95	0.77	0.84		TNFR1
TNFRSF1B	Hs.256278	0.93	0.62	0.66	0.79		TNFR2
TNFRSF3	Hs.1116	0.94	0.73	0.86	1.39		LTBR
TNFRSF4	Hs.129780	0.64	1.66	0.45	1.83		OX40
TNFRSF5	Hs.25648	1.10	0.97	1.03	0.80		CD40
TNFRSF6	Hs.82359	2.44	0.57	1.62	0.77	++	Fas
TNFRSF6	Hs.82359	8.84	0.99	3.12	1.77	+++	Fas
TNFRSF6	Hs.82359	6.82	2.91	1.29	1.54	+++	Fas
TNFRSF6	Hs.82359	0.77	1.88	1.27	2.94		Fas
TNFRSF8	Hs.1314	0.64	0.48	1.15	0.39		CD30
TNFRSF9	Hs.73895	2.34	4.07	7.92	2.26		ILA
TNFRSF10B	Hs.51233	2.26	0.84	1.39	0.94	++	KILLER/ DR5
TNFRSF10C	Hs.119684	1.21	0.69	1.28	0.66		DcR1
TNFRSF10D	Hs.129844	1.33	1.05	1.54	1.42		DcR2
TNFRSF11A	Hs.114676	2.17	0.67	2.34	1.12	+++	RANK
TNFRSF11B	Hs.129844	4.51	0.70	2.80	0.57	+++	OPG
TNFRSF12	Hs.180338	1.37	1.62	2.48	1.25		DR3
TNFRSF12	Hs.180338	1.03	0.89	1.04	0.67		DR3
TNFRSF12	Hs.180338	0.52	1.15	0.40	1.28		DR3
TNFRSF12	Hs.180338	0.61	0.95	1.48	1.67		DR3
TNFRSF13B	Hs.158341	1.47	0.92	1.24	0.69		TACI
TNFRSF14	Hs.279899	1.51	0.74	1.40	1.02	+	HVEM
TNFRSF17	Hs.2556	0.12	1.15	1.99	1.78	+	BCM
TNFRSF21	Hs.159651	0.68	0.85	1.06	1.02		DR6
EDAR	Hs.58346	1.8	ND	3.5	NA	ND	EDAR
ACTB	Hs.288061	1.03	0.90	0.94	0.96		beta-actin
GAPDH	Hs.169476	1.14	0.90	1.06	0.89		GAPDH

ND, not determined
+,++,+++ designate weak, good, & excellent evidence, respectively for p53-dependent regulation

shown that Apo2L/TRAIL mRNA levels are also increased following IR in Jurkat, MOLT-4, and CEM T-cell lines, as well as peripheral blood mononuclear cells (PBMCs). Increased Apo2L/TRAIL protein levels were found in MOLT-4 and Jurkat cells. The response to radiation in MOLT-4 cells was lost when only 430 bp of 5' proximal flanking sequence was maintained *(36)*, pointing to possible regulatory elements required for the radiation response.

Type I interferons (IFNs; predominantly α and β) activate signal transducers and activators of transcription (STATs) *(63)* and, once translocated to the nucleus, bind IFN-stimulated regulatory elements (ISRE) to induce gene expression. Of those IFN-stimu-

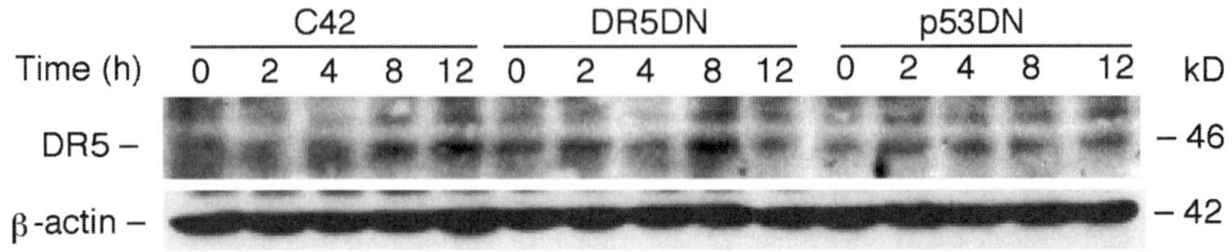

Fig. 1. Treatment with CPT-11 up-regulates DR5 expression in C4-2 cells in a p53-dependent manner. LNCaP C4-2 parental and derivative cells stably expressing DR5 (DR5DN) or p53 (p53DN) dominant-negative mutants, were grown in the absence or presence of 100 ng/mL CPT-11 for the indicated times. Cell lysates were subjected to SDS-PAGE separation and immunoblot analysis using primary antibodies against DR5, or as a control, β-actin. The hybridization signal was revealed using a secondary antibody and ECL. This experiment shows that CPT-11, similar to IR (Table 2, 3), up-regulates DR5 expression in a p53-dependent manner.

lated genes, several were recently reported to be associated with apoptosis. Notable among them is Apo2L/TRAIL, its transcriptional induction being one of the earliest events following IFN administration in MM *(37,53)*. We have cloned the 1.2-kb promoter region upstream of the translation initiation codon of Apo2l/TRAIL and defined its transcription start site. It lacks a recognizable TATA box but contains several putative transcription factor-binding sites. Luciferase reporter constructs, transfected into Jurkat cells, indicated transcriptional regulation by IFNs. Deletion analysis indicates that the Apo2L/TRAIL promoter region controls the expression of the gene following IFN-β treatment *(53)*. Thus, following IFN binding to its receptor, the STAT transcription factors may bind to cis-elements in the human Apo2L/TRAIL promoter (ISRE) and stimulate its transcriptional activity. Our results indicate that Apo2L/TRAIL can be regulated by therapeutic treatments, which may be exploited for future clinical modalities.

Apo2L/TRAIL and Its Cancer Therapeutic Potential

Recombinant soluble Apo2L/TRAIL induces apoptosis in a variety of cancer cell lines regardless of p53 status. Moreover, recent studies suggest that Apo2L/TRAIL is effective at inducing apoptosis in primary tumor samples from patients with MM *(64)* or colon carcinoma *(65)*. In mouse models, Apo2L/TRAIL demonstrated remarkable efficacy against tumor xenografts of colon carcinoma *(66,67)*, breast and ovarian carcinoma *(68,69)*, MM *(64)*, melanoma *(70)*, or glioma *(71,72)*. Moreover, combinations of Apo2L/TRAIL and certain DNA-damaging drugs *(39,66,69)* or radiotherapy *(36,73)* may exert synergistic antitumor activity.

C4-2 human prostate cancer cells are quite resistant to treatment with Apo2L/TRAIL. When combined with the topoisomerase I inhibitor CPT-11, Apo2L/TRAIL exhibits enhanced apoptotic activity in C4-2 cells cultured in vitro as well as xenografted tumors in vivo *(39)*. Previous work has indicated that IR *(36,73)*, etoposide *(74,75)*, or CDDP *(74)* sensitize tumor cells to Apo2L/TRAIL-mediated apoptosis by upregulating the Apo2L/TRAIL receptor DR5. We found that a combination treatment with CPT-11 in CaP induced significantly the expression of DR4, and to a lesser extent, that of DR5. A dominant-negative Apo2L/TRAIL receptor, DR5Δ, was able to block partially Apo2L/TRAIL plus CPT-11-mediated apoptosis both in vitro and in vivo xenografts. This combination treatment needed both the cell-extrinsic and -intrinsic pathways to induce apoptosis in C4-2 cells, as inactivation of DR5 and Bax completely prevented cell death. Our study suggests that the combination of Apo2L/TRAIL plus CPT-11 exerts antitumor activity both in vitro and in vivo. These results, taken together with reports that several chemotherapeutic agents or radiation have a synergistic cytotoxic effect with Apo2L/TRAIL *(66,76,77)*, indicate that a combination therapy using Apo2L/TRAIL with CPT-11, other chemotherapeutic agents, or radiation is likely to be widely applicable and may become a potentially promising, novel antiprostate cancer therapeutic modality.

Apo2L/TRAIL and FasL could utilize distinct pathways to induce apoptosis, since Bid *(78)* and caspase-8 *(79)* knockout mice are resistant to Fas-induced apoptosis in hepatocytes but sensitive to other types of death stimuli, including Apo2L/TRAIL. We reported that U266 MM cells are sensitive to Apo2L/TRAIL but not to Fas agonistic mAbs *(37)*, further suggesting that there are distinct apoptotic pathways activated by FasL and Apo2L/TRAIL. Myeloma cells express FasL, but only some are sensitive to anti-Fas antibody resulting in apoptosis *(80)*.

CONCLUSIONS AND FUTURE DIRECTIONS

Discovery of TNF and its receptors paved the way for investigations into the involvement of these superfamilies of receptors and their ligands in basic biological processes. Clearly, the complexity of receptor-ligand interactions points to the myriad of biological functions they elicit. More recently, once the receptors for Fas and then Apo2L/TRAIL were discovered, more focus has been placed in understanding their role in apoptosis signaling. In particular, signaling by Apo2L/TRAIL, since it acts as a tumor-specific cell ligand, has raised enthusiasm for its potential use in the clinic. Despite extensive work, however, we still do not understand why some tumor cells are resistant to Apo2L/TRAIL. Nevertheless, it has become clear that through a combination therapy approach, many tumors become responsive, making this an attractive approach for treating tumors of various types and origins. How apoptosis is triggered during these therapies, or that following activation of other non-conventional death receptors (e.g., EGFR, DAPK), will be an interesting area of investigation to be pursued in the years to come.

ACKNOWLEDGMENTS

We thank Drs. E.S. Alnemri and S.M. Srinivasula (Thomas Jefferson Univ.) and A. Gudkov (Cleveland Clinic) for the pCDNA3-DR5Δ and GSE56-p53Δ constructs, and Dr. W. Heston (Cleveland Clinic) for the C4-2 cells. Supported in part by research grants from the National Cancer Institute CA81504 and CA82858 to A. Almasan.

REFERENCES

1. Wahl GM, Carr AM. The evolution of diverse biological responses to DNA damage: insights from yeast and p53. Nat Cell Biol 2001; 3:E277–E286.
2. Gong B, Chen Q, Endlich B, Mazumder S, Almasan A. Ionizing radiation-induced, Bax-mediated cell death is dependent on activation of serine and cysteine proteases. Cell Growth Diff. 1999; 10:491–502.
3. Wang X. The expanding role of mitochondria in apoptosis. Genes Dev 2001; 15:2922–2933.
4. Ashkenazi A. Targeting death and decoy receptors of the tumour-necrosis factor superfamily. Nat Rev Cancer 2002; 2:420–430.
5. Almasan A, Ashkenazi A. Apo2L/TRAIL: apoptosis signaling, biology, and potential for cancer therapy. Cytokine Growth Factor Rev 2003;14:337–348.

6. Hohmann HP, Remy R, Brockhaus M, van Loon AP. Two different cell types have different major receptors for human tumor necrosis factor (TNF alpha). J Biol Chem 1989;264:14,927–14,934.
7. Locksley RM, Killeen N, Lenardo MJ. The TNF and TNF receptor superfamilies: integrating mammalian biology. Cell 2001;104:487–501.
8. Chan FK, Chun HJ, Zheng L, Siegel RM, Bui KL, Lenardo MJ. A domain in TNF receptors that mediates ligand-independent receptor assembly and signaling. Science 2000;288:2351–2354.
9. Pitti RM, Marsters SA, Ruppert S, Donahue CJ, Moore A, Ashkenazi A. Induction of apoptosis by Apo-2 ligand, a new member of the tumor necrosis factor cytokine family. J Biol Chem 1996;271:12,687–12,690.
10. Wiley SR, Schooley K, Smolak PJ, et al. Identification and characterization of a new member of the TNF family that induces apoptosis. Immunity 1995;3:673–682.
11. Pan G, O'Rourke K, Chinnaiyan AM, et al. The receptor for the cytotoxic ligand TRAIL. Science 1997;276:111–113.
12. Sheridan JP, Marsters SA, Pitti RM, et al. Control of TRAIL-induced apoptosis by a family of signaling and decoy receptors. Science 1997;277:818–821.
13. Screaton GR, Mongkolsapaya J, Xu XN, Cowper AE, McMichael AJ, Bell JI. TRICK2, a new alternatively spliced receptor that transduces the cytotoxic signal from TRAIL. Curr Biol 1997;7:693–696.
14. MacFarlane M, Ahmad M, Srinivasula SM, Fernandes-Alnemri T, Cohen GM, Alnemri ES. Identification and molecular cloning of two novel receptors for the cytotoxic ligand TRAIL. J Biol Chem 1997;272:25,417–25,420.
15. Chaudhary PM, Eby M, Jasmin A, Bookwalter A, Murray J, Hood L. Death receptor 5, a new member of the TNFR family, and DR4 induce FADD-dependent apoptosis and activate the NF-kappaB pathway. Immunity 1997;7:821–830.
16. Walczak H, Degli-Esposti MA, Johnson RS, et al. TRAIL-R2: a novel apoptosis-mediating receptor for TRAIL. Embo J 1997;16:5386–5397.
17. Schneider P, Bodmer JL, Thome M, Hofmann K, Holler N, Tschopp J. Characterization of two receptors for TRAIL. FEBS Lett 1997;416:329–334.
18. Pan G, Ni J, Wei YF, Yu G, Gentz R, Dixit VM. An antagonist decoy receptor and a death domain-containing receptor for TRAIL. Science 1997;277:815–818.
19. Pai SI, Wu GS, Ozoren N, et al. Rare loss-of-function mutation of a death receptor gene in head and neck cancer. Cancer Res 1998;58:3513–3518.
20. Wu GS, Burns TF, McDonald ERr, et al. KILLER/DR5 is a DNA damage-inducible p53-regulated death receptor gene. Nat Genet 1997;17:141–143.
21. Kischkel FC, Hellbardt S, Behrmann I, et al. Cytotoxicity-dependent APO-1 (Fas/CD95)-associated proteins form a death-inducing signaling complex (DISC) with the receptor. Embo J 1995;14:5579–5588.
22. Kischkel FC, Lawrence DA, Chuntharapai A, Schow P, Kim KJ, Ashkenazi A. Apo2L/TRAIL-dependent recruitment of endogenous FADD and caspase-8 to death receptors 4 and 5. Immunity 2000;12:611–620.
23. Sprick MR, Weigand MA, Rieser E, et al. FADD/MORT1 and caspase-8 are recruited to TRAIL receptors 1 and 2 and are essential for apoptosis mediated by TRAIL receptor 2. Immunity 2000;12:599–609.
24. Bodmer JL, Holler N, Reynard S, et al. TRAIL receptor-2 signals apoptosis through FADD and caspase-8. Nat Cell Biol 2000;2:241–243.
25. Degli-Esposti MA, Smolak PJ, Walczak H, et al. Cloning and characterization of TRAIL-R3, a novel member of the emerging TRAIL receptor family. J Exp Med 1997;186:1165–1170.
26. Mongkolsapaya J, Cowper AE, Xu XN, et al. Lymphocyte inhibitor of TRAIL (TNF-related apoptosis-inducing ligand): a new receptor protecting lymphocytes from the death ligand TRAIL. J Immunol 1998;160:3–6.
27. Marsters SA, Sheridan JP, Pitti RM, et al. A novel receptor for Apo2L/TRAIL contains a truncated death domain. Curr Biol 1997;7:1003–1006.
28. Degli-Esposti MA, Dougall WC, Smolak PJ, Waugh JY, Smith CA, Goodwin RG. The novel receptor TRAIL-R4 induces NF-kappaB and protects against TRAIL-mediated apoptosis, yet retains an incomplete death domain. Immunity 1997;7:813–820.
29. Pan G, Ni J, Yu G, Wei YF, Dixit VM. TRUNDD, a new member of the TRAIL receptor family that antagonizes TRAIL signalling. FEBS Lett 1998;424:41–45.
30. Simonet WS, Lacey DL, Dunstan CR, et al. Osteoprotegerin: a novel secreted protein involved in the regulation of bone density. Cell 1997;89:309–319.
31. Emery JG, McDonnell P, Burke MB, et al. Osteoprotegerin is a receptor for the cytotoxic ligand TRAIL. J Biol Chem 1998;273:14,363–14,367.

32. Holen I, Croucher PI, Hamdy FC, Eaton CL. Osteoprotegerin (OPG) is a survival factor for human prostate cancer cells. Cancer Res 2002;62:1619–1623.
33. Truneh A, Sharma S, Silverman C, et al. Temperature-sensitive differential affinity of TRAIL for its receptors. DR5 is the highest affinity receptor. J Biol Chem 2000;275:23,319–23,325.
34. Karin M, Cao Y, Greten FR, Li ZW. NF-kappaB in cancer: from innocent bystander to major culprit. Nat Rev Cancer 2002;2:301–310.
35. Thalmann GN, Anezinis PE, Chang SM, et al. Androgen-independent cancer progression and bone metastasis in the LNCaP model of human prostate cancer. Cancer Res 1994;54:2577–2581.
36. Gong B, Almasan A. Apo2 ligand/TNF-related apoptosis-inducing ligand and death receptor 5 mediate the apoptotic signaling induced by ionizing radiation in leukemic cells. Cancer Res 2000;60:5754–5760.
37. Chen Q, Gong B, Mahmoud-Ahmed A, et al. Apo2L/TRAIL and Bcl-2-related proteins regulate type I interferon-induced apoptosis in multiple myeloma. Blood 2001;98:2183–2192.
38. Ossovskaya VS, Mazo IA, Chernov MV, et al. Use of genetic suppressor elements to dissect distinct biological effects of separate p53 domains. Proc Natl Acad Sci USA 1996;93:10,309–10,314.
39. Ray S, Almasan A. Apoptosis induction in prostate cancer cells and xenografts by combined treatment with Apo2L/TRAIL and CPT-11. Cancer Res 2003;63:4713–4723.
40. Laabi Y, Gras MP, Carbonnel F, et al. A new gene, BCM, on chromosome 16 is fused to the interleukin 2 gene by a t(4;16)(q26;p13) translocation in a malignant T cell lymphoma. Embo J 1992;11:3897–3904.
41. Gras MP, Laabi Y, Linares-Cruz G, et al. BCMAp: an integral membrane protein in the Golgi apparatus of human mature B lymphocytes. Int Immunol 1995;7:1093–1106.
42. Hatzoglou A, Roussel J, Bourgeade MF, et al. TNF receptor family member BCMA (B cell maturation) associates with TNF receptor-associated factor (TRAF) 1, TRAF2, and TRAF3 and activates NF-kappa B, elk-1, c-Jun N-terminal kinase, and p38 mitogen-activated protein kinase. J Immunol 2000;165:1322–1330.
43. Mackay F, Woodcock SA, Lawton P, et al. Mice transgenic for BAFF develop lymphocytic disorders along with autoimmune manifestations. J Exp Med 1999;190:1697–1710.
44. Morel Y, Schiano de Colella JM, Harrop J, et al. Reciprocal expression of the TNF family receptor herpes virus entry mediator and its ligand LIGHT on activated T cells: LIGHT down-regulates its own receptor. J Immunol 2000;165:4397–4404.
45. Clark EA. CD40: a cytokine receptor in search of a ligand. Tissue Antigens 1990;36:33–36.
46. Mach F, Schonbeck U, Sukhova GK, Atkinson E, Libby P. Reduction of atherosclerosis in mice by inhibition of CD40 signalling. Nature 1998;394:200–203.
47. Kurts C, Carbone FR, Krummel MF, Koch KM, Miller JF, Heath WR. Signalling through CD30 protects against autoimmune diabetes mediated by CD8 T cells. Nature 1999;398:341–344.
48. Horie R, Gattei V, Ito K, et al. Frequent expression of the variant CD30 in human malignant myeloid and lymphoid neoplasms. Am J Pathol 1999;155:2029–2041.
49. Mazumder S, Chen Q, Gong B, Drazba JA, Buchsbaum JC, Almasan A. Proteolytic cleavage of cyclin E leads to inactivation of associated kinase activity and amplification of apoptosis in hematopoietic cells. Mol. Cell. Biol. 2002;22:2398–2409.
50. Mazumder S, Gong B, Almasan A. Cyclin E induction by genotoxic stress leads to apoptosis of hematopoietic cells. Oncogene 2000;19:2828–2835.
51. El-Deiry WS, Tokino T, Velculescu VE, et al. WAF1, a potential mediator of p53 tumor suppression. Cell 1993;75:817–825.
52. Wu GS, Burns TF, Zhan Y, Alnemri ES, El-Deiry WS. Molecular cloning and functional analysis of the mouse homologue of the KILLER/DR5 tumor necrosis factor-related apoptosis-inducing ligand (TRAIL) death receptor. Cancer Res 1999;59:2770–2775.
53. Gong B, Almasan A. Genomic organization and transcriptional regulation of the human Apo2L/TRAIL gene. Biochem Biophys Res Commun 2000;278:747–752.
54. Sheikh MS, Burns TF, Huang Y, et al. p53-dependent and -independent regulation of the death receptor KILLER/DR5 gene expression in response to genotoxic stress and tumor necrosis factor alpha. Cancer Res 1998;58:1593–1598.
55. Sheikh MS, Huang Y, Fernandez-Salas EA, et al. The antiapoptotic decoy receptor TRID/TRAIL-R3 is a p53-regulated DNA damage-inducible gene that is overexpressed in primary tumors of the gastrointestinal tract. Oncogene 1999;18:4153–4159.
56. Kim KM, Kim HW, Kim JO, Baek KM, Kim JG, Kang CY. Induction of 4-1BB (CD137) expression by DNA damaging agents in human T lymphocytes. Immunology 2002;107:472–479.
57. Schwarz H, Blanco FJ, von Kempis J, Valbracht J, Lotz M. ILA, a member of the human nerve growth factor/tumor necrosis factor receptor family, regulates T-lymphocyte proliferation and survival. Blood 1996;87:2839–2845.

58. Chen Q, Ray S, Hussein M, Srkalovic G, Almasan A. Role of Apo2L/TRAIL and Bcl-2-family proteins in apoptosis of multiple myeloma. Leuk Lymp 2003;44:1209–1214.
59. Sordillo EM, Pearse RN. RANK-Fc: a therapeutic antagonist for RANK-L in myeloma. Cancer 2003;97:802–812.
60. Lipton A, Ali SM, Leitzel K, et al. Serum osteoprotegerin levels in healthy controls and cancer patients. Clin Cancer Res 2002;8:2306–2310.
61. Pearse RN, Sordillo EM, Yaccoby S, et al. Multiple myeloma disrupts the TRANCE/ osteoprotegerin cytokine axis to trigger bone destruction and promote tumor progression. Proc Natl Acad Sci USA 2001;98:11,581–11,586.
62. Standal T, Seidel C, Hjertner O, et al. Osteoprotegerin is bound, internalized, and degraded by multiple myeloma cells. Blood 2002;100:3002–3007.
63. Stark GR, Kerr IM, Williams BR, Silverman RH, Schreiber RD. How cells respond to interferons. Annu Rev Biochem 1998;67:227–264.
64. Mitsiades CS, Treon SP, Mitsiades N, et al. TRAIL/Apo2L ligand selectively induces apoptosis and overcomes drug resistance in multiple myeloma: therapeutic applications. Blood 2001;98:795–804.
65. Naka T, Sugamura K, Hylander BL, Widmer MB, Rustum YM, Repasky EA. Effects of tumor necrosis factor-related apoptosis-inducing ligand alone and in combination with chemotherapeutic agents on patients' colon tumors grown in SCID mice. Cancer Res 2002;62:5800–5806.
66. Ashkenazi A, Pai RC, Fong S, et al. Safety and antitumor activity of recombinant soluble Apo2 ligand. J Clin Invest 1999;104:155–162.
67. LeBlanc H, Lawrence D, Varfolomeev E, et al. Tumor cell resistance to death receptor induced apoptosis through mutational inactivation of the proapoptotic Bcl-2 homolog Bax. Nature Medicine 2002;8:274–278.
68. Walczak H, Miller RE, Ariail K, et al. Tumoricidal activity of tumor necrosis factor-related apoptosis-inducing ligand in vivo. Nat Med 1999;5:157–163.
69. Morrison BH, Bauer JA, Hu J, et al. Inositol hexakisphosphate kinase 2 sensitizes ovarian carcinoma cells to multiple cancer therapeutics. Oncogene 2002;21:1882–1889.
70. Chawla-Sarkar M, Bauer JA, Lupica JA, et al. Suppression of NF-kappa B survival signaling by nitrosylcobalamin sensitizes neoplasms to the anti-tumor effects of Apo2L/TRAIL. J Biol Chem 2003;24:24.
71. Pollack IF, Erff M, Ashkenazi A. Direct stimulation of apoptotic signaling by soluble Apo2l/tumor necrosis factor-related apoptosis-inducing ligand leads to selective killing of glioma cells. Clin Cancer Res 2001;7:1362–1369.
72. Fulda S, Wick W, Weller M, Debatin KM. Smac agonists sensitize for Apo2L/TRAIL- or anticancer drug-induced apoptosis and induce regression of malignant glioma in vivo. Nat Med 2002;8:808–815.
73. Chinnaiyan AM, Prasad U, Shankar S, et al. Combined effect of tumor necrosis factor-related apoptosis-inducing ligand and ionizing radiation in breast cancer therapy. Proc Natl Acad Sci USA 2000;97:1754–1759.
74. Nagane M, Pan G, Weddle JJ, Dixit VM, Cavenee WK, Huang HJ. Increased death receptor 5 expression by chemotherapeutic agents in human gliomas causes synergistic cytotoxicity with tumor necrosis factor-related apoptosis-inducing ligand in vitro and in vivo. Cancer Res 2000;60:847–853.
75. Gibson SB, Oyer R, Spalding AC, Anderson SM, Johnson GL. Increased expression of death receptors 4 and 5 synergizes the apoptosis response to combined treatment with etoposide and TRAIL. Mol Cell Biol 2000;20:205–212.
76. Rokhlin OW, Gudkov AV, Kwek S, Glover RA, Gewies AS, Cohen MB. p53 is involved in tumor necrosis factor-alpha-induced apoptosis in the human prostatic carcinoma cell line LNCaP. Oncogene 2000;19:1959–1968.
77. Keane MM, Ettenberg SA, Nau MM, Russell EK, Lipkowitz S. Chemotherapy augments TRAIL-induced apoptosis in breast cell lines. Cancer Res 1999;59:734–741.
78. Yin XM, Wang K, Gross A, et al. Bid-deficient mice are resistant to Fas-induced hepatocellular apoptosis. Nature 1999;400:886–891.
79. Varfolomeev EE, Schuchmann M, Luria V, et al. Targeted disruption of the mouse caspase 8 gene ablates cell death induction by the TNF receptors, Fas/Apo1, and DR3 and is lethal prenatally. Immunity 1998;9:267–276.
80. Shima Y, Nishimoto N, Ogata A, Fujii Y, Yoshizaki K, Kishimoto T. Myeloma cells express Fas antigen/ APO-1 (CD95) but only some are sensitive to anti-Fas antibody resulting in apoptosis. Blood 1995;85:757–764.
81. Drexler HG, Dirks WG, MacLeod RA. False human hematopoietic cell lines: cross-contaminations and misinterpretations. Leukemia 1999;13:1601–1607.

17 Regulation of TRAIL-Induced Apoptosis by Transcriptional Factors

Rüdiger Göke and Youhai H. Chen, MD, PhD

TRAIL AND ITS RECEPTORS

In 1995, tumor necrosis factor (TNF)-related apoptosis-inducing ligand (TRAIL) was identified based on its sequence homology to other TNF family members *(1)*. Among members of the TNF family, TRAIL shares the highest sequence homology with Fas ligand (FasL, CD95L). However, unlike FasL, TRAIL appears to induce apoptosis of tumor cells but not most normal cells *(2)*. To date, five receptors for TRAIL have been cloned: TRAIL-R1 (DR4, Apo2A) *(3)*, TRAIL-R2 (DR5, TRICK, Killer) *(3–8)*, TRAIL-R3 (DcR1, TRID, LIT) *(6–9)*, TRAIL-R4 (DcR2, TRUNDD) *(10)*, and osteoprotegerin (OPG) *(11)*. Unlike other TRAIL receptors, which bind only to TRAIL, osteoprotegerin also binds to osteoprotegerin ligand (OPGL), TRANCE, and RANK ligand (RANKL). TRAIL-R1 and TRAIL-R2 contain intracellular death domains and induce, via coupling with intracellular adaptor proteins, the proteolytic cleavage of caspase-8 *(12)*. Caspase-8 activation initiates the extrinsic and intrinsic apoptotic pathways, resulting in caspase-3 cleavage, which is an irreversible step in a cell's commitment to apoptosis. Other TRAIL receptors do not generate death signals because TRAIL-R3 does not contain a death domain and is attached to the membrane by a glycolipid anchor *(6,9)*, whereas the death domain of TRAIL-R4 is not functional *(10)* and OPG exists only in a soluble form *(11)*. Therefore, TRAIL-R3 and TRAIL-R4 might act as decoy receptors by competing with other TRAIL receptors for TRAIL. The expression pattern of TRAIL receptors on certain cell lines might determine their sensitivity to TRAIL. However, the expression of TRAIL decoy receptors is not always related to a cell's resistance to TRAIL-induced apoptosis *(13)*. Other factors may, therefore, play more decisive roles in determining a cell's sensitivity to TRAIL. In this review, we will focus on NF-κB and PPAR-γ, two transcription factors that were recently found to play important roles in TRAIL-induced apoptosis.

From: *Cancer Drug Discovery and Development: Death Receptors in Cancer Therapy*
Edited by: W. S. El-Deiry © Humana Press Inc., Totowa, NJ

ROLES OF NF-κB IN TRAIL-INDUCED APOPTOSIS

The Rel/NF-κB family of transcription factors regulates a number of biological processes, including cell proliferation and differentiation, apoptosis, immune response, and inflammation *(14–16)*. Rel/NF-κB are normally present in the cytoplasm in association with a family of inhibitors (IκBs) that mask their nuclear localization sequences *(17,18)*. Activation of IκB kinase (IKK) leads to phosphorylation and degradation of IκBs. As a result, Rel/NF-κB are released and translocated to the nucleus, where they bind to DNA and induce the transcription of target genes *(15)*.

Rel/NF-κB induce the expression of a number of anti-apoptotic genes, including cellular inhibitors of apoptosis (cIAPs), mitochondrial proteins of the Bcl_2 family such as Bfl-1/A1 and $Bcl\text{-}X_L$, A20, manganese superoxide dismutase (MnSOD), IEX-1L, caspase 8/FADD-like IL-1β-converting enzyme (FLICE)-inhibitory protein (c-FLIP), TNF receptor-associated factor 1 (TRAF1) and 2 (TRAF2), and TRAIL receptor 3 *(16,19–30)*. Numerous studies exist which demonstrate that Rel/NF-κB inhibit programmed cell death induced by TNF-α, anticancer drugs, and ionizing radiation *(16,31–33)*.

Recently, it has also become clear that Rel/NF-κB regulate TRAIL-induced apoptosis. Thus, treatment of TRAIL-resistant pancreatic cancer cell line L3.6 with TRAIL and the NF-κB inhibitor NBD (NEMO-binding domain) peptide significantly decreased cell viability and increased apoptosis *(34)*. This effect was most likely due to decreased FLIP levels in L3.6 cells as a result of NF-κB inhibition. Prostate cancer cell lines PC3AR and PC3Neo show different TRAIL sensitivities, which are associated with a difference in NF-κB levels in these cells *(35)*. Blocking NF-κB function by adenoviral transfer of mutated IκB increased apoptotic responses, suggesting a direct role for NF-κB in this system.

Multiple myeloma (MM) is an incurable disease. TRAIL might represent a new treatment option, since it kills most MM cell lines and MM cells freshly isolated from patients. Treatment with the NF-κB inhibitor SN50 enhanced TRAIL-induced apoptosis in sensitive cells and reversed resistance of ARH-77 and IM-9 MM cells *(36)*. Interestingly, treatment with SN50 did not sensitize normal B-lymphocytes towards TRAIL-induced apoptosis. Insulin-like growth factor-1 (IGF-1) promotes proliferation of MM cells and protects them against TRAIL-induced apoptosis. In a recent study, IGF-1 was shown to activate NF-κB and upregulate the expression of survival factors FLIP, survivin, cIAP-2, A1/Bfl-1, and XIAP *(37)*. Overexpression of Akt decreased TRAIL sensitivity of MM cells. Interestingly, treatment of cells with an Akt inhibitor abrogated NF-κB activation and prevented the protective effect. These data show that besides NF-κB, the PI-3K/Akt pathway is also involved in the regulation of TRAIL sensitivity. An important role for NF-κB in TRAIL-induced apoptosis has also been demonstrated in lymphoid cell lines. Thus, acute T-cell leukemia cells (CEM, Jurkat) and BJAB cells (Burkitt lymphoma) treated with NF-κB inhibitors showed a significantly increased sensitivity towards TRAIL *(38,39)*.

It has been previously reported that TRAIL, but not other TNF family members, induces apoptosis in the majority of melanoma cell lines *(40–44)*. The mechanisms of TRAIL resistance of some melanoma cells are not well understood. Lack of response to TRAIL was partially due to a loss of TRAIL receptor expression *(41)*. However, a clear correlation between expression of TRAIL decoy receptors and TRAIL resistance could not be established *(13)*. In a recent study, pretreatment of melanoma cell lines with the proteasome inhibitor -acetyl-L-leucinyl-L-leucinyl-L-norleucinal (LLnL), which also inhibits NF-κB, sensitized 10 of 12 cell lines to TRAIL-induced apoptosis *(45)*. Furthermore, TRAIL resistant melanoma cells generated by intermittent TRAIL exposure exhibited elevated levels of activated NF-κB. Resistance in these cell lines could be reversed by LLnL and by a degradation-resistant form of IκBα *(45)*. These results suggest that NF-κB significantly influences TRAIL sensitivity in melanoma cells. Reports on renal cancer cells provide contradictory results. Whereas Pawlowski et al. reported that neither activation nor inhibition of NF-κB signal transduction pathway protected renal carcinoma cells from TRAIL-induced apoptosis *(46)*, a recent report shows that constitutive activation of NF-κB prevents TRAIL-induced apoptosis in these cells *(47)*.

Platelet-activating factor (PAF) is a proinflammatory lipid mediator that acts via a G protein-coupled receptor. Activation of epidermal PAF receptor results in protection against TRAIL-induced apoptosis. Recently, this effect was shown to be NF-κB-dependent since it could be antagonized by a super-repressor form of IκB *(48)*. Therefore, it seems that G protein-coupled receptors like the PAF receptor are able to block TRAIL-induced apoptosis in a NF-κB-dependent manner.

Various subunits of NF-κB can have different effects on the cellular response to TRAIL. Thus, the c-Rel subunit promotes TRAIL-induced cell death by increasing the expression of TRAIL receptors 1 and 2; the Rel-A subunit blocks TRAIL-induced apoptosis by increasing Bcl-X_L expression *(49)*. However, further investigation is needed to establish the specific roles of each NF-κB subunit in TRAIL-induced apoptosis.

ROLES OF PPAR-γ IN TRAIL-INDUCED APOPTOSIS

Peroxisome proliferator-activated receptors (PPARs) are members of the nuclear hormone receptor superfamily of ligand-activated transcription factors. PPARs form a subfamily consisting of PPAR-α, PPAR-Δ, and PPAR-γ *(50)*. PPAR-γ is highly expressed in adipose tissues but also present in intestine, mammary gland, endothelial and smooth muscle cells, monocytes, macrophages, and a number of other cell types *(51–58)*. PPAR-γ exists in two isoforms, PPAR-γ1 and PPAR-γ2, which are produced from a single gene as a result of the utilization of different promoters and alternative splicing *(51)*. PPAR-γ forms a dimer with the retinoid X receptor. This complex binds to the promoter region of specific target genes. Binding of PPAR-γ ligands leads to conformational changes resulting in activation of the target genes. PPAR-γ plays an important role in cell growth and differentiation, lipid metabolism, and inflammation *(59,60)*.

PPAR-γ is highly expressed in several cancer cell lines, including breast cancer *(53,61–63)*, prostate cancer *(64,65)*, pancreatic cancer *(66)*, gastric cancer *(67)*, colon cancer *(68,69)*, liposarcoma *(70)*, bladder cancer *(71)*, lung cancer *(72)*, and related cancer tissues from patients *(64,68,70)*. Activation of PPAR-γ resulted in suppression of cell growth, induction of apoptosis, promotion of terminal differentiation, and morphological changes to a well differentiated and less malignant state *(50,60,73)*.

The mechanisms by which PPAR-γ ligands promote apoptosis are not well understood. PPAR-γ ligands were shown to up-regulate Bax and Bad protein levels and downregulate Bcl_2 *(61,74)*. However, in other studies PPAR-γ ligands had no effect on Bax and Bcl_2 mRNA expressions *(75–77)*. While troglitazone and pioglitazone were shown to increase the expression of cyclin-dependent kinase inhibitors $p21^{WAF/CIP1}$ and $p16^{INK4}$ *(71,78)*, troglitazone did not change $p21^{WAF/CIP1}$ levels in smooth muscle cells *(75)*. Furthermore, PPAR-γ ligand-induced inhibition of NF-κB-dependent transcription might be mediated by PPAR-γ-independent mechanisms *(58,79)*. Thus, further investigations are needed to elucidate the proapoptotic activities of PPAR-γ ligands.

TRAIL holds tremendous promise for cancer therapy because of its ability to selectively kill transformed cells but not normal cells. However, not all tumor cells are equally sensitive to TRAIL-induced apoptosis. Using Jurkat cells, we showed that pioglitazone inhibits cell growth and sensitizes them for TRAIL-induced apoptosis *(39)*. Similar results were obtained in carcinoid cells that are normally resistant to TRAIL-induced apoptosis *(78)*. In carcinoid cells, pioglitazone treatment upregulated $p21^{WAF/CIP1}$ expression. Because overexpression of $p21^{WAF/CIP1}$ by adenoviral gene transfer sensitized cells to TRAIL-induced apoptosis, the proapoptotic effect of pioglitazone might be mediated by $p21^{WAF/CIP1}$ in carcinoid cells. Recently, the sensitizing effect of PPAR-γ ligands on TRAIL-induced apoptosis was also observed in prostate and ovarian cancer cell lines *(80)*. In these cells, PPAR-γ ligands induced ubiquitination and proteasome-dependent degradation of FLIP without affecting FLIP mRNA levels. Interestingly, this effect was not related to NF-κB, independent of PPAR-γ expression, and could be observed even in the presence of a PPAR-γ dominant-negative mutant, indicating a novel PPAR-γ-independent mechanism. This assertion is supported by a recent study in which the PPAR-γ agonist bisphenol A diglycidyl ether (BADGE) induces apoptosis in Jurkat cells independent of PPAR-γ, in both caspase-dependent and -independent manners *(81)*.

In summary, transcription factors NF-κB and PPAR-γ play important roles in the regulation of programmed cell death. Recent studies strongly suggest that while PPAR-γ promotes TRAIL-induced apoptosis, NF-κB inhibits it. Therefore, NF-κB inhibitors and PPAR-γ agonists may be used as enhancers for TRAIL-based cancer therapy.

REFERENCES

1. Wiley SR, Schooley K, Smolak PJ, et al. Identification and characterization of a new member of the TNF family that induces apoptosis. Immunity 1995;3:673–82.
2. Walczak H, Krammer PH. The CD95 (APO-1/Fas) and the TRAIL (APO-2L) apoptosis systems. Exp Cell Res 2000;256:58–66.
3. Pan G, O'Rourke K, Chinnaiyan AM, et al. The receptor for the cytotoxic ligand TRAIL. Science 1997;276:111–113.
4. Walczak H, Degli-Esposti MA, Johnson RS, et al. TRAIL-R2: a novel apoptosis-mediating receptor for TRAIL. EMBO J 1997;16:5386–5397.
5. Sheridan JP, Marsters SA, Pitti RM, et al. Control of TRAIL-induced apoptosis by a family of signaling and decoy receptors. Science 1997;277:818–821.
6. Schneider P, Bodmer JL, Thome M, Hofmann K, Holler N, Tschopp J. Characterization of two receptors for TRAIL. FEBS Letters 1997;416:329–334.
7. Screaton GR, Mongkolsapaya J, Xu XN, Cowper AE, McMichael AJ, Bell JI. TRICK2, a new alternatively spliced receptor that transduces the cytotoxic signal from TRAIL. Curr Biol 1997;7:693–696.
8. Wu GS, Burns TF, McDonald III ER, et al. Killer/DR5 is a DNA damage-inducible p53-regulated death receptor gene. Nat Genet 1997;17:141–143.
9. Degli-Espost MA, Smolak PJ, Walczak H, et al. Cloning and characterization of TRAIL-R3, a novel member of the emerging TRAIL receptor family. J Exp Med 1997;186:1165–1170.
10. Degli-Esposti MA, Dougall WC, Smolak PJ, Waugh JY, Smith CA, Goodwin RG. The novel receptor TRAIL-R4 induces NF-κB and protects against TRAIL-mediated apoptosis, yet retains an incomplete death domain. Immunity 1997;7:813–820.

11. Emery JG, McDonnell P, Burke MB, et al. Osteoprotegerin is a receptor for the cytotoxic ligand TRAIL. J Biol Chem 1998;273:14,363–14,367.
12. Srivastava RK. Intracellular mechanisms of TRAIL and its role in cancer therapy. Mol Cell Biol Res Commun 2000;4:67–75.
13. Griffith TS, Lynch DH. TRAIL: a molecule with multiple receptors and control mechanisms. Curr Opin Immunol 1998;10:559–563.
14. Ghosh S, May MJ, Kopp EB. NF-kappa B and Rel proteins: evolutionarily conserved mediators of immune responses. Ann Rev Immun 1998;16:225–260.
15. Bours V, Bentires AM, Hellin AC, et al. Nuclear factor-kappa B, cancer, and apoptosis. Biochem Pharma 2000;60:1085–1089.
16. Karin M, Lin A. NF-kappaB at the crossroads of life and death. 2002;3:221–227.
17. Verma IM, Stevenson JK, Schwarz EM, Van_Antwerp D, Miyamoto S. Rel/NF-kappa B/I kappa B family: intimate tales of association and dissociation. Genes Dev 1995;9:2723–2735.
18. Karin M. The beginning of the end: IkappaB kinase (IKK) and NF-kappaB activation. J Biol Chem 1999;274:27,339–27,342.
19. Wang CY, Mayo MW, Korneluk RG, Goeddel DV, Baldwin AS. NF-kappaB antiapoptosis: induction of TRAF1 and TRAF2 and c-IAP1 and c-IAP2 to suppress caspase-8 activation. Science 1998;281: 1680–1683.
20. Stehlik C, de Martin R, Kumabashiri I, Schmid JA, Binder BR, Lipp J. Nuclear factor (NF)-kappaB-regulated X-chromosome-linked iap gene expression protects endothelial cells from tumor necrosis factor alpha-induced apoptosis. J Exp Med 1998;188:211–216.
21. Zong WX, Edelstein LC, Chen C, Bash J, Gelinas C. The prosurvival Bcl-2 homolog Bfl-1/A1 is a direct transcriptional target of NF-kappaB that blocks TNFalpha-induced apoptosis. Genes Dev 1999; 13:382–387.
22. Grumont RJ, Rourke IJ, Gerondakis S. Rel-dependent induction of A1 transcription is required to protect B cells from antigen receptor ligation-induced apoptosis. Genes Dev 1999;13:400–411.
23. Chen F, Demers LM, Vallyathan V, Lu Y, Castranova V, Shi X. Involvement of 5'-flanking kappaB-like sites within bcl-x gene in silica-induced Bcl-x expression. J Biol Chem 1999;274:35,591–35,595.
24. Lee HH, Dadgostar H, Cheng Q, Shu J, Cheng G. NF-kappaB-mediated up-regulation of Bcl-x and Bfl-1/A1 is required for CD40 survival signaling in B lymphocytes. Proc Natl Acad Sci USA 1999;96:9136–9141.
25. Tamatani M, Che YH, Matsuzaki H, et al. Tumor necrosis factor induces Bcl-2 and Bcl-x expression through NFkappaB activation in primary hippocampal neurons. J Biol Chem 1999;274:8531–8538.
26. Krikos A, Laherty CD, Dixit VM. Transcriptional activation of the tumor necrosis factor alpha-inducible zinc finger protein, A20, is mediated by kappa B elements. J Biol Chem 1992;267:17,971–17,976.
27. Jones PL, Ping D, Boss JM. Tumor necrosis factor alpha and interleukin-1beta regulate the murine manganese superoxide dismutase gene through a complex intronic enhancer involving C/EBP-beta and NF-kappaB. Mol Cell Biol 1997;17:6970–6981.
28. Wu MX, Ao Z, Prasad KV, Wu R, Schlossman SF. IEX-1L, an apoptosis inhibitor involved in NF-kappaB-mediated cell survival. Science 1998;281:998–1001.
29. Kreuz S, Siegmund D, Scheurich P, Wajant H. NF-kappaB inducers upregulate cFLIP, a cycloheximide-sensitive inhibitor of death receptor signaling. Mol Cell Biol 2001;21:3964–3973.
30. Bernard D, Quatannens B, Vandenbunder B, Abbadie C. Rel/NF-kappaB transcription factors protect against tumor necrosis factor (TNF)-related apoptosis-inducing ligand (TRAIL)-induced apoptosis by up-regulating the TRAIL decoy receptor DcR1. J Biol Chem 2001;276:27,322–27,328.
31. Wang CY, Mayo MW, Baldwin AS. TNF- and cancer therapy-induced apoptosis: potentiation by inhibition of NF-kappaB. Science 1996;274:784–787.
32. Wang CY, Cusack JC, Liu R, Baldwin AS. Control of inducible chemoresistance: enhanced anti-tumor therapy through increased apoptosis by inhibition of NF-kappaB. Nature Med 1999;5:412–417.
33. Karin M, Cao Y, Greten FR, Li ZW. NF-kappaB in cancer: from innocent bystander to major culprit. Nat Rev Cancer 2002;2:301–310.
34. Thomas RP, Farrow BJ, Kim S, May MJ, Hellmich MR, Evers BM. Selective targeting of the nuclear factor-kappaB pathway enhances tumor necrosis factor-related apoptosis-inducing ligand-mediated pancreatic cancer cell death. Surgery 2002;132:127–134.
35. Eid MA, Lewis RW, Abdel_Mageed AB, Kumar MV. Reduced response of prostate cancer cells to TRAIL is modulated by NFkappaB-mediated inhibition of caspases and Bid activation. Internat J Oncol 2002;21:111–117.

36. Mitsiades CS, Treon SP, Mitsiades N, et al. TRAIL/Apo2L ligand selectively induces apoptosis and overcomes drug resistance in multiple myeloma: therapeutic applications. Blood 2001;98:795–804.
37. Mitsiades CS, Mitsiades N, Poulaki V, et al. Activation of NF-kappaB and upregulation of intracellular anti-apoptotic proteins via the IGF-1/Akt signaling in human multiple myeloma cells: therapeutic implications. Oncogene 2002;21:5673–5683.
38. Jeremias I, Herr I, Boehler T, Debatin KM. TRAIL/Apo-2-ligand-induced apoptosis in human T cells. Eur J Immunol 1998;28:143–152.
39. Göke R, Göke A, Göke B, Chen Y. Regulation of TRAIL-induced apoptosis by transcription factors. Cell Immunol 2000;201:77–82.
40. Thomas WD, Hersey P. TNF-related apoptosis-inducing ligand (TRAIL) induces apoptosis in Fas ligand-resistant melanoma cells and mediates CD4 T cell killing of target cells. J Immunol 1998;161:2195–2200.
41. Zhang XD, Franco A, Myers K, Gray C, Nguyen T, Hersey P. Relation of TNF-related apoptosis-inducing ligand (TRAIL) receptor and FLICE-inhibitory protein expression to TRAIL-induced apoptosis of melanoma. Cancer Res 1999;59:2747–2753.
42. Zhang XD, Franco AV, Nguyen T, Gray CP, Hersey P. Differential localization and regulation of death and decoy receptors for TNF-related apoptosis-inducing ligand (TRAIL) in human melanoma cells. J Immun 2000;164:3961–3970.
43. Thomas WD, Smith MJ, Si Z, Hersey P. Expression of the co-stimulatory molecule CD40 on melanoma cells. Internat J Cancer 1996;68:795–801.
44. Thomas WD, Hersey P. CD4 T cells kill melanoma cells by mechanisms that are independent of Fas (CD95). Internat J Cancer 1998;75:384–390.
45. Franco AV, Zhang XD, Van_Berkel E, et al. The role of NF-kappa B in TNF-related apoptosis-inducing ligand (TRAIL)-induced apoptosis of melanoma cells. J Immunol 2001;166:5337–5345.
46. Pawlowski JE, Nesterov A, Scheinman RI, Johnson TR, Kraft AS. NF-kappa B does not modulate sensitivity of renal carcinoma cells to TNF alpha-related apoptosis-inducing ligand (TRAIL). Anticancer Res 2000;20:4243–4255.
47. Oya M, Ohtsubo M, Takayanagi A, Tachibana M, Shimizu N, Murai M. Constitutive activation of nuclear factor-kappaB prevents TRAIL-induced apoptosis in renal cancer cells. Oncogene 2001; 20:3888–3896.
48. Southall MD, Isenberg JS, Nakshatri H, et al. The platelet-activating factor receptor protects epidermal cells from tumor necrosis factor (TNF) alpha and TNF-related apoptosis-inducing ligand-induced apoptosis through an NF-kappa B-dependent process. J Biol Chem 2001;276:45,548–45,554.
49. Ravi R, Bedi GC, Engstrom LW, et al. Regulation of death receptor expression and TRAIL/Apo2L-induced apoptosis by NF-kappaB. Nat Cell Biol 2001;3:409–416.
50. Desvergne B, Wahli W. Peroxisome proliferator-activated receptors: nuclear control of metabolism. Endocrine Rev 1999;20:649–688.
51. Tontonoz P, Hu E, Graves RA, Budavari AI, Spiegelman BM. mPPAR gamma 2: tissue-specific regulator of an adipocyte enhancer. Genes Dev 1994;8:1224–1234.
52. Mansen A, Guardiola_Diaz H, Rafter J, Branting C, Gustafsson JA. Expression of the peroxisome proliferator-activated receptor (PPAR) in the mouse colonic mucosa. Biochem Biophys Res Commun 1996;222:844–851.
53. Mueller E, Sarraf P, Tontonoz P, et al. Terminal differentiation of human breast cancer through PPAR gamma. Mol Cell 1998;1:465–470.
54. Delerive P, Martin-Nizard F, Chinetti G, et al. Peroxisome proliferator-activated receptor activators inhibit thrombin-induced endothelin-1 production in human vascular endothelial cells by inhibiting the activator protein-1 signaling pathway. Circ Res (Online) 1999;85:394–402.
55. Marx N, Schonbeck U, Lazar MA, Libby P, Plutzky J. Peroxisome proliferator-activated receptor gamma activators inhibit gene expression and migration in human vascular smooth muscle cells. Circ Res (Online) 1998;83:1097–1103.
56. Ricote M, Li AC, Wilson TM, Kelly CJ, Glass CK. The peroxisome proliferator-activated receptor-g is a negative regulator of macrophage activation. Nature 1998;391:79–82.
57. Marx N, Sukhova G, Murphy C, Libby P, Plutzky J. Macrophages in human atheroma contain PPARgamma: differentiation-dependent peroxisomal proliferator-activated receptor gamma (PPARgamma) expression and reduction of MMP-9 activity through PPARgamma activation in mononuclear phagocytes in vitro. Am J Pathol 1998;153:17–23.

58. Chinetti G, Griglio S, Antonucci M, et al. Activation of proliferator-activated receptors alpha and gamma induces apoptosis of human monocyte-derived macrophages. J Biol Chem 1998;273:25,573–25,580.
59. Chinetti G, Fruchart JC, Staels B. Peroxisome proliferator-activated receptors (PPARs): nuclear receptors at the crossroads between lipid metabolism and inflammation. Inflam Res 2000;49:497–505.
60. Rosen ED, Spiegelman BM. PPARgamma: a nuclear regulator of metabolism, differentiation, and cell growth. J Biol Chem 2001;276:37,731–37,734.
61. Elstner E, Muller C, Koshizuka K, et al. Ligands for peroxisome proliferator-activated receptorgamma and retinoic acid receptor inhibit growth and induce apoptosis of human breast cancer cells in vitro and in BNX mice. Proc Natl Acad Sci USA 1998;95:8806–8811.
62. Badawi AF, Badr MZ. Chemoprevention of breast cancer by targeting cyclooxygenase-2 and peroxisome proliferator-activated receptor-gamma (Review). Int J Oncol 2002;20:1109–1122.
63. Elstner E, Williamson EA, Zang C, et al. Novel therapeutic approach: ligands for PPARgamma and retinoid receptors induce apoptosis in bcl-2-positive human breast cancer cells. Breast Cancer Res Treat 2002;74:155–165.
64. Mueller E, Smith M, Sarraf P, et al. Effects of ligand activation of peroxisome proliferator-activated receptor gamma in human prostate cancer. Proc Natl Acad Sci USA 2000;97:10,990–10,995.
65. Hisatake JI, Ikezoe T, Carey M, Holden S, Tomoyasu S, Koeffler HP. Down-regulation of prostate-specific antigen expression by ligands for peroxisome proliferator-activated receptor gamma in human prostate cancer. Cancer Res 2000;60:5494–5498.
66. Eibl G, Wente MN, Reber HA, Hines OJ. Peroxisome proliferator-activated receptor gamma induces pancreatic cancer cell apoptosis. Biochem Biophys Res Commun 2001;287:522–529.
67. Takahashi N, Okumura T, Motomura W, Fujimoto Y, Kawabata I, Kohgo Y. Activation of PPARgamma inhibits cell growth and induces apoptosis in human gastric cancer cells. FEBS Lett 1999;455:135–139.
68. Sarraf P, Mueller E, Jones D, et al. Differentiation and reversal of malignant changes in colon cancer through PPARgamma. Nature Med 1998;4:1046–1052.
69. Yang WL, Frucht H. Activation of the PPAR pathway induces apoptosis and COX-2 inhibition in HT-29 human colon cancer cells. Carcinogenesis 2001;22:1379–1383.
70. Tontonoz P, Singer S, Forman BM, et al. Terminal differentiation of human liposarcoma cells induced by ligands for peroxisome proliferator-activated receptor gamma and the retinoid X receptor. Proc Natl Acad Sci USA 1997;94:237–241.
71. Guan YF, Zhang YH, Breyer RM, Davis L, Breyer MD. Expression of peroxisome proliferator-activated receptor gamma (PPARgamma) in human transitional bladder cancer and its role in inducing cell death. Neoplasia 1999;1:330–339.
72. Tsubouchi Y, Sano H, Kawahito Y, et al. Inhibition of human lung cancer cell growth by the peroxisome proliferator-activated receptor-gamma agonists through induction of apoptosis. Biochem Biophys Res Commun 2000;270:400–405.
73. Fujiwara T, Horikoshi H. Troglitazone and related compounds: therapeutic potential beyond diabetes. Life Sci 2000;67:2405–2416.
74. Zander T, Kraus JA, Grommes C, et al. Induction of apoptosis in human and rat glioma by agonists of the nuclear receptor PPARgamma. J Neurochem 2002;81:1052–1060.
75. Okura T, Nakamura M, Takata Y, Watanabe S, Kitami Y, Hiwada K. Troglitazone induces apoptosis via the p53 and Gadd45 pathway in vascular smooth muscle cells. Eur J Pharm 2000;407:227–235.
76. Ohta K, Endo T, Haraguchi K, Hershman JM, Onaya T. Ligands for peroxisome proliferator-activated receptor gamma inhibit growth and induce apoptosis of human papillary thyroid carcinoma cells. J Clin Endocrin Metab 2001;86:2170–2177.
77. Toyoda M, Takagi H, Horiguchi N, et al. A ligand for peroxisome proliferator activated receptor gamma inhibits cell growth and induces apoptosis in human liver cancer cells. Gut 2002;50:563–567.
78. Göke R, Göke A, Göke B, El-Deiry WS, Chen Y. Pioglitazone inhibits growth of carcinoid cells and promotes TRAIL-induced apoptosis by induction of p21waf1/cip1. Digestion 2001;64:75–80.
79. Straus DS, Pascual G, Li M, et al. 15-deoxy-delta 12,14-prostaglandin J2 inhibits multiple steps in the NF-kappa B signaling pathway. Proc Natl Acad Sci USA 2000;97:4844–4849.
80. Kim Y, Suh N, Sporn M, Reed JC. An inducible pathway for degradation of FLIP protein sensitizes tumor cells to TRAIL-induced apoptosis. J Biol Chem 2002;277:22,320–22,329.
81. Fehlberg S, Trautwein S, Göke A, Göke R. Bisphenol A diglycidyl ether induces apoptosis in tumour cells independently of peroxisome proliferator-activated receptor-gamma, in caspase-dependent and -independent manners. Biochem J 2002;362:573–578.

18 Sensitizing Tumor Cells by Targeting Death Receptor Signaling Inhibitors

Christina Voelkel-Johnson, PhD

INTRODUCTION

Therapies aimed at death receptor signaling using FasL or tumor necrosis factor-related apoptosis-inducing ligand (TRAIL) as agonists have become an active area of research in the development of novel anticancer therapies. Systemic delivery of FasL causes hepatotoxicity, limiting its use to local administration *(1)*. In contrast, preclinical studies with TRAIL show that systemic delivery of the soluble form is well tolerated in nonhuman primates *(2–4)*. Exposure of normal human cells to TRAIL was also well tolerated, whereas TRAIL induced apoptosis in numerous malignant cell lines that were analyzed in initial studies *(2,5,6)*. However, as more malignant cell lines and fresh tumor explants were examined, it became clear that TRAIL also fails to induce significant apoptosis in many transformed cells *(7–11)*. Numerous studies have been undertaken to understand mechanisms of death receptor ligand resistance, and strategies to enhance sensitivity or overcome resistance have been devised. In this chapter the role, function, and regulation of the death receptor signaling pathway inhibitors, how they can be targeted therapeutically, and the implications for future cancer therapies will be discussed.

DEATH RECEPTOR-MEDIATED APOPTOSIS

Initiation of death receptor-mediated apoptosis (FasL/CD95L or TRAIL/Apo2L) begins with ligand-receptor binding and formation of the death-inducing signaling complex (DISC). The DISC consists of at least the ligand, receptor, adaptor molecules, and initiator caspases (-8 and/or -10). Initiator caspases that are activated at the DISC cleave and activate downstream targets in a mitochondria-independent or -dependent fashion. During mitochondria-dependent apoptosis (also known as the intrinsic or type II pathway) caspase-8 cleaves Bid, yielding a truncated form called tBid, which inserts into the mitochondrial membrane where it facilitates the release of cytochrome c. This is followed by formation of the apoptosome, which consists of cytochrome c, Apaf-1, and caspase-9. Both caspase-8 and -9 can cleave and activate downstream executioner caspases 3 and 7, which are responsible for cleavage of death substrates.

From: *Cancer Drug Discovery and Development: Death Receptors in Cancer Therapy*
Edited by: W. S. El-Deiry © Humana Press Inc., Totowa, NJ

Intracellularly, apoptosis is negatively regulated at three levels: initiator caspases, executioner caspases, and the mitochondria (Fig. 1). (1) At the DISC, cellular FLICE-inhibitory protein (c-FLIP) binds to initiator caspases, preventing activation and aborting the apoptotic signal. (2) The family of proteins known as "inhibitors of apoptosis proteins" (IAPs) suppresses apoptosis by directly binding to and inhibiting caspases 3, 7, and 9. (3) At the mitochondrial level, apoptosis is negatively regulated by the antiapoptotic members of the Bcl-2 family, which inhibit or prevent the release of cytochrome c and Smac/DIABLO, an inhibitor of IAPs. Survival signaling pathways including NF-κB, Akt (PKB), and PKC also negatively regulate apoptosis, in part by modulating levels or activity of inhibitors in the death receptor signaling pathway.

SENSITIZATION TO DEATH RECEPTOR SIGNALING

Sensitivity to death receptor-mediated apoptosis can be augmented by metabolic inhibitors *(10,12–18)*, chemotherapeutic drugs *(2,19–27)*, radiation *(28,29)*, or other agents *(30–40)* (Table 1). Several of these treatments are proposed to enhance sensitivity to death receptor ligands by upregulation of the corresponding receptors, which may certainly contribute to increased susceptibility following ligand binding if surface expression of the receptors is a limiting factor. However, increased receptor expression is likely ineffective if inhibitors of death receptor signaling are high and prevent transmission of the apoptotic signal. Therefore, this chapter will focus on those agents that target intracellular components of the death receptor signaling pathway.

INHIBITORS OF DEATH RECEPTOR SIGNALING

c-FLIP

c-FLIP (also known as Casper, CLARP, CASH, I-FLICE, Usurpin, FLAME-1, and MRIT) is located on chromosome 2q33-34 near the genes of the initiator caspases 8 and 10. Although multiple mRNA splice variants of the gene have been reported *(41)*, typically two forms of the protein can be detected *(42)*. The long form of c-FLIP (55 kDa) consists of two tandem death effector domains (DEDs) and a caspase-like domain that lacks catalytic activity due to several amino acid substitutions. The short form of c-FLIP (26 kDa) also contains the two DEDs and a short C-terminal portion that is not homologous to c-FLIP$_L$. Both forms of the protein can associate with adapter molecules and/or initiator caspases via the DED.

Elevated levels of c-FLIP have been observed in malignant melanoma lesions but not in surrounding normal melanocytes *(43)*. The prostate cancer cells PC3 and Du145 also express higher levels of c-FLIP than normal prostate stromal or epithelial cells *(44)*. It is believed that elevated levels of c-FLIP allow tumors to escape immune surveillance.

Inhibition of death receptor-mediated signaling by FLIP has been implicated not only in tumor formation but also in resistance to treatment in vivo *(45–48)*.

Activation of Caspase-8 and Inhibition by c-FLIP

According to a recent model, activation of caspase-8 from inactive zymogen to active tetramer (consisting of two p18 and two p10 subunits) occurs via auto- and transcatalytic cleavage of homodimers *(49)*. During the autocatalytic step, the zymogen form is cleaved into p43/41 and p10 subunits, while the transcatalytic step is responsible for the release

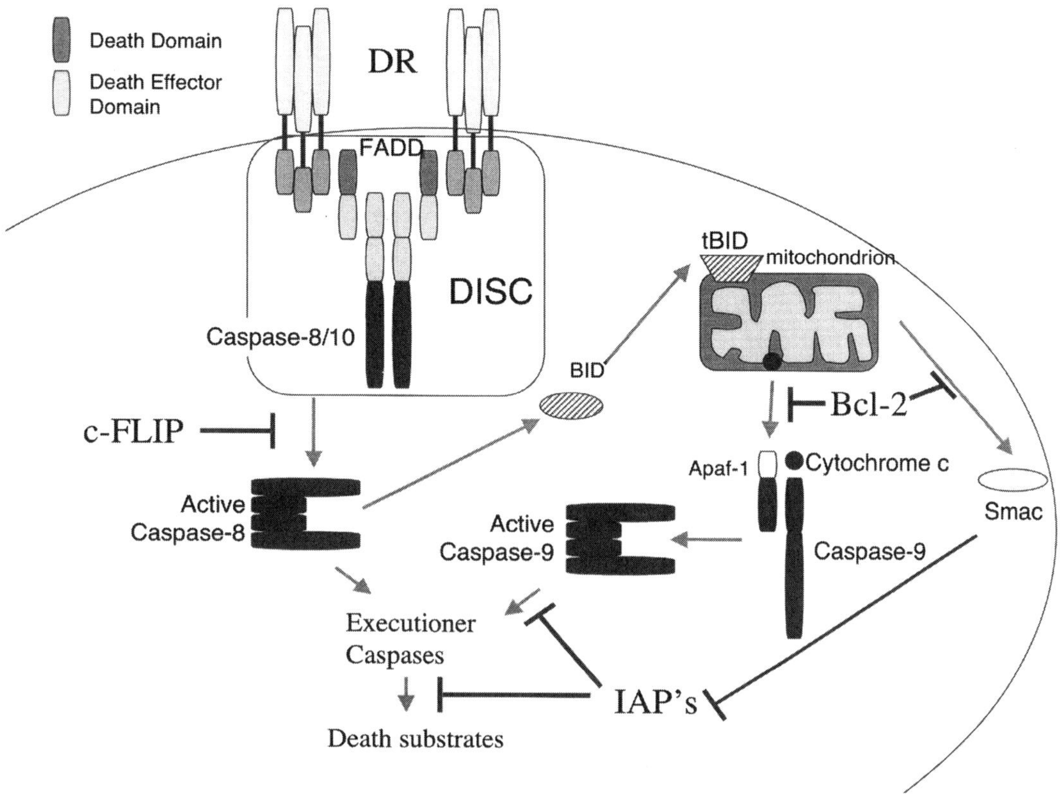

Fig. 1. Death receptor-mediated signaling. For details refer to the text.

of the p18 subunit. Heterodimer association of caspase-8 and c-FLIP$_L$ results in caspase-8 autocatalytic processing, generating the p43/41 and p10 subunits, and in a transcatalytic step cleaving c-FLIP$_L$ into a 41-kDa protein. c-FLIP$_L$, lacking the catalytic center, is unable to transcatalytically cleave the p41/43 caspase-8 into the p18 form, and the apoptotic signal is aborted. No intermediates are generated in caspase-8/c-FLIP$_S$ heterodimers, suggesting that the proximity of a caspase-like domain is required to initiate the autocatalytic step.

c-FLIP/Caspase-8 Ratios

Two studies indicated that high levels of FLIP correlated with TRAIL resistance *(9,10)* but many subsequent studies failed to observe a correlation between susceptibility and c-FLIP expression *(19,50–55)*. Several possibilities for this discrepancy are discussed below.

First, although the stoichiometry of DISC components has not been fully elucidated, the ratio between caspase-8 and c-FLIP seems critical, since full activation of caspase-8 requires homodimer formation. Therefore, a high c-FLIP/caspase-8 ratio or low caspase-8 expression would favor resistance *(56,57)*. In pediatric rhabdomyosarcoma cell lines where

Table 1
Proposed Mechanisms of Sensitizing Agents

Sensitizing agent	*Proposed mechanism*	*Cell type*	*Reference*
ActD, CHX	↓c-FLIP, ↓XIAP	neuroblastoma	*12*
ActD, CHX	↓c-FLIP	colon	*13*
ActD	↓XIAP	prostate	*14,15*
ActD	↓ c-FLIP	melanoma	*10*
ActD	↑ DR, ↓survivin	renal cell carcinoma	*16*
ActD, CHX, BIM	↓c-FLIP, ↓c-IAP-2	multiple myeloma	*17*
CHX	↓ c-FLIP	keratinocytes	*18*
Doxo, etopo, Ara-C	↑ DR	leukemia	*19*
Doxo, etopo, cisplatin, gemcitabine	↑ C9, ↑Apaf1	mesothelioma	*20*
Doxo	↓ c-FLIP	prostate	*21*
Etopo, cisplatin	↑DR	glioma	*22*
Cisplatin	↓ c-FLIP	osteosarcoma	*26*
Cisplatin, 5-FU	↑Bax	renal cells, bladder	*96,97*
Cisplatin, 5FU	↑DR	colon	*27*
9-nitrocamptothecin	↓ c-FLIP	prostate	*25*
Paclitaxel	↑DR	prostate	*23*
Etopo, camptothecin	↑DR, ↑Bak	colon	*101*
Radiation	↑DR	breast, leukemia	*28,29*
Sulindac sulfide	↓ Bcl-XL	colon	*98*
Adenovirus E1A		melanoma, fibrosarcoma	*30*
Adenovirus E1A	↓ c-FLIP	HeLa	*31*
reovirus	↑ C8 activity	lung, breast	*32*
Smac peptides	↓XIAP	glioma	*102*
retinoids	↑DR	lung, prostate	*33,34*
PPAR-γ inhibitors	↓ c-FLIP	colon, ovarian, prostate	*35*
herceptin	↓ erbB2 (Akt)	breast	*36*
Demethylating agents	↑C8	Ewing, brain, melanoma	*37,38*
IFN-γ	↑C8	Ewing sarcoma	*39,40*

Doxo (doxorubicin), etopo (etoposide), ActD (actinomycin D), CHX (cycloheximide), BIM (Bisindolylmeleimide), DR (death receptor), C8 (caspase-8), C9 (caspase-9), IFN-γ (interferon-γ).

expression of c-FLIP did not correlate with TRAIL susceptibility, cell lines that were resistant expressed little or no caspase-8 *(52)* and would therefore be unable to transmit the apoptotic signal. In myeloma cells, TRAIL resistance was associated with high levels of c-FLIP or low levels of caspase-8 *(17)*. Resistance to FasL-induced apoptosis in glioma cell lines also correlated with a high c-FLIP/caspase-8 ratio in the majority of cell lines *(58)*. Comparison of DISC components in HeLa and 293 cells following stimulation with TRAIL revealed that a high c-FLIP/caspase-8 ratio at the DISC may be responsible for higher resistance in 293 cells *(59)*. Second, many studies have utilized antibodies that detect only c-FLIP$_L$. Since both isoforms have been detected at the DISC, where they can interfere with the apoptotic signal, it is important to consider the total c-FLIP content of a cell when assessing ratios. Third, although c-FLIP acts at the apex of the death receptor signaling pathway, there are multiple factors that determine the apoptotic potential of a cell. During our analysis of the glioma cell panel, three cell lines that displayed a resistant phenotype exhibited a c-FLIP/caspase-8 ratio that predicted sensitivity to the death receptor ligand FasL. However, we found that these cell lines had low or no cell-surface expression of FasL receptor, indicating a defect upstream of c-FLIP *(58)*.

While the c-FLIP/caspase-8 ratio is not the only determinant of a cell's apoptotic potential upon treatment with death receptor ligands, c-FLIP does provide resistance at the apex of death receptor-induced apoptosis and would thus be an ideal target to increase susceptibility of tumor cells to death receptor ligands. Altering the cFLIP/caspase-8 ratio can be accomplished by reducing c-FLIP or by increasing caspase-8 expression.

Modulating c-FLIP/Caspase-8 Ratios

About 15 yr ago, several groups observed that metabolic inhibitors such as actinomycin D (ActD) and cycloheximide (CHX), inhibitors of transcription and translation respectively, sensitize resistant cells to TNF-induced apoptosis, leading to the hypothesis that synthesis of a protein with a short half-life was required to maintain resistance *(60,61)*. Three years ago, Fulda and coworkers demonstrated that metabolic inhibitors rapidly decreased levels of both c-FLIP isoforms, thereby inducing susceptibility to FasL-induced apoptosis. Numerous studies using ActD *(10,13,14,62–65)* or CHX *(12,13,17,18)* report sensitization to death-receptor ligands and find a correlation to down-regulation of c-FLIP. Interestingly, one group reported that ActD does not affect levels of c-FLIP *(14,15,20)*. We attribute this result to an antibody that does not appear to be specific for c-FLIP (Fig. 2).

Many tumors are resistant to chemotherapy, and initial studies using combinations of chemotherapy and death receptor ligands were an attempt to bombard cells with multiple apoptotic stimuli. It was the process of examining the mechanism by which chemotherapeutic agents sensitized cells to death receptor ligands that led to the discovery of their effect on c-FLIP. For example, cisplatin sensitized the osteosarcoma cell line MG-63 to FasL-mediated apoptosis, which correlated to reduced levels of $FLIP_L$ *(26)*. In NCI-H358 lung carcinoma cells, doxorubicin and camptothecin decreased levels of c-$FLIP_L$ and augmented TRAIL-induced apoptosis *(54)*. Inhibitors of PPAR-γ also reduce levels of c-$FLIP_L$ by a mechanism that involves increased c-$FLIP_L$ protein turnover following ubiquitination *(35)*. Unfortunately the c-$FLIP_S$ isoform was not analyzed in these studies.

Prostate cancer cells are sensitized to TRAIL by pretreatment with doxorubicin, which correlated with a decrease of c-$FLIP_S$ in all cell lines analyzed. Although c-$FLIP_L$ was reduced in some of the cells following doxorubicin treatment, the effect occurred later, thus not correlating with sensitization to TRAIL *(21)*. Like doxorubicin, the camptothecin 9-NC selectively downregulated c-$FLIP_S$ in DU145 prostate carcinoma cells and sensitized to FasL-mediated apoptosis *(25)*. The adenovirus protein E1A, which sensitizes cells to TNF, FasL, and TRAIL, has also been shown to decrease c-$FLIP_S$ without affecting c-$FLIP_L$ *(31)*.

Because chemotherapeutic agents affect numerous cellular processes, investigators have targeted c-FLIP directly using antisense oligomers or small interfering RNA *(66,67)*. Both approaches sensitize resistant cells to death receptor-mediated apoptosis, indicating that targeting of c-FLIP can be sufficient to overcome resistance.

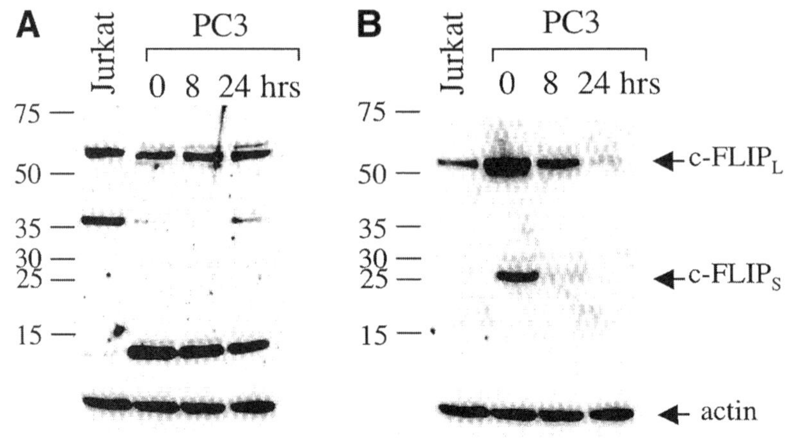

Fig. 2. Comparison of c-FLIP antibodies. Identical lysates from untreated Jurkat or PC3 cells treated with 1 µg/mL doxorubicin for 0, 8, or 24 h, were analyzed with two antibodies against c-FLIP. Jurkat cells were included because it is the recommended postive control for the c-FLIP-CT antibody from Upstate Biotechnology. Western analysis was performed as described (21). (**A**) Lysates were probed with 1 µg/mL c-FLIP-CT followed by 1:50,000 anti-rabbit-HRP while (**B**) was probed with 1:5 dilution of NF- 6 followed by 1:5,000 anti-mouse-HRP. c-FLIP-CT detected a band migrating at about 60 kDa that did not change following doxorubicin treatment. This antibody also reacted with proteins migrating at 37 kDa and below 15 kDa. In contrast, NF-6 detected two bands at 55 kDa and 26 kDa that decrease upon doxorubicin treatment. These results are consistent with those obtained with another c-FLIP monoclonal antibody (Dave-2), indicating that Dave-2 and NF-6 detect c-FLIP$_L$ and c-FLIP$_S$ while c-FLIP-CT is not specific for c-FLIP. Identical lysates were probed with anti-actin to confirm equal loading.

Currently, the role of c-FLIP$_L$ in resistance to death receptor signaling is still being debated, with two recent studies reporting that c-FLIP$_L$ enhances caspase-8 processing *(68,69)*. In our model, TRAIL binding in resistant Du145 and LNCaP cells results in generation of c-FLIP$_L$ cleavage, presumably by c-FLIP$_L$/caspase heterodimer formation, but without concomitant downregulation of c-FLIP$_S$, the apoptotic signal is aborted, yielding only intermediate caspase-8 fragments *(21)*. A similar observation was made in TRAIL-resistant glioma cell lines *(70)*. These results show that cleavage of c-FLIP$_L$ may be necessary but is not sufficient for sensitization, presumably because in resistant cells, levels of c-FLIP$_S$ are high enough to prevent caspase-8 homodimer formation. Therefore, it is possible that two stimuli are required for sensitization. The first stimulus is provided by ligand binding, which causes cleavage of c-FLIP$_L$, and the second stimulus is provided by any agent that reduces levels of c-FLIP$_S$. Alternatively, c-FLIP$_S$ alone may provide resistance to death receptor-mediated apoptosis. In support of this hypothesis, only c-FLIP$_S$ but not c-FLIP$_L$ was selected as a resistance gene in genetic screens *(71,72)*. In addition, Jurkat cells, which are highly susceptible to death receptor-mediated apoptosis, do not express detectable levels of c-FLIP$_S$ (Fig. 2B). Finally, in PC3 cells, c-FLIP$_S$ was detected only in the non-apoptotic but not in the apoptotic population, suggesting that partial susceptibility to TRAIL in these cells may be due to a subpopulation that lacks c-FLIP$_S$ expression *(21)*. Generation of antisense oligomers or small interfering RNAs that selectively target c-FLIP$_L$ or c-FLIP$_S$ may address the role of each c-FLIP isoform in resistance to death receptor-mediated apoptosis.

In addition to decreasing c-FLIP, upregulation of caspase-8 can also reduce the c-FLIP/caspase-8 ratio and restore susceptibility. In pediatric tumors, resistance to TRAIL-mediated apoptosis has been shown to correlate with loss of caspase-8 expression due to methylation of the caspase-8 promoter region *(73–75)*. Treatment with the demethylating agent 5-aza-2-deoxycytidine restored caspase-8 expression and sensitized the cells to death receptor-mediated apoptosis *(37,38)*. The cytokine interferon-γ also increased caspase-8 expression via the Stat-1 pathway and augmented TRAIL-mediated apoptosis *(39,76,77)*. Interferon-γ also inhibited TRAIL-induced upregulation of c-IAP *(78)*.

IAPs

Members of the family of IAPs (inhibitors of apoptosis proteins) are characterized by the presence of at least one BIR (baculovirus IAP repeat) domain and the ability to inhibit apoptosis when overexpressed in cells. Although IAPs (cIAP1, cIAP2, XIAP, and survivin) do not interfere with the initiator caspases, they can prevent mitochrondrial amplification of the apoptotic signal by binding to and inhibiting caspase-9 and progression by binding to and inhibiting the activity of caspase-3/7 *(79)*.

Survivin is overexpressed in many human tumors and has therefore been explored as a therapeutic target *(80)*. Although survivin can bind to caspases it may not play a major role in resistance to death receptor-mediated apoptosis. Cotransfection experiments with Fas revealed that survivin only partially inhibited cell death, whereas other IAP members completely blocked apoptosis *(81)*. The most potent inhibitor of caspases is XIAP *(79)*.

XIAP provides resistance to death receptor signals downstream of c-FLIP. For example, in human melanoma cells, TRAIL induced activation of caspase-3, but resistant cells failed to show cleavage of caspase-3 targets *(82)*. Transfection of resistant cells with Smac/DIABLO, an inhibitor of XIAP, resulted in conversion to a sensitive phenotype, while transfection of XIAP into TRAIL-sensitive melanoma cells resulted in a resistant phenotype *(82)*. Therefore, some cells may exhibit defects downstream of c-FLIP and would benefit from targeting IAPs.

Targeting IAPs

Chemotherapeutic agents such as taxol, cisplatin, and doxorubicin do not alter protein levels of IAP-1, IAP-2, or XIAP *(20,23,26)*, although one study reported an inhibitory effect of cisplatin on levels of survivin mRNA *(83)*. Wen demonstrated that caspase activity induced by etoposide and Ara-C was associated with decreases in XIAP and survivin.

Pretreatment with these agents enhanced TRAIL-mediated apoptosis, but the effect was only additive and the drug concentrations used were above subtoxic levels *(19)*. Therefore, there is no convincing evidence that chemotherapeutic agents can be used to target IAPs.

Metabolic inhibitors reduce levels of survivin and XIAP, but as discussed above, ActD and CHX also decrease c-FLIP protein *(12)*. In TRAIL-resistant renal cells that expressed higher levels of survivin than sensitive cells, ActD treatment resulted in sensitization and reduction in survivin protein *(16)*. In CL-1 cells, ActD has been reported to reduce XIAP but not c-FLIP *(14,15)*. If XIAP solely provided resistance in CL-1 cells, one would predict that cleavage of caspase-8 occurs in TRAIL-treated cells in the absence or presence of ActD, while PARP would be cleaved only when both agents are added. However, neither caspase-8 nor PARP is cleaved in TRAIL-treated cells, while both are cleaved in the presence of ActD and TRAIL, suggesting that ActD affects death-receptor signaling inhibitors upstream of XIAP.

The proteasome inhibitor MG-132 sensitizes enterocytes to Fas-induced apoptosis by preventing Fas-mediated upregulation of c-IAP-1 and c-IAP-2 *(84)*. Keratinocytes are sensitized to TRAIL by the proteasome inhibitor MG-115. MG-115 did not affect DISC composition or the NF-κB pathway, but reduced levels of XIAP by a yet undefined mechanism that may involve the mitochondria *(85)*.

Bcl-2 Family

Members of the Bcl-2 family are either pro- (i.e., Bax, Bak, Bad) or antiapoptotic (i.e., Bcl-2, Bcl-XL). The stoichiometry and interaction between pro- and antiapoptotic members determines whether a cell survives or undergoes apoptosis *(86)*. Although the exact mechanism is still being debated, the proapoptotic proteins of the family are responsible for pore formation in the mitochondria, which allows factors such as cytochrome c (apoptosome component) and Smac/DIABLO (IAP inhibitor) to escape.

The antiapoptotic members negatively regulate mitochondrial permeability. Like other negative regulators of apoptosis, Bcl-2 is overexpressed in certain tumors and may thus provide additional resistance to apoptotic stimuli *(87,88)*. For example, in neuroblastoma cells, downregulation of c-FLIP and Bcl-2 by antisense oligomers was necessary to achieve Fas-mediated apoptosis, suggesting that in these cells apoptosis is blocked at the DISC and the mitochondria *(89)*. Overexpression of anti-apoptotic molecules of the Bcl-2 family would affect death receptor-mediated apoptosis only in cells that utilize the mitochondria-dependent pathway. This may explain why several studies report inhibition of TRAIL-induced apoptosis by Bcl-2 or Bcl-XL overexpression *(90,91)* while others do not *(92,93)*.

Not only overexpression of anti-apoptotic but also lack of proapoptotic members of the Bcl-2 family can impair progression of the apoptotic signal. Mutations in Bax have been detected in both colon and gastric cancers *(94)*. Cells deficient in Bax can activate caspase-8 following TRAIL stimulation but exhibit a block at caspase-3 processing due to XIAP binding. Bax is required for the release of Smac/DIABLO from the mitochondria, which downregulates XIAP and allows apoptosis to progress *(95,96)*. Therefore, stimuli that activate Bax can also be used to target cells in which apoptosis is inhibited by IAPs.

Modulating Ratios of Pro- and Antiapoptotic Members of the Bcl-2 Family

Cancer cells in which overexpression of Bcl-2 or Bcl-XL inhibits death receptor-mediated apoptosis are best targeted by altering the ratio of pro- and antiapoptotic proteins. However, chemotherapeutic agents that sensitize cells to death receptor-induced apoptosis do not appear to reduce levels of Bcl-2 and Bcl-XL *(20,21,97,98)*. Only sulindac sulfide, a non-steroidal anti-inflammatory drug that reduces NF-κB activity, and ActD have been shown to reduce Bcl-XL *(62,99)*. In contrast, chemotherapeutic agents positively affect the pro-apoptotic proteins of the family. Cisplatin and 5-fluorouracil (5-FU), which sensitize bladder and renal cell carcimonas to TRAIL, respectively, increase levels of Bax, thereby changing the Bcl-2/Bax ratio toward apoptosis *(97,98)*. Doxorubicin does not affect overall levels of Bax, Bcl-2, or Bcl-XL *(21)* but can induce Bax and Bak to assume their active conformation *(100)*. In addition, doxorubicin can alter the subcellular distribution of Bax, leading to a more proapoptotic phenotype *(101)*. Etoposide and camptothecin elevate not only DR5 expression but also levels of Bak *(102)*.

Expression of Smac/DIABLO or its peptides can also bypass a Bcl-2 block in the mitochondria. Administration of Smac peptides sensitized malignant cells to TRAIL not only in vitro but also in vivo *(103)*. Using an intracranial malignant glioma model, Fulda and co-workers were able to demonstrate that treatment with Smac peptides and TRAIL eradicated established tumors without toxicity to normal brain tissue.

REGULATION OF DEATH RECEPTOR INHIBITORS BY SURVIVAL PATHWAYS

Signals that regulate death receptor inhibitors can also serve as targets for therapy. Several pathways, including NF-κB, Akt, and PKC, have been demonstrated to affect c-FLIP levels or activity, IAP expression, or progression of apoptosis at the mitochondria.

NF-κB

NF-κB is a transcription factor that is retained in the cytoplasm through interaction with inhibitory molecules called IκBs. Various stimuli can lead to degradation of IκB, allowing dimerization and translocation of NF-κB to the nucleus, where it activates transcription of target genes. Inhibition of NF-κB has been shown to enhance TRAIL-mediated apoptosis in a variety of cancer cell lines, including breast *(104)* and renal cells *(105)*, pancreatic adenocarcinoma *(106,107)*, hepatoma cells *(108)*, and multiple myeloma *(109)*. c-FLIP has recently been identified as a target gene of NF-κB signaling *(110,111)*. Therefore, it is tempting to speculate that inhibition of NF-κB activity in the aforementioned studies lead to sensitization by reducing levels of c-FLIP. In CL-1 tumor cells, 5-FU has been shown to inhibit NF-κB activity and reduce levels of c-FLIP *(112)*.

Direct evidence for NF-κB-mediated regulation of c-FLIP and modulation of death receptor ligand susceptibility was demonstrated in pancreatic carcinoma cells. NF-κB activity was inhibited using a peptide against the NEMO binding domain (NEMO is a regulatory subunit of IκB that when disrupted results in NF-κB unresponsiveness) or an adenovirus expressing an IκB mutant, both of which led to a decrease in levels of c-FLIP and enhanced susceptibility to TRAIL *(107)*. Some members of the IAP family are also regulated by NF-κB. For example, in multiple myeloma cells, inhibition of the NF-κB pathway by SN-50 not only decreased levels of c-FLIP but also survivin, c-IAP-2, and XIAP *(109)*, while stimulation of NF-κB with IGF-1 had the opposite effect *(17)*.

Akt (PKB)

Akt (PKB) serves as a hub for kinase pathways and is involved in signaling that determines survival or cell death *(113)*. Constitutive Akt activity results in resistance to death receptor ligands, which can be reversed by inhibitors of the Akt pathway *(114,115)*. Panka demonstrated that inhibition of Akt by LY294002 reduces levels of c-FLIP in all four cancer cell lines tested *(116)*. Inhibitor studies were corroborated by infecting cells with an adenovirus expressing dominant-negative Akt, which downregulated c-FLIP, and an adenovirus expressing a constitutively active Akt, which resulted in increased c-FLIP expression *(116)*. In T-cells, inhibition of Akt allows cleavage of caspase-8 to proceed from the intermediate p41/43 to the active form, suggesting that when Akt is active, caspase intermediates may be bound to c-FLIP *(117)*. Glucose deprivation causes transient dephosphorylation of Akt on Ser473 and downregulates c-FLIP protein, which enhances TRAIL-mediated apoptosis in Du145 cells *(118)*.

The EGF survival response also involves activation of Akt and can be blocked by Herceptin®, an antibody to the EGF receptor *(119)*. Herceptin has been demonstrated to downregulate the EGF-receptor and enhance TRAIL-mediated apoptosis in cells that overexpress erbB-2 by decreasing Akt activity *(36)*. The effect of Herceptin on inhibitors of death receptor signaling has not yet been examined. Inhibition of Akt can also relieve a mitochondrial block during apoptosis. In resistant NSCLC cells, Akt does not inhibit caspase-8 activity but Bid cleavage, indicating that apoptosis is inhibited downstream of c-FLIP *(120)*. Since Akt can phosphorylate and inactivate Bad, a pro-apoptotic member of the Bcl-2 family, it is possible that constitutive activation of Akt prevents progression of apoptosis at the mitochondrial level.

PKC

Protein kinase C isoforms are activated by a variety of stimuli that lead to a number of cellular responses, including proliferation. Activation of PKC protects pancreatic and breast cancer cells from death receptor-mediated apoptosis *(106,121)*. Shinohara and colleagues reported that a dominant-negative form of PKC epsilon augmented TRAIL-induced apoptosis *(122)*. Bisindolylmaleimides (BIM) originally described as inhibitors of PKC also sensitize to death receptor-induced apoptosis *(17,123)*. However, only BIM VIII and IX were shown to potentiate FasL-induced apoptosis, while other derivatives, despite effective inhibition of PKC, did not *(124)*. Therefore, reduction in levels of c-FLIP following BIM treatment appears to be independent of PKC inhibition *(17,123)* and may involve inhibition of transcription *(125)*. Higuchi and coworkers recently demonstrated that bile acids sensitize a human liver cell line to TRAIL by a mechanism that involved PKC-mediated phosphorylation of c-FLIP. Phosphorylated c-FLIP failed to be recruited to the DISC *(126)*. In glioma cells, PKC-mediated phosphorylation of PED/PEA15, another anti-apoptotic protein, also has a protective effect against death receptor-mediated apoptosis *(53)*. Therefore, the phosphorylation status of anti-apoptotic proteins may also be important in determining their activity.

THERAPEUTIC IMPLICATIONS OF DEATH RECEPTOR INHIBITOR TARGETING

One important question that needs to be addressed prior to targeting inhibitors of death receptor signaling pathways is the mechanism by which normal cells maintain resistance. If death receptor ligand-resistant tumor cells and normal cells rely on identical mechanisms of protection, selective sensitization of tumor cells via systemic administration will be impossible due to toxicity in normal tissues.

Animal Studies With Sensitizing Agents

Information about effects of combination of death-receptor ligands and chemotherapeutic agents in vivo is limited to TRAIL plus 5-FU, cisplatin, or camptothecin *(2,27,127)*. Combination therapy with these agents in athymic mice carrying human xenografts was more effective in reducing tumor growth than either agent alone, and did not result in toxicity. In vitro, these drugs have been reported to increase TRAIL receptor expression and/or downregulate c-FLIP *(22,24–27,112)*. 5-FU also elevates levels of Bak, a proapoptotic member of the Bcl-2 family *(102)*. However, the mechanism by which these agents enhance tumor reduction in vivo remains to be established. Fulda and co-workers were able to combine TRAIL with Smac peptides to eradicate human glioma xenografts without side effects to normal tissue *(103)*. Currently there is little information on the regulation of inhibitory proteins of death receptor signaling in normal mouse cells. Only if death receptor signaling inhibitors of mouse and human origin are regulated and affected similarly by sensitizing agents, will mice serve as useful models in determining the effects of combination therapy.

Studies with Primary Human Cultures

Several studies have included cultures of primary cells in their analysis of agents that down-regulate inhibitors of death receptor signaling. For example, inhibitors of PPAR-γ in combination with TRAIL induced apoptosis in a variety of cancer cells but not in monkey hepatocytes or human umbilical vein endothelial cells *(35)*. Similarly, bone cells do not appear to be sensitized to TRAIL by chemotherapeutic agents *(128,129)*. However, doxorubicin did not selectively sensitize malignant cells from breast, prostate, and the mesothelium to TRAIL *(7,11,130)*. These observations suggest that resistance in normal cells may be mediated by different mechanisms. In support of this hypothesis, one study found that the TRAIL decoy receptor DcR1 (TRAIL-R3) is important for resistance in endothelial cells, while lack of death receptor cell-surface expression and inhibitors downstream of caspase-3 play a role in protection in melanocytes and fibroblasts *(131)*.

A study using normal (TRAIL-resistant) and transformed (TRAIL-sensitive) keratinocytes showed that these normal cells are protected by XIAP *(85)*. Normal enterocytes also resist death receptor signaling by IAP expression *(84)*. Further investigation of resistance mechanisms in normal human cells will be needed to make educated decisions about targeting death receptor signaling inhibitors.

CONCLUSIONS

Targeting of death-receptor signaling inhibitors can be accomplished by metabolic inhibitors, chemotherapeutic agents, or inhibition of survival pathways. Alternatively, antisense oligomers, small interfering RNAs, or peptides can be used to target inhibitors with higher specificity. It appears that reducing c-FLIP is sufficient in most cells, since this inhibitor prevents transmission of the apoptotic signal at the apex of the pathway. Cells that have additional downstream defects may benefit from using sensitizing drugs with broader effects or specific agents that target multiple inhibitors. Whether this can be achieved in a tumor-selective manner in humans remains to be determined and may depend on the agent used. Future studies that elucidate mechanisms of resistance and regulation of death-receptor signaling inhibitors in normal cells are crucial in developing approaches to selectively kill tumor cells.

ACKNOWLEDGMENT

The author would like to thank Dr. Marcus E. Peter for the NF-6 antibody and Dr. Margaret M. Kelly for careful reading of the manuscript.

REFERENCES

1. Aoki K, Akyurek L, San H, Leung K, Parmacek M, Nabel E, and N GJ, Restricted Expression of an Adenoviral Vector encoding Fas Ligand (CD95L) Enhances Safety for Cancer Gene Therapy. Mol Ther 2000;1:555–565.
2. Ashkenazi A, Pai RC, Fong S, S Leung, DA Lawrence, SA Marsters, C Blackie, L Chang, AE McMurtrey, A Hebert, L DeForge, IL Koumenis, D Lewis, L Harris, J Bussiere, H Koeppen, Z Shahrokh, and RH Schwall, Safety and antitumor activity of recombinant soluble Apo2 ligand. J Clin Invest 1999;104(2):155–162.
3. Lawrence D, Shahrokh Z, Marsters S, et al. Differential hepatocyte toxicity of recombinant Apo2L/TRAIL versions. Nat Med 2001;7(4):383–385.
4. Kelley SK, Harris LA, Xie D, L Deforge, K Totpal, J Bussiere, and JA Fox, Preclinical studies to predict the disposition of Apo2L/tumor necrosis factorrelated apoptosis-inducing ligand in humans: Characterization of in vivo efficacy, pharmacokinetics, and safety. J Pharmacol Exp Ther 2001;299(1):31–38.
5. Pitti RM, Marsters SA, Ruppert S, Donahue CJ, Moore A, and Ashkenazi A, Induction of apoptosis by Apo-2 ligand, a new member of the tumor necrosis factor cytokine family. J Biol Chem 1996; 271(22):12,687–12,690.
6. Wiley SR, Schooley K, Smolak PJ, et al. Identification and characterization of a new member of the TNF family that induces apoptosis. Immunity 1995;3(6):673–682.
7. Keane MM, Ettenberg SA, Nau MM, Russell EK, Lipkowitz S. Chemotherapy augments TRAIL-induced apoptosis in breast cell lines. Cancer Res 1999;59(3):734–741.
8. Dejosez M, Ramp U, Mahotka C, et al. Sensitivity to TRAIL/APO-2L-mediated apoptosis in human renal cell carcinomas and its enhancement by topotecan. Cell Death Differ 2000;7(11):1127–1136.
9. Kim KH, Fisher MJ, Xu SQ, El-Deiry WS. Molecular determinants of response to TRAIL in killing of normal and cancer cells. Clin Cancer Res 2000;6(2):335–346.
10. Griffith TS, Chin WA, Jackson GC, Lynch DH, Kubin MZ. Intracellular regulation of TRAIL-induced apoptosis in human melanoma cells. J Immunology 1998;161(6):2833–2840.
11. Voelkel-Johnson C, King DL, Norris JS. Resistance of prostate cancer cells to soluble TNF-related apoptosis-inducing ligand (TRAIL/Apo2L) can be overcome by doxorubicin or adenoviral delivery of full-length TRAIL. Cancer Gene Ther 2002;9(2):164–172.
12. Fulda S, Meyer E, Debatin KM. Metabolic inhibitors sensitize for CD95 (APO-1/Fas)-induced apoptosis by down-regulating Fas-associated death domain-like interleukin 1-converting enzyme inhibitory protein expression. Cancer Res 2000;60(14):3947–3956.
13. Hernandez A, Wang QD, Schwartz SA, Evers BM. Sensitization of human colon cancer cells to TRAIL-mediated apoptosis. J Gastroint Surg 2001;5(1):56–65.
14. Ng CP, Zisman A, Bonavida B. Synergy is achieved by complementation with Apo2L/TRAIL and actinomycin D in Apo2 L/TRAIL-mediated apoptosis of prostate cancer cells: Role of XIAP in resistance. Prostate 2002;53(4):286–299.
15. Ng CP, Bonavida B. X-linked inhibitor of apoptosis (XIAP) blocks Apo2 ligand/tumor necrosis factor-related apoptosis-inducing ligand-mediated apoptosis of prostate cancer cells in the presence of mitochondrial activation: sensitization by overexpression of second mitochondria-derived activator of caspase/direct IAP-binding protein with low pl (Smac/DIABLO). Mol Cancer Ther 2002;1(12):1051–1058.
16. Griffith TS, Fialkov JM, Scott DL, et al. Induction and regulation of tumor necrosis factorrelated apoptosis-inducing ligand/Apo-2 ligand-mediated apoptosis in renal cell carcinoma. Cancer Res 2002;62(11):3093–3099.
17. Mitsiades N, Mitsiades CS, Poulaki V, Anderson KC, Treon SP. Intracellular regulation of tumor necrosis factor-related apoptosis-inducing ligand-induced apoptosis in human multiple myeloma cells. Blood 2002;99(6):2162–2171.
18. Leverkus M, Neumann M, Mengling T, et al. Regulation of tumor necrosis factor-related apoptosis-inducing ligand sensitivity in primary and transformed human keratinocytes. Cancer Res 2000;60(3):553–559.
19. Wen J, Ramadevi N, Nguyen D, Perkins C, Worthington E, Bhalla K. Antileukemic drugs increase death receptor 5 levels and enhance Apo-2L-induced apoptosis of human acute leukemia cells. Blood 2000;96(12):3900–3906.
20. Jazirehi AR, Ng CP, Gan XH, Schiller G, Bonavida B. Adriamycin sensitizes the adriamycin-resistant 8226/Dox40 human multiple myeloma cells to Apo2L/tumor necrosis factor-related apoptosis-inducing ligand-mediated (TRAIL) apoptosis. Clin Cancer Res 2001;7(12):3874–3883.

21. Kelly MM, Hoel BD, Voelkel-Johnson C. Doxorubicin pretreatment sensitizes prostate cancer cell lines to TRAIL induced apoptosis which correlates with the loss of c-FLIP expression. Cancer Biol Ther 2002;1(5):520–527.
22. Nagane M, Pan GH, Weddle JJ, Dixit VM, Cavenee WK, Huang HJS. Increased death receptor 5 expression by chemotherapeutic agents in human gliomas causes synergistic cytotoxicity with tumor necrosis factor-related apoptosis-inducing ligand in vitro and in vivo. Cancer Res 2000;60(4):847–853.
23. Nimmanapalli R, Perkins CL, Orlando M, O'Bryan E, Nguyen D, Bhalla KN. Pretreatment with paclitaxel enhances Apo-2 ligand tumor necrosis factor-related apoptosis-inducing ligand-induced apoptosis of prostate cancer cells by inducing death receptors 4 and 5 protein levels. Cancer Res 2001;61(2):759–763.
24. Xiang H, Fox JA, Totpal K, et al. Enhanced tumor killing by Apo2L/TRAIL and CPT-11 co-treatment is associated with p21 cleavage and differential regulation of Apo2L/TRAIL ligand and its receptors. Oncogene 2002;21(22):3611–3619.
25. Chatterjee D, Schmitz I, Krueger A, et al. Induction of apoptosis in 9-nitrocamptothecin-treated DU145 human prostate carcinoma cells correlates with de novo synthesis of CD95 and CD95 ligand and down-regulation of c-FLIPshort. Cancer Res 2001;61(19):7148–7154.
26. Kinoshita H, Yoshikawa H, Shiiki K, Hamada Y, Nakajima Y, Tasaka K. Cisplatin (CDDP) sensitizes human osteosarcoma cell to Fas/CD95-mediated apoptosis by down-regulating FLIP-L expression. Int J Cancer 2000;88(6):986–991.
27. Naka T, Sugamura K, Hylander BL, Widmer MB, Rustum YM, Repasky EA. Effects of tumor necrosis factor-related apoptosis-inducing ligand alone and in combination with chemotherapeutic agents on patients' colon tumors grown in SCID mice. Cancer Res 2002;62(20):5800–5806.
28. Chinnaiyan AM, Prasad U, Shankar S, et al. Combined effect of tumor necrosis factor-related apoptosis-inducing ligand and ionizing radiation in breast cancer therapy. Proc Natl Acad Sci USA 2000;97(4): 1754–1759.
29. Gong B, Almasan A. Apo2 ligand/TNF-related apoptosis-inducing ligand and death receptor 5 mediate the apoptotic signaling induced by ionizing radiation in leukemic cells. Cancer Res 2000;60(20):5754–5760.
30. Routes JM, Ryan JC, Ryan S, Nakamura M. MHC class I molecules on adenovirus E1A-expressing tumor cells inhibit NK cell killing but not NK cell-mediated tumor rejection. Int Immunol 2001;13(10):1301–1307.
31. Perez D, White E. E1A sensitizes cells to tumor necrosis factor alpha by downregulating c-$FLIP_S$. J Virol 2003;77(4):2651–2662.
32. Clarke P, Meintzer SM, Spalding AC, Johnson GL, Tyler KL. Caspase 8-dependent sensitization of cancer cells to TRAIL-induced apoptosis following reovirus-infection. Oncogene 2001;20(47):6910–6919.
33. Sun SY, Yue P, Lotan R. Implication of multiple mechanisms in apoptosis induced by the synthetic retinoid CD437 in human prostate carcinoma cells. Oncogene 2000;19(39):4513–4522.
34. Sun SY, Yue P, Hong WK, Lotan R. Augmentation of tumor necrosis factor-related apoptosis-inducing ligand (TRAIL)-induced apoptosis by the synthetic retinoid 6-[3-(1-adamantyl)-4-hydroxyphenyl]-2-naphthalene carboxylic acid (CD437) through up-regulation of TRAIL receptors in human lung cancer cells. Cancer Res 2000;60(24):7149–7155.
35. Kim Y, Suh N, Sporn M, Reed JC. An inducible pathway for degradation of FLIP protein sensitizes tumor cells to TRAIL-induced apoptosis. J Biol Chem 2002;277(25):22,320–22,329.
36. Cuello M, Ettenberg SA, Clark AS, et al. Down-regulation of the erbB-2 receptor by trastuzumab (herceptin) enhances tumor necrosis factor–related apoptosis-inducing ligand-mediated apoptosis in breast and ovarian cancer cell lines that overexpress erbB-2. Cancer Res 2001;61(12):4892–4900.
37. Eggert A, Grotzer MA, Zuzak TJ, et al. Resistance to tumor necrosis factor-related apoptosis-inducing ligand (TRAIL)-induced apoptosis in neuroblastoma cells correlates with a loss of caspase-8 expression. Cancer Res 2001;61(4):1314–1319.
38. Fulda S, Kufer MU, Meyer E, van Valen F, Dockhorn-Dworniczak B, Debatin KM. Sensitization for death receptor- or drug-induced apoptosis by reexpression of caspase-8 through demethylation or gene transfer. Oncogene 2001;20(41):5865–5877.
39. Fulda S, Debatin KM. IFN gamma sensitizes for apoptosis by upregulating caspase-8 expression through the Stat1 pathway. Oncogene 2002;21(15):2295–2308.
40. Kontny HU, Hammerle K, Klein R, Shayan P, Mackall CL, Niemeyer M. Sensitivity of Ewing's sarcoma to TRAIL-induced apoptosis. Cell Death Differ 2001;8(5):506–514.

41. Djerbi M, Darreh-Shori T, Zhivotovsky B, Grandien A. Characterization of the human FLICE-inhibitory protein locus and comparison of the antiapoptotic activity of four different FLIP isoforms. Scand J Immunol 2001;54(1–2):180–189.
42. Irmler M, Thome M, Hahne M, et al. Inhibition of death receptor signals by cellular FLIP. Nature 1997;388(6638):190–195.
43. Bullani RR, Huard B, Viard-Leveugle I, et al. Selective expression of FLIP in malignant melanocytic skin lesions. J Invest Dermatol 2001;117(2):360–364.
44. Voelkel-Johnson C. An antibody against DR4 (TRAIL-R1) in combination with doxorubicin selectively kills malignant but not normal prostate cells. Cancer Biol Ther 2003;2(3):283–290.
45. Djerbi M, Screpanti V, Catrina AI, Bogen B, Biberfeld P, Grandien A. The inhibitor of death receptor signaling, FLICE-inhibitory protein defines a new class of tumor progression factors. J Exp Med 1999;190(7):1025–1031.
46. French LE, Tschopp J. Inhibition of death receptor signaling by FLICE-inhibitory protein as a mechanism for immune escape of tumors. J Exp Med 1999;190:891–894.
47. Medema J, de Jong J, van Hall T, Melief C, Offringa R. Immune escape of tumors in vivo by expression of cellular FLICE-inhibitory protein. J Exp Med 1999;190:1033–1038.
48. Tepper C, Seldin M. Modulation of caspase-8 and FLICE-inhibitory protein expression as a potential mechanism of Epstein-Barr virus tumorigenesis in Burkitt's lymphoma. Blood 1999;94:1727–1737.
49. Krueger A, Baumann S, Krammer PH, Kirchhoff S. FLICE-inhibitory proteins: Regulators of death receptor-mediated apoptosis. Mol Cell Biol 2001;21(24):8247–8254.
50. Clodi K, Wimmer D, Li Y, et al. Expression of tumour necrosis factor (TNF)-related apoptosis-inducing ligand (TRAIL) receptors and sensitivity to TRAIL-induced apoptosis in primary B-cell acute lymphoblastic leukaemia cells. Brit J Haemat 2000;111(2):580–586.
51. Pawlowski JE, Nesterov A, Scheinman RI, Johnson TR, Kraft AS. NFkappa B does not modulate sensitivity of renal carcinoma cells to TNF alpha-related apoptosis-inducing ligand (TRAIL). Anticancer Res 2000;20(6B):4243–4255.
52. Petak I, Douglas L, Tillman DM, Vernes R, Houghton JA. Pediatric rhabdomyosarcoma cell lines are resistant to Fas-induced apoptosis and highly sensitive to TRAIL-induced apoptosis. Clin Cancer Res 2000;6(10):4119–4127.
53. Hao C, Beguinot F, Condorelli G, et al. Induction and intracellular regulation of tumor necrosis factor-related apoptosis-inducing ligand (TRAIL) mediated apotosis in human malignant glioma cells. Cancer Res 2001;61(3):1162–1170.
54. Frese S, Brunner T, Gugger M, Uduehi A, Schmid RA. Enhancement of Apo2L/TRAIL (tumor necrosis factor-related apoptosis-inducing ligand)-induced apoptosis in non–small cell lung cancer cell lines by chemotherapeutic agents without correlation to the expression level of cellular protease caspase-8 inhibitory protein. J Thorac Cardiovasc Surg 2002;123(1):168–174.
55. Mitsiades N, Poulaki V, Mitsiades C, Tsokos M. Ewing's sarcoma family tumors are sensitive to tumor necrosis factor-related apoptosis-inducing ligand and express death receptor 4 and death receptor 5. Cancer Res 2001;61(6):2704–2712.
56. Shivapurkar N, Reddy J, Matta H, et al. Loss of expression of death-inducing signaling complex (DISC) components in lung cancer cell lines and the influence of MYC amplification. Oncogene 2002;21(55): 8510–8514.
57. Maggio EM, van den Berg A, de Jong D, Diepstra A, Poppema S. Low frequency of FAS mutations in Reed-Sternberg cells of Hodgkin's lymphoma. Am J Pathol 2003;162(1):29–35.
58. Wang D, Rubinchik S, Ding R, et al. Adenoviral vector delivery of FasL-GFP fusion gene is lethal to a majority of glioma cell lines, with Fas pathway defects rather than transduction efficiency being the major determinants of resistance. In preparation.
59. Harper N, Farrow SN, Kaptein A, Cohen GM, MacFarlane M. Modulation of tumor necrosis factor apoptosis-inducing ligand-induced NFkappa B activation by inhibition of apical caspases. J Biol Chem 2001;276(37):34743–34752.
60. Nophar Y, Holtmann H, Ber R, Wallach D. Dominance of resistance to the cytocidal effect of tumor necrosis factor in heterokaryons formed by fusion of resistant and sensitive cells. J Immunology 1988;140:3456–3460.
61. Ruggiero V, Latham K, Baglioni C. Cytostatic and cytotoxic activity of tumor necrosis factor on human cancer cells. J Immunology 1987;138:2711–2717.
62. Mori S, Murakami-Mori K, Nakamura S, Ashkenazi A, Bonavida B. Sensitization of AIDS-Kaposi's sarcoma cells to Apo-2 ligand-induced apoptosis by actinomycin D. J Immunology 1999;162(9):5616–5623.

63. Kleeff J, Kornmann M, Sawhney H, Korc M. Actinomycin D induces apoptosis and inhibits growth of pancreatic cancer cells. Int J Cancer 2000;86(3):399–407.
64. Olsson A, Diaz T, Aguilar-Santelises M, et al. Sensitization to TRAIL-induced apoptosis and modulation of FLICE-inhibitory protein in B chronic lymphocytic leukemia by actinomycin D. Leukemia 2001;15(12):1868–1877.
65. Matsuzaki H, Schmied BM, Ulrich A, et al. Combination of tumor necrosis factor-related apoptosis-inducing ligand (TRAIL) and actinomycin D induces apoptosis even in TRAIL-resistant human pancreatic cancer cells. Clin Cancer Res 2001;7(2):407–414.
66. Hyer ML, Sudarshan S, Kim Y, et al. Downregulation of c-FLIP sensitizes DU145 prostate cancer cells to Fas-mediated apoptosis. Cancer Biol Ther 2002;1 (4):401–406.
67. Siegmund D, Hadwiger P, Pfizenmaier K, Vornlocher HP, Wajant H. Selective inhibition of FLICE-like inhibitory protein (FLIP) expression with small interfering RNA oligonucleotides (siRNAs) is sufficient to sensitize tumor cells for TRAIL-induced apoptosis. Mol Med 2002;8(11):725–732.
68. Chang DW, Xing Z, Pan Y, et al. c-FLIPL is a dual function regulator for caspase-8 activation and CD95-mediated apoptosis. EMBO J 2002;21(14):3704–3714.
69. Micheau O, Thome M, Schneider P, et al. The long form of FLIP is an activator of caspase-8 at the Fas death-inducing signaling complex. J Biol Chem 2002;277(47):45,162–45,171.
70. Xiao C, Yang BF, Asadi N, Beguinot F, Hao CH. Tumor necrosis factor-related apoptosis-inducing ligand-induced death-inducing signaling complex and its modulation by c-FLIP and PED/PEA-15 in glioma cells. J Biol Chem 2002;277(28):25020–25025.
71. Burns TF, El-Deiry WS. Identification of inhibitors of TRAIL-induced death (ITIDs) in the TRAIL-sensitive colon carcinoma cell line SW480 using a genetic approach. J Biol Chem 2001;276(41):37,879– 37,886.
72. Bin LH, Li XY, Xu LG, Shu HB. The short splice form of Casper/c-FLIP is a major cellular inhibitor of TRAIL-induced apoptosis. FEBS Lett 2002;510(1–2):37–40.
73. Grotzer MA, Eggert A, Zuzak TJ, et al. Resistance to TRAIL-induced apoptosis in primitive neuroectodermal brain tumor cells correlates with a loss of caspase-8 expression. Oncogene 2000;19(40):4604–4610.
74. Zuzak TJ, Steinhoff DF, Sutton LN, Phillips PC, Eggert A, Grotzer MA. Loss of caspase-8 mRNA expression is common in childhood primitive neuroectodermal brain tumour/medulloblastoma. Eur J Cancer 2002;38(1):83–91.
75. Harada K, Toyooka S, Shivapurkar N, et al. Deregulation of caspase 8 and 10 expression in pediatric tumors and cell lines. Cancer Res 2002;62(20):5897–5901.
76. Langaas V, Shahzidi S, Johnsen JI, Smedsrod B, Sveinbjornsson B. Interferon-gamma modulates TRAIL-mediated apoptosis in human colon carcinoma cells. Anticancer Res 2001;21(6A):3733–3738.
77. Varela N, Munoz-Pinedo C, Ruiz-Ruiz C, Robledo G, Pedroso M, Lopez-Rivas A. Interferon-gamma sensitizes human myeloid leukemia cells to death receptor-mediated apoptosis by a pleiotropic mechanism. J Biol Chem 2001;276(21):17,779–17,787.
78. Park SY, Billiar TR, Seol DW. IFN-gamma inhibition of TRAIL-induced IAP-2 upregulation, a possible mechanism of IFN-gamma-enhanced TRAIL-induced apoptosis. Biochem Biophys Res Commun 2002;291(2):233–236.
79. Deveraux Q, Reed JC. IAP family proteins: suppressors of apoptosis. Genes Dev 1999;13:239–252.
80. Zaffaroni N, Daidone M. Survivin expression and resistance to anticancer treatments: perspectives for new therapeutic interventions. Drug Resist Upd 2002;5(2):65–72.
81. Tamm I, Wang Y, Sausville E, et al. IAP-family protein survivin inhibits caspase activity and apoptosis induced by Fas (CD95), Bax, caspases, and anticancer drugs. Cancer Res 1998;58:p. 5315–5320.
82. Zhang XD, Zhang XY, Gray CP, Nguyen T, Hersey P. Tumor necrosis factor-related apoptosis-inducing ligand-induced apoptosis of human melanoma is regulated by Smac/DIABLO release from mitochondria. Cancer Res 2001;61(19):7339–7348.
83. Ikeguchi M, Kaibara N. Changes in survivin messenger RNA level during cisplatin treatment in gastric cancer. Int J Mol Med 2001;8(6):661–666.
84. Ruemmele F, Beaulieu J, O'Connell J, Bennett M, Seidman E, Lentze M. The susceptibility to Fas-induced apoptosis in normal enterocytes is regulated on the level of cIAP1 and 2. Biochem Biophys Res Commun 2002;290(4):1308–1314.
85. Leverkus M, Sprick M, Wachter T, et al. Proteasome inhibition results in TRAIL sensitization of primary keratinocytes by removing the resistance-mediating block of effector caspase maturation. Mol Cell Biol 2003;23(3):777–790.
86. Finkel E. The mitochondrion: is it central to apoptosis. Science 2001;292:624–626.

87. Yang Q, Sakurai T, Yoshimura G et al. Expression of Bcl-2 but not Bax or p53 correlates with in vitro resistance to a series of anticancer drugs in breast carcinoma. Breast Cancer Res Treat 2000;61:211–216.
88. Catz S, Johnson J. BCL-2 in prostate cancer: a minireview. Apoptosis 2003;8(1):29–37.
89. Poulaki V, Mitsiades N, Romero M, Tsokos M. Fas-mediated apoptosis in neuroblastoma requires mitochondrial activation and is inhibited by FLICE inhibitor protein and bcl-2. Cancer Res 2001;61:4864–4872.
90. Hinz S, Trauzold A, Boenicke L, et al. Bcl-XL protects pancreatic adenocarcinoma cells against CD95- and TRAIL-receptor-mediated apoptosis. Oncogene 2000;19(48):5477–5486.
91. Munshi A, Pappas G, Honda T, et al. TRAIL (APO-2L) induces apoptosis in human prostate cancer cells that is inhibitable by Bcl-2. Oncogene 2001;20(29):3757–3765.
92. Walczak H, Bouchon A, Stahl H, Krammer PH. Tumor necrosis factor-related apoptosis-inducing ligand retains its apoptosis-inducing capacity on Bcl- 2- or Bcl-xL-overexpressing chemotherapy-resistant tumor cells. Cancer Res 2000;60(11):3051–3057.
93. Keogh SA, Walczak H, Bouchier-Hayes L, Martin SJ. Failure of Bcl-2 to block cytochrome c redistribution during TRAIL-induced apoptosis. FEBS Lett 2000;471(1):93–98.
94. Ionov Y, Yamamoto H, Krajewski S, Reed J, Perucho M. Mutational inactivation of the proapoptotic gene BAX confers selective advantage during tumor clonal evolution. Proc Natl Acad Sci USA 2000;97:10,872–10,877.
95. Deng YB, Lin YH, Wu XW. TRAIL-induced apoptosis requires Bax-dependent mitochondria release of Smac/DIABLO. Genes Dev 2002;16(1):33–45.
96. Kim JY, Kim YH, Chang I, et al. Resistance of mitochondrial DNA-deficient cells to TRAIL: role of Bax in TRAIL-induced apoptosis. Oncogene 2002;21(20):3139–3148.
97. Mizutani Y, Nakanishi H, Yoshida O, Fukushima M, Bonavida B, Miki T. Potentiation of the sensitivity of renal cell carcinoma cells to TRAIL-mediated apoptosis by subtoxic concentrations of 5-fluorouracil. Eur J Cancer 2002;38(1):167–176.
98. Mizutani Y, Nakao M, Ogawa O, Yoshida O, Bonavida B, Miki T. Enhanced sensitivity of bladder cancer cells to tumor necrosis factor related apoptosis inducing ligand mediated apoptosis by cisplatin and carboplatin. J Urol 2001;165(1):263–270.
99. Ravi R, Bedi A. Requirement of BAX for TRAIL/Apo2L-induced apoptosis of colorectal cancers: Synergism with sulindac-mediated inhibition of Bcl-x(L). Cancer Res 2002;62(6):1583–1587.
100. Panaretakis T, Pokrovskaja K, Shoshan M, Grander D. Activation of Bak, Bax, and BH3-only proteins in the apoptotic response to doxorubicin. J Biol Chem 2002;277(46):44317.
101. Ruiz de Almodovar C, Ruiz-Ruiz C, Munoz-Pinedo C, Robledo G, Lopez-Rivas A. The differential sensitivity of Bcl-2-overexpressing human breast tumor cells to TRAIL or doxorubicin-induced apoptosis is dependent on Bcl-2 protein levels. Oncogene 2001;20:7128–7133.
102. LeBlanc H, Lawrence D, Varfolomeev E, et al. Tumor-cell resistance to death receptor-induced apoptosis through mutational inactivation of the proapoptotic Bcl-2 homolog Bax. Nat Med 2002;8(3):274–281.
103. Fulda S, Wick W, Weller M, Debatin KM. Smac agonists sensitize for Apo2L/TRAIL- or anticancer drug-induced apoptosis and induce regression of maligant glioma in vivo. Nat Med 2002;8(8):808–815.
104. Keane MM, Rubinstein Y, Cuello M, et al. Inhibition of NF-kappaB activity enhances TRAIL mediated apoptosis in breast cancer cell lines. Breast Cancer Res Treat 2001;64(2):211–219.
105. Oya M, Ohtsubo M, Takayanagi A, Tachibana M, Shimizu N, Murai M. Constitutive activation of nuclear factor-kappa B prevents TRAIL-induced apoptosis in renal cancer cells. Oncogene 2001;20(29):3888–3896.
106. Trauzold A, Wermann H, Arlt A, et al. CD95 and TRAIL receptor-mediated activation of protein kinase C and NF-kappa B contributes to apoptosis resistance in ductal pancreatic adenocarcinoma cells. Oncogene 2001;20(31):4258–4269.
107. Thomas RP, Farrow BJ, Kim S, May MJ, Hellmich MR, Evers BM. Selective targeting of the nuclear factor-kappa B pathway enhances tumor necrosis factor-related apoptosis-inducing ligand-mediated pancreatic cancer cell death. Surgery 2002;132(2):127–134.
108. Kim YS, Schwabe RF, Qian T, Lemasters JJ, Brenner DA. TRAIL-mediated apoptosis requires NF-kappa B inhibition and the mitochondrial permeability transition in human hepatoma cells. Hepatology 2002;36(6):1498–1508.
109. Mitsiades N, Mitsiades CS, Poulaki V, et al. Biologic sequelae of nuclear factor–kappa B blockade in multiple myeloma: therapeutic applications. Blood 2002;99(11):4079–4086.

110. Kreuz S, Siegmund D, Scheurich P, Wajant H. NF-kappa B inducers upregulate cFLIP, a cycloheximide-sensitive inhibitor of death receptor signaling. Mol Cell Biol 2001;21(12):3964–3973.
111. Micheau O, Lens S, Gaide O, Alevizopoulos K, Tschopp J. NF-kappaB signals induce the expression of c-FLIP. Mol Cell Biol 2001;21(16):5299–5305.
112. Azuma M, Yamashita T, Aota K, Tamatani T, Sato M. 5-Fluorouracil suppression of NF-kappa B is mediated by the inhibition of I kappa B kinase activity in human salivary gland cancer cells. Biochem Biophys Res Commun 2001;282(1):292–296.
113. Franke T, Cantley L. Apoptosis. A Bad kinase makes good. Nature 1997;390:116–117.
114. Thakkar H, Chen XF, Tyan F, et al. Pro-survival function of Akt/protein kinase B in prostate cancer cells—relationship with trail resistance. J Biol Chem 2001;276(42):38361–38369.
115. Nesterov A, Lu XJ, Johnson M, Miller GJ, Ivashchenko Y, Kraft AS. Elevated Akt activity protects the prostate cancer cell line LNCaP from TRAIL-induced apoptosis. J Biol Chem 2001;276(14): 10,767–10,774.
116. Panka DJ, Mano T, Suhara T, Walsh K, Mier JW. Phosphatidylinositol 3-kinase/Akt activity regulates c-FLIP expression in tumor cells. J Biol Chem 2001;276(10):6893–6896.
117. Varadhachary A, Peter ME, Perdow S, Krammer PH, Salgame P. Selective Upregulation of phosphatidylinositol 3'-kinase activity in Th2 cells inhibits caspase-8 cleavage at the death-inducing complex: a mechanism for Th2 resistance from Fas-mediated apoptosis. J Immunology 1999;163: 4772–4779.
118. Nam SY, Amoscato AA, Lee YJ. Low glucose-enhanced TRAIL cytotoxicity is mediated through the ceramide-Akt-FLIP pathway. Oncogene 2002;21(3):337–346.
119. Gibson EM, Henson ES, Haney N, Villanueva J, Gibson SB. Epidermal growth factor protects epithelial-derived cells from tumor necrosis factor-related apoptosis-inducing ligand-induced apoptosis by inhibiting cytochrome c release. Cancer Res 2002;62(2):488–496.
120. Kandasamy K, Srivastava RK. Role of the phosphatidylinositol 3'- kinase/PTEN/Akt kinase pathway in tumor necrosis factor-related apoptosisinducing ligand-induced apoptosis in non-small cell lung cancer cells. Cancer Res 2002;62(17):4929–4937.
121. Sarker M, Ruiz-Ruiz C, Robledo G, Lopez-Rivas A. Stimulation of the mitogen-activated protein kinase pathway antagonizes TRAIL-induced apoptosis downstream of BID cleavage in human breast cancer MCF-7 cells. Oncogene 2002;21(27):4323–4327.
122. Shinohara H, Kayagaki N, Yagita H, et al. A protective role of PKC epsilon against TNF-related apoptosis-inducing ligand (TRAIL)-induced apoptosis in glioma cells. Biochem Biophys Res Commun 2001;284(5):1162–1167.
123. Poulaki V, Mitsiades CS, Kotoula V, et al. Regulation of Apo2L/tumor necrosis factor–related apoptosis-inducing ligand-induced apoptosis in thyroid carcinoma cells. Am J Pathol 2002;161(2):643–654.
124. Zhou T, Song L, Yang P, Wang Z, Lui D, Jope R. Bisindolylmaleimide VIII facilitates Fas-mediated apoptosis and inhibits T cell-mediated autoimmune diseases. Nat Med 1999;5:42–48.
125. Rokhlin OW, Glover RA, Taghiyev AF, et al. Bisindolylmaleimide IX facilitates tumor necrosis factor receptor family-mediated cell death and acts as an inhibitor of transcription. J Biol Chem 2002;277(36):33,213–33,219.
126. Higuchi H, Bronk SF, Taniai M, Canbay A, Gores GJ. Cholestasis increases tumor necrosis factor-related apoptotis-inducing ligand (TRAIL)- R2/DR5 expression and sensitizes the liver to TRAIL-mediated cytotoxicity. J Pharmacol Exp Ther 2002;303(2):461–467.
127. Gliniak B, Le T. Tumor necrosis factor-related apoptosis-inducing ligand's antitumor activity in vivo is enhanced by the chemotherapeutic agent CPT-11. Cancer Res 1999;59(24):6153–6158.
128. Atkins GJ, Bouralexis S, Evdokiou A, et al. Human osteoblasts are resistant to Apo2L/TRAIL-mediated apoptosis. Bone 2002;31(4):448–456.
129. Evdokiou A, Bouralexis S, Atkins GJ, et al. Chemotherapeutic agents sensitize osteogenic sarcoma cells, but not normal human bone cells, to Apo2L/TRIAL-induced apoptosis. Int J Cancer 2002;99(4):491–504.
130. Liu WH, Bodle E, Chen JY, Gao MX, Rosen GD, Broaddus VC. Tumor necrosis factor-related apoptosis-inducing ligand and chemotherapy cooperate to induce apoptosis in mesothelioma cell lines. American Journal of Respiratory Cell & Molecular Biology 2001;25(1):111–118.
131. Zhang XD, Franco AV, Nguyen T, Gray CP, Hersey P. Differential localization and regulation of death and decoy receptors for TNF-related apoptosis-inducing ligand (TRAIL) in human melanoma cells. J Immunology 2000;164(8):3961–3970.

19 Ceramide, Ceramidase, and FasL Gene Therapy in Prostate Cancer

James S. Norris, PhD*, David H. Holman,* BS*,*
Marc L. Hyer, PhD*, Alicja Bielawska,* PhD*,*
Ahmed El-Zawahry, MD*, Charles Chalfant,* PhD*,*
Charles Landen, MD*, Stephen Tomlinson,* PhD*,*
Jian-Yun Dong, MD*,* PhD*, Lina M. Obeid,* MD*,*
and Yusuf A. Hannun, MD

THE ROLE OF CERAMIDE IN APOPTOSIS AND STRESS RESPONSES

Glycerolipid-derived second messengers such as diacylglycerol, phosphatidylinositides, and eicosanoids are now well-established mediators of signal transduction. Sphingolipids, which are even more structurally complex than glycerophospholipids, are also appreciated to serve as potential reservoirs for bioactive lipids *(1–9)*. Thus, regulation of sphingolipid metabolism appears involved in regulation of cell growth, differentiation, senescence, and programmed cell death, and possibly, as proposed herein, favoring growth of a subset of prostate cancers.

CERAMIDE AND APOPTOSIS

In most cancer cells, including prostate cancer (PCa), ceramide elevation results in apoptosis. At a biochemical level, ceramide causes activation of caspases, DNA fragmentation, and other characteristics and hallmarks of apoptosis, induction of the stress-activated protein kinases (SAPK/JNK), inhibition of phospholipase D, dephosphorylation and inactivation of protein kinase C (PKC), enhanced release of mitochondrial reactive oxygen species, release of cytochrome c, and activation of PP1, which dephosphorylates SR proteins leading to a more proapoptotic phenotype *(10–21)*.

From: *Cancer Drug Discovery and Development: Death Receptors in Cancer Therapy*
Edited by: W. S. El-Deiry © Humana Press Inc., Totowa, NJ

Mechanistically, studies are beginning to allow a coordinated picture of cell growth regulation involving ceramide and other key regulators of cell-cycle progression and apoptosis. Thus, the formation of ceramide in response to tumor necrosis factor (TNF) and other, but not all, inducers requires activation of upstream caspases (e.g., caspase-8) which are inhibited by YVAD and by Crm A *(22,23)*. However, inhibitors of downstream caspases fail to prevent ceramide formation and yet ceramide activates downstream caspases (e.g., caspase-3) but not upstream caspases *(22,24)*. Moreover, the ability of ceramide to induce apoptosis is blocked by inhibitors of the executioner caspases but not effector caspases, placing ceramide formation between the two sets of enzymes. Also, studies with Bcl-2 show that Bcl-2 is downstream of ceramide in the same pathway *(13,19)*. Thus, ceramide regulates phosphorylation of Bcl-2, and the action of ceramide on cell death is inhibited by Bcl-2 overexpression *(5,13,19,25)*. Recent data also implicate ceramide in the capping process (DISC formation) in response to FasL and Fas-agonistic antibodies, and reveal a potential early role in Fas signal transduction *(26)*.

In all these actions, short-chain ceramides exhibit a level of potency consistent with levels of endogenous ceramides *(12,14)*. The action of ceramide analogs exhibits significant specificity. For example, the closely related neutral lipid DAG not only does not mimic the action of ceramide, but more often antagonizes it *(11,12,14,17)*. Studies by Bielawska et al. showed that dihydroceramide, which is the metabolic precursor to ceramide and differs from it only in that it lacks the 4-5 trans double bond, exhibits no activity in these cellular studies, although it shows similar levels of uptake *(27,28)*.

In contrast, short-chain ceramides are poor effectors of other key actions associated with TNF and other inducers of ceramide formation *(29)*. Notably, ceramide is not active in inducing NF-κB, a transcription factor that plays a role in the inflammatory and antiapoptotic function of TNF *(29)*. Also, ceramide is a poor activator of erk members of the MAP kinase family, especially when compared with sphingosine and sphingosine-1-phosphate. This restricted action of short-chain ceramides to a subset of biochemical targets in cytokine responses provides further impetus to the emerging hypothesis of a more specific function for ceramide in the regulation of apoptosis in cancer.

FAS LIGAND

Fas ligand (CD95L or APO-1L) is a 40-kDa type II membrane protein belonging to the TNF family. Its receptor, Fas (CD95 or APO-1) is a 45-kDa type I membrane protein belonging to the TNF/nerve growth factor (NGF) superfamily of receptors *(30,31)*. Following engagement with its ligand, Fas functions to initiate an apoptotic signal. This signal originates at the death-inducing signaling complex (DISC) and is believed to form on the cytoplasmic face of the plasma membrane around the cytoplasmic domain of Fas. The DISC, in part, is composed of Fas, an adapter molecule (FADD/MORT), receptor-interacting protein (RIP), and procaspase-8 (FLICE/MACH) *(32)*. Upon Fas stimulation, FADD and procaspase 8 are recruited to Fas, enabling procaspase-8 to become autocatalytically activated *(33)*. Active caspase-8, in turn, cleaves and/or activates several downstream substrates, including the effector caspases 3 and 7 *(34)* (type I pathway) or Bid, which acts through the mitochondrial type II pathway to amplify programmed cell death (PCD) signals. Both pathways have been described *(35)*. The mitochondrial pathway may involve ceramide formation *(36)*. Cellular FLICE- inhibitory protein (c-FLIP) acts at the level of the DISC to block apoptosis, while inhibitors of apoptosis (IAP) act downstream.

Fas is a widely expressed protein found on the plasma membrane in most tissues, including the prostate. FACS analysis has been used to detect membrane Fas expression on all human PCa cell lines examined to date *(37–42)*. Membrane Fas expression has also been detected on the surface of both benign *(40)* and malignant human prostate tissue samples *(42)* using immunohistochemistry. In contrast, FasL expression appears to be more tightly regulated on the plasma membrane. Membrane FasL (mFasL) expression has been detected in immune privileged tissue—for example, testis *(43)*, retina *(44)*, cornea *(45)*, and in T- and natural killer (NK)-cells *(46–48)*. Several reports suggest that mFasL expression also occurs in both normal and malignant prostate, although these data remain controversial *(42,49)*.

Despite the inconsistencies regarding surface FasL expression in prostate, several experiments both in vitro and in vivo demonstrate that a functional Fas-mediated apoptotic pathway exists in PCa cells. For example, in vitro studies of PPC-1 and ALVA-31 reveal sensitivity to Fas-mediated apoptosis when challenged with a Fas agonist *(40)*. Other PCa cell lines such as DU145, ND1, PC-3, and LNCaP cells *(37,39–41)* are resistant to Fas agonist antibodies or recombinant soluble FasL. Resistance is overcome by pretreatment with subtoxic concentrations of cyclohexamide, doxorubicin, cis-diamminedichloroplatinum (II) (CDDP), VP-16, adriamycin (ADR), or camptothecin *(37,39–41,50)*. These chemotherapeutic drugs have different mechanisms of action, but presumably function to remove a block (possibly c-FLIP) *(51,52)* in the Fas-mediated pathway and allow the death signal to proceed. However, both sensitive and resistant PCa lines became uniformly sensitive to Fas-mediated apoptosis following treatment with our AdGFPFasL adenovirus *(37)*. Collectively, these data demonstrate that a Fas-mediated pathway is functional in all PCa cells tested so far by our laboratory. The role of ceramide in sensitization of resistant cells will be discussed below.

FAS-FASL AND CERAMIDE

Multiple lines of evidence point to a role for ceramide in mediating Fas-induced apoptosis. First, ceramide generation has been demonstrated to be an integral part of Fas-induced apoptosis *(26,53–56)*. Second, Fas activation has been shown to activate acid sphingomyelinase, which was demonstrated to be involved in propagation of Fas-generated apoptotic signaling *(54,57–61)*. Third, Fas-induced ceramide formation acts in conjunction with caspase activation and is not a consequence of apoptosis *(62)*. Fourth, Fas-resistant cells demonstrate insignificant changes in ceramide levels yet have normal receptor expression and intact downstream signaling (*[63]* and our unpublished data). Fifth, a role for *de novo* ceramide synthesis has also been established in Fas-induced apoptosis *(21,64)*, suggesting two possible "pools" of ceramide can affect Fas signal transduction. Sixth, acidic sphingomyelinase (aSMase)-null hepatocytes are insensitive to Fas-induced capping *(26)* but are sensitized with a 25 n*M* dose of C16-ceramide. Thus, a role for the lipid second messenger, ceramide, in mediating Fas-induced apoptosis is now established.

CERAMIDASE ELEVATION IN PROSTATE CANCER

The family of ceramidases includes acid, neutral, and alkaline species *(65–69)*. Human acid ceramidase maps to 8p22, which is frequently altered in PCa *(69)*. This enzyme catalyses the hydrolysis of ceramide to sphingosine and free fatty acids *(65)*, the overall effect of which is downregulation of ceramide signaling (i.e., decreased apoptosis) and increased pools of sphingosine, which can be phosphorylated by sphingosine kinase to generate sphingosine 1 phosphate (S1P). S1P interacts with the endothelial differentiation gene family (Edg/S1P receptors) to promote endothelial cell migration and angiogenesis *(70)*. Thus, a cell or tumor overexpressing ceramidase generates an antiapoptotic phenotype and a potential increase in angiogenesis in its microenvironment.

The PCa cell lines DU145, PC3, and LNCaP all show elevated levels of ceramidase mRNA by Northern blotting *(69)*. Prostate tumors obtained from radical prostatectomies, when analyzed for acid ceramidase expression by a competitive PCR approach, demonstrated that 41.6% had increased levels of acid ceramidase mRNA, 55.5% had no change, and 2.7% had a decrease *(69)*. Thus, a significant fraction of prostate tumors have the potential to assume an antiapoptotic phenotype and possibly to promote growth and angiogenesis. We have preliminary data that overexpression of sphingosine kinase in DU145 cells promotes significantly better xenograft growth in nude mice (unpublished data).

Although not necessarily directly causative for prostate cancer development, acid ceramidase elevation in 41% of human tumors (60% of Gleeson grade 7 and only 38% of grade 6 tumors) would suggest that its expression provides a selective advantage for tumor growth *(69)*. The mechanism likely manifests itself in two ways. First, reduced levels of ceramide have an antiapoptotic effect, and inhibition of apoptosis is clearly a hallmark of some cancers, including the prostate. Second, S1P production, via increased sphingosine kinase, has an angiogenic and growth effect as well as promoting endothelial cell migration in the prostate. We hypothesized that if we inhibited acid ceramidase activity, we expect our prostate cancer models to become more sensitive to AdGFPFasL virus, because AdGFPFasL elevates ceramide levels via *de novo* (myriocin-dependent) synthesis in all prostate cancer cell lines tested thus far (unpublished data). Figure 1 demonstrates that an acid ceramidase inhibitor (LCL102) at subtoxic doses increases the ability of AdGFPFasL to kill tumor cells in vitro by fourfold. Also of note, 75 mg/kg of LCL102 is nontoxic to mice, via IP injection (unpublished data, JSN, AELZ, AB). We have developed over 200 analogs of ceramide and ceramidase inhibitors based on the structure of ceramide *(71)*. The usefulness of these compounds in a mouse tumor model has been demonstrated as a marked reduction in liver metastatic disease in nude mice injected with two highly aggressive colon cancer cell lines *(72)*. Of note, B-13 (LCL4) was used in these in vivo experiments and was well tolerated by the nude mice at a maximum dose of 75 mg/kg (IP) *(72)*. We envision that if we combine this class of inhibitors with virus in vivo, we may achieve increased success in deleting tumor xenografts under preclinical conditions. These studies are underway, and should our hypothesis be proven correct, this sets the stage for examining such therapies in a phase I clinical trial format.

SR PROTEINS

Since the late 1980s, a family of highly conserved, serine-arginine-rich binding proteins (SR proteins) has been intensely studied for their role in RNA splicing *(73,74)*. Alternative splicing has already been determined to be regulated by both SR protein phosphorylation status and by the ratio of SR protein to hnRNP A/B family members *(73,74)*. SR proteins are targeted to nuclear sub-regions (speckles) with numerous other

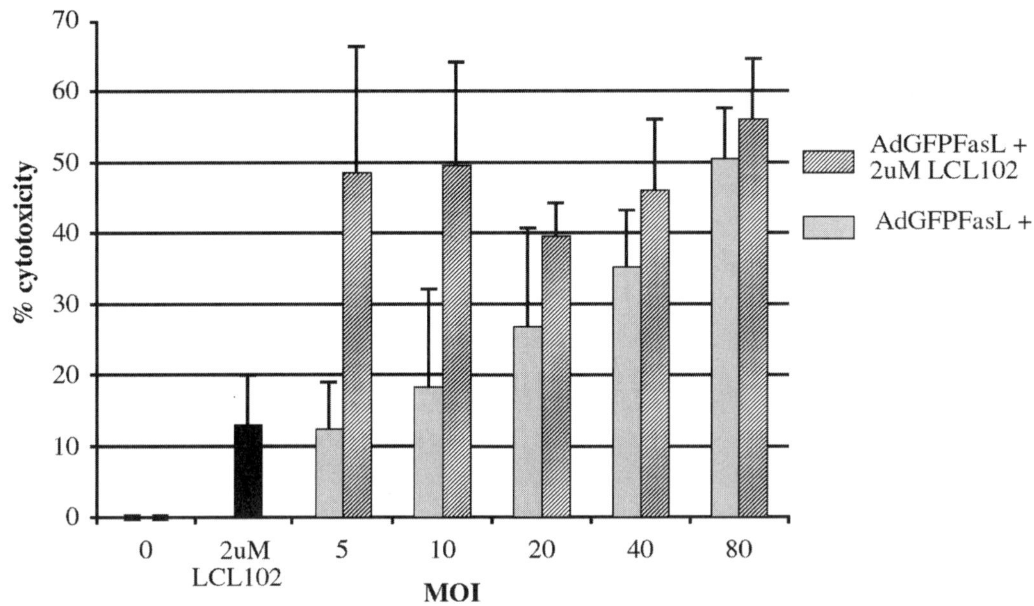

Fig. 1. DU145 cells growing in 96-well plates at 1×10^4 cells/well were treated with either media alone or 2 μ*M* LCL102 *(71)* for 48 h followed by AdGFPFasL for 24 h at the indicated MOIs. Cell death was assayed by the MTS assay as previously described *(37)*.

proteins and small RNAs, and cycle between these domains and the spliceosome *(75)*. Splicing of both major U12 (AT-AG)- and minor U2 (AT-AC)-dependent pathways involve SR proteins *(76)*. Cytoplasmic to nuclear shuttling of some SR proteins has been observed *(73,76)*. One factor, transportin, has also been shown to escort SR proteins to sub-nuclear domains *(77)*.

The issue of SR protein phosphorylation has been addressed by many investigators *(74)*. At least six different protein kinases are involved in SR phosphorylation, including SRPKs *(78)*, CLK/STY *(79–81)*, and cdc2 kinase *(82)*. A protein phosphatase 1 (PP1) subunit, NIPP1, can be demonstrated to co-localize with SR proteins in the spliceosome, and, when activated, PP1 dephosphorylates SR proteins *(83)*. Of note, PP1 has been shown to be a ceramide-activated protein phosphatase (CAPP). Chalfant et al. *(78,84)* have demonstrated in vitro that PP1 activation by gemcitabine or exogenous C6-ceramide results in SR protein dephosphorylation, resulting in a more proapoptotic phenotype in A549 cells. SR protein dephosphorylation is also observed in prostate cancer cell lines infected with AdGFPFasL adenovirus (unpublished data).

ALTERNATIVELY SPLICED GENES INVOLVED IN APOPTOSIS

There are a growing number of alternatively spliced genes (54 variants) *(85)* involved in apoptosis, including: Bax, Bim, caspases-1, -2, -8, -9, Fas, Bcl-x, c-FLIP, and IAP family members (livin and survivin). In many cases alternative splice products have different functions. For example, caspase-9b interacts with Apaf and functions as a dominant-negative, while the proapoptotic splice variant caspase-9, which also interacts with Apaf, is able to undergo catalytic cleavage to its active form *(78)*. In other cases, such as caspase-8a/8b, both alternatively spliced components seem to be required for apoptosis *(86)*. A thorough study of Ich-1 (caspase-2) splicing demonstrated that the SR protein (SC35) promoted exon skipping to favor the long proapoptotic form of caspase-2, while hnRNP A1 promoted exon inclusion and an increase in the antiapoptotic form of the molecule *(85)*. CD95 (Fas receptor) is alternatively spliced with at least three splice variants observed in a T-cell lymphoma *(87,88)*. In these papers, the authors observed a secreted Fas protein, which blocked apoptosis, and a truncated membrane-localized Fas receptor lacking the intracellular death-signaling domain, which functioned as a dominant-negative. The latter splicing variant arose due to a mutation.

INHIBITORS OF APOPTOSIS (IAP)

IAP family members (seven at last count) are evolutionarily related, and characterized by having one or multiple repeats of an amino acid domain (70 amino acids each) called the baculovirus IAP repeat (BIR). At least two of them, livin and survivin, are alternatively spliced *(89–92)*, and with respect to livin, the alpha splice variant has a more inhibitory effect than the beta form against certain chemotherapeutic agents *(90,92)*. Some IAP members function by interacting with caspases to block their activation. Typically, they do not act on caspase-8 but target downstream executioner caspases 3 and 7 *(93–100)*. A second pathway of inhibition has also been described by Sanna et al. *(101)*. In this study, the authors demonstrate that XIAP and NAIP function through TAK1 MAP kinase to activate JNK1, and that this pathway is independent of caspase inhibition. They also showed XIAP and NAIP directly associates with TAK1 to mediate the functional interaction with JNK1. Other IAPs, such as c-IAP1, c-IAP2, and survivin do not appear to act through JNK1.

IAP family members, including XIAP, c-IAP1 and c-IAP2, undergo proteasome-dependent degradation when monocytes are induced to enter apoptosis by etoposide *(102,103)*. Of particular interest, these proteins have E3 ligase activity and can undergo ubiquitination auto-catalytically. Kroesen et al. have demonstrated that *de novo* ceramide is required for proteolysis of XIAP *(104)*, further linking ceramide to generation of a proapoptotic phenotype. Another IAP member, BRUCE, is a giant 530 kd protein with a BIR repeat that contains ubiquitin-conjugating activity *(105)*. The human version of this gene is called apollon *(103)*. c-IAP1 will ubiquitinate caspases 3 and 7 but not caspase-1 under in vitro conditions *(102)*.

C-FLIP

c-FLIP is an alternatively spliced gene with important antiapoptotic functions via its interaction with caspase-8 (FLICE) in the DISC. c-FLIP is cleaved to p43 by caspase-8, but complete caspase-8 processing into the active p20/p18 and p10 subunits is blocked by the p43 of c-FLIP. Thus, when c-FLIP concentration exceeds that of caspase-8, it efficiently blocks caspase-8 activation *(106)*. c-FLIP$_S$ prevents the first caspase-8 cleavage step to p43/p41 and blocks induction of apoptosis by FasL in a number of human cell lines *(106,107)*. There are 11 possible alternatively spliced forms of c-FLIP (see Djerbi et al. *[108]*). How many of these are important in PCa is not known, but our data *(109)* and those of Kim et al. *(110)* clearly implicate a role for c-FLIP in inhibiting Fas and TNF-related apoptosis-inducing ligand (TRAIL) signaling in PCa.

Panka et al. *(111)* described the role of protein kinase B/AKT in c-FLIP expression in several cancer cell lines, including prostate (DU145 and PC3). DU145 cells are $PTEN^+$ (phosphorylated AKT is downregulated) while PC3 cells are $PTEN^-$, although phosphorylated AKT is still not as high as in the $PTEN^-$LNCaP cell line (unpublished, JSN). Panka et al. *(111)* observed that the MEK1 inhibitor PD98059 had no effect on prostate cell lines. However, disruption of PI3 kinase activity using LY294002 reduced AKT phosphorylation and also downregulated c-FLIP at both the protein and mRNA level. The mechanism for this is unknown. Since one target of phosphorylated AKT is the Forkhead transcription factor family, which effectively blocks transcriptional activation of apoptosis-inducing genes such as Fas and FasL (i.e., creating a more antiapoptotic phenotype), one can surmise from Panka's data that c-FLIP expression might be added to the growing list of indirect AKT targets. The primers used to determine RNA levels in Panka et al. do not discriminate between c-$FLIP_L$ and c-$FLIP_S$, so no conclusions about alternative splicing of FLIP mRNA could be drawn. There is no evidence for an AKT role in SR protein phosphorylation that we are aware of (personal communication, Lewis C. Cantley, PhD). There have been several reports *(112,113)* that NFκB upregulates c-FLIP expression, and Fulda et al. *(114)* report that several metabolic inhibitors of either transcription or translation downregulate c-FLIP. The latter report suggests mRNA stability may be involved in c-FLIP expression *(115)*, although there is no easily discernable AUUU degradation targeting sequence *(115,116)*. Thus, c-FLIP regulation remains a complicated issue in tumor cells, although there is mounting evidence for its importance in resistance to FasL and TRAIL signaling. We have examined this issue in Fig. 2, which demonstrates that doxorubicin downregulates c-$FLIP_S$ protein levels without affecting mRNA levels, suggesting an effect on translation or proteasome targeting, of which the latter is most likely *(110)*.

In CD3-activated T–cells, Fas signaling leads to proliferation. Apparently, c-FLIP is involved in this by a two-step process involving blockade of caspase-8 activation, and by providing a platform for assembly of TNF receptor-associated factor (TRAF)1, TRAF2, IκB kinase (IKK)α, IKKβ, Iκβα, NEMO, or IKAP and RIP *(22)*. This complex leads to activation of NFκB. Specifically, c-FLIP recruits RIP and TRAF1-3, likely via its caspase-like domain. The net result is activation of a proliferation response including activation of the MAP-kinase Erk. Activation of caspase activity is not required for these effects. Although it is not known specifically whether the pathway functions in tumor cells, we have anecdotal evidence for CH-11 (Fas agonistic antibody) stimulating growth of some of our resistant PCa lines (unpublished data). We have not examined these lines for NF-κB activation in response to the FasL agonists. The subject of c-FLIP has been recently reviewed *(117)*.

LACK OF SYSTEMIC EFFECTS FROM ORTHOTOPIC DELIVERY OF FASL-EXPRESSING ADENOVIRUSES

Pilot studies in our laboratory (data not shown) have demonstrated that direct intratumor injection of up to 5×10^9 MOI of AdGFPFasL was safe in a 25-g nude mouse, which is equivalent to 1.36×10^{13} particles in a 150-pound human. Safety is a potential issue when using FasL in gene therapy due to FasL's toxic effect on the liver. To ameliorate

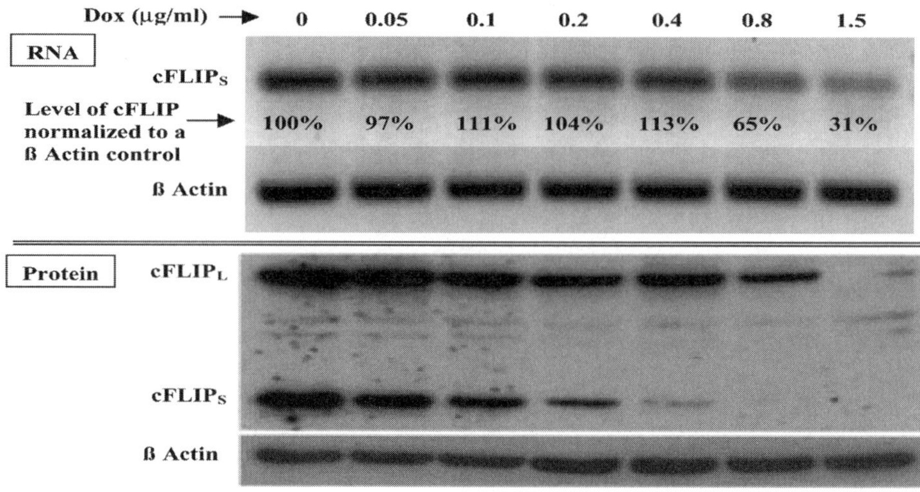

Fig. 2. Replicate DU145 cell cultures were treated for 24 h with various concentrations of doxorubicin (dox) in medium containing 2% FBS, and then harvested for either total RNA or protein. Total RNA was reverse transcribed to cDNA using random primers, and gene-specific primers were used for PCR. PCR products were resolved by agarose gel electrophoresis, and quantified by ethidium bromide fluorescence on a Fluorimager. PCR using β actin primers was used as a normalizing control. For protein analysis, a Western blot was probed with the anti-c-FLIP monoclonal antibody NF6 (kindly provided by Marcus Peter), followed by a β actin antibody as a normalizing control. The results demonstrate that at doses such as 0.4 μg /mL dox, the c-$FLIP_S$ mRNA is unaffected while the protein has disappeared.

this safety concern, we have successfully developed adenoviral vectors with prostate-restricted expression that can be administered systemically to mice without side effects *(118,119)*. These new, improved vectors can be injected intravenously into mice without ill effects, which is direct evidence that using FasL as a therapeutic molecule in vivo is a reasonable possibility if mouse safety data translate to humans. Further, our new vectors are designed to be regulated by doxycycline *(118,120)*, providing a second level of control. If a patient should experience an adverse reaction to FasL expression, addition or withdrawal of doxycycline (depending upon the virus) will stop production of FasL, which is surmised to allow the patient to recover.

THE BYSTANDER EFFECT

We have used the viruses described in Rubinchik et al. *(118)* under in vivo conditions to treat prostate cancer xenografts. Figure 3 demonstrates that following administration of 1.5×10^9 pfu of AdGFPFasL to PPC1 (prostate cancer) xenografts, 50% of tumors regress or fail to grow. Since viral delivery is at most 25% efficient, complete regression of an injected tumor suggests that a bystander effect is operative *(121)*. We have unpublished preliminary data that the immune system is also engaged in tumor eradication (JSN, ST, CL). These observations are important because one of the limitations in PCa gene therapy is delivery of the therapeutic gene to every cell in the tumor. One way to

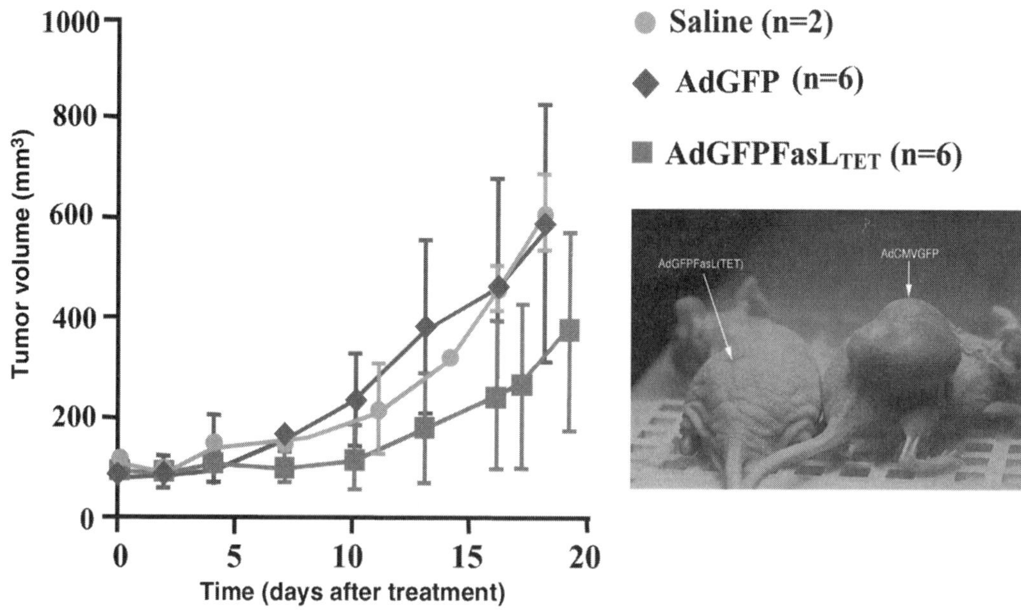

Fig. 3. Xenografts were developed by injection of 6.2×10^6 PPC1 cells subcutaneously in 300 µL of PBS. Tumors reached 70–100 mm^3 by 10 d. 1.5×10^9 IU of AdGFPFasL$_{TET}$ or AdCMVGFP in a final volume of 100 µL was perfused into the tumor over 10 min using a Harvard perfusion pump. This equates to an approximate MOI of 20.9 (75 mm^3 tumor estimated to contain 1.43×10^8 cells). Three animals in the AdGFPFasL-treated group had no tumor growth, while three animals had growing tumors. We frequently see this and attribute it to variable viral administration. Tumor size is monitored every 2–3 d and volume is calculated using the formula length $\times$ (width)^2/0.52.

overcome this is to amplify the response to the delivered gene. Understanding why and how to combine FasL therapy with chemo- or immunotherapy has the potential to address this problem by taking advantage of the bystander effect. The bystander effect is defined as a situation in which the number of cells undergoing PCD in the tumor bed is greater than the number of cells transduced. This mechanism is the foundation of both prodrug therapy and virally expressed p53 therapy *(122)*. Prodrug therapy is based upon the concept that a prodrug, formulated to undergo a specific metabolic conversion to a toxic metabolite, can be administered to a patient whose tumor has been previously treated with a vector expressing a unique enzyme (e.g., herpes-based thymidine kinase, or cytosine diaminase) capable of performing the enzymatic conversion *(123–127)*. Virally expressed wild-type p53 is capable of inducing apoptosis in many types of cancer cells and is reported to have bystander activity by inducing localized FasL expression, which recruits neutrophils infiltration that is believed to play a critical role in the bystander mechanism *(118,120,128)*. In a clinical setting, the bystander effect can result in regression of a solid tumor in spite of the physician's inability to deliver, by virus or liposome, a therapeutic gene to every cell. In vitro or in vivo bystander activity has been demonstrated for FasL, TRAIL, and p53 *(121,128,129)*.

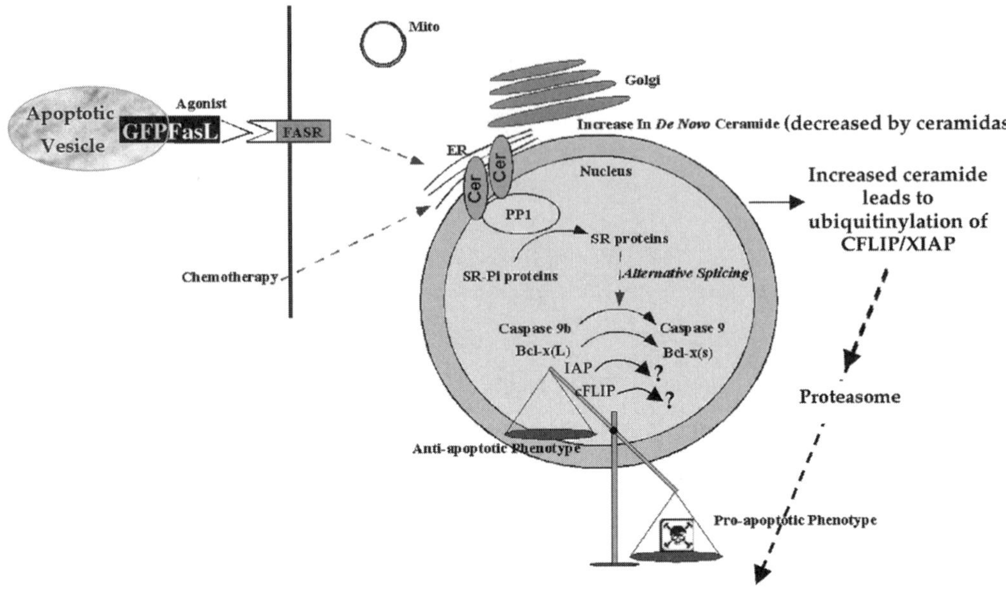

Fig. 4. This carton depicts how small-molecule therapy with conventional chemotherapy drugs or our new class of ceramidase inhibitors augments tumor cell death in vivo via a mechanism involving *de novo* ceramide synthesis, which activates protein phosphatase I, alters splicing of anti-apoptotic genes, and promotes proteasome function to tip the scales in favor of a proapoptotic phenotype that responds to bystander-induced cell death. Cells overexpressing ceramidase would be less likely to respond due to decreased ceramide.

SUMMARY

The recent availability of the human genome sequence and continued development of bioinformatic tools leads one to believe that our understanding of the causes of cancer will expand in the near future and will define and/or refine signaling pathway components as targets for cancer therapy. Relative to cancer gene therapy, the difficulty will lie not in the choice of therapeutic genes *per se*, but in our ability to deliver or amplify a corrective signal to every cell in the cancer. Thus, studies on delivery of therapeutic genes, as well as studies on methods to amplify delivery systems, are urgently required. In the DU145 model of prostate cancer, we have determined that resistance to the induction of apoptosis through the Fas receptor signaling pathway is due to overexpression of apoptotic resistance genes, including c-FLIPs *(30)*. We went on to demonstrate that expression of a FasL-GFP fusion gene overcomes resistance in infected cells *(37)*, kills the cell apoptotically, and produces apoptotic vesicles that also can signal Fas to induce apoptosis in adjacent cells (i.e., bystander activity) *(121)*. However, expression of apoptotic resistance genes in some cancers, including in the DU145 model, makes the cells relatively insensitive to vesicle-mediated bystander activity *(121)*. To overcome this, we have examined a number of different chemotherapeutic drugs and other small molecules for their effect on apoptotic resistance mechanisms. As presented in Fig. 2, doxorubicin (0.2 μg/mL) will decrease expression of c-FLIP protein without a concomitant decrease in levels of FLIP mRNA. This decrease in protein levels may be due to proteasomal degradation or a translational block. Under these conditions, a 20% increase in sensitivity of apoptotic vesicles is observed with 0.2 μg/mL doxorubicin (unpublished data). However, 0.2 μg/mL doxorubicin is itself toxic to DU145 cells at 48–72 h, which in this case obscures the role of the bystander vesicles in promoting apoptosis. We have also examined LCL102, a ceramidase inhibitor, which acts to increase intracellular ceramide levels by elevating ceramide. This molecule is highly efficient at activating cell death in DU145 cells at nontoxic doses if combined with AdGFPFasL virus at MOIs achievable in vivo (Fig. 1). A depiction of this process of anti- vs proapoptotic status of a cancer cell is provided in Fig. 4. We envision that small-molecule inhibitors of the antiapoptotic phenotype, promoting a proapoptotic phenotype with lower systemic toxicity like LCL102, can be used to shift cancer cells to the apoptotic phenotype and allow increased bystander sensitivity and the immune system to prevail. Therapeutic approaches such as these are likely to become increasingly important in cancer gene therapy.

REFERENCES

1. Hannun YA. Functions of ceramide in coordinating cellular responses to stress. Science 1996;274: 1855–1859.
2. Hannun YA, Bell RM. Functions of sphingolipids and sphingolipid breakdown products in cellular regulation [comment]. Science 1989;243:500–507.
3. Hannun YA, Linardic CM. Sphingolipid breakdown products: anti-proliferative and tumor-suppressor lipids. Biochim Biophys Acta 1993;1154:223–236.
4. Merrill AH Jr, Wang E, Gilchrist DG, Riley RT. Fumonisins and other inhibitors of de novo sphingolipid biosynthesis. Adv Lipid Res1993;26:215–234.
5. Ruvolo PP, Deng X, Ito T, Carr BK, May WS. Ceramide induces Bcl2 dephosphorylation via a mechanism involving mitochondrial PP2A. J Biol Chem 1999;274:20,296–20,300.
6. Pinto WJ, Srinivasan B, Shepherd S, Schmidt A, Dickson RC, Lester RL. Sphingolipid long-chain-base auxotrophs of Saccharomyces cerevisiae: genetics, physiology, and a method for their selection. J Bacteriol 1992;174:2565–2574.
7. Hanada K, Nishijima M, Kiso M, et al. Sphingolipids are essential for the growth of Chinese hamster ovary cells. Restoration of the growth of a mutant defective in sphingoid base biosynthesis by exogenous sphingolipids. J Biol Chem 1992;267:23,527–23,533.
8. Spiegel S, Merrill AH Jr. Sphingolipid metabolism and cell growth regulation. FASEB J 1996;10: 1388–1397.
9. Spiegel S, Merrill AH. Jr. (1996). Sphingolipid metabolism and cell growth regulation. FASEB Journal 10, 1388–1397.
10. Lee JY, Hannun YA, Obeid LM. Ceramide inactivates cellular protein kinase Calpha. J Biol Chem 1996;271:13,169–13,174.
11. Jayadev S, Liu B, Bielawska AE, et al. Role for ceramide in cell cycle arrest. J Biol Chem 1995;270: 2047–2052.
12. Venable ME, Lee JY, Smyth MJ, Bielawska A, Obeid LM. Role of ceramide in cellular senescence. J Biol Chem 1995;270:30,701–30,708.
13. Zhang J, Alter N, Reed JC, Borner C, Obeid LM, Hannun YA. Bcl-2 interrupts the ceramide-mediated pathway of cell death. Proc Natl Acad Sci USA 1996;93:5325–5328.
14. Obeid LM, Linardic CM, Karolak LA, Hannun YA. Programmed cell death induced by ceramide. Science 1993;259:1769–1771.
15. Cifone MG, De Maria R, Roncaioli P, et al. Apoptotic signaling through CD95 (Fas/Apo-1) activates an acidic sphingomyelinase. J Exp Med 1994;180:1547–1552.
16. Quintans J, Kilkus J, McShan CL, Gottschalk AR, Dawson G. Ceramide mediates the apoptotic response of WEHI 231 cells to anti-immunoglobulin, corticosteroids and irradiation. Biochem Biophys Res Commun 1994;202:710–714.
17. Jarvis WD, Fornari FA, Traylor RS, et al. Induction of apoptosis and potentiation of ceramide-mediated cytotoxicity by sphingoid bases in human myeloid leukemia cells. J Biol Chem 1996;271:8275–8284.
18. Mizushima N, Koike R, Kohsaka H, et al. Ceramide induces apoptosis via CPP32 activation. FEBS Lett 1996;395:267–271.

19. Smyth MJ, Perry DK, Zhang J, Poirier GG, Hannun YA, Obeid LM. prICE: a downstream target for ceramide-induced apoptosis and for the inhibitory action of Bcl-2. Biochem J 1996;316:25–28.
20. Westwick JK, Bielawska AE, Dbaibo G, Hannun YA, Brenner DA. Ceramide activates the stress-activated protein kinases. J Biol Chem 1995;270:22,689–22,692.
21. Chalfant CE, Ogretmen B, Galadari S, Kroesen BJ, Pettus BJ, Hannun YA. FAS activation induces dephosphorylation of SR proteins; dependence on the de novo generation of ceramide and activation of protein phosphatase 1. J Biol Chem 2001;276:44,848–44,855.
22. Kataoka T, Budd RC, Holler N, et al. The caspase-8 inhibitor FLIP promotes activation of NF-kappaB and Erk signaling pathways. Curr Biol 2000;10:640–648.
23. Zhuang S, Lynch MC, Kochevar IE. Caspase-8 mediates caspase-3 activation and cytochrome c release during singlet oxygen-induced apoptosis of HL-60 cells. Exp Cell Res 1999;250:203–212.
24. Cuvillier O, Rosenthal DS, Smulson ME, Spiegel S. Sphingosine 1-phosphate inhibits activation of caspases that cleave poly(ADP-ribose) polymerase and lamins during Fas- and ceramide-mediated apoptosis in Jurkat T lymphocytes. J Biol Chem 1998;273:2910–2916.
25. Ruvolo PP, Deng X, Carr BK, May WS. A functional role for mitochondrial protein kinase Calpha in Bcl2 phosphorylation and suppression of apoptosis. J Biol Chem 1998;273:25,436–25,442.
26. Cremesti A, Paris F, Grassme H, et al. Ceramide enables fas to cap and kill. J Biol Chem 2001;276: 23,954–23,961.
27. Bielawska A, Crane HM, Liotta D, Obeid LM, Hannun YA. Selectivity of ceramide-mediated biology. Lack of activity of erythro-dihydroceramide. J Biol Chem 1993;268:26,226–26,232.
28. Bielawska A, Linardic CM, Hannun YA. Ceramide-mediated biology. Determination of structural and stereospecific requirements through the use of N-acyl-phenylaminoalcohol analogs. J Biol Chem 1992;267:18,493–18,497.
29. Jayadev S, Hayter HL, Andrieu N, et al. Phospholipase A2 is necessary for tumor necrosis factor alpha-induced ceramide generation in L929 cells. J Biol Chem 1997;272:17,196–17,1203.
30. Suda T, Nagata S. Purification and characterization of the Fas-ligand that induces apoptosis. J Exp Med 1994;179:873–879.
31. Takahashi T, Tanaka M, Inazawa J, Abe T, Suda T, Nagata S. Human Fas ligand: gene structure, chromosomal location and species specificity. Int Immunol 1994;6:1567–1574.
32. Ashkenazi A, Dixit VM. Death receptors: signaling and modulation. Science 1998;281:1305–1308.
33. Medema JP, Scaffidi C, Kischkel FC, et al. FLICE is activated by association with the CD95 death-inducing signaling complex (DISC). EMBO J 1997;16:2794–2804.
34. Muzio M, Salvesen GS, Dixit VM. FLICE induced apoptosis in a cell-free system. Cleavage of caspase zymogens. J Biol Chem 1997;272:2952–2956.
35. Scaffidi C, Fulda S, Srinivasan A, et al. Two CD95 (APO-1/Fas) signaling pathways. EMBO J 1998;17:1675–1687.
36. Krammer PH. (1999). CD95(APO-1/Fas)-mediated apoptosis: live and let die. Advances in Immunology. 71, 163–210.
37. Hyer ML, Voelkel-Johnson C, Rubinchik S, Dong J, Norris JS. Intracellular Fas ligand expression causes Fas-mediated apoptosis in human prostate cancer cells resistant to monoclonal antibody-induced apoptosis. Mol Ther 2000;2:348–358.
38. Hedlund TE, Duke RC, Schleicher MS, Miller GJ. Fas-mediated apoptosis in seven human prostate cancer cell lines: correlation with tumor stage. Prostate 1998;36:92–101.
39. Frost P, Ng CP, Belldegrun A, Bonavida B. Immunosensitization of prostate carcinoma cell lines for lymphocytes (CTL, TIL, LAK)-mediated apoptosis via the Fas-Fas-ligand pathway of cytotoxicity. Cell Immunol 1997;180:70–83.
40. Rokhlin OW, Bishop GA, Hostager BS, et al. Fas-mediated apoptosis in human prostatic carcinoma cell lines. Cancer Res 1997;57:1758–1768.
41. Uslu R, Borsellino N, Frost P, et al. Chemosensitization of human prostate carcinoma cell lines to anti-fas-mediated cytotoxicity and apoptosis. Clin Cancer Res 1997;3:963–972.
42. Sasaki Y, Ahmed H, Takeuchi T, Moriyama N, Kawabe K. Immunohistochemical study of Fas, Fas ligand and interleukin-1 beta converting enzyme expression in human prostatic cancer. Br J Urol 1998;81:852–855.
43. Bellgrau D, Gold D, Selawry H, Moore J, Franzusoff A, Duke RC. A role for CD95 ligand in preventing graft rejection. Nature 1995;377:630–632.
44. Griffith TS, Brunner T, Fletcher SM, Green DR, Ferguson TA. Fas ligand-induced apoptosis as a mechanism of immune privilege. Science 1995;270:1189–1192.

45. Stuart PM, Griffith TS, Usui N, Pepose J, Yu X, Ferguson TA. CD95 ligand (FasL)-induced apoptosis is necessary for corneal allograft survival. J Clin Invest 1997;99:396–402.
46. Arase H, Arase N, Saito T. Fas-mediated cytotoxicity by freshly isolated natural killer cells. J Exp Med 1995;181:1235–1238.
47. Rouvier E, Luciani MF, Golstein P. Fas involvement in Ca(2+)-independent T cell-mediated cytotoxicity. J Exp Med 1993;177:195–200.
48. Stalder T, Hahn S, Erb P. Fas antigen is the major target molecule for CD4+ T cell-mediated cytotoxicity. J Immunol 1994;152:1127–1133.
49. Liu QY, Rubin MA, Omene C, Lederman S, Stein CA. (1998). Fas ligand is constitutively secreted by prostate cancer cells in vitro. Clin Cancer Res. 4, 1803–1811.
50. Costa-Pereira AP, Cotter TG. Camptothecin sensitizes androgen-independent prostate cancer cells to anti-Fas-induced apoptosis. Br J Cancer 1999;80:371–378.
51. Kim CW, Lee HM, Lee TH, Kang CH, Kleinman HK, Gho YS. Extracellular membrane vesicles from tumor cells promote angiogenesis via sphingomyelin. Cancer Res 2002;62:6312–6317.
52. Kelly MM, Hoel BD, Voelkel-Johnson C. Doxorubicin pretreatment sensitizes prostate cancer cell lines to TRAIL induced apoptosis, which correlates with the loss of c-FLIP expression. Cancer Biol Ther 2002;1(5):520–527.
53. Grullich C, Sullards MC, Fuks Z, Merrill AH Jr, Kolesnick R. CD95(Fas/APO-1) signals ceramide generation independent of the effector stage of apoptosis. J Biol Chem 2000;275:8650–8656.
54. Raisova M, Bektas M, Wieder T, et al. Resistance to CD95/Fas-induced and ceramide-mediated apoptosis of human melanoma cells is caused by a defective mitochondrial cytochrome c release. FEBS Lett 2000;473:27–32.
55. Kim JH, Yoon YD, Shin I, Han JS. Effects of ceramide, the Fas signal intermediate, on apoptosis and phospholipase D activity in mouse ovarian granulosa cells in vitro. IUBMB Life 1999;48:445–452.
56. Foghi A, Ravandi A, Teerds KJ, Van Der Donk H, Kuksis A, Dorrington J. Fas-induced apoptosis in rat thecal/interstitial cells signals through sphingomyelin-ceramide pathway. Endocrinology 1998;139:2041–2047.
57. Brenner B, Ferlinz K, Grassme H, et al. Fas/CD95/Apo-I activates the acidic sphingomyelinase via caspases. Cell Death & Differentiation 1998;5:29–37.
58. Lin T, Genestier L, Pinkoski MJ, et al. Role of acidic sphingomyelinase in Fas/CD95-mediated cell death. J Biol Chem 2000;275:8657–8663.
59. Lepple-Wienhues A, Belka C, Laun T, et al. Stimulation of CD95 (Fas) blocks T lymphocyte calcium channels through sphingomyelinase and sphingolipids. Proc Natl Acad Sci USA 1999;96:13,795–13,800.
60. Hebestreit H, Dibbert B, Balatti I, et al. Disruption of fas receptor signaling by nitric oxide in eosinophils. J Exp Med 1998;187:415–425.
61. De Maria R, Rippo MR, Schuchman EH, Testi R. Acidic sphingomyelinase (ASM) is necessary for fas-induced GD3 ganglioside accumulation and efficient apoptosis of lymphoid cells. J Exp Med 1998;187:897–902.
62. Tepper AD, Cock JG, de Vries E, Borst J, van Blitterswijk WJ. CD95/Fas-induced ceramide formation proceeds with slow kinetics and is not blocked by caspase-3/CPP32 inhibition. J Biol Chem 1997;272:24,308–24,312.
63. Tepper CG, Jayadev S, Liu B, et al. Role for ceramide as an endogenous mediator of Fas-induced cytotoxicity. Proc Natl Acad Sci USA 1995;92:8443–8447.
64. Cuvillier O, Edsall L, Spiegel S. Involvement of sphingosine in mitochondria-dependent Fas-induced apoptosis of type II Jurkat T cells. J Biol Chem 2000;275:15,691–15,700.
65. Koch J, Gartner S, Li CM, et al. Molecular cloning and characterization of a full-length complementary DNA encoding human acid ceramidase. Identification Of the first molecular lesion causing Farber disease. J Biol Chem 1996;271:33,110–33,115.
66. Mao C, Xu R, Szulc ZM, Bielawska A, Galadari SH, Obeid LM. Cloning and characterization of a novel human alkaline ceramidase. A mammalian enzyme that hydrolyzes phytoceramide. J Biol Chem 2001;276:26,577–26,588.
67. El Bawab S, Bielawska A, Hannun YA. Purification and characterization of a membrane-bound nonlysosomal ceramidase from rat brain. J Biol Chem 1999;274:27,948–27,955.
68. El Bawab S, Cungui M, Obeid LM, Hannun YA. Ceramidases in the regulation of ceramide levels and function. In: Quinn PJ, Kagan VE (eds), Subcellular Biochemistry: Phospholipid Metabolism in Apoptosis, Vol. 36. Kluwer Academic/Plenum Publishers, New York: 2002;187–205. .

69. Seelan RS, Qian C, Yokomizo A, Bostwick DG, Smith DI, Liu W. Human acid ceramidase is overexpressed but not mutated in prostate cancer. Genes Chromosomes Cancer 2000;29:137–146.
70. Birbes H, El Bawab S, Obeid LM, Hannun YA. Mitochondria and ceramide: intertwined roles in regulation of apoptosis. Adv Enzyme Regul 2002;42:113–129.
71. Usta J, El Bawab S, Roddy P, Szulc ZM, Hannun YA, Bielawska A. Structural requirements of ceramide and sphingosine based inhibitors of mitochondrial ceramidase. Biochemistry 2001;40:9657–9668.
72. Selzner M, Bielawska A, Morse MA, et al. Induction of apoptotic cell death and prevention of tumor growth by ceramide analogues in metastatic human colon cancer. Cancer Res 2001;61:1233–1240.
73. Hastings ML, Krainer AR. Pre-mRNA splicing in the new millennium. Curr Opin Cell Biol 2001;13: 302–309.
74. Zahler AM, Lane WS, Stolk JA, Roth MB. SR proteins: a conserved family of pre-mRNA splicing factors. Genes Dev 1992;6:837–847.
75. Misteli T, Spector DL. Serine/threonine phosphatase 1 modulates the subnuclear distribution of pre-mRNA splicing factors. Mol Biol Cell 1996;7:1559–1572.
76. Hastings ML, Krainer AR. Functions of SR proteins in the U12-dependent AT-AC pre-mRNA splicing pathway. RNA 2001;7:471–482.
77. Lai MC, Lin RI, Tarn WY. Transportin-SR2 mediates nuclear import of phosphorylated SR proteins. Proc Natl Acad Sci USA 2001;98:10,154–10,159.
78. Chalfant CE, Rathman K, Pinkerman RL, et al. De novo ceramide regulates the alternative splicing of caspase 9 and Bcl-x in A549 lung adenocarcinoma cells. Dependence on protein phosphatase-1. J Biol Chem 2002;277:12,587–12,595.
79. Siebel CW, Feng L, Guthrie C, Fu XD. Conservation in budding yeast of a kinase specific for SR splicing factors. Proc Natl Acad Sci USA 1999;96:5440–5445.
80. Colwill K, Pawson T, Andrews B, et al. The Clk/Sty protein kinase phosphorylates SR splicing factors and regulates their intranuclear distribution. EMBO J 1996;15:265–275.
81. Prasad J, Colwill K, Pawson T, Manley JL. The protein kinase Clk/Sty directly modulates SR protein activity: both hyper- and hypophosphorylation inhibit splicing. Mol Cell Biol 1999;19:6991–7000.
82. Okamoto Y, Onogi H, Honda R, et al. cdc2 kinase-mediated phosphorylation of splicing factor SF2/ASF. Biochem Biophys Res Commun 1998;249:872–878.
83. Boudrez A, Beullens M, Groenen P, et al. NIPP1-mediated interaction of protein phosphatase-1 with CDC5L, a regulator of pre-mRNA splicing and mitotic entry. J Biol Chem 2000;275:25,411–25,417.
84. Chalfant CE, Kishikawa K, Mumby MC, Kamibayashi C, Bielawska A, Hannun YA. Long chain ceramides activate protein phosphatase-1 and protein phosphatase-2A. Activation is stereospecific and regulated by phosphatidic acid. J Biol Chem 1999;274:20,313–20,317.
85. Jiang ZH, Wu JY. Alternative splicing and programmed cell death. Proc Soc Exp Biol Med 1999;220: 64–72.
86. Scaffidi C, Schmitz I, Krammer PH, Peter ME. The role of c-FLIP in modulation of CD95-induced apoptosis. J Biol Chem 1999;274:1541–1548.
87. Cascino I, Fiucci G, Papoff G, Ruberti G. Three functional soluble forms of the human apoptosis-inducing Fas molecule are produced by alternative splicing. J Immunol 1995;154:2706–2713.
88. Cascino I, Papoff G, De Maria R, Testi R, Ruberti G. Fas/Apo-1 (CD95) receptor lacking the intracytoplasmic signaling domain protects tumor cells from Fas-mediated apoptosis. J Immunol 1996;156:13–17.
89. Conway EM, Pollefeyt S, Cornelissen J, et al. Three differentially expressed survivin cDNA variants encode proteins with distinct antiapoptotic functions. Blood 2000;95:1435–1442.
90. Ashhab Y, Alian A, Polliack A, Panet A, Ben Yehuda D. Two splicing variants of a new inhibitor of apoptosis gene with different biological properties and tissue distribution pattern. FEBS Lett 2001;495:56–60.
91. Kasof GM, Gomes BC. Livin, a novel inhibitor of apoptosis protein family member. J Biol Chem 2001;276:3238–3246.
92. Mahotka C, Wenzel M, Springer E, Gabbert HE, Gerharz CD. Survivin-deltaEx3 and survivin-2B: two novel splice variants of the apoptosis inhibitor survivin with different antiapoptotic properties. Cancer Research 1999;59:6097–6102.
93. Deveraux QL, Leo E, Stennicke HR, Welsh K, Salvesen GS, Reed JC. Cleavage of human inhibitor of apoptosis protein XIAP results in fragments with distinct specificities for caspases. EMBO J 1999;18:5242–5251.

94. Deveraux QL, Roy N, Stennicke HR, et al. IAPs block apoptotic events induced by caspase-8 and cytochrome c by direct inhibition of distinct caspases. EMBO J 1998;17:2215–2223.
95. Shin S, Sung BJ, Cho YS, et al. An anti-apoptotic protein human survivin is a direct inhibitor of caspase-3 and -7. Biochemistry 2001;40:1117–1123.
96. Deveraux QL, Takahashi R, Salvesen GS, Reed JC. X-linked IAP is a direct inhibitor of cell-death proteases. Nature 1997;388:300–304.
97. Tamm I, Wang Y, Sausville E, et al. IAP-family protein survivin inhibits caspase activity and apoptosis induced by Fas (CD95), Bax, caspases, and anticancer drugs. Cancer Res 1998;58:5315–5320.
98. Suzuki A, Ito T, Kawano H, et al. Survivin initiates procaspase 3/p21 complex formation as a result of interaction with Cdk4 to resist Fas-mediated cell death. Oncogene 2000;19:1346–1353.
99. Takahashi R, Deveraux Q, Tamm I, et al. A single BIR domain of XIAP sufficient for inhibiting caspases. J Biol Chem 1998;273:7787–7790.
100. Roy N, Deveraux QL, Takahashi R, Salvesen GS, Reed JC. The c-IAP-1 and c-IAP-2 proteins are direct inhibitors of specific caspases. EMBO J 1997;16:6914–6925.
101. Sanna MG, da Silva Correia J, Ducrey O, et al. IAP suppression of apoptosis involves distinct mechanisms: the TAK1/JNK1 signaling cascade and caspase inhibition. Mol Cell Biol 2002;22:1754–1766.
102. Yang Y, Fang S, Jensen JP, Weissman AM, Ashwell JD. Ubiquitin protein ligase activity of IAPs and their degradation in proteasomes in response to apoptotic stimuli. Science 2000;288:874–877.
103. Yang YL, Li XM. The IAP family: endogenous caspase inhibitors with multiple biological activities. Cell Res 2000;10:169–177.
104. Kroesen B-J, Jacobs S, Pettus BJ, et al. BcR-induced apoptosis involves differential regulation of C16 and C24-ceramide formation and sphingolipid-dependent activation of the proteasome. J Biol Chem 2003;278:14723–14731.
105. Hauser HP, Bardroff M, Pyrowolakis G, Jentsch S. A giant ubiquitin-conjugating enzyme related to IAP apoptosis inhibitors. J Cell Biol 1998;141:1415–1422.
106. Krueger A, Schmitz I, Baumann S, Krammer PH, Kirchhoff S. Cellular FLICE-inhibitory protein splice variants inhibit different steps of caspase-8 activation at the CD95 death-inducing signaling complex. J Biol Chem 2001;276:20,633–20,640.
107. Houghton JA. Apoptosis and drug response. Curr Opin Oncol 1999;11:475–481.
108. Djerbi M, Darreh-Shori T, Zhivotovsky B, Grandien A. Characterization of the human FLICE-inhibitory protein locus and comparison of the anti-apoptotic activity of four different flip isoforms. Scand J Immunol 2001;54:180–189.
109. Hyer ML, Sudarshan S, Kim Y, et al. Downregulation of c-FLIP sensitizes DU145 prostate cancer cells to fas-mediated apoptosis. Cancer Biol Ther 2002;1:401–406.
110. Kim Y, Suh N, Sporn M, Reed JC. An inducible pathway for degradation of FLIP protein sensitizes tumor cells to TRAIL-induced apoptosis. J Biol Chem 2002;277:22320–22329.
111. Panka DJ, Mano T, Suhara T, Walsh K, Mier JW. Phosphatidylinositol 3-kinase/Akt activity regulates c-FLIP expression in tumor cells. J Biol Chem 2001;276:6893–6896.
112. Kreuz S, Siegmund D, Scheurich P, Wajant H. NF-kappaB inducers upregulate cFLIP, a cycloheximide-sensitive inhibitor of death receptor signaling. Mol Cell Biol 2001;21:3964–3973.
113. Micheau O, Lens S, Gaide O, Alevizopoulos K, Tschopp J. NF-kappaB signals induce the expression of c-FLIP. Mol Cell Biol 2001;21:5299–5305.
114. Fulda S, Meyer E, Debatin KM. Metabolic inhibitors sensitize for CD95 (APO-1/Fas)-induced apoptosis by down-regulating Fas-associated death domain-like interleukin 1-converting enzyme inhibitory protein expression. Cancer Res 2000;60:3947–3956.
115. Tschopp J, Irmler M, Thome M. Inhibition of Fas death signals by FLIPs. Curr Opin Immunol 1998;10:552–558.
116. Shaw G, Kamen R. A conserved AU sequence from the 3' untranslated region of GM-CSF mRNA mediates selective mRNA degradation. Cell 1986;46:659–667.
117. Krueger A, Baumann S, Krammer PH, Kirchhoff S. FLICE-inhibitory proteins: regulators of death receptor-mediated apoptosis. Mol Cell Biol 2001;21:8247–8254.
118. Rubinchik S, Wang D, Yu H, et al. A complex adenovirus vector that delivers FASL-GFP with combined prostate-specific and tetracycline-regulated expression. Mol Ther 2001;4:416–426.

119. Lowe SL, Rubinchik S, Honda T, McDonnell TJ, Dong JY, Norris JS. Prostate-specific expression of Bax delivered by an adenoviral vector induces apoptosis in LNCaP prostate cancer cells. Gene Ther 2001;8:1363–1371.
120. Rubinchik S, Ding R, Qiu AJ, Zhang F, Dong J. Adenoviral vector which delivers FasL-GFP fusion protein regulated by the tet-inducible expression system. Gene Ther 2000;7:875–885.
121. Hyer ML, Sudarshan S, Schwartz DA, Hannun YA, Dong J-Y, Norris JS. Quantification and characterization of the bystander effect in prostate cancer cells following adenovirus-mediated FasL expression. Cancer Gene Ther 2003;10:330–339.
122. Roth JA, Grammer SF, Swisher SG, et al. p53 gene replacement for cancer—interactions with DNA damaging agents. Acta Oncologica 2001;40:739–744.
123. Moolten FL. Tumor chemosensitivity conferred by inserted herpes thymidine kinase genes: paradigm for a prospective cancer control strategy. Cancer Res 1986;46:5276–5281.
124. Reid R, Mar EC, Huang ES, Topal MD. Insertion and extension of acyclic, dideoxy, and ara nucleotides by herpesviridae, human alpha and human beta polymerases. A unique inhibition mechanism for 9-(1,3-dihydroxy-2-propoxymethyl)guanine triphosphate. J Biol Chem 1988;263:3898–3904.
125. Uckert W, Kammertons T, Haack K, et al. Double suicide gene (cytosine deaminase and herpes simplex virus thymidine kinase) but not single gene transfer allows reliable elimination of tumor cells in vivo. Hum Gene Ther 1998;9:855–865.
126. Shand N, Weber F, Mariani L, et al. A phase 1–2 clinical trial of gene therapy for recurrent glioblastoma multiforme by tumor transduction with the herpes simplex thymidine kinase gene followed by ganciclovir. GLI328 European-Canadian Study Group. Hum Gene Ther 1999;10:2325–2335.
127. Seino K, Kayagaki N, Okumura K, Yagita H. Antitumor effect of locally produced CD95 ligand. Nature Med 1997;3:165–170.
128. Waku T, Fujiwara T, Shao J, et al. Contribution of CD95 ligand-induced neutrophil infiltration to the bystander effect in p53 gene therapy for human cancer. J Immunol 2000;165:5884-5890.
129. Kagawa S, He C, Gu J, et al. Antitumor activity and bystander effects of the tumor necrosis factor-related apoptosis-inducing ligand (TRAIL) gene. Cancer Res 2001;61:3330–3338.
130. Hyer ML, Sudarshan S, Kim Y, Reed JC, Dong JY, Schwartz DA, Norris JS. Downregulation of c-FLIP sensitizes DU145 prostate cancer cells to Fas-mediated apoptosis. Cancer Biol Ther 2002;1(4):407–408.

20 Gene Therapy Targeting Receptor-Mediated Cell Death to Cancers

Lidong Zhang, MD *and Bingliang Fang,* MD

SUMMARY

Research has demonstrated that delivery of genes encoding tumor necrosis factor (TNF)-α, Fas ligand (FasL), and TNF-related apoptosis-inducing ligand (TRAIL) to tumors can elicit apoptosis in cancer cells and can induce local inflammatory response, leading to regression of cancers. Constitutively active death receptors or chimeric death receptors that can be activated by other ligands, such as vascular endothelial growth factor, have also been exploited for cancer gene therapy. Systemic toxicity of death ligands can be prevented by using genes encoding membrane-bound death ligands and by targeted transgene expression through either targeted transduction or targeted transcription. Improvements have been made for tumor-selective transgene expressions. Various studies have demonstrated that the human telomerase reverse transcriptase promoter, whose gene is active in over 85% of cancers but not in normal cells, can drive tumor-specific transgene expression in a variety of cancer types. Moreover, transgene expression from a tumor-specific promoter can be augmented via transcriptional factors without loss of specificity. Thus far, reported data have shown that targeted expression of TRAIL, FasL, and TNF-α effectively suppressed tumor growth with minimal systemic toxicity. Challenges remain for treatment of metastatic diseases and for overcoming resistances. Here we summarize recent advances in targeted cancer gene therapy with receptor-mediated death pathways.

INTRODUCTION

At least 18 genes have been identified that encode type II transmembrane proteins that have a common extracellular C-terminal domain named *tumor necrosis factor* (TNF), the homology domain of the TNF ligand family *(1)*. This trimeric domain can bind to cysteine-rich domains of TNF receptors, eliciting a wide range of different functions that regulate immune response, inflammation, gene expression, cell differentiation, and cell

From: *Cancer Drug Discovery and Development: Death Receptors in Cancer Therapy*
Edited by: W. S. El-Deiry © Humana Press Inc., Totowa, NJ

death. TNF-α, FasL, and TRAIL are the three members of the TNF ligand family that are known to promote cell death by activating a receptor-mediated death pathway, one of two major pathways that drive cells into programmed death, or apoptosis. The interaction of death receptors and their ligands leads to recruitment of adapter proteins such as Fas-associated death-domain protein (FADD) and TNF receptor-associated death-domain protein (TRADD) inside of cells, activating caspases and triggering apoptosis *(2,3)*. In certain cases, necrosis can be induced upon the interaction of death receptors and their ligands.

Because initiation of cell death by a receptor pathway occurs on the cell surface, it is not necessary to deliver ligand proteins into cells in order to induce their biological functions. Thus, death-receptor ligands are excellent candidates of anticancer agents. For this reason, each discovery and cloning of the genes encoding TNF-α, FasL, and TRAIL has been hailed for its potential value as an anticancer agent; however, clinical trials with TNF *(4,5)* and preclinical study with agonistic antibody against Fas *(6)* have revealed intolerable systemic toxicity of TNF-α and FasL, including severe hepatotoxicity and cytokine release syndrome, casting dark shadows on these agents and preventing them from being used in systemic clinical applications. Similarly, a recent finding that hepatocytes from humans but not from animals are susceptible to recombinant, soluble TRAIL *(7)* has raised serious concerns about the potential risk for liver toxicity with TRAIL. Recombinant TRAIL-induced cell death has also been observed in neurons, oligodendrocytes, astrocytes, and microglial cells in normal living brain sections and in erythropoietic cells *(8,9)*. Although some of the observed toxicity could be caused by tagged histidine or leucine in the recombinant TRAIL proteins *(10)*, clinical trials with soluble TRAIL must be conducted cautiously because of reported toxicity in normal cells.

Gene therapy may allow the use of therapeutic agents that are otherwise not tolerable in patients, because local intratumoral expression of desired therapeutic proteins can reduce systemic toxicity while providing a constant therapeutic effect at the cancer site. Therefore, targeted gene therapy with molecules involved in the death receptor pathway may be advantageous if their expression can be limited to cancer cells by either targeted transduction via tropism-modified vectors, or targeted transcription via tumor-specific promoters. Preclinical studies with these gene-based approaches have generated promising data that indicate potential application of receptor-mediated cell death for cancer therapy in the near future.

TARGETED TRANSDUCTION

Intralesional and local-regional delivery of genes are the most common approaches used in current clinical trials of anticancer gene therapy*(11)*. Whereas local or local-regional delivery of therapeutic genes can be used to minimize systemic toxicity, local administration in the clinical setting has limited application and is applicable only in situations in which local, unresectable tumor is the major clinical problem (e.g., situations seen in some head, neck, lung, brain, pancreatic, and liver cancers). Thus, many investigators have tried to develop vectors that can specifically transduce cancer cells.

Vector targeting can be achieved, to a limited extent, by taking advantage of the natural determinants of the virus–host cell interactions or the presence of specific receptors on the cell surface responsible for specific uptake of a vector *(12,13)*. Different types of cells vary greatly in their susceptibility to different vectors. For example, adenoviral vectors that are efficient at transducing epithelial cells are quite inefficient at transducing hematopoietic cells, which are susceptible instead to retrovirus or adeno-associated virus vectors. Herpes simplex virus is most efficient at infecting and mediating prolonged gene expression in neuronal cells.

Ample studies have been aimed at controlling tissue tropism by modification of surface molecules of various vectors. Viral particles can be modified by reshaping preformed vector particles with bispecific conjugates or by manipulating the genes encoding the viral capsid or coating proteins, resulting in viral particles with modified surface proteins or incorporated ligands *(14,15)*. Bispecific conjugates are molecules that can bridge vector and target cells by binding specifically to surface molecules on vectors and on target cells. Various forms of bispecific conjugates have been reported. For example, antiadenovirus knob antibody or its Fab fragment conjugated with folate*(16)*, with growth factor *(17,18)*, or with antibodies against growth factor receptor *(19,20)* has been used for targeting adenovectors to various cell types. Recombinant fusion proteins containing single-chain antibody (scFV) against knob and epidermal growth factor (EGF) or antigrowth factor receptor scFv have also been reported for retargeting adenovectors *(19,21–23)*.

Vector targeting can also be achieved by modification of genes encoding the viral capsid or coating proteins, resulting in viral particles with modified surface proteins or incorporated ligands. Evidence has demonstrated that fibers of adenovectors can be modified to redirect vector tropism. Adenoviral vector that contains a chimeric fiber of serotypes 3 and 5 is reported to enhance the transduction efficiency in certain cell lines *(24)*. Replacing Ad5 fiber with Ad35 fiber led to increased tropism for hematopoietic cells *(25)*. Moreover, ligands can be added to adenoviral fiber genetically. For example, adding polylysine to the fiber by erasing the stop codon targets viral vector to broadly expressed, heparin-containing cellular receptors *(26)*. This vector can effectively transduce a variety of cell types that are coxsackie virus and adenovirus receptor (CAR)-defective or refractory to commonly used Ad2 or Ad5 vectors *(26,27)*. Alternatively, peptides containing arginine-glycine-aspartatic acid (RGD) sequences can be added to the knob of adenoviral fiber. Adenovectors with an RGD fiber can effectively bind αv integrin-positive cells, leading to enhanced transduction of endothelials, dendritic cells, smooth muscle cells, and various cancer cells in vitro and in vivo *(28–31)*.

Retroviral vectors have also been engineered to incorporate a cell-specific ligand into the viral envelope *(32–34)*. Cell-surface molecules that are overexpressed in malignant cells, such as members of the EGF receptor family, have been considered vector-cell-specific binding devices and tested for tumor-specific gene delivery. The fusion of EGF with an envelope protein resulted in retroviral particles that could bind to EGFR *(35)*. Similar approaches have been employed for targeting nonviral vectors. The ligands used for cell-specific gene delivery include folate to promote delivery into cells that overexpress the folate receptor (e.g., ovarian carcinoma cells), and EGF to cancer cells overexpressing EGF receptors *(36)*.

Whereas various studies have demonstrated the feasibility of redirected vector tropism by vector modification, there are also hurdles and obstacles to be solved. One major problem in targeted transduction for cancer therapy is the paucity of candidate receptors that are present specifically in cancer cells. Although some tumor antigens, folate receptors, or growth-factor receptors may be overexpressed in certain types of cancer cells, they are also present in a variety of normal cells. Several groups have used phage display libraries and other techniques to identify peptides that can specifically bind to cancer cells or cancer vasculature *(37–40)*. Arap et al. showed that RGD-4C and NGR motifs can specifically bind to tumor blood vessels *(37)*. These peptides are able to home in on specific organs or tissues by specific binding to receptors that are differentially expressed in vascular endothelial cells. For example, RGD-4C binds to αv integrins *(41)*, whereas NGR peptide binds to aminopeptidase N (CD13) *(42)*. Adenovectors with RGD-4C incorporated in fiber can effectively target primary tumor cells *(29)*. Retroviral vectors tagged with NGR specifically enhance the transduction efficiency of human endothelial cells in culture *(43)*. Another issue in vector targeting is that incorporation of targeting ligand may increase transduction in refractory cells but is not necessary to block natural tropism of a vector. For example, adding polylysine or RGD to adenoviral fiber may increase transduction in some refractory cells, and it may also increase transduction in cells that are susceptible to unmodified Ad5- or Ad2-based vectors. Several reasons may account for this. First, ligand for natural tropism is not abolished by the modification in the targeting vector *(44)*. Second, vector–host cell interaction may not completely depend on ligand-receptor interaction. Nonspecific adsorption of targeted vector particles to cells could be sufficient for transduction *(45)*. Finally, in vivo distribution and tropism of a vector are largely dependent on bioavailability of the vector in a specific site or organ. Passing through blood vessels and reaching target cells impose a major limit for in vivo targeting via vector transduction. The large molecular size of gene-based medicines decreases their extravasation from blood into tissues and increases their clearance by macrophages, immunoglobulins, and complements. Thus, even with adenovectors that are ablated of their capacity to bind CAR, their in vivo distribution is quite similar to those of commonly used Ad5 vectors, the majority of which end in the liver *(46)*.

TARGETED TRANSCRIPTION

Use of tissue- or tumor-specific promoters for selective transgene expression after nonselective gene delivery has also been zealously pursued in cancer gene therapy *(47,48)*. A number of promoters have been identified as being more active in cancer cells than in their normal counterparts. These include the carcinoembryonic antigen (CEA) promoter for colon and pancreatic cancers*(49,50)*, α-feto-protein promoter for hepatic cancers *(51,52)*, probasin promoter and prostate-specific antigen promoter for prostate carcinoma *(53,54)*, MUC1 promoter for mucin-secreting adenocarcinoma *(55)*, and the E2F promoter for cancers with a defective retinoblastoma gene *(56)*. Completion of the human genome project and development of new technologies will lead to identification of more genes that are overexpressed in cancer cells and whose promoters can be employed for targeted cancer gene therapy.

These promoters have several limitations, however. First, most selective promoters are limited to specific histologic types of tumors and cannot be broadly applied to tumors of various origins. Second, most of these promoters are much weaker than commonly used viral promoters, and it is difficult to achieve therapeutic levels of transgene expression with them. Fortunately, these limitations can be overcome by using promoters that are active in a variety of cancer types and by using transcriptional factors to augment transgene expression.

Human Telomerase Reverse Transcriptase (hTERT) Promoter as Universal Tumor-Specific Promoter

Telomerase is a specialized type of reverse transcriptase that is responsible for the replication of chromosomal ends, or telomeres *(57,58)*. This enzyme is composed of a template RNA, a catalytic peptide, and several associated proteins. In most human somatic cells, telomerase activity cannot be detected, and telomeres shorten with successive cell divisions *(59)*. However, telomerase is highly active in immortalized cell lines and in 85% of human cancer cells *(60–62)*. For this reason, telomerase has recently become a popular target in anticancer therapy and has been used as a marker of cancer.

It is now known that the catalytic subunits of telomerase (telomerase reverse transcriptase, or TERT) is the rate-limiting component of telomerase *(63)*. Human TERT (hTERT) (GenBank AF015950) encodes a 1,132-amino-acid polypeptide with a predicted molecular mass greater than 100 kDa *(63)*. This gene is expressed at high levels in primary tumors, cancer cell lines, and telomerase-positive tissues but is undetectable in telomerase-negative cell lines and differentiated telomerase-negative tissues. The expression of hTERT is mainly regulated at the transcriptional level, and there is no difference in its expression levels during cell cycles (G_1, S, G_2, and M phases) in telomerase-positive cells. However, telomerase activity is dramatically repressed when these cells become quiescent (G_0) or enter terminal differentiation *(64)*. Nevertheless, telomerase is never detected in ordinarily telomerase-negative cells, regardless of their growth status.

Forced expression of exogenous hTERT is sufficient to reconstitute telomerase activity in telomerase-negative normal human cells and can extend the life span of these cells *(65,66)*. Moreover, evidence has demonstrated that forced expression of hTERT, together with the SV40 early region and an oncogenic *ras* gene, can transform normal human fibroblasts, kidney epithelial cells, and mammary epithelial cells into tumorigenic cells *(67,68)*.

Because the hTERT gene is highly active in immortalized cell lines and in 85% of human cancer cells but undetectable in normal, differentiated tissues, the hTERT promoter may be used as a universal tumor-specific promoter for targeted cancer gene therapy after nonspecific gene delivery. The promoter region of hTERT has been cloned (GenBank AB016767) *(69–71)*. The promoter is GC rich and lacks both TATA and CAAT boxes. Deletion analysis of the hTERT promoter identified the 181-bp core promoter region upstream of the transcription start side that contains a binding site for an E box (CACGTG) binding factor and Sp1. Overexpression of c-Myc results in a significant increase in transcriptional activity of the core promoter.

Using the hTERT promoter for targeted cancer gene therapy has been tested by several groups, including us *(72–74)*. Using the *lacZ* gene as a reporter and adenovirus as a gene transfer vector, we have tested hTERT promoter activities in vitro and in vivo. The in vitro studies showed that the hTERT promoter is highly active in human and murine cancer cells derived from carcinomas of lung, colon, liver, breast, ovary, and brain *(73,75–79)*. The hTERT promoter is not active in normal human fibroblasts*(73)*; normal human epithelial cells from trachea*(73)*, mammary *(79)*, and ovary *(77)*; normal human primary hepatocytes *(78)*; normal human CD34$^+$ progenitor cells *(75)*; normal mouse fibroblasts *(75)*; and normal mouse livers *(73,78)*. In cancer cells, the differences in promoter activity between cytomegalovirus (CMV) promoter and hTERT were 2- to

20-fold, whereas in normal cells, the differences were more than 500-fold. In all cells tested, hTERT promoter activity was significantly higher in cancer cells than in normal cells, usually by more than 100-fold. In the in vivo study, high levels of β-galactosidase activity were detected in the livers and spleens of animals treated with Ad/CMV-LacZ, whereas mice treated with Ad/TERT-LacZ had no detectable β-galactosidase activity in any organs, suggesting that the hTERT promoter is indeed dormant in adult somatic tissues *(73,75)*.

Furthermore, expression of the Bax gene from the hTERT promoter elicited tumor-specific apoptosis and suppressed tumor growth in both xenographic human cancers and syngeneic mouse tumors, in vitro and in vivo. Expression of the *Bax* gene from the hTERT promoter also prevented the toxicity of the *Bax* gene in vitro and in vivo. In addition to the *Bax* gene, hTERT promoter has been used for targeted cancer gene therapy with *caspase-8 (80)*, *rev-caspase-6 (74)*, *FADD (81)*, the bacterium diphtheria toxin A *(72)*, and *TRAIL (78,79)*. Together, these published reports demonstrated that the hTERT promoter is highly tumor selective, indicating its potential application in targeted cancer gene therapy.

Augmenting Transgene Expression With Transcription Factors

Like other tissue- or tumor-specific promoters, the hTERT promoter is still relatively weak when compared with commonly used viral promoters such as the CMV promoter. Weak transcription activity that frequently leads to low therapeutic efficacy is a common feature of most tissue- or tumor-specific promoters. To solve this problem, several research groups have recently used the Cre/loxP system to enhance transgene expression from the CEA and thyroglobulin promoters *(82,83)*. In this system, a stuffer DNA flanked by a loxP sequence was placed between the transgene and a strong upstream viral promoter, such as CMV. After transfection with a second vector expressing a *Cre* gene driven by a tumor-specific promoter, such as the CEA or thyroglobulin promoters, the stuffer DNA was removed to permit expression of the transgene from its upstream viral promoter. However, this approach requires rearrangement of vectors and is limited by the transcriptional activity of the upstream promoter, which could be weak in some cancer cells. Nettelbeck et al. *(84)* devised an alternative solution to the problem. They established a positive feedback loop in which a cell-type-specific promoter is used to drive the simultaneous expression of the desired effector/reporter gene product and a strong artificial transcriptional activator via an internal ribosome entry sequence *(85)*. The binding sequences of the transcriptional activator are placed upstream of the cell-type-specific promoter, and the transcriptional activator expressed from the promoter stimulates transcription through appropriate binding sites in the promoter. However, this method leads to a simultaneous increase in the expression of both the therapeutic gene and the transcription factor gene.

We hypothesize that a small amount of a potent transcriptional factor, such as GAL4/VP16 *(86)* and tetR/VP16 (tTA) *(87)* fusion proteins, expressed from a tumor-specific promoter, would be sufficient to activate their target promoters upstream of a transgene, and so increase transgene expression. To test this hypothesis, we compared transgene expression directly from the CEA promoter and from the CEA promoter via the GAL4 gene regulatory system in cultured cells and in subcutaneous tumors after intratumoral administration *(88)*. Our results showed that transgene expression from the CEA promoter can be augmented up to 100-fold, whether in vitro or in vivo, without the loss of its specificity *(88)*. The increment of the transgene expression was more dramatic in CEA-positive cells than in CEA-negative cells, suggesting that this method not only can increase the levels of transgene expression but also widen the so-called therapeutic window of a gene. To test whether the levels of transgene expression from the hTERT promoter also can be increased by using this method, we compared the levels of *lacZ* gene expression directly from the hTERT promoter with that from the hTERT promoter via the GAL4 components after adenovirus-mediated gene transfer. In all cells tested, the levels of *lacZ* gene expression from the hTERT promoter via the GAL4 system were consistently higher than those directly from the hTERT promoter. The levels of β-galactosidase activity in cancer cells treated with the vectors expressing the *lacZ* gene from the hTERT promoter via GAL4/VP16 were more than 150-fold higher than in cancer cells treated with Ad/hTERT-LacZ. In normal fibroblasts, however, the increase in β-galactosidase activity by the GAL4 system was less than 38-fold, much less than that seen in cancer cells. This result suggests that transgene expression from the hTERT promoter can be increased with transcriptional factors without losing its specificity.

TARGETED TRAIL GENE THERAPY

TRAIL, first identified by searching an expressed sequence tag (EST) database with a conserved sequence contained in many TNF family members *(89,90)*, appears to induce apoptotic cell death only in tumorigenic or transformed cells and not in most normal cells *(89,91,92)*. Evidence has shown that repeated intravenous injection of a recombinant, biologically active TRAIL protein induces tumor-cell apoptosis, suppresses tumor progression, and improves the survival of animals bearing solid tumors without causing any detectable toxicity in nonhuman primates *(91,92)*. Furthermore, TRAIL cooperated synergistically with the chemotherapeutic drugs 5-fluorouracil and CPT-11 in causing substantial tumor regression or complete tumor ablation *(92)*. Therefore, it appears that TRAIL may act as a potent anticancer agent without causing significant toxicity to most normal tissues.

Using adenovirus-mediated gene transfer, we and others have recently demonstrated that direct introduction of the *TRAIL* gene into cancer cells can elicit apoptosis and suppress tumor growth in vitro and in vivo *(93)*. In vitro transfer of the full-length TRAIL coding sequence elicited massive apoptosis in various cancer cells without apparent toxicity to normal human fibroblasts. The intratumoral delivery of the TRAIL gene also elicited tumor-cell apoptosis and suppressed tumor growth, whereas systemic administration of the TRAIL-expressing adenovector did not elicit noticeable liver toxicity in mouse. Furthermore, our study demonstrated that overexpressing the *TRAIL* gene elicited the bystander effect. This bystander effect can be visualized by using a green fluorescent protein (GFP)-TRAIL fusion construct and is mediated by membrane-bound TRAIL but not with soluble or diffusible factors *(94)*.

As a type II membrane protein, TRAIL is reportedly cleaved by a cysteine protease to form soluble TRAIL *(95,96)*. However, the resulting soluble form seems to be too small to retain a functional TNF homology domain *(1)*. In our study with TRAIL gene therapy, we found that no detectable soluble TRAIL was present in media of normal and malignant cells transduced with a full-length TRAIL coding sequence. The enzyme-linked immunosorbent assay used in this study can easily detect 5 ng of recombinant soluble TRAIL suspended in medium *(78,94)*. Moreover, the bystander apoptotic effect of the *TRAIL* gene is not transferable with medium of the TRAIL-expressing cell culture *(94)*. Furthermore, this bystander effect was prevented when TRAIL-transduced and nontransduced cells were cultured in separated compartments of Transwell plates with a pore size up to 3.0 μm in diameter. These results collectively suggest that spontaneous cleavage of membrane-bound TRAIL is either extremely low, or cleavage soluble TRAIL is extremely unstable and/or not functional.

The report on the toxicity of recombinant soluble TRAIL protein in normal human primary hepatocytes (NHPH) *(7)* prompted us to evaluate the effect of the *TRAIL* gene on these cells. Our results showed that expressing full-length membrane-bound TRAIL elicits massive apoptosis in NHPH *(78)*. Because cultured primary hepatocytes are dramatically different from hepatocytes *in situ (97)*, the significance of the hepatocyte toxicity of full-length, membrane-bound TRAIL we observed is not yet clear. However, because the liver is a complex organ composed of multiple cell types *(97)*, and because the *TRAIL* gene is normally not expressed in human liver, the issue of liver toxicity resulting from *TRAIL* gene overexpression should not be overlooked. Therefore, in order to limit TRAIL gene expression to cancer cells, we constructed a bicistronic adenoviral vector expressing GFP-TRAIL fusion protein driven by the hTERT promoter via GAL4 gene regulatory components (designated Ad/gTRAIL). The GAL4 gene regulatory system is incorporated into this vector because it can augment transgene expression from a tumor-specific promoter without loss of specificity *(88)*.

In vitro studies have shown that treatment with Ad/gTRAIL resulted in high expression levels of GFP/TRAIL and induced apoptosis in human lung, breast, colon, liver, and ovary cancer cells *(77–79)*, including a caspase-3-defective breast cancer cell line MCF7 *(98)*, suggesting that deficiency of caspase-3 is not sufficient to block TRAIL-mediated apoptosis . Furthermore, treatment with Ad/gTRAIL was effective in killing breast cancer cell lines resistant to doxorubicin or resistant to soluble TRAIL protein *(79)*, suggesting that membrane-bound TRAIL is more effective than soluble recombinant TRAIL in apoptosis induction. This is consistent with a recent report by Voelkel-Johnson et al. that prostate cancer cells resistant to soluble TRAIL were susceptible to adenoviral delivery of full-length TRAIL *(99)*.

The intratumoral administration of Ad/gTRAIL significantly suppressed the growth of subcutaneous tumors derived from colon and breast cancer cell lines and prolonged the survival of tumor-bearing animals *(78,79)*. Specifically, about 50% of animals bearing doxorubicin-sensitive and doxorubicin–resistant breast cancer xenografts showed complete tumor regression and remained tumor free for over 200 d. In contrast, all animals treated with saline or control vector Ad/CMV-GFP died from the tumor burden within 90 d. These data suggest that Ad/gTRAIL is a potent antitumor agent for both chemosensitive and chemoresistant tumors.

Transgene expression and apoptosis induction by Ad/gTRAIL was minimal in normal human fibroblasts, normal human primary hepatocytes (NHPHs), mammary epithelial cells, and ovary epithelial cells in culture *(77–79)*. For example, fluorescent activated cell sorting analysis showed that treatment of NHPHs with the same dose of Ad/CMV-GFP resulted in more than 50% GFP-positive NHPHs, whereas treatment with Ad/gTRAIL resulted in less than 1% GFP-positive cells, similar to the percentage seen after treatment with either saline or control vectors. Although treatment with vectors expressing the

TRAIL gene from the PGK promoter led to a dramatic increase in apoptotic cells and loss of cell viability, treatment with Ad/gTRAIL resulted in only a background level of cell death, similar to that seen in cells treated with saline or control vector *(78)*. These data demonstrate that NHPHs are susceptible to full-length human *TRAIL* molecules and that the hTERT promoter can be used to prevent expression of therapeutic genes in normal human hepatocytes, thereby preventing possible normal tissue toxicity. In an in vivo study, systemic administration of Ad/CMV-GFP resulted in high levels of GFP expression in livers. In contrast, transgene expression was not detectable in mouse liver after systemic administration of Ad/gTRAIL, suggesting that the hTERT promoter can prevent expression of the *GFP/TRAIL* gene in liver after systemic administration of Ad/gTRAIL, consistent with our observations that the hTERT promoter prevents *LacZ* and *Bax* gene expression after systemic administration of adenovectors expressing these genes *(73)*.

TARGETED EXPRESSION OF TNF, FASL, AND THEIR RECEPTORS

Several groups have demonstrated that direct transfer of the *FasL* gene to tumor cells promotes tumor regression through apoptosis or inflammation *(100–104)*; in Fas+ tumor cells, transfer of FasL leads to activation of apoptosis via FasL and Fas interaction. In Fas- tumors, transfer of FasL resulted in elimination of tumors by neutrophil infiltration and inflammation *(100,102)*. Similarly, there are also ample reports of the use of the *TNF*-α gene for cancer therapy. In general, delivery of the *TNF*-α gene can induce apoptosis in various types of cancer cells and suppress tumor growth in vivo *(105–110)*.

In addition to direct transfer of the *TNF*-α or *FasL* gene to tumor cells, cell-mediated delivery of TNF and FasL gene therapy have also been reported. Gautam et al. showed that bone marrow-derived primary hematopoietic progenitors expressing the *TNF*-α gene can be used to inhibit the development of leukemia in mice without noticeable systemic toxicity *(111)*. Primary myoblasts, defective in Fas but genetically engineered to express FasL, were shown to be remarkably potent in destruction of solid tumors in vivo, much more effective than well characterized cytotoxic antibodies to Fas *(112)*.

Whereas spontaneous cleavage of wild-type TRAIL is still controversial, cleavage of membranous TNF and FasL are well documented. The extracellular part of TNF and FasL proteins can form soluble homotrimeric molecules upon cleavage by the membrane metalloproteinases disintegrin and matrilysin, respectively *(113–115)*.

Theoretically, systemic toxicity may not be prevented by targeted gene therapy if the therapeutic gene product is a secreting protein, because the protein will enter the blood stream and circulate to other parts of the body. Thus, toxicity from shedding of soluble TNF and FasL could be challenging *(4,5,116)*. Nevertheless, it has been reported that the apoptotic-inducing capacity of naturally processed soluble FasL was reduced by more than 1000-fold compared with membrane-bound FasL, and injection of high doses of recombinant sFasL in mice did not induce liver failure *(117)*. However, soluble human FasL is active in inducing apoptosis in vitro and in vivo, and its deleterious effect may be strengthened in patients who are suffering from bacterial infection *(118)* or in the presence of crosslinking antibodies *(117)*.

Fortunately, systemic toxicity from shedding of soluble factors of TNF and FasL can be prevented by using noncleavable, membrane-bound TNF or FasL via deletion of a segment containing the cleavage site *(101)*. Aoki et al. reported that FasL with a deletion of 34 aa spanning the metalloproteinase cleavage site (residues 103–136) rendered an increase in FasL expression on the cell surface and a decrease in release of soluble FasL *(101)*. Adenovector expressing this FasL mutant from a smooth-muscle-specific promoter, SM22apha, suppressed the growth of leiomyosarcomas in vivo without significant hepatic injury or systemic toxicity in mice, and the maximum tolerated dose was increased by 10- to 100-fold. Marr et al. *(119)* compared antitumor activity and toxic effects of adenovectors expressing wild-type murine TNF and a mutant nonsecreted (membrane-bound) form, respectively. Whereas both vectors induced efficient cell-surface expression of TNF-α and substantial disruption of tumor pathology, only the vector that expresses the wild type induced high levels of TNF-α secretion in transduced cells and high serum concentrations of mTNF-α in vivo. The wild-type TNF vector was highly toxic, whereas membrane-bound TNF vector was not, indicating that the use of a nonsecreted form of TNF alpha can minimize systemic toxicity without reducing antitumor activity. These membrane-bound, noncleavable *TNF* and *FasL* genes should be useful for targeted gene therapy.

In addition to the muscle-specific promoter, SM22apha *(101)*, other tissue-specific promoters have been used for targeted expression of *FasL* and *TNF* genes. For example, Rubinchik et al. constructed an adenovector expressing FasL-GFP fusion gene under the control of a prostate-specific ARR2PB promoter via the tetracycline transactivator *(120)*. The FASL-GFP expression and apoptosis-induction from this vector is restricted to prostate cancer cells and can be regulated by doxycycline *(120)*. An in vivo study with this vector also showed that it was well tolerated at doses that were lethal for the vector in which the FASL-GFP is driven by the CMV promoter. Moreover, higher levels of prostate-specific FASL-GFP expression were generated by this approach than by driving the FASL-GFP expression directly with ARR2PB, suggesting that use of the tetracycline transactivator also enhanced transgene expression from a tumor- or tissue-specific promoter.

Targeted TNF gene therapy has also been reported with promoters responding to irradiation *(105,121)* or chemotherapeutic agents *(109)*, or to hypoxia and cytokines *(122)*. For example, treatment with adenovector expressing the TNF gene driven by the promoter of early growth response (Egr)-1 gene *(123)* combined with radiation produced occlusion of tumor microvessels without significant normal-tissue damage *(121)*.

In addition to targeted death ligands gene therapy, there are also several reports that have used constitutively active or chimeric death receptors for cancer gene therapy. Bazzoni et al. showed that chimeric receptors containing the extracellular domain of the mouse erythropoietin receptor and transmembrane and cytoplasmic domains of the mouse TNF receptors exerted a constitutive cytotoxic effect *(124)*. Adenovector expressing the constitutively active version of the 55-kDa TNF receptor driven by a melanoma-specific promoter/enhancer element elicits a high level of transgene expression and triggers apoptosis in melanoma cell lines but not in other cell types *(125)* . Alternatively, Quinn et al. constructed a chimeric receptor (VEGFR2Fas) consisting of the extracellular and transmembrane domains of vascular endothelial growth factor (VEGF) receptor and the cytoplasmic domain of Fas *(126)*. A similar chimeric receptor (Flk-1/Fas) was constructed by Carpenito et al. that is composed of the extracellular domain of the VEGF receptor Flk-1/KDR fused to the transmembrane and cytoplasmic domain of Fas *(127)*. When these receptors were stably expressed in endothelial cells in vitro, treatment with VEGF rapidly induced cell death with features characteristic of Fas-mediated apoptosis.

These findings raise the possibility that introduction of chimeric receptors of VEGF and FasL into tumor endothelium or tumor cells in vivo may convert tumor-derived VEGF from an angiogenic factor into an anticancer agent.

FUTURE PERSPECTIVE

The bystander effect and local inflammatory response elicited by death ligands and their receptors suggest that targeted expression of molecules involved in the receptor-mediated death pathway represent an interesting approach for cancer therapy, because it does not require that the therapeutic gene be delivered to 100% of malignant cells. Substantial data have revealed that systemic toxicity of death ligands can be minimized by targeted, tumor-selective transgene expression. However, much has to be improved before gene therapy can be used to benefit patients, especially those with metastatic tumors. Vectors for effective systemic gene delivery are not yet available. Thus, most current clinical trial protocols in cancer gene therapy used local and local-regional gene delivery that rarely affects metastatic tumors. Moreover, we have recently found that, like conventional chemotherapy and radiotherapy, repeated application of gene therapy may lead to development of resistance *(128)*. Resistance to vector transduction or to therapeutic gene products can all be associated. Thus, characterizing the mechanisms of resistance and developing strategies to overcome resistance are essential to ensure success of anticancer therapy with gene-based approaches. It is expected that developments in molecular biology and biotechnology will improve the efficacy of gene therapy by enhancing transduction efficiency, increasing target specificity, and overcoming resistance. Nevertheless, combination with other treatment modalities, including chemotherapy, radiotherapy, immunotherapy, and antiangiogenesis, is expected to be necessary for better clinical outcomes with gene therapy.

ACKNOWLEDGMENT

We thank Vickie J. Williams for editorial review and Carrie A Langford for assistance in preparation of this manuscript. This work was supported in part by grants from the NIH (RO1 CA92487-01A1) and from the American Cancer Society (RPG-00-274-01-MGO).

REFERENCE:

1. Bodmer JL, Schneider P, Tschopp J. The molecular architecture of the TNF superfamily. Trend Biochem Sci 2002;27:19–26.
2. Locksley RM, Killeen N, Lenardo MJ. The TNF and TNF receptor superfamilies: integrating mammalian biology. Cell 2001;104:487–501.
3. Chen G, Goeddel DV. TNF-R1 signaling: a beautiful pathway. Science 2002;296:1634–1635.
4. Brown TD, Goodman P, Fleming T, Macdonald JS, Hersh EM, Braun TJ. A phase II trial of recombinant tumor necrosis factor in patients with adenocarcinoma of the pancreas: a Southwest Oncology Group study. J Immunother 1991;10:376–378.
5. Kemeny N, Childs B, Larchian W, Rosado K, Kelsen D. A phase II trial of recombinant tumor necrosis factor in patients with advanced colorectal carcinoma. Cancer 1990;66:659–663.
6. Ogasawara J, Watanabe-Fukunaga R, Adachi M, et al. Lethal effect of the anti-Fas antibody in mice. Nature 1993;364:806–809.
7. Jo M, Kim TH, Seol DW, et al. Apoptosis induced in normal human hepatocytes by tumor necrosis factor-related apoptosis-inducing ligand. Nat Med 2000;6:564–567.

8. Nitsch R, Bechmann I, Deisz RA, et al. Human brain-cell death induced by tumour-necrosis-factor-related apoptosis-inducing ligand (TRAIL). Lancet 2000;356:827–828.
9. Zamai L, Secchiero P, Pierpaoli S, et al. TNF-related apoptosis-inducing ligand (TRAIL) as a negative regulator of normal human erythropoiesis. Blood 2000;95:3716–3724.
10. Lawrence D, Shahrokh Z, Marsters S, et al. Differential hepatocyte toxicity of recombinant Apo2L/TRAIL versions. Nat Med 2001;7:383–385.
11. Roth JA, Grammer SF, Swisher SG, et al. Gene therapy approaches for the management of non-small cell lung cancer. Seminar Oncol 2001;28:50–56.
12. Smith AE. Viral vectors in gene therapy. Ann Rev Microbiol 1995;49:807–838.
13. Kovesdi I, Brough DE, Bruder JT, Wickham TJ. Adenoviral vectors for gene transfer. Cur Opinion Biotech 1997;8:583–589.
14. Wickham TJ. Targeting adenovirus. Gene Ther 2000;7:110–114.
15. Barnett BG, Crews CJ, Douglas JT. Targeted adenoviral vectors. Biochim Biophys Acta 2002;1575:1–14.
16. Douglas JT, Rogers BE, Rosenfeld ME, Michael SI, Feng M, Curiel DT. Targeted gene delivery by tropism-modified adenoviral vectors. Nat Biotech 1996;14:1574–1578.
17. Gu DL, Gonzalez AM, Printz MA, et al. Fibroblast growth factor 2 retargeted adenovirus has redirected cellular tropism: evidence for reduced toxicity and enhanced antitumor activity in mice. Cancer Res 1999;59:2608–2614.
18. Goldman CK, Rogers BE, Douglas JT, et al. Targeted gene delivery to Kaposi's sarcoma cells via the fibroblast growth factor receptor. Cancer Res 1997;57:1447–1451.
19. Van Beusechem VW, Grill J, Mastenbroek DC, et al. Efficient and selective gene transfer into primary human brain tumors by using single-chain antibody-targeted adenoviral vectors with native tropism abolished. J Virol 2002;76:2753–2762.
20. Miller CR, Buchsbaum DJ, Reynolds PN, et al. Differential susceptibility of primary and established human glioma cells to adenovirus infection: targeting via the epidermal growth factor receptor achieves fiber receptor-independent gene transfer. Cancer Res 1998;58:5738–5748.
21. Nettelbeck DM, Miller DW, Jerome V, et al. Targeting of adenovirus to endothelial cells by a bispecific single-chain diabody directed against the adenovirus fiber knob domain and human endoglin (CD105). Mol Ther 2001;3:882–891.
22. Wesseling JG, Bosma PJ, Krasnykh V, et al. Improved gene transfer efficiency to primary and established human pancreatic carcinoma target cells via epidermal growth factor receptor and integrin-targeted adenoviral vectors. Gene Ther 2001;8:969–976.
23. Dmitriev I, Kashentseva E, Rogers BE, Krasnykh V, Curiel DT. Ectodomain of coxsackievirus and adenovirus receptor genetically fused to epidermal growth factor mediates adenovirus targeting to epidermal growth factor receptor-positive cells. J Virol 2000;74:6875–6884.
24. Stevenson SC, Rollence M, Marshall-Neff J, McClelland A. Selective targeting of human cells by a chimeric adenovirus vector containing a modified fiber protein. J Virol 1997;71:4782–4790.
25. Yotnda P, Onishi H, Heslop HE, et al. Efficient infection of primitive hematopoietic stem cells by modified adenovirus. Gene Ther 2001;8:930–937.
26. Wickham TJ, Roelvink PW, Brough DE, Kovesdi I. Adenovirus targeted to heparan-containing receptors increases its gene delivery efficiency to multiple cell types. Nat Biotech 1996;14:1570–1573.
27. Pearson AS, Koch PE, Atkinson N, et al. Factors limiting adenovirus-mediated gene transfer into human lung and pancreatic cancer cell lines. Clin Cancer Res 1999;5:4208–4213.
28. Wickham TJ, Tzeng E, Shears LL 2nd, et al. Increased in vitro and in vivo gene transfer by adenovirus vectors containing chimeric fiber proteins. J Virol 1997;71:8221–8229.
29. Dmitriev I, Krasnykh V, Miller CR, et al. An adenovirus vector with genetically modified fibers demonstrates expanded tropism via utilization of a coxsackievirus and adenovirus receptor-independent cell entry mechanism. J Virol 1998;72:9706–9713.
30. Lamfers ML, Grill J, Dirven CM, et al. Potential of the conditionally replicative adenovirus Ad5-Delta24RGD in the treatment of malignant gliomas and its enhanced effect with radiotherapy. Cancer Res 2002;62:5736–5742.
31. Asada-Mikami R, Heike Y, Kanai S, et al. Efficient gene transduction by RGD-fiber modified recombinant adenovirus into dendritic cells. Japan J Cancer Res 2001;92:321–327.
32. Kasahara N, Dozy AM, Kan YW. Tissue-specific targeting of retroviral vectors through ligand-receptor interactions. Science 1994;266:1373–1376.
33. Gollan TJ, Green MR. Selective targeting and inducible destruction of human cancer cells by retroviruses with envelope proteins bearing short peptide ligands. J Virol 2002;76:3564–3569.

34. Martin F, Chowdhury S, Neil S, Phillipps N, Collins MK. Envelope-targeted retrovirus vectors transduce melanoma xenografts but not spleen or liver. Mol Ther 2002;5:269–274.
35. Cosset FL, Morling FJ, Takeuchi Y, Weiss RA, Collins MK, Russell SJ. Retroviral retargeting by envelopes expressing an N-terminal binding domain. J Virol 1995;69:6314–6322.
36. Wolschek MF, Thallinger C, Kursa M, et al. Specific systemic nonviral gene delivery to human hepatocellular carcinoma xenografts in SCID mice. Hepatol 2002;36:1106–1114.
37. Arap W, Pasqualini R, Ruoslahti E. Cancer treatment by targeted drug delivery to tumor vasculature in a mouse model. Science 1998;279:377–380.
38. Koivunen E, Arap W, Valtanen H, et al. Tumor targeting with a selective gelatinase inhibitor. Nat Biotech 1999;17:768–774.
39. Nicklin SA, White SJ, Watkins SJ, Hawkins RE, Baker AH. Selective targeting of gene transfer to vascular endothelial cells by use of peptides isolated by phage display. Circulation 2000;102:231–237.
40. Kolonin M, Pasqualini R, Arap W. Molecular addresses in blood vessels as targets for therapy. Curr Opinion Chem Biol 2001;5:308–313.
41. Pasqualini R, Koivunen E, Ruoslahti E. A peptide isolated from phage display libraries is a structural and functional mimic of an RGD-binding site on integrins. J Cell Biol 1995;130:1189–1196.
42. Pasqualini R, Koivunen E, Kain R, et al. Aminopeptidase N is a receptor for tumor-homing peptides and a target for inhibiting angiogenesis. Cancer Res 2000;60:722–727.
43. Liu L, Anderson WF, Beart RW, Gordon EM, Hall FL. Incorporation of tumor vasculature targeting motifs into moloney murine leukemia virus env escort proteins enhances retrovirus binding and transduction of human endothelial cells. J Virol 2000;74:5320–5328.
44. Roelvink PW, Mi LG, Einfeld DA, Kovesdi I, Wickham TJ. Identification of a conserved receptor-binding site on the fiber proteins of CAR-recognizing adenoviridae. Science 1999;286:1568–1571.
45. Pizzato M, Blair ED, Fling M, et al. Evidence for nonspecific adsorption of targeted retrovirus vector particles to cells. Gene Ther 2001;8:1088–1096.
46. Leissner P, Legrand V, Schlesinger Y, et al. Influence of adenoviral fiber mutations on viral encapsidation, infectivity and in vivo tropism. Gene Ther 2001;8:49–57.
47. Nettelbeck DM, Jerome V, Muller R. Gene therapy: designer promoters for tumour targeting. Trend Genet 2000;16:174–181.
48. Clary BM, Lyerly HK. Transcriptional targeting for cancer gene therapy. Surg Oncol Clinic North Am 1998;7:565–574.
49. Osaki T, Tanio Y, Tachibana I, et al. Gene therapy for carcinoembryonic antigen-producing human lung cancer cells by cell type-specific expression of herpes simplex virus thymidine kinase gene. Cancer Res 1994;54:5258–5261.
50. Richards CA, Austin EA, Huber BE. Transcriptional regulatory sequences of carcinoembryonic antigen: identification and use with cytosine deaminase for tumor-specific gene therapy. Hum Gene Ther 1995;6:881–893.
51. Ido A, Nakata K, Kato Y, et al. Gene therapy for hepatoma cells using a retrovirus vector carrying herpes simplex virus thymidine kinase gene under the control of human alpha-fetoprotein gene promoter. Cancer Res 1995;55:3105–3109.
52. Kaneko S, Hallenbeck P, Kotani T, et al. Adenovirus-mediated gene therapy of hepatocellular carcinoma using cancer-specific gene expression. Cancer Res 1995;55:5283–5287.
53. Andriani F, Nan B, Yu J, et al. Use of the probasin promoter ARR2PB to express Bax in androgen receptor-positive prostate cancer cells. J Natl Cancer Inst 2001;93:1314–1324.
54. Gotoh A, Ko SC, Shirakawa T, et al. Development of prostate-specific antigen promoter-based gene therapy for androgen-independent human prostate cancer. J Urol 1998;160:220–229.
55. Chen L, Chen D, Manome Y, Dong Y, Fine HA, Kufe DW. Breast cancer selective gene expression and therapy mediated by recombinant adenoviruses containing the DF3/MUC1 promoter. J Clin Invest 1995;96:2775–2782.
56. Parr MJ, Manome Y, Tanaka T, et al. Tumor-selective transgene expression in vivo mediated by an E2F-responsive adenoviral vector. Nat Med 1997;3:1145–1149.
57. Morin GB. The human telomere terminal transferase enzyme is a ribonucleoprotein that synthesizes TTAGGG repeats. Cell 1989;59:521–529.
58. Blackburn EH. Telomerases. Ann Rev Biochem 1992;61:113–129.
59. Harley CB, Futcher AB, Greider CW. Telomeres shorten during ageing of human fibroblasts. Nature 1990;345:458–460.

60. Kim NW, Piatyszek MA, Prowse KR, et al. Specific association of human telomerase activity with immortal cells and cancer. Science 1994;266:2011–2015.
61. Counter CM, Avilion AA, LeFeuvre CE, et al. Telomere shortening associated with chromosome instability is arrested in immortal cells which express telomerase activity. EMBO J 1992;11:1921–1929.
62. Shay JW, Bacchetti S. A survey of telomerase activity in human cancer. European Journal of Cancer 1997;33:787–791.
63. Nakamura TM, Morin GB, Chapman KB, et al. Telomerase catalytic subunit homologs from fission yeast and human. Science 1997;277:955–959.
64. Holt SE, Aisner DL, Shay JW, Wright WE. Lack of cell cycle regulation of telomerase activity in human cells. Proc Natl Acad Sci USA 1997;94:10,687–10,692.
65. Bodnar AG, Ouellette M, Frolkis M, et al. Extension of life-span by introduction of telomerase into normal human cells. Science 1998;279:349–352.
66. Toouli CD, Huschtscha LI, Neumann AA, et al. Comparison of human mammary epithelial cells immortalized by simian virus 40 T-antigen or by the telomerase catalytic subunit. Oncogene 2002;21:128–139.
67. Elenbaas B, Spirio L, Koerner F, et al. Human breast cancer cells generated by oncogenic transformation of primary mammary epithelial cells. Gene Develop 2001;15:50–65.
68. Hahn WC, Counter CM, Lundberg AS, Beijersbergen RL, Brooks MW, Weinberg RA. Creation of human tumour cells with defined genetic elements. Nature 1999;400:464–468.
69. Takakura M, Kyo S, Kanaya T, et al. Cloning of human telomerase catalytic subunit (hTERT) gene promoter and identification of proximal core promoter sequence essential for transcriptional activation in immortalized and cancer cells. Cancer Res 1999;59:551–557.
70. Horikawa I, Cable PL, Afshari C, Barrett JC. Cloning and characterization of the promoter region of human telomerase reverse transcriptase gene. Cancer Res 1999;59:826–830.
71. Wu KJ, Grandori C, Amacker M, et al. Direct activation of TERT transcription by c-MYC. Nat Genet 1999;21:220–224.
72. Abdul-Ghani R, Ohana P, Matouk I, et al. Use of transcriptional regulatory sequences of telomerase (hTER and hTERT) for selective killing of cancer cells. Mol Ther 2000;2:539–544.
73. Gu J, Kagawa S, Takakura M, et al. Tumor-specific transgene expression from the human telomerase reverse transcriptase promoter enables targeting of the therapeutic effects of the *Bax* gene to cancers. Cancer Res 2000;60:5359–5364.
74. Komata T, Kondo Y, Kanzawa T, et al. Treatment of malignant glioma cells with the transfer of constitutively active caspase-6 using the human telomerase catalytic subunit (human telomerase reverse transcriptase) gene promoter. Cancer Res 2001;61:5796–5802.
75. Gu J, Andreeff M, Roth JA, Fang B. hTERT promoter induces tumor-specific *Bax* gene expression and cell killing in syngenic mouse tumor model and prevents systemic toxicity. Gene Ther 2002;9:30–37.
76. Gu J, Zhang L, Huang X, et al. A novel single tetracycline-regulative adenoviral vector for tumor-specific Bax gene expression and cell killing in vitro and in vivo. Oncogene 2002;21:4757–4764.
77. Huang X, Lin T, Gu J, et al. Combined TRAIL and Bax gene therapy prolonged survival in mice with ovarian cancer xenograft. Gene Ther 2002;9:1379–1386.
78. Lin T, Gu J, Zhang L, et al. Targeted expression of green fluorescent protein/tumor necrosis factor-related apoptosis-inducing ligand fusion protein from human telomerase reverse transcriptase promoter elicits antitumor activity without toxic effect on primary human hepatocytes. Cancer Res 2002;62:3620–3625.
79. Lin T, Huang X, Gu J, et al. Long-term tumor-free survival from treatment with the GFP-TRAIL fusion gene expressed from the hTERT promoter in breast cancer cells. Oncogene 2002;21:8020–8028.
80. Koga S, Hirohata S, Kondo Y, et al. A novel telomerase-specific gene therapy: gene transfer of caspase-8 utilizing the human telomerase catalytic subunit gene promoter. Hum Gene Ther 2000;11:1397–1406.
81. Koga S, Hirohata S, Kondo Y, et al. FADD gene therapy using the human telomerase catalytic subunit (hTERT) gene promoter to restrict induction of apoptosis to tumors in vitro and in vivo. Anticancer Res 2001;21:1937–1943.
82. Nagayama Y, Nishihara E, Iitaka M, Namba H, Yamashita S, Niwa M. Enhanced efficacy of transcriptionally targeted suicide gene/prodrug therapy for thyroid carcinoma with the Cre-loxP system. Cancer Res 1999;59:3049–3052.
83. Ueda K, Iwahashi M, Nakamori M, Nakamura M, Yamaue H, Tanimura H. Enhanced selective gene expression by adenovirus vector using Cre/loxP regulation system for human carcinoembryonic antigen-producing carcinoma. Oncology 2000;59:255–265.

84. Nettelbeck DM, Jerome V, Muller R. A strategy for enhancing the transcriptional activity of weak cell type-specific promoters. Gene Ther 1998;5:1656–1664.
85. Borovjagin AV, Ezrokhi MV, Rostapshov VM, Ugarova TY, Bystrova TF, Shatsky IN. RNA-protein interactions within the internal translation initiation region of encephalomyocarditis virus RNA. Nucleic Acid Res 1991;19:4999–5005.
86. Sadowski I, Ma J, Triezenberg S, Ptashne M. GAL4-VP16 is an unusually potent transcriptional activator. Nature 1988;335:563–564.
87. Gossen M, Bujard H. Tight control of gene expression in mammalian cells by tetracycline-responsive promoters. Proc Natl Acad Sci USA 1992;89:5547–5551.
88. Koch P, Guo ZS, Kagawa S, Gu J, Roth JA, Fang B. Augmenting transgene expression from carcinoembryonic antigen (CEA) promoter via a GAL4 gene regulatory system. Mol Ther 2001;3: 278–283.
89. Wiley SR, Schooley K, Smolak PJ, et al. Identification and characterization of a new member of the TNF family that induces apoptosis. Immunity 1995;3:673–682.
90. Pitti RM, Marsters SA, Ruppert S, Donahue CJ, Moore A, Ashkenazi A. Induction of apoptosis by Apo-2 ligand, a new member of the tumor necrosis factor cytokine family. J Biol Chem 1996;271:12,687–12,690.
91. Walczak H, Miller RE, Ariail K, et al. Tumoricidal activity of tumor necrosis factor-related apoptosis-inducing ligand in vivo. Nat Med 1999;5:157–163.
92. Ashkenazi A, Pai RC, Fong S, et al. Safety and antitumor activity of recombinant soluble Apo2 ligand. J Clin Invest 1999;104:155–162.
93. Griffith TS, Anderson RD, Davidson BL, Williams RD, Ratliff TL. Adenoviral-mediated transfer of the TNF-related apoptosis-inducing ligand/Apo-2 ligand gene induces tumor cell apoptosis. J Immunol 2000;165:2886–2894.
94. Kagawa S, He C, Gu J, et al. Antitumor activity and bystander effects of the tumor necrosis factor-related apoptosis-inducing ligand (*TRAIL*) gene. Cancer Res 2001;61:3330–3338.
95. Mariani SM, Matiba B, Armandola EA, Krammer PH. Interleukin 1 beta-converting enzyme related proteases/caspases are involved in TRAIL-induced apoptosis of myeloma and leukemia cells. J Cell Biol 1997;137:221–229.
96. Mariani SM, Krammer PH. Differential regulation of TRAIL and CD95 ligand in transformed cells of the T and B lymphocyte lineage. Eur J Immunol 1998;28:973–982.
97. Gores GJ, Kaufmann SH. Is TRAIL hepatotoxic? Hepatol 2001;34:3–6.
98. Kagawa S, Gu J, Honda T, et al. Deficiency of caspase-3 in MCF7 cells blocks Bax-mediated nuclear fragmentation but not cell death. Clin Cancer Res 2001;7:1474–1480.
99. Voelkel-Johnson C, King DL, Norris JS. Resistance of prostate cancer cells to soluble TNF-related apoptosis-inducing ligand (TRAIL/Apo2L) can be overcome by doxorubicin or adenoviral delivery of full-length TRAIL. Cancer Gene Ther 2002;9:164–172.
100. Seino K, Kayagaki N, Okumura K, Yagita H. Antitumor effect of locally produced CD95 ligand. Nat Med 1997;3:165–170.
101. Aoki K, Akyurek LM, San H, et al. Restricted expression of an adenoviral vector encoding Fas ligand (CD95L) enhances safety for cancer gene therapy. Mol Ther 2000;1:555–565.
102. Arai H, Gordon D, Nabel EG, Nabel GJ. Gene transfer of Fas ligand induces tumor regression in vivo. Proc Natl Acad Sci USA 1997;94:13,862–13,867.
103. Hyer ML, Voelkel-Johnson C, Rubinchik S, Dong J, Norris JS. Intracellular Fas ligand expression causes Fas-mediated apoptosis in human prostate cancer cells resistant to monoclonal antibody-induced apoptosis. Mol Ther 2000;2:348–358.
104. Rubinchik S, Ding R, Qiu AJ, Zhang F, Dong J. Adenoviral vector which delivers FasL-GFP fusion protein regulated by the tet-inducible expression system. Gene Ther 2000;7:875–885.
105. Chung TD, Mauceri HJ, Hallahan DE, et al. Tumor necrosis factor-alpha-based gene therapy enhances radiation cytotoxicity in human prostate cancer. Cancer Gene Ther 1998;5:344–349.
106. Jerome V, Muller R. Tissue-specific, cell cycle-regulated chimeric transcription factors for the targeting of gene expression to tumor cells. Hum Gene Ther 1998;9:2653–2659.
107. Mizuguchi H, Nakagawa T, Toyosawa S, et al. Tumor necrosis factor alpha-mediated tumor regression by the in vivo transfer of genes into the artery that leads to tumors. Cancer Res 1998;58:5725–5730.
108. Staba MJ, Mauceri HJ, Kufe DW, Hallahan DE, Weichselbaum RR. Adenoviral TNF-alpha gene therapy and radiation damage tumor vasculature in a human malignant glioma xenograft. Gene Ther 1998;5:293–300.

109. Walther W, Wendt J, Stein U. Employment of the mdr1 promoter for the chemotherapy-inducible expression of therapeutic genes in cancer gene therapy. Gene Ther 1997;4:544–552.
110. Wright P, Braun R, Babiuk L, et al. Adenovirus-mediated TNF-alpha gene transfer induces significant tumor regression in mice. Cancer Biother Radiopharm 1999;14:49–57.
111. Gautam SC, Xu YX, Pindolia KR, Yegappan R, Janakiraman N, Chapman RA. TNF-alpha gene therapy with myeloid progenitor cells lacks the toxicities of systemic TNF-alpha therapy. J Hematother 1999;8:237–245.
112. Hofmann A, Blau HM. Death of solid tumor cells induced by Fas ligand expressing primary myoblasts. Som Cell Mol Genet 1997;23:249–257.
113. Gearing AJ, Beckett P, Christodoulou M, et al. Processing of tumour necrosis factor-alpha precursor by metalloproteinases. Nature 1994;370:555–557.
114. Black RA, Rauch CT, Kozlosky CJ, et al. A metalloproteinase disintegrin that releases tumour-necrosis factor-alpha from cells. Nature 1997;385:729–733.
115. Powell WC, Fingleton B, Wilson CL, Boothby M, Matrisian LM. The metalloproteinase matrilysin proteolytically generates active soluble Fas ligand and potentiates epithelial cell apoptosis. Curr Biol 1999;9:1441–1447.
116. Hersh EM, Metch BS, Muggia FM, et al. Phase II studies of recombinant human tumor necrosis factor alpha in patients with malignant disease: a summary of the Southwest Oncology Group experience. J Immunother 1991;10:426–431.
117. Schneider P, Holler N, Bodmer JL, et al. Conversion of membrane-bound Fas(CD95) ligand to its soluble form is associated with downregulation of its proapoptotic activity and loss of liver toxicity. J Exp Med 1998;187:1205–1213.
118. Tanaka M, Suda T, Yatomi T, Nakamura N, Nagata S. Lethal effect of recombinant human Fas ligand in mice pretreated with Propionibacterium acnes. J Immunol 1997;158:2303–2309.
119. Marr RA, Addison CL, Snider D, Muller WJ, Gauldie J, Graham FL. Tumour immunotherapy using an adenoviral vector expressing a membrane-bound mutant of murine TNF alpha. Gene Ther 1997;4:1181–1188.
120. Rubinchik S, Wang D, Yu H, et al. A complex adenovirus vector that delivers FASL-GFP with combined prostate-specific and tetracycline-regulated expression. Mol Ther 2001;4:416–426.
121. Mauceri HJ, Hanna NN, Wayne JD, Hallahan DE, Hellman S, Weichselbaum RR. Tumor necrosis factor alpha (TNF-alpha) gene therapy targeted by ionizing radiation selectively damages tumor vasculature. Cancer Res 1996;56:4311–4314.
122. Modlich U, Pugh CW, Bicknell R. Increasing endothelial cell specific expression by the use of heterologous hypoxic and cytokine-inducible enhancers. Gene Ther 2000;7:896–902.
123. Datta R, Rubin E, Sukhatme V, et al. Ionizing radiation activates transcription of the EGR1 gene via CArG elements. Proc Natl Acad Sci USA 1992;89:10,149–10,153.
124. Bazzoni F, Alejos E, Beutler B. Chimeric tumor necrosis factor receptors with constitutive signaling activity. Proc Natl Acad Sci USA 1995;92:5376–5380.
125. Bazzoni F, Regalia E. Triggering of antitumor activity through melanoma-specific transduction of a constitutively active tumor necrosis factor (TNF) R1 chimeric receptor in the absence of TNF-alpha. Cancer Res 2001;61:1050–1057.
126. Quinn TP, Soifer SJ, Ramer K, Williams LT, Nakamura MC. A receptor for vascular endothelial growth factor that stimulates endothelial apoptosis. Cancer Res 2001;61:8629–8637.
127. Carpenito C, Davis PD, Dougherty ST, Dougherty GJ. Exploiting the differential production of angiogenic factors within the tumor microenvironment in the design of a novel vascular-targeted gene therapy-based approach to the treatment of cancer. Int J Rad Oncol Biol Phys 2002;54:1473–1478.
128. Zhang L, Gu J, Lin T, Huang X, Roth JA, Fang B. Mechanisms involved in development of resistance to adenovirus-mediated proapoptotic gene therapy in DLD1 human colon cancer cell line. Gene Ther 2002;9:1262–1270.

21 Combination of Chemotherapy and Death Ligands in Cancer Therapy

Simone Fulda, MD,
and Klaus-Michael Debatin, MD

SUMMARY

Killing of cancer cells by diverse cytotoxic therapies including chemotherapy, γ-irradiation, or immunotherapy is predominantly mediated by induction of apoptosis, the cell's intrinsic death program. Failure to undergo apoptosis in response to anticancer therapy may result in resistance. Signaling through death receptors has been implicated to contribute to the efficacy of cancer therapy. Importantly, combined treatment with chemotherapy together with death ligands resulted in enhanced antitumor activity and may even overcome some forms of resistance. Understanding the molecular events that regulate apoptosis induced by anticancer therapy or by death ligands may provide new opportunities for drug development. Thus, novel strategies targeting tumor cell resistance will be based on further insights into the molecular mechanisms of cell death.

INTRODUCTION

Apoptosis, a distinct, intrinsic cell-death program, occurs in various physiological and pathological situations and has an important regulatory function in tissue homeostasis and immune regulation *(1,2)*. Apoptosis is characterized by typical morphological and biochemical hallmarks including cell shrinkage, nuclear DNA fragmentation, and membrane blebbing. Various stimuli can trigger an apoptosis response, e.g., withdrawal of growth factors or stimulation of cell-surface receptors *(1,2)*. Also, killing of tumor cells by diverse cytotoxic strategies, such as anticancer drugs, γ-irradiation, or immunotherapy, has been shown to involve induction of apoptosis in target cells *(3–9)*. The mechanisms responsible for triggering apoptosis in response to cytotoxic treatments may differ for different stimuli, and have not exactly been delineated. However, damage to DNA or to other critical molecules is considered to be a common primary event, which initiates a cellular stress response *(10)*. Various stress-inducible molecules, including JNK, MAPK/

From: *Cancer Drug Discovery and Development: Death Receptors in Cancer Therapy*
Edited by: W. S. El-Deiry © Humana Press Inc., Totowa, NJ

ERK, NFκB, or ceramide, have been implicated in the regulation of apoptosis *(10–13)*. Also, T-cells or natural killer (NK) cells may release cytotoxic compounds such as granzyme B that can directly initiate apoptosis effector pathways inside the cell *(2)*. Proteolytic enzymes called caspases are important effector molecules of different forms of cell death *(14,15)*. Apoptosis pathways are tightly controlled by a number of inhibitory and promoting factors *(16)*. The antiapoptotic mechanisms regulating apoptotic cell death have also been implicated in conferring drug resistance to tumor cells *(4)*. Importantly, combinations of anticancer agents together with death-inducing ligands have been shown to synergize in triggering apoptosis in cancer cells and may even overcome some forms of drug resistance *(3–7)*. Further insights into the mechanisms controlling tumor cell death in response to cytotoxic therapies or death receptor ligation will provide a molecular basis for novel strategies targeting death pathways in apoptosis-resistant forms of cancer.

APOPTOSIS SIGNALING PATHWAYS IN CANCER THERAPY

In most cases, anticancer therapies eventually result in activation of caspases, a family of cysteine proteases that act as common death effector molecules in various forms of cell death *(14,15)*. Caspases are synthesized as inactive proforms, and upon activation, they cleave next to aspartate residues *(14,15)*. The fact that caspases can activate each other by cleavage at identical sequences results in amplification of caspase activity through a protease cascade *(14,15)*.

Caspases cleave a number of different substrates in the cytoplasm or nucleus, leading to many of the morphologic features of apoptotic cell death *(14,15)*. For example, polynucleosomal DNA fragmentation is mediated by cleavage of inhibitor of caspase-activated DNase (ICAD), the inhibitor of the endonuclease caspase-activated DNase (CAD) that cleaves DNA into the characteristic oligomeric fragments *(17)*. Likewise, proteolysis of several cytoskeletal proteins such as actin or fodrin leads to loss of overall cell shape, while degradation of lamin results in nuclear shrinking *(1)*.

Activation of caspases can be initiated from different angles, e.g., at the plasma membrane upon ligation of death receptor (receptor pathway) or at the mitochondria (mitochondrial pathway) *(18)*. Stimulation of death receptors of the tumor necrosis factor (TNF) receptor superfamily, such as CD95 (APO-1/Fas) or TNF-related apoptosis-inducing ligand (TRAIL) receptors, results in activation of the initiator caspase-8, which can propagate the apoptosis signal by direct cleavage of downstream effector caspases such as caspase-3 *(19)*. The mitochondrial pathway is initiated by the release of apoptogenic factors such as cytochrome c, apoptosis inducing factor (AIF), Smac/DIABLO, Omi/HtrA2, endonuclease G, caspase-2, or caspase-9 from the mitochondrial intermembrane space *(20)*. The release of cytochrome c into the cytosol triggers caspase-3 activation through formation of the cytochrome c/Apaf-1/caspase-9-containing apoptosome complex, while Smac/DIABLO and Omi/HtrA2 promote caspase activation through neutralizing the inhibitory effects to IAPs *(20)*.

Links between the receptor and the mitochondrial pathway exist at different levels *(21,22)*. Upon death receptor triggering, activation of caspase-8 may result in cleavage of Bid, a Bcl-2 family protein with a BH3 domain only, which in turn translocates to mitochondria to release cytochrome c, thereby initiating a mitochondrial amplification loop *(21)*. In addition, cleavage of caspase-6 downstream of mitochondria may feed back to the receptor pathway by cleaving caspase-8 *(22)*.

DEATH RECEPTORS AND THEIR LIGANDS

Death receptors belong to the TNF/nerve growth factor (NGF) superfamily of cell-surface receptors, which is defined by several similar, cysteine-rich extracellular domains *(2,19,23–25)*. They also contain a homologous cytoplasmic protein motif, termed the *death domain*, which typically enables death receptors to engage the cell's apoptotic machinery *(23–25)*. Death receptors play an essential role in cell turnover and tissue homeostasis through the regulation of apoptosis *(23–25)*. Currently, six different death receptors have been identified, including CD95 (APO-1/Fas), TNF receptor type I (TNFRI), death receptor (DR)3 (TRAMP), TRAIL-R1 (DR4), TRAIL-R2 (DR5), and DR6 *(23–25)*. The CD95, TNF, and TRAIL receptors have been studied extensively, while the role of DR3 and DR6 has not exactly been defined *(23–25)*.

Death receptors are activated upon binding by their cognate ligands *(2,19,23–25)*. Death receptor ligands include CD95L, TRAIL, TNF-α and lymphotoxinα (both binding to TNFRI), and TWEAK, which activates DR3 *(23–25)*. One common feature of death-receptor ligands is that all ligands except lymphotoxin-α are type II transmembrane proteins that are synthesized as membrane-bound molecules and can be cleaved by specific metalloprotesases to generate soluble ligands *(2,23–25)*.

CD95

The CD95 receptor/CD95 ligand system has been described as a key signaling pathway involved in the regulation of apoptosis in several different cell types *(2,19)*. CD95, a 48-kDa type I transmembrane receptor, is expressed in activated lymphocytes, in a variety of tissues of lymphoid or nonlymphoid origin, as well as in tumor cells *(2,19)*. CD95L, a 40-kDa type II transmembrane molecule, occurs in a membrane-bound and in a soluble form generated through cleavage by specific metalloprotesases *(2)*. CD95L is produced by activated T-cells and plays a crucial role in the regulation of the immune system by triggering autocrine suicide or paracrine death in neighboring lymphocytes or other target cells *(2)*. Also, constitutive expression of CD95L on cancer cells has been implicated as a mechanism of immune escape of tumors *(26,27)*. By constitutive expression of death receptor ligands such as CD95L on the cell's surface, tumors may adopt a killing mechanism from cytotoxic lymphocytes to delete the attacking antitumor T-cells through induction of apoptosis via CD95/CD95L interaction *(27)*. However, this model of tumor counterattack has also been challenged, since no study has so far conclusively demonstrated that tumor counterattack by CD95L expression is a relevant immune escape mechanism in vivo *(27)*.

TRAIL

TRAIL is constitutively expressed in many tissues, as are the agonistic TRAIL receptors TRAIL-R1 and TRAIL-R2 *(19,28–30)*. Similar to CD95L, TRAIL rapidly triggers apoptosis in many tumor cell lines. The TRAIL ligand and its signaling pathway is of special interest for cancer therapy, since TRAIL has been shown to predominantly kill cancer cells, while sparing normal cells *(19,28–30)*. The underlying mechanisms for this differential sensitivity of malignant versus non-malignant cells have not exactly been defined. One possible mechanism of protection of normal tissues may be based on a set of antagonistic decoy receptors, which compete with the agonistic TRAIL receptors TRAIL-R1 and TRAIL-R2 for binding to TRAIL *(28,29)*. However, screening of various tumor cell types and normal cells did not reveal a consistent association between TRAIL sensitivity and TRAIL receptor expression *(28,29)*. Therefore, susceptibility for TRAIL-induced cytotoxicity has been suggested to be regulated intracellularly by distinct patterns of pro- and antiapoptotic molecules.

DEATH RECEPTOR SIGNALING

Ligation of death receptors such as CD95 or TRAIL receptors by their cognate ligands or agonistic antibodies results in receptor trimerization, clustering of the receptors' death domains, and recruitment of adaptor molecules such as Fas-associated death domain protein (FADD) through homophilic interaction mediated by the death domain *(2,19,23–25,28–31)*. FADD in turn recruits caspase-8 to the activated CD95 receptor to form the CD95 death-inducing signaling complex (DISC) *(24)*. Oligomerization of caspase-8 upon DISC formation drives its activation through self-cleavage *(24)*. Caspase-8 then activates downstream effector caspases such as caspase-3. In addition to activation at the DISC, caspase-8 can also be activated downstream of mitochondria, e.g., by caspase-6, depending on the cell type and/or apoptotic stimulus *(24)*. For the CD95 signaling pathway, two distinct prototypic cell types have been identified *(32)*. In type I cells, caspase-8 is activated upon death receptor ligation at the DISC in quantities sufficient to directly activate downstream effector caspases such as caspase-3 *(32)*. In type II cells, however, the amount of active caspase-8 generated at the DISC is insufficient to activate caspase-3 *(32)*. In these cells, a mitochondrial amplification loop is required for full activation of caspases, involving Bid, which translocates to mitochondria upon cleavage by caspase-8 to trigger the release of apoptogenic proteins such as cytochrome c from mitochondria into the cytosol *(32)*. Accordingly, CD95-induced apoptosis is blocked by overexpression of Bcl-2 or Bcl-X_L, which inhibit mitochondrial alterations only in type II, but not in type I cells *(32)*.

DEATH RECEPTORS IN CANCER AND CANCER THERAPY

The idea to specifically target death receptors to trigger apoptosis in tumor cells is attractive for cancer therapy, since death receptors have a direct link to the cell's death machinery. In addition, apoptosis upon death receptor ligation has been reported to occur independent of the p53 tumor suppressor gene, which is deleted or inactivated in more than half of human tumors *(30)*. However, the clinical application of CD95L or TNFα is hampered by severe toxic side effects *(23,25)*. Systemic administration of TNF-α or CD95L causes a severe inflammatory response syndrome or massive liver-cell apoptosis, respectively. In contrast, TRAIL appears to be a relatively safe and promising death ligand for clinical application, although some concerns about potential toxic side effects on human hepatocytes or brain tissue have recently been raised *(28,29)*.

CD95 and Cancer Therapy

The CD95 system has been implicated in chemotherapy-induced tumor cell death in a number of studies *(33–47)*. Expression of CD95L was found to be up-regulated upon treatment with anticancer drugs *(33–42,46)*. In turn, CD95L then triggered the CD95 pathway in an autocrine or paracrine manner by binding to its receptor, CD95. In support of this concept, an increase of CD95L mRNA and protein expression was found in a variety of different tumor cell lines derived from leukemia, neuroblastoma, malignant brain tumors, hepatoma, colon, breast, or small lung cell carcinoma cells in vitro *(33–42)*. Upregulation of CD95L upon chemotherapy was also observed ex vivo in primary, patient-derived tumor cells *(33,36)*. Various anticancer agents with different primary intracellular targets have been used in these studies, including DNA-damaging agents such as doxorubicin, etoposide, cisplatin, or bleomycin *(33–42)*. The increase in CD95L transcription and mRNA levels by cytotoxic drugs was related to activation of the transcription factors AP-1 and NF-κB *(44,45)*. AP-1 and NF-κB binding sites were identified in the human CD95L promoter, which respond to DNA damage or inhibition of DNA metabolism by upregulating NF-κB activity *(44,45)*. In addition, CD95 expression on the cell's surface increased upon drug treatment, in particular in cells harboring wild-type p53 *(41,42)*. Accordingly, p53-responsive elements were identified in the first intron of the CD95 gene, as well as three putative p53-binding sites within the CD95 promoter, which showed limited homology with the p53 consensus binding site *(41)*. Also, rapid transport of presynthesized CD95 receptor molecules, which were stored in vesicles in the cytoplasm, to the cell membrane upon activation of p53 may contribute to upregulation of CD95 receptor surface expression in response to chemotherapy *(48)*. Moreover, soluble antagonistic CD95 receptors, antagonistic CD95L antibodies, or DN-FADD were found to reduce drug-induced apoptosis under certain circumstances *(33,34,42)*. Also, CD95L-independent activation of the CD95 pathway through CD95 receptor oligomerization has been reported, e.g., by ultraviolet (UV) irradiation or suicide gene therapy using the herpes simplex thymidine kinase (HSV/TK) system *(49,50)*. Furthermore, resistance to CD95-triggered apoptosis has been associated with cross-resistance to various anticancer agents in some leukemia and solid tumor cell lines *(34,51)*. This indicates that cell-death signaling upon physiological stimuli such as CD95 triggering and chemotherapy required, at least in part, pathways similar to the CD95 system.

Despite the reproducibility of these findings in a variety of different model systems, other reports challenged the concept that CD95 signaling is involved in drug-mediated cell death *(52–56)*. To that end, antagonistic antibodies against CD95L or CD95 did not confer protection against apoptosis induced by cytotoxic drugs in other cell lines *(54–56)*. Although splenocytes from lpr mice showed decreased sensitivity to γ-irradiation, thymocytes of these mice did not show increased proliferation upon γ-irradiation or cytotoxic drugs *(57)*. Enforced expression of FLICE-inhibitory protein (FLIP), DN-FADD, or the serpin crmA did not inhibit drug-induced apoptosis, although it inhibited caspase-8 activation *(54–56,58)*. Also, targeted disruption of genes involved in death receptor signaling conferred no protection against cytotoxic drug treatment, at least in nontransformed cells. $FADD^{-/-}$ and caspase-$8^{-/-}$ fibroblasts were sensitive to cytotoxic drugs, while they remained resistant to death receptor stimulation *(59,60)*. In contrast, caspase-$9^{-/-}$ embryonic stem cells and Apaf-$1^{-/-}$ thymocytes were sensitive to death receptor triggering, but remained resistant to cytotoxic drugs *(61,62)*.

How can these divergent findings be reconciled? The discrepancies in findings may be related to the relative contribution of the death receptor vs the mitochondrial pathway to drug-induced apoptosis, depending on the anticancer agent, dose, and kinetics or on cell-type-specific differences. To this end, a cell-type-dependent signaling following treatment with cytotoxic drugs has been described, similar to the cell-type-dependent organization of the CD95 pathway *(63)*. In type I cells, both the receptor and the mitochondrial pathway were activated upon drug treatment, since blockade of either the receptor pathway by overexpression of dominant-negative FADD (FADD-DN) or of the mitochondrial pathway by overexpression of Bcl-X_L only partially inhibited apoptosis *(63)*. In contrast, in type II cells, apoptosis was predominantly controlled by mitochondria, since overexpression of Bcl-2 completely blocked drug-induced apoptosis, while overexpression of FADD-DN had no protective effect *(63)*.

The discrepancies in data may also be explained by differences in blocking reagents used to inhibit CD95/CD95L interaction. The quality of CD95/CD95L blocking agents—e.g., anti-CD95 antibody, anti-CD95L antibody, or soluble decoy CD95-Fc receptor constructs—may vary significantly depending on their origin and preparation. Importantly, CD95/CD95L neutralizing agents may not be effective because they simply cannot gain access to their proposed targets. Experiments with adenoviral delivery of a CD95L-GFP construct showed that CD95 and CD95L are stored intracellularly and colocalize to the same intracellular compartments, e.g., the Golgi and/or endoplasmatic reticulum *(64)*. An anti-CD95 blocking antibody did not inhibit CD95L-induced cell death, suggesting that CD95L may trigger CD95 within the same intracellular compartment and that these two molecules may already interact prior to surface presentation *(64)*. Under those circumstances, the lack of efficacy of CD95/CD95L neutralizing agents may be explained by the inaccessibility of their targets. Moreover, some studies that challenge an involvement of the CD95 system in chemotherapy of tumor cells are based on experiments performed in nontransformed cells, e.g., embryonic fibroblasts, but not in cancer cells. However, the mechanisms regulating apoptosis in non-malignant cells may vary considerably from those in malignant tumor cells, which is highlighted by the differential sensitivity of these cell types to various death stimuli.

Despite the involvement of the CD95 system in anticancer drug-induced apoptosis under certain circumstances, most cytotoxic drugs are considered to primarily initiate cell death by triggering a cytochrome c/Apaf-1/caspase-9-dependent pathway linked to mitochondria *(5)*. Collectively, these data point to a crucial role of the mitochondrial pathway in drug-induced apoptosis, while the CD95 system may amplify drug-induced apoptosis under certain conditions. Importantly, this amplification of the chemoresponse may have important clinical implications, since it may critically affect the time required for execution of the death program *(65)*. However, the model of mitochondria being the key initiator to integrate stress stimuli into an apoptotic response has also been challenged by recent evidence demonstrating that a functional apoptosome is dispensable for stress-induced apoptosis *(66,67)*. Remarkably, activation of caspases, e.g., caspase-2, following cellular stress, was found to be required for mitochondrial perturbation rather than vice versa *(66)*. In addition, Bcl-2 was shown to regulate a caspase activation program that did not depend on the cytochrome c/caspase-9/Apaf-1-containing apoptosome complex *(67)*. These recent studies indicate that mitochondria may act as amplifiers rather than initiators of death upon cellular stress. Thus, key components of apoptosis pathways may yet have to be reconsidered.

In addition to the CD95 system being involved in chemotherapy-triggered cell death, numerous studies have shown that anticancer agents or irradiation can synergize with CD95L or agonistic CD95 antibodies to signal through CD95 *(68–71)*. Importantly, chemotherapy or irradiation can even sensitize resistant tumor cells for CD95 triggering by modulating several components of the CD95 signaling pathway. Multiple molecular mechanisms may underlie defects in the CD95 system *(16,46,72)*. For example, death receptor expression may vary among different cell types and can be downregulated or absent in resistant tumor cells, which has been assumed to contribute to immune escape of tumor cells from negative growth control *(2,27)*. Drug-resistant leukemia or neuroblastoma cells showed strong downregulation of CD95 expression, suggesting that critical levels of CD95 expression may have an impact on drug sensitivity *(51)*. Impaired transmembrane expression of CD95 may be caused by promoter hypermethylation, histone acetylation, transcriptional repression, inactivating CD95 mutations, or alternative mRNA splicing to generate soluble CD95 receptors lacking a transmembrane anchor *(72,73)*. Also, drug-resistant tumor cells were found to be deficient in upregulation of CD95L in response to treatment with cytotoxic drugs that were involved in drug response in chemosensitive tumor cells *(51)*. CD95 signaling can also be negatively regulated by proteins that associate with their cytoplasmic domains, e.g., FLIP, which prevents the interaction between the adaptor molecule FADD and procaspase-8 *(74)*. Importantly, several mechanisms may account for the synergistic interaction between chemotherapy and the CD95 system. For example, upregulation of CD95 or CD95L upon treatment with DNA-damaging drugs occurred in a p53-dependent manner *(41,42)*. As described above, wild-type p53 can transcriptionally activate CD95L or CD95 and/or can stimulate the translocation of presynthesized molecules from intracellular stores, e.g., the Golgi compartment, to the cell membrane *(41,42,48)*. Also, treatment with cytotoxic drugs has been reported to modulate expression of anti- and proapoptotic components of the CD95 DISC *(75)*. Upregulation of FADD and procaspase-8 by cisplatin or doxorubicin was observed in colon carcinoma cells *(75)*. In addition, enhanced recruitment of FADD and caspase-8 to form the CD95 DISC was found upon treatment with cytotoxic drugs in type I cells *(63)*. Treatment with actinomycin D or cisplatin sensitized neuroblastoma or osteosarcoma cells for CD95 triggering by downregulating FLIP expression *(76,77)*. However, the impact of FLIP on apoptosis sensitivity towards cytotoxic drugs may vary among cell types, since overexpression of FLIP did not confer protection against cytotoxic drugs in T-cell leukemia cells *(58)*. A recent study has provided further evidence that CD95/CD95 ligand interactions are important in the control of tumor growth and treatment response *(78)*. In tumors with epigenetically silenced CD95, restoration of CD95 expression by histone deacetylase inhibitors resulted in suppression of tumor growth and restoration of chemosensitivity in an NK cell-dependent manner *(78)*. These findings demonstrated that the level of CD95 expression and the intact function of the CD95 system has an important impact on chemosensitivity and on immune surveillance by CD95L-expressing NK cells.

TRAIL and Cancer Therapy

Although most tumor cells express both agonistic TRAIL receptors, many resistant tumors remain refractory towards treatment with TRAIL, which has been related to the dominance of anti-apoptotic signals, e.g., those delivered by NF-κB, AKT, or by inhibitor of apoptosis proteins (IAPs) *(28,29)*. Importantly, numerous studies have shown that TRAIL together with cytotoxic drugs or γ-irradiation strongly synergized to achieve antitumor activity in various cancers, including malignant glioma, melanoma, leukemia, breast, colon, or prostate carcinoma *(79–82)*. Remarkably, TRAIL and anticancer agents also cooperated to suppress tumor growth in different mouse models of human cancers

(83,84). In addition, agonistic antibodies targeting TRAIL-R1 or TRAIL-R2 showed promising antitumor activity, alone or in combination with anticancer agents *(85,86)*. The molecular mechanisms that account for this synergistic interaction may include transcriptional up-regulation of the agonistic TRAIL receptors TRAIL-R1 and –R2, which occurred in a p53-dependent or p53-independent manner *(28–30,79–83)*. Also, downregulation of anti-apoptotic proteins such as Bcl-2, Bcl-X_L, or FLIP, as well as upregulation of pro-apoptotic molecules including FADD or caspase-8 upon treatment with cytotoxic drugs, may sensitize tumor cells for TRAIL. In addition, biological response modifiers such as interferon (IFN)-γ strongly enhanced the cytotoxic activity of TRAIL by upregulating caspase-8 expression in a STAT-1-dependent manner *(87)* Transcriptional upregulation of caspase-8 or caspase-3 upon cytotoxic drug treatment was also reported to occur independently of STAT-1 *(88)*. Since caspase-8 expression is frequently impaired by hypermethylation in several tumors, including neuroblastoma, Ewing tumors, malignant brain tumors, or melanoma, administration of TRAIL together with IFNγ may overcome some forms of resistance towards TRAIL, e.g., in tumors with impaired caspase-8 expression *(89,90)*. Also, small molecules may serve as molecular targeted therapeutics to enhance TRAIL sensitivity of resistant cancers *(91)*. To this end, Smac agonists have recently been reported to potentiate the efficacy of TRAIL treatment by antagonizing the inhibitory effect of IAPs, which are overexpressed in many tumors *(91)*. Importantly, Smac peptides synergized with TRAIL to eradicate malignant glioma in an orthotopic mouse model, without any detectable toxicities to the normal brain tissue *(91)*.

Furthermore, there is mounting evidence for an important role of TRAIL in tumor surveillance *(92–94)*. To this end, tumor formation induced by carcinogens was found to be enhanced in the presence of antagonistic TRAIL antibodies *(92)*. Also, TRAIL-deficient mice were more susceptible to tumor metastasis than wild-type mice *(93)*. These data are in accordance with studies showing an important role of NK cells, which constitutively express TRAIL, in the control of tumor metastasis *(94)*. Together, these findings point to a critical role of TRAIL in NK cell-dependent tumor surveillance.

CONCLUSIONS

Numerous reports over the last years have provided evidence that anticancer therapies primarily act by triggering apoptosis in cancer cells. Key elements of the basic apoptosis machinery, including death receptors and their ligands or mitochondria, have been inferred to play a critical role in cancer therapy as well as in surveillance of tumor formation. In addition, studies on the regulation of apoptosis signaling pathways upon cancer therapy gave substantial insights into the molecular mechanisms regulating the response of cancer cells towards current treatment regimens. Defects in apoptosis programs may result in treatment resistance of cancers. Remarkably, synergistic interaction between cytotoxic therapies such as anticancer drugs or γ-irradiation and death ligands to trigger tumor cell death has been reported in a variety of cancers. Most importantly, combined treatment with chemotherapy together with death ligands was found to be even effective against resistant tumors, and may thus overcome some forms of resistance. However, detailed studies of the therapeutic potential of death ligands combined with chemotherapy in preclinical in vivo mouse models and in primary patient-derived tumor cells are far from being complete. This approach may hopefully lead to novel therapeutic strategies targeting apoptosis-resistant forms of cancers.

REFERENCES

1. Hengartner MO. The biochemistry of apoptosis. Nature 2000;407:770–777.
2. Krammer PH. CD95's deadly mission in the immune system. Nature 2000;407:789–795.
3. Debatin KM. The role of the CD95 system in chemotherapy. In: Broxterman HJA (ed), Drug Resistance Updates. Churchill Livingstone, Edinburgh: 1999:85–90.
4. Herr I, Debatin KM. Cellular stress response and apoptosis in cancer therapy. Blood 2001;98:2603–2614.
5. Debatin KM, Poncet D, Kroemer G. Chemotherapy: targeting the mitochondrial cell death pathway. Oncogene 2002;21:8786–8803.
6. Kaufmann SH, Earnshaw WC. Induction of apoptosis by cancer chemotherapy. Exp Cell Res 2000;256:42–49.
7. Solary E, Droin N, Bettaieb A, Corcos L, Dimanche-Boitrel MT, Garrido C. Positive and negative regulation of apoptotic pathways by cytotoxic agents in hematological malignancies. Leukemia 2000;14:1833–1849.
8. Lowe SW, Lin AW. Apoptosis in cancer. Carcinogenesis 2000;21:485–495.
9. Johnstone RW, Ruefli AA, Lowe SW. Apoptosis: a link between cancer genetics and chemotherapy. Cell 2002;108:153–164.
10. Rich T, Allen RL, Wyllie AH. Defying death after DNA damage. Nature 2000;407, 777–783.
11. Leppa S, Bohmann D. Diverse functions of JNK signaling and c-Jun in stress response and apoptosis. Oncogene 1999;18:6158–6162.
12. Davis RJ. Signal transduction by the JNK group of MAP kinases. Cell 2000;103:239–252.
13. Karin M, Cao Y, Greten FR, Li ZW. NF-kappaB in cancer: from innocent bystander to major culprit. Nat Rev Cancer 2002;2:301–310.
14. Thornberry N, Lazebnik Y. Caspases: enemies within. Science 1998;281:1312–1316.
15. Earnshaw WC, Martins LM, Kaufmann SH. Mammalian caspases: structure, activation, substrates, and functions during apoptosis. Annu Rev Biochem 1999;68:383–424.
16. Igney FH, Krammer PH. Death and anti-death: tumour resistance to apoptosis. Nat Rev Cancer 2002;2:277–288.
17. Nagata S. Apoptotic DNA fragmentation. Exp Cell Res 2000;256:12–18.
18. Fulda S, Debatin KM. Caspase activation in cancer therapy. In: Los M, Walczak H (eds), Caspases—Their Role in Cell Death and Cell Survival. Kluwer Academic Press: 2002;185–196.
19. Walczak H, Krammer PH. The CD95 (APO-1/Fas) and the TRAIL (APO-2L) apoptosis systems. Exp Cell Res 2000;256:58–66.
20. van Loo G, Saelens X, van Gurp M, MacFarlane M, Martin SJ, Vandenabeele P. The role of mitochondrial factors in apoptosis: a Russian roulette with more than one bullet. Cell Death Differ 2002;9:1031–1042.
21. Roy S, Nicholson DW. Cross-talk in cell death signaling. J Exp Med 2000;192:21–26.
22. Cowling V, Downward J. Caspase-6 is the direct activator of caspase-8 in the cytochrome c-induced apoptosis pathway: absolute requirement for removal of caspase-6 prodomain. Cell Death Differ 2002;9:1046–1056.
23. Ashkenazi A, Dixit VM. Death receptors: signaling and modulation. Science 1998;281:1305–1308.
24. Schulze-Osthoff K, Ferrari D, Los M, Wesselborg S, Peter ME. Apoptosis signaling by death receptors. Eur J Biochem 1998;4:439–459.
25. Ashkenazi A. Targeting death and decoy receptors of the tumour-necrosis factor superfamily. Nat Rev Cancer 2002;2:420–430.
26. Green DR, Ferguson TA. The role of Fas ligand in immune privilege. Nat Rev Mol Cell Biol 2001;2: 917–924.
27. Igney FH, Krammer PH. Immune escape of tumors: apoptosis resistance and tumor counterattack. J Leukoc Biol 2002;71:907–920.
28. Wajant H, Pfizenmaier K, Scheurich P. TNF-related apoptosis inducing ligand (TRAIL) and its receptors in tumor surveillance and cancer therapy. Apoptosis 2002;7:449–459.
29. Nagane M, Huang HJ, Cavenee WK. The potential of TRAIL for cancer chemotherapy. Apoptosis 2001;6:191–197.
30. El-Deiry WS. Insights into cancer therapeutic design based on p53 and TRAIL receptor signaling. Cell Death Differ 2000;8:1066–1075.
31. Wajant H. The Fas signaling pathway: more than a paradigm. Science 2002;296:1635–1636.
32. Scaffidi C, Fulda S, Srinivasan A, et al. Two CD95 (APO-1/Fas) signaling pathways. EMBO J 1998;17:1675–1687.

33. Friesen C, Herr I, Krammer PH, Debatin KM. Involvement of the CD95 (APO-1/FAS) receptor/ligand system in drug-induced apoptosis in leukemia cells. Nat Med 1996;2:574–577.
34. Fulda S, Sieverts H, Friesen C, Herr I, Debatin KM. The CD95 (APO-1/Fas) system mediates drug-induced apoptosis in neuroblastoma cells. Cancer Res 1997;7:3823–3829.
35. Fulda S, Los M, Friesen C, Debatin KM. Chemosensitivity of solid tumor cells is associated with activation of the CD95 system. Int J Cancer 1998;76:105–114.
36. Fulda S, Scaffidi C, Pietsch T, Krammer PH, Peter ME, Debatin KM. Activation of the CD95 (APO-1/Fas) pathway in drug- and γ-irradiation-induced apoptosis of brain tumor cells. Cell Death Differ 1998;5:884–893.
37. Fulda S, Susin SA, Kroemer G, Debatin KM. Molecular ordering of apoptosis induced by anticancer drugs in neuroblastoma cells. Cancer Res 1998;58:4453–4460.
38. Fulda S, Strauss G, Meyer E, Debatin KM. Functional CD95 ligand and CD95 DISC in activation-induced cell death and doxorubicin-induced apoptosis in leukemic T cells. Blood 2000;95:301–308.
39. Herr I, Wilhelm D, Bohler T, Angel P, Debatin KM. Activation of CD95 (APO-1/Fas) signaling by ceramide mediates cancer therapy-induced apoptosis. EMBO J 1997;16:6200–6208.
40. Houghton JA, Harwood FG, Tillman DM. Thymineless death in colon carcinoma cells is mediated via fas signaling. Proc Natl Acad Sci USA 1997;94:8144–8149.
41. Muller M, Wilder S, Bannasch D, et al. p53 activates the CD95 (APO-1/Fas) gene in response to DNA damage by anticancer drugs. J Exp Med 1998;188:2033–2045.
42. Muller M, Strand S, Hug H, et al. Drug-induced apoptosis in hepatoma cells is mediated by the CD95 (APO-1/Fas) receptor/ligand system and involves activation of wild-type p53. J Clin Invest 1997;99:403–413.
43. Reap EA, Roof K, Maynor K, Borrero M, Booker J, Cohen PL. Radiation and stress-induced apoptosis: a role for Fas/Fas ligand interactions. Proc Natl Acad Sci USA 1997;94:5750–5755.
44. Kasibhatla S, Brunner T, Genestier L, Echeverri F, Mahboubi A, Green DR. DNA damaging agents induce expression of Fas ligand and subsequent apoptosis in T lymphocytes via the activation of NF-kappa B and AP-1. Mol Cell 1998;1:543–551.
45. Eichhorst ST, Muller M, Li-Weber M, Schulze-Bergkamen H, Angel P, Krammer PH. A novel AP-1 element in the CD95 ligand promoter is required for induction of apoptosis in hepatocellular carcinoma cells upon treatment with anticancer drugs. Mol Cell Biol 2000;20:7826–7837.
46. Poulaki V, Mitsiades CS, Mitsiades N. The role of Fas and FasL as mediators of anticancer chemotherapy. Drug Resist Updat 2001;4:233–242.
47. Mo YY, Beck WT. DNA damage signals induction of fas ligand in tumor cells. Mol Pharmacol 1999; 55:216–222.
48. Bennett M, Macdonald K, Chan SW, Luzio JP, Simari R, Weissberg P. Cell surface trafficking of Fas: a rapid mechanism of p53-mediated apoptosis. Science 9;282:290–293.
49. Beltinger C, Fulda S, Kammertoens T, Meyer E, Uckert W, Debatin KM. Herpes simplex virus thymidine kinase/ganciclovir-induced apoptosis involves ligand-independent death receptor aggregation and activation of caspases. Proc Natl Acad Sci USA 1999;96:8699–8704.
50. Rehemtulla A, Hamilton CA, Chinnaiyan AM, Dixit VM. Ultraviolet radiation-induced apoptosis is mediated by activation of CD-95 (Fas/APO-1). J Biol Chem 1997;272:25,783–25,786.
51. Friesen C, Fulda S, Debatin KM. Deficient activation of the CD95 (APO-1/Fas) system in drug-resistant cells. Leukemia 1997;11:1833–1841.
52. Landowski TH, Shain KH, Oshiro MM, Buyuksal I, Painter JS, Dalton WS. Myeloma cells selected for resistance to CD95-mediated apoptosis are not cross-resistant to cytotoxic drugs: evidence for independent mechanisms of caspase activation. Blood 1999;94:265–274.
53. Eischen CM, Kottke TJ, Martins LM, et al. Comparison of apoptosis in wild-type and Fas-resistant cells: chemotherapy-induced apoptosis is not dependent on Fas/Fas ligand interactions. Blood 1997; 90:935–943.
54. Villunger A, Egle A, Kos M, et al. Drug-induced apoptosis is associated with enhanced Fas (Apo-1/CD95) ligand expression but occurs independently of Fas (Apo-1/CD95) signaling in human T-acute lymphatic leukemia cells. Cancer Res 1997;57:3331–3334.
55. Wesselborg S, Engels IH, Rossmann E, Los M, Schulze-Osthoff K. Anticancer drugs induce caspase-8/FLICE activation and apoptosis in the absence of CD95 receptor/ligand interaction. Blood 1999;93:3053–3063.
56. Glaser T, Wagenknecht B, Groscurth P, Krammer PH, Weller M. Death ligand/receptor-independent caspase activation mediates drug-induced cytotoxic cell death in human malignant glioma cells. Oncogene 1999;18:5044–5053.

57. Reap EA, Roof K, Maynor K, Cohen PL. Markedly diminished radiation-induced lymphocyte apoptosis in lpr mice suggests a role for Fas in eliminating damaged cells. Ann NY Acad Sci 1997;815:116–118.
58. Kataoka T, Schroter M, Hahne M, et al. FLIP prevents apoptosis induced by death receptors but not by perforin/granzyme B, chemotherapeutic drugs, and gamma irradiation. J Immunol 1998;161:3936–3942.
59. Yeh WC, Pompa JL, McCurrach ME, et al. FADD: essential for embryo development and signaling from some, but not all, inducers of apoptosis. Science 1998;279:1954–1958.
60. Varfolomeev EE, Schuchmann M, Luria V, et al. Targeted disruption of the mouse Caspase 8 gene ablates cell death induction by the TNF receptors, Fas/Apo1, and DR3 and is lethal prenatally. Immunity 1998;9:267–276.
61. Hakem R, Hakem A, Duncan GS, et al. Differential requirement for caspase 9 in apoptotic pathways in vivo. Cell 1998;94:339–352.
62. Yoshida H, Kong YY, Yoshida R, et al. Apafl is required for mitochondrial pathways of apoptosis and brain development. Cell 1998;94:739–750.
63. Fulda S, Meyer E, Susin SA, Kroemer G, Debatin KM. Cell type specific activation of death receptor and mitochondrial pathways in drug-induced apoptosis. Oncogene 2000;20:1063–1075.
64. Hyer ML, Voelkel-Johnson C, Rubinchik S, Dong J, Norris JS. Intracellular Fas ligand expression causes Fas-mediated apoptosis in human prostate cancer cells resistant to monoclonal antibody-induced apoptosis. Mol Ther 2000;2:348–358.
65. Tang D, Lahti JM, Kidd VJ. Caspase-8 activation and bid cleavage contribute to MCF7 cellular execution in a caspase-3-dependent manner during staurosporine-mediated apoptosis. J Biol Chem 2000;275:9303–9307.
66. Lassus P, Opitz-Araya X, Lazebnik Y. Requirement for caspase-2 in stress-induced apoptosis before mitochondrial permeabilization. Science 2002;297:1352–1354.
67. Marsden VS, O'Connor L, O'Reilly LA, et al. Apoptosis initiated by Bcl-2-regulated caspase activation independently of the cytochrome c/Apaf-1/caspase-9 apoptosome. Nature 2002;419:634–637.
68. Posovszky C, Friesen C, Herr I, Debatin KM. Chemotherapeutic drugs sensitize pre-B ALL cells for CD95- and cytotoxic T-lymphocyte-mediated apoptosis. Leukemia 1999;13:400–409.
69. Roth W, Fontana A, Trepel M, Reed JC, Dichgans J, Weller M. Immunochemotherapy of malignant glioma: synergistic activity of CD95 ligand and chemotherapeutics.Cancer Immunol Immunother 1997;44:55–63.
70. Micheau O, Solary E, Hammann A, Martin F, Dimanche-Boitrel MT. Sensitization of cancer cells treated with cytotoxic drugs to fas-mediated cytotoxicity. J Natl Cancer Inst 1997;89:783–789.
71. Wu XX, Mizutani Y, Kakehi Y, Yoshida O, Ogawa O. Enhancement of Fas-mediated apoptosis in renal cell carcinoma cells by adriamycin. Cancer Res 2000;60:2912–2918.
72. Owen-Schaub L, Chan H, Cusack JC, Roth J, Hill LL. Fas and Fas ligand interactions in malignant disease. Int J Oncol 2000;17:5–12.
73. Owen-Schaub LB. Fas function and tumor progression: use it and lose it. Cancer Cell 2002;2:95–96.
74. Tschopp J, Irmler M, Thome M. Inhibition of fas death signals by FLIPs. Curr Opin Immunol 1998;10:552–558.
75. Micheau O, Solary E, Hammann A, Dimanche-Boitrel MT. Fas ligand-independent, FADD-mediated activation of the Fas death pathway by anticancer drugs. J Biol Chem 1999;274:7987–7992.
76. Kinoshita H, Yoshikawa H, Shiiki K, Hamada Y, Nakajima Y, Tasaka K. Cisplatin (CDDP) sensitizes human osteosarcoma cell to Fas/CD95-mediated apoptosis by down-regulating FLIP-L expression. Int J Cancer 2000;88:986–991.
77. Fulda S, Meyer E, Debatin KM. Metabolic inhibitors sensitize for CD95 (APO-1/Fas)-induced apoptosis by down-regulating Fas-associated death domain-like interleukin 1-converting enzyme inhibitory protein expression. Cancer Res 2000;60:3947–3956.
78. Maecker HL, Yun Z, Maecker HT, Giaccia AJ. Epigenetic changes in tumor Fas levels determine immune escape and response to therapy. Cancer Cell 2002;2:139–148.
79. Belka C, Schmid B, Marini P, et al. Sensitization of resistant lymphoma cells to irradiation-induced apoptosis by the death ligand TRAIL. Oncogene 2001;20:2190–2196.
80. Keane MM, Ettenberg SA, Nau MM, Russell EK, Lipkowitz S. Chemotherapy augments TRAIL-induced apoptosis in breast cell lines. Cancer Res 1999;59:734–741.
81. Nagane M, Pan G, Weddle JJ, Dixit VM, Cavenee WK, Huang HJ. Increased death receptor 5 expression by chemotherapeutic agents in human gliomas causes synergistic cytotoxicity with tumor necrosis factor-related apoptosis-inducing ligand in vitro and in vivo. Cancer Res 2000;60:847–853.

82. Lacour S, Hammann A, Wotawa A, Corcos L, Solary E, Dimanche-Boitrel MT. Anticancer agents sensitize tumor cells to tumor necrosis factor-related apoptosis-inducing ligand-mediated caspase-8 activation and apoptosis. Cancer Res 2001;61:1645–1651.
83. Dejosez M, Ramp U, Mahotka C, et al. Sensitivity to TRAIL/APO-2L-mediated apoptosis in human renal cell carcinomas and its enhancement by topotecan. Cell Death Differ 2000;7:1127–1136.
84. Walczak H, Miller RE, Ariail K, et al. Tumoricidal activity of tumor necrosis factor-related apoptosis-inducing ligand in vivo. Nat Med 1999;5:157–163.
85. Chuntharapai A, Dodge K, Grimmer K, et al. Isotype-dependent inhibition of tumor growth in vivo by monoclonal antibodies to death receptor 4. J Immunol 2001;166:4891–4898.
86. Ichikawa K, Liu W, Zhao L, et al. Tumoricidal activity of a novel anti-human DR5 monoclonal antibody without hepatocyte cytotoxicity. Nat Med 2001;7:954–960.
87. Fulda S, Debatin KM. IFNγ sensitizes for apoptosis by upregulating caspase-8 expression through the Stat1 pathway. Oncogene 2002;21:2295–2308.
88. Micheau O, Hammann A, Solary E, Dimanche-Boitrel MT. STAT-1-independent upregulation of FADD and procaspase-3 and -8 in cancer cells treated with cytotoxic drugs. Biochem Biophys Res Commun 1999;256:603–607.
89. Teitz T, Wie T, Valentine MB, et al. Caspase 8 is deleted or silenced preferentially in childhood neuroblastomas with amplification of MYCN. Nat Med 2000;6:529–535.
90. Fulda S, Kufer MU, Meyer E, van Valen F, Dockhorn-Dworniczak B, Debatin KM. Sensitization for death receptor- or drug-induced apoptosis by re-expression of caspase-8 through demethylation or gene transfer. Oncogene 2001;20:5865–5877.
91. Fulda S, Wick W, Weller M, Debatin KM. Smac agonists sensitize for Apo2L/TRAIL- or anticancer drug-induced apoptosis and induce regression of malignant glioma in vivo. Nat Med 2002;8:808–815.
92. Takeda K, Hayakawa Y, Smyth MJ, et al. Involvement of tumor necrosis factor-related apoptosis-inducing ligand in surveillance of tumor metastasis by liver natural killer cells. Nat Med 2001;7:94–100.
93. Cretney E, Takeda K, Yagita H, Glaccum M, Peschon JJ, Smyth MJ. Increased susceptibility to tumor initiation and metastasis in TNF-related apoptosis-inducing ligand-deficient mice. J Immunol 2002;168:1356–1361.
94. Smyth MJ, Cretney E, Takeda K, et al. Tumor necrosis factor-related apoptosis-inducing ligand (TRAIL) contributes to interferon gamma-dependent natural killer cell protection from tumor metastasis. J Exp Med 2001;193:661–670.

Index